HUMAN DISEASE AND HEALTH PROMOTION

HUMAN DISEASE AND HEALTH PROMOTION

Leslie Beale

WILEY

Published by John Wiley & Sons, Inc., Hoboken, New Jersey.
Published simultaneously in Canada.

For general information on our other products and services, please contact our Customer Care Department within the U.S. at 800-956-7739, outside the U.S. at 317-572-3986, or fax 317-572-4002.

Wiley publishes in a variety of print and electronic formats and by print-on-demand. Some material included with standard print versions of this book may not be included in e-books or in print-on-demand. If this book refers to media such as a CD or DVD that is not included in the version you purchased, you may download this material at http://booksupport.wiley.com. For more information about Wiley products, visit www.wiley.com.

Library of Congress Cataloging-in-Publication Data

Names: Beale, Leslie, author.
Title: Human disease and health promotion / Leslie Beale.
Description: Hoboken, New Jersey : Jossey-Bass & Pfeiffer/Wiley, [2017] |
    Includes bibliographical references and index.
Identifiers: LCCN 2016055929 (print) | LCCN 2016057037 (ebook) | ISBN
    9780470589083 (paper) | ISBN 9781118220580 (pdf) | ISBN 9781118234136 (epub)
Subjects: | MESH: Health Promotion | Health Literacy | Patient Education as
    Topic | Cultural Diversity
Classification: LCC RA427.8 (print) | LCC RA427.8 (ebook) | NLM WA 590 | DDC
    362.1–dc23
LC record available at https://lccn.loc.gov/2016055929

Cover Design: Wiley
Cover Illustration: © David Marchal/iStockphoto

Printed in the United States of America

FIRST EDITION

PB Printing   10 9 8 7 6 5 4 3 2 1

CONTENTS

This textbook's introduction speaks to those most interested in reading *Human Disease and Health Promotion.* There are notes to students who want to know what the textbook has to offer them and how it can help them in their chosen careers. There are also notes to instructors who want to know why they should use this textbook as part of their course syllabus.

Notes to Students

Are you a student seeking a job in health care, but finding that learning about human diseases is a challenge? Are you put off or discouraged about learning this subject? Do you find that human disease textbooks are too difficult to read because of medical jargon? *Human Disease and Health Promotion* is student-friendly and written in easy-to-understand language. It is designed to help you understand human diseases, health promotion, and how to work with patients. It gives you the knowledge and skills needed to get a job in health care.

    Human Disease and Health Promotion has 21 chapters organized into two parts. Part 1 (Chapters 1 through 9) sets up a framework for health promotion and describes health care. Chapters 10 through 21 are organized by body systems. Each chapter starts with an explanation of how the body system works, then follows with a description of related common diseases. All 21 chapters include learning objectives, chapter summaries, review questions, key terms with definitions, and chapter activities.

Notes to Instructors

When one is writing a textbook for a diverse audience, the question arises, "How do you organize content to meet the needs of your readers?" *Human Disease and Health Promotion* answers this question by keeping in mind the need for flexibility. Chapters can be seen as building blocks of information. Each block is included or excluded depending on course goals and outcome measures. All chapters can be taught over two semesters or taught in consecutive courses. Part 1 and Part 2 can each stand alone. Chapter sequence can be altered or some chapters omitted, depending on students' needs. Some chapters can be required, whereas others can be treated as suggested readings. *Human Disease and Health Promotion* is designed to be flexible to support instructors' pedagogy and students' educational needs.

    Not all human diseases are discussed in this textbook. The emphasis is on common rather than rare diseases. Although rare diseases are interesting to study, becoming acquainted with the more common diseases is what helps students in their career. For the diseases chosen, only an overview is given and not a detailed physiological explanation. The textbook explains complex medical concepts in easy-to-understand language when possible. This does not mean that the textbook lacks academic rigor; rather, information is presented to be understandable and useful to students.

This textbook is dedicated in loving memory of my parents,
Frederick F. Beale, MD, and Anna V. Beale.
I have been most fortunate to receive their gifts of love,
inspiration, and encouragement.

Human Disease and Health Promotion presents a new approach to learning about human disease. Students who read this textbook improve their understanding of human disease through a body systems approach and gain health promotion knowledge and skills.

Medical and technological advances of the 21st century continue to challenge what we know about human diseases. These challenges have made increasing demands on health care providers. To meet these demands, those seeking to work in health care can be trained in new and developing nonclinical careers that support and assist physicians in a variety of health care settings.

This textbook is intended for students who seek nonclinical professional careers in health care—for example, health promotion specialists, health educators, public health workers, health care administrators, allied health professionals, medical assistants, nursing assistants and aides, medical secretaries, and patient navigators. In fact, I hope this textbook is useful to anyone who wants to work with and for patients.

It can be academically demanding to study the basic concepts related to diseases. This is particularly true when textbooks use complex medical jargon. This textbook, in contrast, offers a student-friendly experience because it is written in easy-to-understand language. When a textbook makes information easy to understand, readers are more likely to use it. Students who read this textbook gain the information they need to get a health care job.

Presenting health promotion and human disease in one textbook places special demands on the reader. In response, the textbook has two parts. The first part examines issues related to health promotion and health care. The second part describes each of the body's organ systems along with associated common diseases.

ACKNOWLEDGMENTS

For this author, the task of writing a textbook took many years to complete. The task however was not completed without social support. I gratefully acknowledge and wish to give thanks to the following institutions and individuals for their support, assistance, and understanding.

I begin by thanking Springfield College, the School of Health, Physical Education, and Recreation, and the Department of Physical Education and Health Education. Many thanks to Stephen Coulon, Chair of the Department of Physical Education and Health Education, who supported my writing by allocating time and resources. I would also like to thank my undergraduate and graduate students who listened to my lectures, engaged in critical thinking and class discussions, and challenged my assumptions.

To my dearest friend and closest colleague for 20-odd years, Dr. Gordon Robinson. Due to his sudden death in 2016, he sadly did not receive a signed hardcopy of this textbook, as promised. My colleagues, professors Bridget Halpern and Diane Lorenzo, who listened patiently to my never-ending saga of yet another chapter revision completed.

Other acknowledgements go to my first editor at Wiley, Andy Pasternack. Andy understood the contributions this textbook makes to the field of health promotion. I miss our discussions and our mutual dedication for health equity. His death was not just a loss for me but for many other public health authors.

Seth Schwartz direction and patient support helped me to complete the textbook. Melinda Noack's assistance guided me in following Wiley's publishing format.

The final Wiley team that deserves special thanks are Justin Frahm, Tisha Rossi, and Monica Rogers as well as the copyeditor Michele Jones and proofreader Diane Turso. Their hard work, dedication, and talents challenged me to be a better writer. I have been fortunate to work with such a gifted team of professionals.

Many people offered their comments, assistance and support including Warren Liebesman, Marc Willems, Ray McManus, and Dimana Todorova.

Thank you Steve Buckley for taking care of and sharing in the love of the Pointer Sisters, Chamois, Zoe, Billie Holiday, Roxie, and Lola; and for being the best next-door neighbor and dear friend.

Last but certainly not least, a special thanks to my brother, John Beale, for his love and unwavering confidence in my ability to complete this task.

Leslie Beale, MEd, EdD, is a full professor in the Physical Education Health Education Department and program coordinator for the Health Promotion Program at Springfield College, Springfield, Massachusetts. Beale holds a BA in sociology from the University of Massachusetts and an MEd and EdD in community health education from Boston University. Beale has over 30 years of experience as a health promotion specialist. She was one of the first health educators hired by the Massachusetts Department of Public Health Regional Prevention Centers and wrote the Massachusetts Department of Public Health's state plan for substance abuse prevention. As the adolescent health educator for the City of Boston, she conducted urban hospital, school, and community health education programs. As a health promotion specialist, Beale has worked extensively with school, community, health, higher education, nonprofit, and law enforcement personnel on issues related to substance abuse, sexual assault, violence prevention, HIV/AIDS infection, adolescent depression, school phobia, asthma, vaccinations, peer education, patient advocacy, program planning and evaluation, health literacy, and the American Disabilities Act (ADA).

HUMAN DISEASE AND HEALTH PROMOTION

PART 1

FOUNDATIONS OF HUMAN HEALTH AND HEALTH PROMOTION

OVERVIEW OF HEALTH

CHAPTER OBJECTIVES

- Define health and wellness.

- Identify the two aspects of health: physical and mental.

- Describe and give examples of health determinants.

- Compare and contrast risk factors and protective factors that influence health.

- Explain how the three P's—population, poverty, and pollution—influence health.

- Summarize why health is a basic human right.

This chapter introduces concepts of health and wellness. It also explains how determinants as well as risk and protective factors influence health. Some determinants such as the three P's—poverty, population, and pollution—cause many health problems for people at the local, national, and global levels. The chapter also offers a rationale for why health is a human right.

Health Defined

Health is not easy to define. To some people, health is a sense of well-being, of "feeling good." For others, health means not being sick, and if sick, healing quickly.

For still others, health is a moral issue; that is, sickness is a result of a person's having done something "bad" or "wrong." For most of us, however, health means doing what we want to do with little or no pain.

The definition of health has changed several times over the course of Western history. In the past, it was limited to the "absence of disease." Now, this definition includes not only an absence of disease but also how health is influenced by other factors, such as lifestyle, genetic makeup, and the environment. For example, the most often quoted definition of health was developed in 1948 by the World Health Organization (WHO): "The state of complete physical, mental, and social well-being and not merely the absence of disease or infirmity."

The WHO 1948 definition recognizes that multiple factors influence health. Health is more than a physical condition and more than just the absence of disease.

The WHO definition defines health more as a *holistic* state; that is, health is multidimensional and is affected by multiple factors.

In the 1986 Ottawa Charter for Health Promotion, WHO expanded the definition of health: "a resource for everyday life, not the objective of living. Health is a positive concept emphasizing social and personal resources, as well as physical capacities." This expanded definition means that health is not just a state of physical, mental, and social well-being but also the ability to develop personal and social resources that are necessary to adapt to changes in one's environment. Health helps us function daily, reach our goals, and be active in family, community, school, and work activities (Corbin, Pangrazi, & Franks, 2005).

The 1948 and the 1986 WHO definitions recognize the holistic state of health. However, there are differences among cultures, ages, genders, and socioeconomic statuses that make it difficult to establish a universal definition of health. These differences include the following:

Culture differences Purnell (2003) expands the WHO 1948 and 1986 definitions by adding that health is "a state of wellness that includes physical, mental, and spiritual states and is defined by individuals within their cultural group."

Age differences Older adults may define health as mobility and independence. Middle-aged adults may define health as an inner strength and the ability to handle life's challenges. Young adults and adolescents may define health as good physical condition, energy, and personal attractiveness. Children may define health as physical strength. In other words, views of health change as we grow older. *Health across the lifespan* means that physical, mental, and social factors are interconnected and that health is a life-course process that requires a changing definition as we age (Manderscheid et al., 2010) (see Figure 1.1).

Gender differences The different roles for men and women have negative as well as positive impacts on health. Work, parenthood, marriage, and aging, for example, create gender-specific physiological and psychological stresses that affect health.

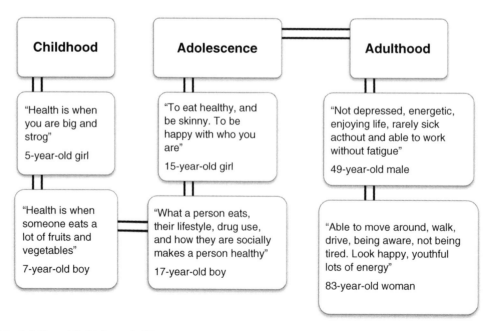

Figure 1.1 Definitions of Health Across the Lifespan

Socioeconomic status (SES) Those who have a high SES may view health as enjoying life, and those who have a low SES may view health as meeting basic needs of food, shelter, and safety.

Adding to the complex influences of culture, age, gender, and SES, health and disease can coexist in a person. For example, a person can have asthma, but if she takes her medications as prescribed and adjusts her lifestyle to manage the disease, she can still experience physical, mental, and social health.

In summary, health is a holistic state and includes many factors beyond just freedom from physical disease and pain. Historically, the definition of health evolved from a limited view that focused on the absence of disease to a view that is multidimensional and includes many different influences on health (Office of Disease Prevention and Health Promotion, 2014).

Two Aspects of Health: Physical and Mental

Regardless of a person's culture, age, gender, and SES, most people accept that there are two aspects of health: physical (body) and mental (mind). *Physical health* or *physical well-being* concerns our bodies and is associated with being physically fit due to healthy choices related to exercise, nutrition, sleep, and relaxation.

Fitness contributes to physical health and it reflects cardiorespiratory endurance, muscle strength, flexibility, and body composition. Other contributors to physical health include appropriate weight, responsible sexual behavior, and hygiene.

Mental health or *mental well-being* is intellectual and emotional well-being. According to the National Mental Health Information Center (2015), mental health includes

> our emotional, psychological, and social well-being. It affects how we think, feel, and act. It also helps determine how we handle stress, relate to others and make choices. Mental health is important at every stage of life, from childhood and adolescence through adulthood.

Most people also agree that mental health includes the ability to enjoy life, bounce back from stressful events, achieve balance, be flexible, and feel safe.

Many of us see mental health defined as a biomedical term: the "absence of mental illness." For some, this definition is not enough because it adds little to understanding the person and the factors that lead to health or illness. The goal of treatment in mental health is to understand as much about a person's emotions, thoughts, and behaviors as about the signs and the symptoms of a disease (Manderscheid et al., 2010). As William Osler (1849–1919), an icon of modern medicine, stated, "It is much more important to know what sort of person has a disease than what sort of disease a patient has."

Wellness Defined

Health and wellness are related terms. Both focus on balancing the physical, social, and emotional aspects of a person's life. *Wellness* is an active, lifelong process of becoming aware of healthy choices and making decisions that promote a more balanced and fulfilling *quality of life*—that is, a general sense of happiness and satisfaction with one's life and environment. Simply put, wellness is the degree to which a person feels positive and enthusiastic about life and has developed the ability to manage feelings and behaviors.

There are two aspects to quality of life. The first is a person's general quality of life, which involves such factors as health, recreation, culture, and values, and the environments that support these factors. The second is health-related quality of life, which involves a personal sense of physical and mental well-being and the ability to engage in healthy behaviors.

Risk and Protective Factors That Influence Health

A person's health is shaped by biological factors, such as genes, age, and gender. However, these biological factors are generally not sufficient to ensure that someone will be healthy. Both health and illness can also be caused by social, economic, educational, cultural, and political factors, ranging from the availability of food to personal responsibility to quality of health care (Doll, 1992; Institute of Medicine, 2001; UN Committee on Economic, Social and Cultural Rights [CESCR], 2000; World Health Organization, 2008).

Those factors associated with illness are referred to as risk factors. *Risk factors* are certain conditions or habits that make a person more likely to develop an illness. They can also increase the chances that an existing illness will get worse. It is important to understand that although risk factors increase the chances of developing an illness, they do not necessarily cause it. Examples of risk factors are obesity, unsafe sex, substance abuse, lack of hygiene, and high blood pressure. *Risk reduction* is a strategy or action that decreases the risk of getting an illness. For example, a risk reduction strategy for heart disease is to exercise or to manage stress.

Protective factors have the opposite effect of risk factors. They decrease the chances of a person developing an illness and lessen the likelihood of negative consequences from exposure to risk. Protective factors may decrease a person's chances of developing an illness, but they do not necessarily prevent someone's getting the illness. Examples of protective factors are clean water, access to quality health care, regular exercise, and healthy foods.

Health Determinants

A way to promote health or to prevent illness is to develop strategies against certain risk factors. *Health determinants* are situations or environments that allow risk and protective factors to directly influence a person's health and illness (Baun, Begin, Houweiling, & Taylor, 2009; Wilkinson & Marmot, 2003; Winklestein, 1992) (see Figure 1.2). It can be confusing to know the differences between risk and protective factors and health determinants because sometimes these terms can be used to mean the same thing.

A person's physical and mental health is influenced by one or more of the following determinants:

Socioeconomic status (SES) Money or lack of money is critical to health. Poverty reduces people's access to health care and resources, resulting in health problems that go untreated.

Employment and work environment Steady employment and a healthy work environment contribute to health.

Education Education provides people with knowledge and skills to make healthy choices and to access quality health care.

Health literacy To be able to obtain, read, understand, and act on health information affects health.

Physical environment Air, noise and water-quality control, toxic waste removal, housing, and community safety all support health.

Family, social, and community support networks Support from families, friends, and communities helps people deal with illness.

Access to quality health care The availability of preventive and primary care services is important in promoting and maintaining health.

Health policies Governmental policies affect the health of individuals, their loved ones, their family, and their community. Examples include antismoking campaigns, immunizations, and gun control laws.

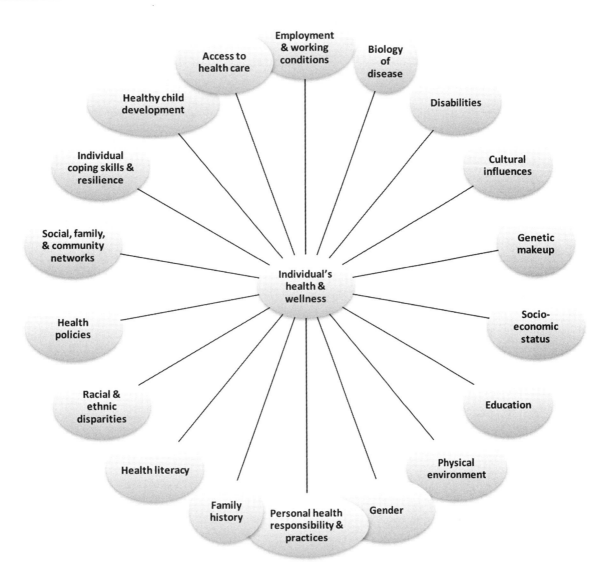

Figure 1.2 Determinants of Health

Genetic makeup Inherited genetic makeup plays a role in health and the chances of getting certain illnesses.

Family history Family health and medical history beyond genetic makeup affects health.

Biology of the disease The type of disease and its signs, symptoms, and prognosis affect health.

Gender Gender differences affect health, including men's shorter life expectancy and women's higher rates of illness.

Healthy child development Prenatal and early childhood experiences have a significant effect on later health.

Racial and ethnic disparities Minority populations often experience illness at higher rates than the majority population because of socioeconomic factors, income disparities, and problems with health care accessibility.

Cultural influences How a culture views health and illness and a culture's health care practices influence people's health.

Disabilities Persons with disabilities are those who have activity limitation, who use assistance, or who see themselves as having a disability. They tend to report more anxiety, pain, and other health issues than people without a disability. They also experience lower rates of physical activity and higher rates of obesity. Many persons with disabilities lack access to quality health care.

Personal health responsibility and practices Being responsible for one's health and making healthy choices play a major role in preventing illness.

Individual coping skills and resilience Coping skills help a person be self-reliant, solve problems, and make healthy choices.

Following extensive research to understand how much of a role determinants play in health and illness, the Robert Wood Johnson (RWJ) Foundation published a 2009 report titled *Health Is More Than Health Care.* The findings in the report focused on why some Americans experience poor health and have shorter lives than others:

- Although health care is important for relieving suffering and curing illness, only an estimated 10 to 15 percent of preventable deaths are caused by issues related to health care.

- A person's health and chances of becoming sick and dying at a young age are strongly influenced by determinants such as education, income, and the quality of community environments.

- American college graduates can expect to live at least five years longer than Americans who have not completed high school.

- Persons with low SES are more than three times as likely as persons with upper-middle SES to suffer physical limitations from a chronic illness.

- Upper-middle SES persons can expect to live more than six years longer than low SES persons.

- People of middle SES are less healthy and can expect to live shorter lives than those with higher SES—even when they are insured.

The RWJ Foundation report also showed that good health depends on personal choice and responsibility. No government or private business program can take the place of a person making healthy choices. It is realistic and beneficial to expect a person to take responsibility for his or her own health by eating a healthy diet, doing regular physical exercises, and avoiding risky health behaviors such as smoking.

The report concluded that the following are major contributors to health and illness:

- *Health care.* Health care is central to reducing suffering and to improving health. Health care also extends the lives of people once they are sick. Equal access to quality health care for all persons is a fundamental human right. However, there should be a focus on keeping people healthy—preventing illness. This focus requires attention and resources that decrease risk factors and increase protective factors.

- *Poor nutrition and lack of physical activity.* These factors are related to almost half of preventable deaths in the United States and are known risk factors for diabetes, heart disease, and stroke, and may contribute to some cancers.

- *Risky behaviors.* Smoking and other forms of substance abuse are among the leading causes of preventable death in the United States. Most people are aware of the health risks associated with these risky behaviors but continue to engage in them. Support from loved ones, family members, and others can provide motivation for someone to stop his or her risky behavior. Environmental changes—in schools, workplaces, and communities—can also promote healthier choices.

- *Early life experiences.* These impact a lifetime of health-related choices. Brain, cognitive, and behavioral development early in life are linked to many common health problems later in life, including cardiovascular disease and stroke, diabetes, obesity, smoking, and depression.

- *Communities.* Disparities in health care due to race, ethnicity, income, or education must be reduced. Community conditions can contribute to disease, such as asthma and lead poisoning, as well as limit the opportunity for healthy behaviors.

- *Income.* Higher income can mean easy access to resources such as health care, healthy foods, quality child care, and housing free of toxins. Lower income can mean that everyday life is a financial struggle, leaving little opportunity to access the resources available to people with higher incomes.

- *Education.* People who lack education have more difficulty understanding how their behaviors affect their health, coping with chronic health problems, and undergoing complex medical treatments. Higher levels of education provide opportunities for higher-paying jobs, which bring better health insurance benefits and healthier working environments. Better education, higher income, and improved health are directly linked.

The Three P's: Population, Poverty, and Pollution

There are many theories that explain the complex influences that shape health. One theory states that to understand these complex influences on health means taking into consideration not only the whole person but also whole populations and the environments they live in. This theory views the "three P's"—population, poverty, and pollution—as intertwined with health (see Figure 1.3). Population growth is associated with poverty, and both poverty and population growth are associated with pollution. Population, poverty, and pollution have a negative impact on health.

The three P's theory of health is rooted in the early 1970s environmental movement, which focused on pollution concerns, such as poor air quality, contaminated water, and toxic waste. From these concerns grew awareness of overpopulation and its impact on the environment. In response to overpopulation, organizations such as Planned Parenthood works toward reducing birth rates, especially in developing countries. The birth control strategies of these organizations do eventually reduce population growth and cut poverty rates in many countries.

The birth rate has dropped in the United States and many other countries, but the global population continues to grow—the current global population of approximately 7 billion people is expected to reach 8–10 billion sometime in the 21st century (Clark, 2005; CESCR, 2000). Population growth is closely linked to poverty, as it reduces economic growth and also drains the environment of resources.

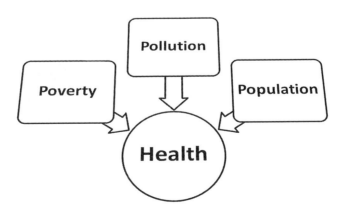

Figure 1.3 Three P's of Health

Associated with population growth is not only the problem of poverty but also the problem of pollution (Worldwatch Institute, 2015). Whereas the wealthy use more resources and produce more pollution, those who are poor bear a greater share of the burden of pollution. Poor people, for example, live without adequate food, housing, clean water, clean air, or basic health care. Because of the increasing numbers of people who continue to increase their levels of consumption, the global and national gains made in pollution control have been threatened.

Unfortunately, many of the same environmental problems of the 1970s are still with us and will continue to be for a long time to come. Doll (1992) identified why the three P's are hazardous. One, pollution of the atmosphere by greenhouse gases causes climate change, which ultimately has major consequences for health. Second, the worldwide population growth rate is now 26 persons every 10 seconds. If this rate continues, there will eventually be a population twice the carrying capacity of the earth even if "we all had a vegetarian diet and shared our food equally" (p. 933). In other words, if we continue to reproduce at the current rate, the earth will no longer be able to provide for the human population. Third, poverty causes illness. Those who live in poverty are more likely to suffer from a variety of chronic health problems, both psychological and physical. At the current rate, poverty will increase along with overpopulation. Increased overpopulation and poverty mean that scarce global resources will be available only to those who can afford to buy them.

Health as a Basic Human Right

In 1948, the United Nations stated in its Universal Declaration of Human Rights, "Everyone has the right to a standard of living adequate for the health and well-being of himself and his family, including food, clothing, housing, and medical care." Then and now, health is a basic human right. Health has universal importance to every person because it is necessary for joy, productivity, and creativity. Persons with physical and mental health socialize, work, and engage in activities that add meaning to their lives. Every person wants to be healthy, to have the best physical and mental health possible, even when he or she experiences an illness. Health is such a basic need that not to have it impacts life, liberty, and the pursuit of happiness. Unfortunately, the majority of people living today do not experience this basic human right.

The right to health includes access to healthy foods and nutrition, housing, adequate sanitation, safety, and positive working environments. It also includes freedoms and opportunities—freedoms meaning the right to control one's health and body and the right to be free from torture and from nonconsensual medical treatment and experimentation; opportunities meaning the right to a health care system that provides access to quality care for all (CESCR, 2000).

Yet the right to health does not mean a right to be healthy. A nation cannot guarantee that all its citizens will be healthy. However, health as a human right is the right to the use of a variety of facilities, goods, services, and environments necessary for a person to reach his or her highest possible level of health.

Chapter Summary

- During the Ottawa Charter for Health Promotion in 1986, WHO expanded its definition of health to "a resource for everyday life, not the objective of living. Health is a positive concept emphasizing social and personal resources, as well as physical capacities."

- Health and wellness are related terms. Both terms focus on balancing physical, emotional, and social aspects of one's life.

- Risk factors increase the chances of contracting an illness. Protective factors decrease the chances of becoming ill.

- Health determinants are situations or environments that allow risk and protective factors to directly influence a person's health and illness.

- The theory known as the three P's of health states that to understand health, you need to consider the whole person and whole populations and the environments they live in.

- In its Universal Declaration of Human Rights of 1948, the United Nations stated, "Everyone has the right to a standard of living adequate for the health and well-being of himself and his family, including food, clothing, housing and medical care." Then, and now, health is a basic human right; unfortunately, many people living today—even in the wealthiest of countries, including the United States—are unable to experience this right.

REVIEW QUESTIONS

1. Identify some of the multiple factors that influence health. How do these factors influence health?

2. What is the difference between health and wellness?

3. What role does fitness play in health?

4. How does health across the lifespan affect a person's well-being?

5. What are the differences among a risk factor, a protective factor, and a health determinant?

6. What is risk reduction, and why is it important to health and wellness?

7. List and describe at least five health determinants. Explain how each of these determinants affects a person's health.

8. What are the three P's of health? How do these three P's influence a person's health?

9. Summarize the Universal Declaration of Human Rights of 1948.

10. Why is health a basic human right?

KEY TERMS

Fitness: Cardio-respiratory endurance, muscular strength, flexibility, and body composition

Health across the lifespan: Physical, mental, and social aging over a lifespan

Health determinant: A situation or environment that allows risk and protective factors to directly influence a person's health and illness

Holistic: Multidimensional and affected by multiple factors

Mental health or mental well-being: How a person thinks, feels, and acts when faced with life's situations and challenges

Physical health or physical well-being: Concerns our bodies and is associated with being physically fit due to healthy choices related to exercise, nutrition, sleep, and relaxation

Protective factor: A factor that decreases the chances of developing a disease, but does not guarantee that a person will not get the disease

Quality of life: A general sense of happiness and satisfaction with one's life and environment

Risk factor: A factor that increases the chances of developing a disease, but does not necessarily cause a disease

Risk reduction: A strategy or action that a person takes to decrease the chances of getting a disease

Wellness: An active, lifelong process of becoming aware of choices and making decisions for a more balanced and fulfilling quality of life

CHAPTER ACTIVITIES

1. Prepare to interview family members, friends, and neighbors who represent health across the lifespan. (For example, interview a child, an adolescent, a young adult, an adult, and an older adult.) Ask each person to tell you his or her definition of health. After conducting the interview, identify how the definitions differ across the lifespan. Write down the interview responses with your analysis and be prepared to discuss your findings in terms of health across the lifespan.

2. Identify and list five to seven health determinants. For each determinant, describe at least one or two risk factors, one or two protective factors, and one or two risk reduction strategies.

3. Go to the World Health Organization's website (http://www.who.int/gho/en/) for information on the Global Health Observatory (GHO) data. Review the links that show health issues at the global level. In small groups, brainstorm impressions of current global health issues. For example, which countries have the longest life expectancy? Which have the shortest? Once you brainstorm impressions, identify the health determinants that explain why specific health problems exist in certain countries while not in others.

4. If health is a human right, identify ways in which the US health care system violates that right and ways that it supports that right. Write your analysis in two columns to compare and contrast your ideas.

5. Develop a two-page case study that addresses health across the lifespan. The case study selection can be based on gender, sexual orientation, or race and ethnicity. Be ready to present your case study during class discussion. The class discussions need to address the issue of how considerations related to health across the lifespan are not the same for everyone.

Bibliography and Works Cited

Baun, F., Begin, M., Houweling, T., & Taylor, S. (2009). Changes not for the fainthearted: Reorienting health care systems toward health equity through action on the social determinants of health. *American Journal of Public Health*, 99, 1967–1973.

Clark, N. M. (2005). Population health and the environment. *Environmental Health Perspectives, 113*(8), 138.

Collins, C. A., Decker, S. I., & Esquibel, K. A. (2004). Definitions of health: Comparison of Hispanic and African-American elders. *Journal of Multicultural Nursing & Health, 10*(3), 13–18.

Corbin, C. B., Pangrazi, R. P., & Franks, G. D. (2005). *Toward a better understanding of physical fitness and activity: Selected topics, volume two.* Scottsdale. AZ; Holcomb Hathaway.

Doll, R. (1992). Health and the environment in the 1990s. *American Journal of Public Health*, 82, 933.

Institute of Medicine. (2001). *Health and behavior: The interplay of biological, behavioral, and societal influences.* Washington, DC: National Academies Press.

Institute of Medicine. (2003). *The future of the public's health in the 21st century.* Washington, DC: National Academies Press.

Manderscheid, R. W., Ryff, C. D., Freeman, E. J., McKnight-Eily, L. R., Dhingra, S., & Strine, T. (2010). Evolving definitions of mental illness and wellness. *Preventing Chronic Disease.* Retrieved from http://www.ncbi.nlm.nih.gov/pmc/articles/PMC2811514/

Miller, W., Simon, P., & Maleque, S. (2009). *Beyond health care: New directions to a healthier America.* Princeton, NJ: Robert Wood Johnson Foundation Commission to Build a Healthier America.

National Mental Health Information Center. (2015). What is mental health? Retrieved from https://www.mentalhealth.gov/basics/what-is-mental-health/index.html

Office of Disease Prevention and Health Promotion. (2014). Determinants of health. *Healthy People 2020.* Retrieved from http://www.healthypeople.gov/2020/about/foundation-health-measures/Determinants-of-Health

Purnell, L. (2003). Transcultural diversity and health care. In L. Purnell and B. Pulanka (Eds.), *Transcultural health care: A culturally; competent approach* (2nd ed., pp. 1–7). Philadelphia, PA: F. A. Davis.

UN Committee on Economic, Social and Cultural Rights. (2000, August 11). *General comment No. 14: The right to the highest attainable standard of health* (Art. 12 of the Covenant), E/C.12/2000/4. Available at http://www .refworld.org/docid/4538838d0.html

Winklestein, W. (1992). Determinants of worldwide health. *American Journal of Public Health, 82,* 931.

World Health Organization. (2008). *Closing the gap in a generation: Health equity through action on the social determinants of health.* Geneva, Switzerland: WHO Commission on the Social Determinants of Health. Retrieved from http://whqlibdocwho.int/publications/2008/9789241563703_eng.pdf

Worldwatch Institute. (2015). *Confronting hidden threats to sustainability.* Washington, DC: Author.

CHAPTER 2

OVERVIEW OF WESTERN MEDICAL PRACTICES

CHAPTER OBJECTIVES

- Summarize milestones in the history of Western medical practices.

- Identify and explain five medical theories on the cause of diseases.

- Summarize disability, disablement, and the disablement process.

- Compare and contrast infectious and noninfectious diseases.

- Give examples of the components of disease prevention: health promotion and health education.

- Explain the social-ecological model.

- Discuss how the goals of Healthy People 2020 improve the nation's health.

This chapter includes an overview of Western medical practices. A discussion follows on how past medical discoveries contributed to today's medical practices and how we view the causes of disease.

The chapter analyzes how the sciences of microbiology, bacteriology, and epidemiology were created in response to overcrowded living conditions during the Industrial Revolution. In addition, it offers an overview of the elements of disability as well as disease prevention. The chapter also looks at the Healthy People 2020 national agenda for disease prevention.

Brief History of Western Medical Practices

Western medical practices evolved from superstitions to a science. This evolution has taken place over thousands of years, each generation building on the knowledge of earlier times (Bynum, 2008; Leavitt, 1990; Loudon, 1997).

Please note that every culture has its own history of medical practices. The original peoples of North America, Africa, Australia, Asia, Southeast Asia, Siberia, and elsewhere have medical practices that reflect their cultural beliefs. These practices are passed from one generation to the next by oral, written, or visual traditions (Winkelman, 2009). In this chapter, however, the focus is on Western medical practices.

8000 BCE: Prehistoric Ages

Archaeologists have found cave paintings in Europe which suggest that the earliest humans believed that spirits and supernatural forces cured diseases. Animals, stars, earth, and dead ancestors inhabited the spirit world and influenced people's health. Specially trained individuals known as *spirit healers* or *shamans* called upon the spirit world for guidance on healing. These spirit healers were the first physicians, performing ceremonies and casting spells to treat diseases. They also used the first herbal medicines.

There was even prehistoric brain surgery, known as *trepanning*. Prehistoric skulls have been found with holes bored into them. These skulls show that the wounds healed and the bones grew back, meaning that the patients often survived. Trepanning was performed to let evil spirits out through the skull. It was done while the person was awake.

Although Western medicine no longer depends on the spirit world as a healing power, spirit healing is still practiced by some. Many people still visit faith healers or shamans or follow alternative therapies that claim to tap into the spirit world.

2000 BCE: Egyptians

Ancient Egyptians had physicians who specialized in treating particular parts of the body as well as researched the benefits of herbal medicines. The Egyptians kept detailed records of symptoms and treatments, creating the first medical textbooks. They also were the first pharmacists who prepared prescriptions used to treat specific diseases.

Physicians were priests who communicated with those gods responsible for the health of different parts of the body. However, instead of just relying on the gods, these physicians used herbal medicines and simple surgical procedures as part of treatment.

450 BCE to 300 CE: Greeks and Romans

The Greek philosopher Hippocrates (460–370 BCE) is considered the father of modern medicine. His name was given to the Hippocratic Oath that physicians are still required to uphold when practicing medicine.

Hippocrates separated medical practice from religion and saw disease as the body's failure to balance four "humors": blood, phlegm, black bile, and yellow bile. If a person was sick, it meant that there was an imbalance in his or her humors. Hippocrates's approach took medical practices away from the spirit or god world and moved toward a bodily explanation for disease.

Once medical practices were no longer dominated by the spirit or god world, ancient Greek physicians talked to their patients and took case histories. They also performed a physical exam on patients to make a diagnosis before recommending treatment.

When ancient Romans conquered the Greeks, they put many of the Greek medical practices to use. In addition, ancient Roman physicians gained much of their surgical knowledge by treating casualties in wars. They had hospitals to treat soldiers, and army surgeons became experts in amputations and stitching wounds.

The ancient Romans also were the first to link dirt and lack of hygiene with disease. To improve public health, they built water canals to supply clean drinking water, and sewers to remove wastes. Improved canals and sewers led to better personal hygiene, which helped reduce infectious diseases.

500–1400: The Middle Ages

With the fall of their empire, many of the ancient Roman public health practices were lost, and the "Dark Ages" of medicine began. The Middle Ages in Europe saw most people without access to clean drinking water, regular bathing, or a sewage system. The lack of public health practices meant that diseases spread more easily.

Although the Middle Ages are often known as the Dark Ages, some of the medical practices of that time are still used today. Laws were enacted that allowed only trained, registered people to practice medicine. Schools and universities began to educate wealthy individuals in medicine. Although surgical instruments were basic, complicated operations such as amputations were common. Opium was used as an anesthetic, and wounds were cleaned with alcohol to prevent infections.

700–1500: Middle East

While the medical practices of Europe during the Middle Ages focused on religious superstitions, the Middle East was the center of medical knowledge. Middle Eastern medical practices focused on universal health care, in that hospitals were not just for the wealthy—they treated rich and poor alike. Hospitals had medical and surgical wards as well as operating theaters and pharmacies. By the 10th century, Middle Eastern hospitals employed trained and licensed physicians and pharmacists. Medicines were certified as safe, and officials visited pharmacists for quality control of prescriptions.

One of the most important medical books of this period was *Laws of Medicine*, written by the physician Avicenna (980–1037). Completed around 1030, this encyclopedia of medicine contained five books detailing the formulas for medicines, diagnosis of diseases, and treatment.

1400–1700: The Renaissance

Leonardo da Vinci (1452–1519) drew the first anatomical drawings based on human dissection. Leonardo's drawings were a medical breakthrough because they helped identify organs and systems of the human body.

Physicians during the Renaissance based their diagnoses on the five senses, including tasting a urine sample. Urine tasting was a way that physicians determined what was wrong with a patient, assigning differences in colors and smells to specific diseases.

Barbers, not physicians, performed minor operations and treated wounds. The red-, white-, and blue-striped barber pole is a symbol that originated in the Renaissance period. The pole's red stripe represented blood; the white, bandages; and the blue, veins—marking the barber as a surgeon.

Renaissance pharmacists experimented with new plants brought from the Americas by Christopher Columbus and other explorers. For example, the leaves of the tobacco plant were thought to be so powerful a medicine that tobacco was called "God's remedy," used to help cure respiratory diseases.

1700–1800: The Industrial Revolution

The Industrial Revolution of the 18th and 19th centuries saw a change in the way people lived. Many people moved from small villages to find work in cities. They often lived in dirty, overcrowded housing with poor sanitation. Many people who lived in these conditions died from infectious diseases, such as cholera, tuberculosis, and pneumonia, which spread quickly.

Physicians during the Industrial Revolution did not understand the causes of most infectious diseases, nor did they know how to prevent them (Loudon, 1997). In the attempt to address the problem of infectious disease, three sciences emerged that helped explain the causes of infectious diseases and how they spread. The first is *microbiology*, the study of microbes, or germs. The second is *bacteriology*, the study of bacteria. These two sciences explain causes of diseases and their spread from a biological or medical perspective.

The third science, epidemiology, is the foundation of public health. *Epidemiology* is a science that identifies the causes of diseases and how they spread, but does so from a different perspective than that of microbiology and bacteriology. This science identifies and measures the physical, social, and cultural factors associated with diseases.

1900–2000: Advances in Medical Practices

In the 19th century, diseases that caused diarrhea were the biggest killer of children, and tuberculosis was the leading cause of death in adults today. In 1901, the average life expectancy in the United States was 47 years. By the year 2000, it had risen to 77 years. New medicines, improved air quality, and better public hygiene contributed to this 64% increase in life expectancy today. The sciences in the 20th century continued to build on the discoveries of the past and made major advances in medical practices. These advances include, to list a few, the development of antibiotics, aspirin, blood transfusions, chemotherapies, dialysis, genetic testing, the Human Genome Project, medical imaging, organ transplants, stem cell therapies, and vaccines.

Many of the medical advances made in the 20th century not only improved people's lives but also created ethical concerns—for patients, for health care providers, and for political leaders. For example, advanced treatments such as genetic engineering are used to treat a range of diseases. However, many of these treatments are expensive and are available only to those who have the money to pay. The wealthier a person is, the more likely it is that he or she has access not only to quality health care but also to medical advances that possibly save lives. The ethical concerns related to medical advances and who has access continue to challenge us.

2100 and Beyond: Medical Technologies

The 21st century has seen further advances in medical research and treatment. One example is *robotic surgery*. This type of surgery allows surgeons to perform complex procedures with more precision and control than is possible with conventional techniques. Robotic surgery enables minimally invasive procedures to be performed through tiny incisions. Patients who undergo robotic surgery have smaller scars, heal faster, and experience less pain than with regular surgery (Bynum, 2008).

Another example is precision medicine. *Precision medicine* is the practice of developing targeted medical treatments based on a person's environment, genetics, and lifestyle. Targeting the right treatment to the right patient reduces cost, decreases side effects, and improves health outcomes.

Yet, regardless of new technologies, it is still impossible to prevent all diseases. Bacteria evolves and become resistance to antibiotics. Viruses mutate to cause new infections. In addition, as people live longer, there are new challenges in treating an aging population.

The main shift in today's medical practices as compared to those used in the past has to do with not just the merits of discoveries but also how these discoveries affect patients (Baun, Begin, Houweling, & Taylor, 2009). We now see physicians and other health care providers in partnership with patients. The patients themselves have varying degrees of control over their health. This partnership has become crucial to understanding and delivering health care (Sarafino, 2008).

Theories on the Causes of Disease

Along with the evolution of Western medical practices have come changes in the theories explaining what causes disease. This chapter limits the discussion of what causes disease to five major theories (Turshen, 1989):

1. *Germ theory.* Germs such as bacteria or viruses cause diseases.

2. *Genetic abnormality theory.* Personal genetic makeup or genes cause diseases.

3. *Lifestyle theory.* Personal lifestyle choices and behaviors cause diseases.

4. *Multi-causes theory.* Diseases have multiple causes, many of which are rooted in physical, psychological, and social environments.

5. *Social production theory.* Diseases are socially produced.

Germ Theory

Germ theory is one of the oldest explanations for what causes diseases. Louis Pasteur (1822–1895), among others, identified multiple bacteria, viruses, and other infectious agents and developed the germ theory.

The germ theory's logic is that by killing germs such as a virus, or by making germs harmless, the disease can be cured and can be stopped from spreading. An example of the germ theory in action is when a person with a cold washes his or her hands to stop the spread of the cold virus to other people.

The germ theory was highly controversial when it was first proposed. Now it is one of the foundations of Western medical practice, which incorporates the use of antibiotics, antiviral medicines, vaccinations, and good hygiene practices.

There are, however, three weaknesses to the germ theory. The first is that it relies solely on the medical causes of diseases, ignoring individual, environmental, and socioeconomic causes. The second weakness is that it gives false hope that once the "germ" that caused the disease is identified, then the disease can be controlled, which is not true. There are many infectious diseases, such as HIV/AIDS, Lyme, and Zika, that are not controlled despite our knowledge of the cause. The third weakness is that the germ theory neglects to explain the causes of noninfectious diseases, such as cancer or heart disease.

Genetic Abnormality Theory

Genetic abnormality theory states that problems with a person's genetic makeup are the cause of diseases. Faulty genes can be the direct cause of a disease such as sickle cell anemia. Diseases can also be caused indirectly by faulty genes; for example, exposure to toxic waste puts some people with faulty genes more at risk for cancer than others.

This theory is based on the importance of identifying those who are more at risk for specific diseases due to their genes. Genetic screening, genetic counseling, and genetic engineering are examples of how the genetic abnormality theory is part of today's medical practices.

The genetic abnormality theory does lead to a better understanding of the causes of certain diseases. However, factors like income, education, and environment are not part of the genetic abnormality theory. Its focus is "something is wrong with the person." This theory can foster a "survival of the fittest" approach because there is not much you can do for people with "bad" genes. The theory sets up a dynamic between those with "good" genes versus those with "bad." As an example of how the genetic abnormality theory was used for destructive purposes, during World War II, the Nazis killed those who were deemed to have inferior genetic makeup, such as gypsies, homosexuals, Jews, and people with disabilities.

Lifestyle Theory

According to the *lifestyle theory*, diseases are a consequence of personal choices and behavior, for which each individual is responsible. A person gets a disease because he or she lacks information or behaves irresponsibly. This theory embraces the concept that with a healthy lifestyle, a person can reduce the chances of getting a disease.

The lifestyle theory is often clouded with a "blaming the victim" stance; that is, if only a person lived "right," then he would not get a disease. For example, according to the lifestyle theory, if a person knew how to manage his stress—avoiding making unhealthy choices and engaging in unhealthy behaviors that lead to stressful situations—then he would not get heart disease.

Research that supports the lifestyle theory is limited. A person can make healthy choices and engage in healthy behaviors yet still get any number of diseases. Healthy lifestyle choices and behaviors can reduce the risk of getting some diseases, but they are no guarantee.

Multi-Causes Theory

The *multi-causes theory* does not abandon the germ, genetic abnormality, or lifestyle theories. Instead, it adds a broader explanation. The multi-causes theory recognizes the complex causes of a disease.

That is, factors such as germs, genetics, lifestyle, income, and environment can all contribute to causing a disease (Office of Disease Prevention and Health Promotion, 2015).

The multi-causes theory is widely held and is supported by US public health policies. It is noteworthy, however, that although this theory explains the cause of diseases, there has been little progress made in reducing overall death rates in the United States (Goodman, Posner, Huang, Parekh, & Koh, 2013). Even when we know the causes of a disease and can treat it, better diagnosis and treatment can only go so far. According to the Office of Disease Prevention and Health Promotion (2015), although death rates from heart disease, stroke, and diabetes have slowed in recent years, there needs to be more emphasis on how to prevent these diseases in the first place. If we were to apply what we know about preventing chronic diseases such as cancer, heart disease, stroke, and diabetes, we could reduce deaths by half. In addition, regardless of the cause of chronic diseases, there is no cure. The multi-causes theory only explains how people get diseases—it does not offer the cure.

Social Production Theory

The social production theory claims that it is more important to understand the circumstances of illness (where people live and work) than the biological information related to a disease. The way in which goods and services such as housing, food, and income are distributed affects our health—and puts us at risk for diseases.

According to this theory, health and disease are products of the way that society is organized in terms of how goods and services as well as surplus are made and distributed. Surplus is that part of goods and services that is not necessary for survival. For example, company profits and owning a second home are two forms of surplus.

This theory suggests that the only way to prevent diseases is through social reorganization, including the ways surplus is distributed to those who are not wealthy. The answer to the question of what is the cause of disease involves a shift in focus from the individual to social class and to the way goods and services are distributed.

Although health care is important for identifying and treating diseases, what is also as important is social organization. Diseases are different from place to place not only because of geography but also because of the way that goods and services are distributed in those places. If we know the answers to "Who gets what? When? How? Why? And how much?" then we can better understand the causes of diseases.

Measuring Health and Disease

How health and disease are measured has evolved with Western medical practices and theories. Health is measured in terms of the absence of disease or of the body's ability to maintain equilibrium, known as *homeostasis*. A way to measure health is to look at a population's health status (Durch, Bailey, & Stoto, 1997). *Health status* is the health description of a population.

The measure of health status includes the death rate, known as *mortality*. It can also include the illness, injury, or disability rate, known as *morbidity*. A growing trend in measuring the health of a population is to use the terms mortality and morbidity rather than health status.

Diseases are what physicians and biologists study. A *disease* is an abnormal condition in physiological and biological factors or an abnormal homeostasis status. The cause, or *etiology*, of a disease can be known or unknown. When the etiology is unknown, the disease is referred to as *idiopathic*.

Signs, such as elevated blood pressure, are the evidence of a disease and are measured during a physical exam. *Symptoms* are what a patient reports to be experiencing but cannot be measured. Examples of symptoms are dizziness, lack of sleep, and itching.

Table 2.1   Comparison of Infectious and Noninfectious Diseases

Infectious Diseases	Noninfectious Diseases
For certain infectious diseases such as seasonal flu, a person's risk is greatly affected by the disease status of others, including whether the people the person meets have been vaccinated.	A person's risk of getting a noninfectious disease is not influenced by the disease status of others.
For certain infectious diseases, such as measles, once a person has had the disease, he or she will never get it again.	For most noninfectious risk factors, such as toxins in the drinking water, there are levels at which all individuals exposed will eventually become ill.
With outbreaks of some infectious diseases, such as Ebola or Zika, the time frame for investigation and preventive action is short, often a matter of hours or days.	Many noninfectious diseases are subject to the impact of environmental (e.g., lead exposure) and behavioral (e.g., smoking) risk factors that require long-term disease prevention strategies.
For many infectious diseases, the cause and characteristics of transmission are well known; this leads to clear targets for disease prevention strategies.	For noninfectious diseases such as obesity and heart disease, the cause and impact of risk factors such as diet and exercise on disease prevention remains a matter of debate.

A disease can be either chronic or acute. There is more than one definition of chronic disease. In light of the multiple definitions, this textbook limits the definition of a *chronic disease or chronic condition* to one that begins slowly and lasts for longer than 3 months, or it can persist for a year or more. Included in both of these definitions is the recognition that a chronic disease requires ongoing medical attention. Chronic diseases generally cannot be cured, but they are not immediately fatal. Examples of chronic diseases are asthma, type 2 diabetes, and multiple sclerosis.

Acute diseases are those that come on quickly but last for a short time, usually less than 3 months. These diseases tend to have severe symptoms. Examples of acute diseases are influenza, measles, and the seasonal flu.

A *disorder* is a functional disturbance that is categorized as mental, physical, genetic, emotional, or behavioral. Disorder is a term used by some people rather than the term disease because it is seen to have less social stigma. A *medical condition* is a broad term for all diseases and disorders, but also can refer to a healthy state such as pregnancy or menopause.

A *syndrome* is a group of simultaneous, multiple signs and symptoms. Examples include chronic fatigue syndrome and Down syndrome.

Chronic and acute diseases can be either infectious or noninfectious. *Infectious diseases* occur because a person has contact with specific viruses, fungi, parasites, bacteria, or toxic product. There are two types of infectious diseases: *communicable,* meaning that a person can give the infectious disease to another person (for example, herpes, SARS, or the flu); and *noncommunicable,* meaning that a person cannot give the infectious disease to another person (for example, rabies, cholera, and Lyme disease). For a more detailed comparison between infectious and noninfectious diseases, see Table 2.1.

The *epidemiologic triangle* is a model that scientists use to understand infectious diseases and to measure how they spread. As shown in Figure 2.1, the epidemiologic triangle has three corners: the *agent* or microbe that causes the disease (the What of the triangle); the *host,* or the organism that carries the disease (the Who of the triangle); and the *environment,* or the external factors that allow a disease to spread (the Where of the triangle).

In the center of the triangle is time. Time relates to the measure of three different situations, depending on what scientists are looking for. The first is the *incubation period*—the time between when the host is infected and when disease symptoms appear. The second is the amount of time a person can be sick before death or recovery occurs. The third is the period from when an infection occurs to the beginning of an epidemic. An *epidemic* is a situation in which there are more cases of a

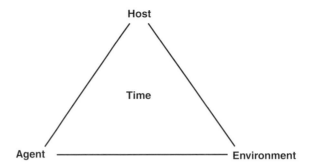

Figure 2.1 Epidemiologic Triangle

particular disease than expected in a given area or among a specific group of people over a particular period of time.

Diseases also are measured by categories—for example, infectious, genetic, psychiatric, genital, cardiovascular, metabolic, and occupational. Syphilis, for example, is a chronic, infectious, communicable, genital disease.

Medical Concepts of Disease and Disability

The terms *health care consumer, client,* and *patient* are often used to mean the same thing, but although these terms are similar, they are not identical. A health care consumer is someone who buys health services or products. A client is someone who uses professional health services. A health care consumer and client may or may not be sick or have a disease or a condition.

Please note that the term *patient* is used in this textbook to describe someone waiting for or using health care services. He or she is most often sick and needs the services of a physician or other health care providers.

The term *health care providers* as used in this textbook is adapted from the 2010 World Health Organization (WHO) definition of *health professionals.* Health care providers "study, advise on or provide preventive, curative, rehabilitative and promotional health services based on theoretical and factual knowledge in diagnosis and treatment of disease and other health problems" (p. 1). According to WHO, health care providers include those who are clinically trained, such as physicians, dentists, physician assistants, nurses, and pharmacists. Health care providers can also be people who are not necessarily clinically trained, such as health education specialists, patient navigators, peer educators, community health workers, psychologists, health advocates, social workers, home health aides, and a wide variety of other professionals trained to provide some type of health care service.

Like the terms *health* and *disease, disability* is defined in a variety of ways. For the purposes of this textbook, *disability* is defined as the inability to perform and to participate in socially defined activities and roles expected of a person within a social or a physical environment (Carmelo & Donatella, 2008). The definition reflects a complex interaction between the health of a person with his or her environment. Disability is measured by how much the person can participate in his or her world. People with disabilities are identified as persons have difficulty doing daily life activities, who use assistance, or who see themselves as having a disability (Carmelo & Donatella, 2008; Masala & Petretto, 2008).

Disablement is the transition from health to disability. The term represents the interaction between the person who has a disease and his or her environment (see Figure 2.2). Disablement happens when a person gets sick and experiences restrictions in basic physical and mental activities within his or her environment.

There are also terms that measure the patient's experience. *Illness* is the personal experience of not feeling well. *Sickness* is being ill but also experiencing the social responses to a disease or illness. For

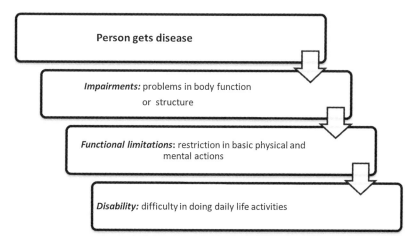

Figure 2.2 The Disablement Process

example, those with a mental health disorder may be described by others as having a "sickness." The *sick role* focuses on social expectations for the behaviors of a person with a disease—for instance, taking sick time off from work.

How the terms *disease, disorder, medical condition, illness, sickness,* and *sick role* are viewed depends on a person's social, racial, and cultural environment. For example, depending on the culture, AIDS carries such a heavy social stigma that a person who has this disease may be too afraid to seek treatment.

Disease Prevention, Health Promotion, and Health Education

The 20th and 21st centuries have seen improvements in disease prevention. The world is now a place where many people live longer and often have healthier lives than they did in earlier periods. The Office of Disease Prevention and Health Promotion (2015) report that this increase in life expectancy and quality of life is due not to medical technology but to disease prevention.

Health promotion is the major strategy of disease prevention (WHO, 1998). The 1998 WHO definition of health promotion is "the process of enabling people to increase control over their health and its determinants, and thereby improve their health." By this definition, health promotion does not focus only on the individual but also on the influences that affect a person's health.

There are two parts to health promotion: (a) health education and (b) environmental strategies that support healthy lifestyles (WHO, 1998). *Health education* is the basis for health promotion; that is, you cannot engage in health promotion without health education (Gold & Miner, 2002). Health education is a specialized field that uses planned strategies based on educational theories. It provides opportunities for individuals, groups, and communities to learn information and develop skills that are necessary for healthy decisions and lifestyles.

Health promotion strategies are put to use at three levels: primary, secondary, and tertiary (Office of Disease Prevention and Health Promotion, 2015).

Primary prevention strategies prevent or stop a person from getting a specific disease. These strategies target healthy people. Primary prevention includes efforts to reduce causes or risk factors associated with a disease. Examples include vaccinations, smoke-free workplaces, and prenatal care.

Secondary prevention strategies try to prevent a disease from getting worse. These strategies try to stop a disease from progressing once a person is exposed to it or at risk of becoming ill. Examples include screenings that detect disease at an early stage. *Screenings* find people who are likely to have a disease, or they look for factors that put a person at risk for disease.

Tertiary prevention strategies soften the negative effects of having a disease. Strategies include services that minimize illness and improve outcomes once someone has a disease. Examples are

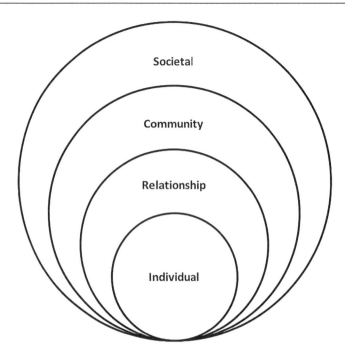

Figure 2.3 The Social-Ecological Model for Health Promotion

rehabilitation services like physical therapy, occupational therapy, or Alcoholics Anonymous (AA) support groups.

These levels of health promotion are based on an understanding that there are multiple factors that influence the likelihood of an individual getting a disease. The *social-ecological model* identifies these factors as individual, relationship, community, and societal (National Center for Injury Prevention and Control, 2015). It also explains how these factors protect people from getting a disease or put them at risk. It is the role of health promotion strategies to positively affect these factors (see Figure 2.3). Health promotion targets these factors at multiple levels and at the same time.

Individual The first level aims at the biological and personal history factors that increase risk. Some of these factors are age, education, income, race, and family history. Strategies at this level target attitudes, beliefs, and behaviors that promote healthy decisions and lifestyles.

Relationship The second level aims at the personal relationships that increase the risk of getting a disease. Strategies at this level target those who influence the health of others, such as peers, loved ones, and family members.

Community The third level aims at the settings—schools, workplaces, and neighborhoods—where people engage in social relationships. Strategies at this level impact the social and physical environment.

Societal The fourth level aims at the societal factors that affect healthy decisions and lifestyles. These factors include the health, economic, educational, and public policies that maintain inequalities between groups in society.

Healthy People 2020

Healthy People is an initiative of the US government that issues national objectives for promoting health and preventing diseases. Every 10 years for the last three decades, Healthy People has provided a national framework for disease prevention.

The US Department of Health and Human Services (HHS) gathers scientific information from the past decade, along with new knowledge of current data, trends, and innovations. It then creates a document to report its findings. *Healthy People 2020* is the most recent initiative, leading the way to increase quality of care, promote years of healthy life, and remove health disparities.

When Healthy People was first developed, the process relied heavily on experts. Now the process relies on public input at every step. The Healthy People 2020 process is inclusive; its strength is in its collaboration across federal, state, and local agencies as well as its reliance on input from community members. There have been thousands of citizens helping shape it at every step along the way.

The vision for Healthy People 2020 is "A society in which all people live long, healthy lives." Its mission is "To improve health through strengthening policy and practice." Its goals are as follows:

1. Eliminate preventable disease, disability, injury, and premature death

2. Achieve health equity, eliminate health disparities, and improve the health of all groups

3. Create social and physical environments that promote good health for all

4. Promote healthy development and healthy behaviors across every stage of life

Healthy People 2020 defines *health equity* as a desirable goal that requires special efforts to improve the health of those who have experienced social or economic disadvantage. *Health disparity* is the health difference between individuals or groups that is unfair because it is caused by social or economic disadvantage. *Social environments* are the social, economic, and cultural institutions, norms, patterns, beliefs, and processes that influence the life of an individual or community. *Physical environments* are both the natural and built environments and how those environments affect health.

Chapter Summary

• Western medical practices have evolved over thousands of years. Each generation has built on the knowledge of earlier times.

• The leading cause of death for an adult in the 19th century was infectious disease; in the 21st century, chronic diseases are the leading cause of death. The specific challenges for the future in disease prevention are linked to risk factors related to chronic diseases, such as lifestyle, environments, and the aging process.

• There are five major theories explaining what causes diseases: Germ theory states that germs such as bacteria or viruses are responsible for diseases. Genetic abnormality theory posits that personal genetic makeup is responsible for diseases. Lifestyle theory argues that lifestyle choices and behaviors are responsible for diseases. Multi-causes theory acknowledges that diseases have multiple causes. According to social production theory, diseases are socially produced.

• People with disabilities are identified as persons who have an activity limitation, who use assistance, or who see themselves as having a disability.

• Health promotion is the major strategy of disease prevention. According to the World Health Organization (WHO), health promotion is "the process of enabling people to increase control over their health and its determinants, and thereby improve their health."

• Health education is the basis for health promotion; that is, there is no health promotion without health education. It is a specialized field that uses planned strategies based on educational theories.

• There are three main levels of health promotion strategies: primary, secondary, and tertiary.

• The social-ecological model recognizes the complex interplay among individual, relationship, community, and societal factors.

• The vision of Healthy People 2020 is "A society in which all people live long, healthy lives." The mission is "To improve health through strengthening policy and practice."

REVIEW QUESTIONS

1. What contributions did the ancient Egyptians make to Western medical practices?

2. Who is the Greek philosopher Hippocrates, and what did he contribute to Western medical practices?

3. What contributions did the ancient Romans make to public health?

4. What is epidemiology, and why is it important to public health?

5. Identify and explain the five theories on what causes diseases discussed in this chapter.

6. What are four differences between infectious and noninfectious diseases?

7. Define disability and explain the disablement process.

8. What is the difference between health promotion and health education?

9. What is the social-ecological model, and why is it important to disease prevention?

10. What is the significance of Healthy People 2020? What is the difference between health equity and health disparity?

KEY TERMS

Acute diseases: Diseases that come on quickly but last less than 3 to 6 months

Agent: Microbe or microorganism that causes an infectious disease

Bacteriology: The study of bacteria

Chronic disease or chronic condition: A disease or condition that begins slowly and lasts anywhere from 3 months to a year or longer, has no cure, limits what a person can do, and requires ongoing care

Communicable infectious diseases: Infectious diseases that one person can give to another

Disability: The inability to perform and participate in socially defined activities and roles expected of a person within a social or a physical environment

Disablement: The transition over time from health to disability

Disease: An abnormal condition in physiological and biological factors or an abnormal homeostatic state

Disorder: Functional disturbance that can be categorized into mental, physical, genetic, emotional, and behavioral

Environment: In the context of health, external factors that cause or allow a disease to spread

Epidemic: Situation that exists when there are more cases of a particular disease than expected in a given area, or among a specific group of people, over a particular period of time

Epidemiologic triangle: A model that scientists use for identifying and understanding infectious diseases and how they spread

Epidemiologist: A scientist who works in the field of epidemiology

Epidemiology: The study of the distribution of deaths, diseases, and other health problems in a population

Etiology: The cause of a disease

Functional limitations: Restrictions in basic physical and mental activities

Health disparity: A health difference between individuals or groups that is unfair because it is caused by social or economic disadvantage

Health education: A field within health promotion that uses planned learning strategies based on educational theories

Health equity: A goal that requires special efforts to improve the health of those who have experienced social or economic disadvantage

Health promotion: The process of enabling people to increase control over their health and its determinants, and thereby improve their health

Health status: The health description of an individual or population

Healthy People 2020: A national framework to address risk factors, determinants of health, diseases, and disorders that affect communities

Homeostasis: The body's ability to maintain equilibrium or a steady state

Idiopathic: Term used to describe a disease whose etiology (cause) is unknown

Illness: A personal experience of not feeling "well" or of suffering that may be the result of a specific disease or caused by cultural beliefs

Impairments: Problems in body function or structure

Incubation period: The time between when the host is infected and when disease symptoms appear

Infectious diseases: Diseases caused by infection with specific viruses, fungi, parasites, bacteria, or toxin

Medical condition: A broad term for all diseases and disorders, but also can mean a healthy state such as pregnancy or menopause

Microbiology: The study of microbes or microorganisms

Microorganism: Specific agent, such as a virus, that is responsible for disease

Morbidity: Illness, injury, or disability

Mortality: Death

Noncommunicable infectious diseases: Infectious diseases that are not passed from one person to another

Physical environments: In terms of health, both the natural and built environments and how those environments affect health

Precision medicine: The practice of developing targeted medical treatments based on a person's environment, genetics, and lifestyle

Prevention: Any action or strategy aimed at eradicating, eliminating, or minimizing the impact of disease and disability

Primary prevention: Efforts to reduce risk factors associated with certain diseases, including efforts to control the causes of a disease

Robotic surgery: Minimally invasive surgical procedures performed through tiny incisions made by robots

Screening: Medical test used to detect the presence of a specific disease, to find people who are likely to have a disease, or to detect factors that put a person at risk for disease

Secondary prevention: Efforts to prevent an existing disease from progressing to long-term illness

Sick role: Social expectations for the behaviors of a person diagnosed with a disease or illness

Sickness: State of being ill but also experiencing the social responses to a disease or illness

Signs: The evidence of a disease as observed during a physical examination

Social-ecological model: A health promotion model that considers the complex interplay between individual, relationship, community, and societal factors in disease prevention

Social environment: The social, economic, and cultural institutions, norms, patterns, beliefs, and processes that influence the life of an individual or community

Spirit healers/shamans: Practitioners who contact the spirit world for guidance on healing

Symptoms: What a person reports to be experiencing and can't be measured by medical procedures

Syndrome: Simultaneous, multiple signs and symptoms associated with a disease

Tertiary prevention: Efforts of rehabilitation and special educational services that minimize illness and improve outcomes once there is a disease

Trepanning: Prehistoric brain surgery

CHAPTER ACTIVITIES

1. Review the five major theories for causes of diseases and identify at least three diseases associated with each theory. Be prepared to discuss and explain your list in group discussions.

2. In pairs, present the epidemiologic triangle in class and show how it helps organize information about a specific disease. This is the same technique that epidemiologists use when they are researching the outbreak of a disease. You will use the example of *Escherichia coli (E. coli)* in describing the three corners of the epidemiologic triangle. See the CDC's website (www.cdc.gov) for information on *E. coli* and how it spreads. After this in-class introduction, gather information about measles by using the epidemiologic triangle and report back to the class on what you have learned. See the CDC's website for information on measles and how it spreads.

3. You have been recently hired as a school health educator for the City of Springfield School System. Your job responsibility is to develop health education strategies at the primary, secondary, and tertiary levels. The topic is tobacco use prevention. Develop two to three learning strategies for each of the three grade groups: grades 1–5 (primary strategies), grades 6–8 (secondary strategies), and grades 9–12 (tertiary strategies).

4. With a partner, brainstorm and list two examples of health promotion strategies addressing adolescent illegal drug use at each level of the social-ecological model.

5. In groups of three to four, develop your own time line for the history of medicine, identifying accomplishments not discussed in this chapter. The time line can be limited to a specific century, a historical period, or a non-Western medical tradition, such as Chinese medicine and practices.

Bibliography and Works Cited

Baun, F., Begin, M., Houweling, T., & Taylor, S. (2009). Changes not for the fainthearted: Reorienting health care systems toward health equity through action on the social determinants of health. *American Journal of Public Health, 99,* 1967–1973.

Bynum, W. F. (2008). *The history of medicine: A very short introduction.* New York, NY: Oxford University Press.

Carmelo, M., & Donatella, R. (2008). From disablement to enablement: Conceptual models of disability in the 20th century. *Disability and Rehabilitation, 30,* 1233–1244.

Clark, N. M. (2005). Population health and the environment. *Environmental Health Perspectives, 113*(8), 138.

Collins, C. A., Decker, S. I., & Esquibel, K. A. (2004). Definitions of health: Comparison of Hispanic and African-American elders. *Journal of Multicultural Nursing & Health, 10*(3), 13–18.

Durch, J., Bailey, L., & Stoto, M. (1997). *Improving health in the community: A role for performance monitoring.* Washington, DC: National Academies Press.

Friis, R. (2007). *Essentials of environmental health.* Sudbury: MA: Jones and Bartlett.

Gold, R. S., & Miner, K. R. (2002). Report of the 2000 Joint Committee on Health Education and Promotion Terminology. *Journal of School Health, 72*(1), 3–7. doi:10.1111/j.1746-1561.2002.tb06501

Goodman, R. A., Posner, S. F., Huang, E. S., Parekh, A. K., & Koh, H. K. (2013). Defining and measuring chronic conditions: Imperatives for research, policy, program, and practice. *Preventing Chronic Disease.* doi: 10:120239

Last, J. M. (1998). *Public health and human ecology* (2nd ed.) Stamford, CT: Appleton & Lange.

Last, J. M. (Ed.) (2006). *A dictionary of public health.* New York, NY: Oxford University Press.

Lawrence, R. H., & Jette, A. M. (1996). Disentangling the disablement process. *Journals of Gerontology, Series B, Psychological Sciences and Social Sciences, 51*(4), 173–182.

Leavitt, J. W. (1990). Medicine in context: A review essay of the history of medicine. *American Historical Review, 95,* 1471–1484.

Loudon, I. (1997). *Western medicine: An illustrated history.* New York, NY: Oxford University Press.

Masala, C., & Petretto, D. R. (2008). From disablement to enablement: Conceptual models of disability in the 20th century. *Disability and Rehabilitation, 30,* 1233–1244.

McGill, N. (2015, September). Public health, prevention to play role in precision medicine: Interventions aimed at individual risks. *Nation's Health.* Retrieved from www.thenationshealth.org

National Center for Injury Prevention and Control, Department of Violence Prevention. (2015). The social-ecological model: A framework for prevention. Retrieved from http://www.cdc.gov/violenceprevention /overview/social-ecologicalmodel.html

Ng, L.K.Y., & Davis, D. L. (1981). *Strategies for public health: promoting health and preventing disease.* Reinhold, NY: Van Nostrand.

Office of Disease Prevention and Health Promotion. (2015). Determinants of health. *Healthy People 2020.* Retrieved from http://www.healthypeople.gov/2020/about/foundation-health-measures/Determinants-of -Health

Patrick, D., & Erikson, P. (1993). *Health status and health policy: Quality of life in evaluation and resource allocation.* New York, NY: Oxford University Press.

Purnell, L. D., & Paulanka, B. J. (2003). *Transcultural health care: A culturally competent approach* (2nd ed.) Philadelphia, PA: F. A. Davis.

Sarafino, E. P. (2008). *Health psychology: Biopsychosocial interactions* (6th ed.) Hoboken, NJ: Wiley.

Turnock, B. J. (2011). *Essentials of public health* (2nd ed.) Sudbury: MA.: Jones and Bartlett.

Turshen, M. (1989). *The politics of public health.* Brunswick, NJ: Rutgers University Press.

Winkelman, M. (2009). *Culture and health: Applying medical anthropology.* San Francisco: CA: Jossey-Bass.

World Health Organization. (1998). Health promotion glossary. *Health Promotion International, 13,* 349–364.

World Health Organization. (2010). Classifying health workers: Mapping occupations to the international standard classification. Retrieved from http://www.who.int/hrh/statistics/Health_workers_classification .pdf?ua=1

OVERVIEW OF CHRONIC DISEASES

CHAPTER OBJECTIVES

- Discuss how chronic diseases are the leading causes of morbidity and mortality in the United States.

- Identify risk factors for noninfectious chronic diseases.

- Explain the Chronic Care Model.

- Describe the chain of infection.

- Compare the differences among the types of palliative care.

This chapter is an overview of chronic diseases. According to the Centers for Disease Control and Prevention (CDC), chronic diseases are among the most common, costly, and preventable of all health problems in the United States. Some chronic diseases are major killers and are responsible for roughly 70% of all deaths and for 86% of our health care dollar.

The Chronic Care Model addresses the rising health care demands of chronic diseases. The goal of this model is to improve the quality and cost-effectiveness of care for patients.

In addition, this chapter describes the different types of palliative care and the need to make a quality end-of-life plan before a medical crisis arises.

Defining Chronic Diseases

In the 21st century, we can expect to live longer than any previous generation. However, there are more than 133 million people—almost one out of every two adults—living with at least one chronic disease (Anderson, 2007, 2010). For many, having a chronic disease means living with an illness for years if not a lifetime. It can also limit a person's daily activities and require ongoing medical care.

As defined in Chapter 2, a *chronic disease or chronic condition* begins slowly and lasts anywhere from more than 3 months to a year or more. Included in this definition is the recognition that having a chronic disease requires ongoing medical attention or limits the activities of daily living. Chronic diseases generally are not immediately fatal, but they are also rarely completely cured.

Chronic condition is a term used to describe a person's experience of a chronic disease. Some people use the term *chronic condition* instead of *chronic disease* because there is social stigma associated with having a "disease." For purposes of this textbook, the terms chronic disease and chronic condition are the same or equal terms. Regardless of which term is used, having a chronic disease is a health condition that requires ongoing care, limits what the person does, and can last a lifetime.

Many chronic diseases are caused by genetic makeup; some are the result of long exposure to environmental factors; still others may be caused by lifestyle choices.

Chronic diseases usually develop over a long time—often at first without causing signs and symptoms. When signs and symptoms do develop, there may be times when the illness gets worse, and, for some chronic diseases, it can be fatal. These diseases are usually more common as we age, when it is more difficult to fully recover; consequently, they can lead to some form of disability.

Some patients with a chronic disease experience major changes to their lives. Their physical and mental health, their social and family life, and their employment status may need adjustment. Certain chronic diseases, such as multiple sclerosis, can be highly disabling; whereas others, such as allergies, are less so. Some chronic diseases, such as diabetes, may not disable a person at first, but can cause severe disabilities if not treated early. Some people return to former levels of daily activity after receiving treatment; others are not as fortunate, growing more and more dependent on others. Many of these diseases allow people to live meaningful and rewarding lives; other diseases cause severe disabilities, depression, and lasting physical pain.

There are two categories of chronic diseases: infectious and noninfectious. However, categorization is often not so clear. For example, some chronic diseases originally thought to be noninfectious, such as cervical cancer and some forms of arthritis, are now seen as having infectious causes (Wylie-Rosett & Karanja, 2009).

Causes of Noninfectious Chronic Diseases

Many *noninfectious chronic diseases*—for example, sickle cell anemia and cystic fibrosis—are caused by genetic makeup or when there is a family history of the disease. Other noninfectious chronic diseases, such as alcoholism and type 2 diabetes, can be caused by lifestyle risk factors. Diseases caused by lifestyle risk factors can be more easily controlled than those caused by genetic makeup.

There are many risk factors for chronic diseases. There are four leading lifestyle risk factors: lack of physical activity, poor dietary choices, tobacco use, and excessive alcohol use (National Center for Chronic Disease Prevention and Health Promotion, 2009; National Health Council, 2014). These risk factors cause much of the *morbidity* (illness) and early *mortality* (death) related to chronic diseases (National Center for Chronic Disease Prevention and Health Promotion, 2016). What is unfortunate is that the chronic diseases caused by these risks factors are preventable.

Regular physical activity is one of the most important things a person can do to stay healthy. Physical activity not only increases the chances of living longer but also helps control weight, reduces the risks for heart diseases and type 2 diabetes, strengthens bones and muscles, improves mental health, and increases a person's ability to perform daily activities like walking and climbing stairs.

Making healthy diet choices lowers the risk for many chronic diseases, including stroke, type 2 diabetes, and osteoporosis. For example, eating fresh fruits and vegetables helps a person maintain a healthy weight and reduce the risk for heart diseases, type 2 diabetes, and certain cancers.

Since 1964, the surgeon general's reports on smoking and health have warned that tobacco use is the single most avoidable cause of disease, disability, and death in the United States. The use of tobacco products, such as cigarettes, cigars, and dip, is linked to cancer, heart diseases, respiratory disorders, sexual dysfunction, and gum disease.

Excessive alcohol use is the third leading lifestyle-related cause of death. It is linked to many chronic diseases, including depression, hypertension, liver disease, osteoporosis, and cancers.

According to the National Center for Health Statistics (2013, 2015), millions of people in the United States engage in behaviors related to these four lifestyle risk factors:

- In 2011, more than half (52%) of adults age 18 years or older did not meet recommendations for physical activity.

- Obesity is a serious health concern in the United States, with about 78.6 million adults obese. Nearly one in five youths ages 2 to 19 years is obese.

- More than 42 million adults said they currently smoked cigarettes in 2012. Cigarette smoking is the leading preventable cause of death and is responsible for about 480,000 deaths per year.

- Drinking too much alcohol is responsible for 88,000 deaths each year, more than half of which are due to binge drinking. Yet most binge drinkers are not alcohol dependent. One does not need to be an alcoholic to have problems with alcohol. Even occasional alcohol abuse can lead to criminal activity, violence, and injury.

Common Noninfectious Chronic Diseases

Persons with noninfectious chronic diseases represent all ages, races, cultures, and levels of socio-economic status. There is the child with asthma, the college student with depression, the coworker with heart disease, the neighbor with lung cancer, the elderly woman with Alzheimer's disease, the friend with bipolar disorder. As the number of people with chronic diseases continues to grow, nearly everyone is likely to know someone whose life is affected by one or more of these diseases.

As we continue further into the 21st century, noninfectious chronic diseases are and will be the major reason for mortality and morbidity in the United States (National Center for Chronic Disease Prevention and Health Promotion, 2016). Forty-five percent of all Americans live with a chronic disease, such as hypertension, epilepsy, depression, or cancer. By 2030, that percentage is expected to grow to more than 50% (National Health Council, 2014).

There are many reasons why so many people are living with these diseases. According to the Robert Wood Johnson Foundation (2010), one is that medical advances in technology are effective in treating and managing many chronic diseases. Another is that more people are being screened for chronic diseases, making *early detection* and treatment possible. Still another, more direct reason for the increasing numbers is the aging of the US population. As people get older, the likelihood of having at least one chronic disease increases. As the baby boomers age, the number of people living with at least one chronic disease will also grow. More significant, women tend to live longer than men. So, over time, we can expect to see a rise in the number of older women living with at least one chronic disease. To add to their own health burdens, many of these older women are caregivers to family members and friends with chronic diseases (Robert Wood Johnson Foundation, 2010).

According to the National Center for Health Statistics (2015), with at least 133 million Americans living with at least one chronic disease and with millions of new cases each year, an even greater number of people suffer from disabilities. Chronic, disabling diseases cause major limitations in daily activities for one in four individuals who have one or more of these diseases:

- *Arthritis,* or chronic joint symptoms, is the most common cause of disability, affecting at least one of every five adults.

- *Asthma* causes 400,000 to 500,000 hospitalizations, 14 million missed school days, and 100 million days of restricted activity each year.

- *Cancer* affects at least 11 million Americans who live with a previous diagnosis of cancer, and that number is on the rise. The most commonly diagnosed cancers are prostate, female breast, lung and bronchus, and colorectal cancers.

- *Diabetes* is the leading cause of kidney failure and of new blindness in adults. Nearly 24 million Americans have diabetes. An estimated 57 million American adults have prediabetes, placing them at increased risk for developing type 2 diabetes.

- *Heart disease* and *stroke* have left millions of people with disabilities; many can no longer perform daily tasks, such as walking or bathing, without help. These diseases remain the first and third leading causes of death, accounting for more than 30% of all mortality, and are among the leading causes of disability.

Disease Prevention for Noninfectious Chronic Diseases

Prevention strategies for chronic diseases are used at multiple levels. These strategies are directed at individuals and their families, their communities, their schools and workplaces, and across their life span. Health promotion strategies are part of chronic disease prevention. These strategies include early detection efforts, such as *screenings* (medical tests that detect the presence of a disease), and disease management. *Disease management* is a multidisciplinary approach that improves the quality and cost-effectiveness of care for patients suffering from chronic diseases. The goal of disease management is to identify persons at risk for one or more chronic diseases, to promote self-management by patients, and to provide effective and efficient health care (Schrijvers, 2009).

In its landmark report *Power of Prevention,* the National Center for Chronic Disease Prevention and Health Promotion (2009) states that the benefits of early detection and disease management include saving lives and lowering health care costs. The following are examples of these benefits:

- Regular screening for some cancers (e.g., colorectal cancer) can reduce the number of people who die from this disease.

- For women who have been sexually active and have a cervix, screening with a Pap test reduces illness and death from cervical cancer.

- Among people with diabetes, annual eye and foot exams can reduce vision loss and lower-extremity amputations.

- Early diagnosis and management of arthritis, including self-management, can help people with arthritis decrease pain, improve function, and stay productive.

- The health benefits of quitting smoking are many and can be experienced rapidly. Within 2 weeks to 3 months after quitting, a person's heart attack risk begins to drop, and lung function begins to improve. Ten years after quitting, the lung cancer death rate is about half that of a current smoker. Fifteen years after quitting, an ex-smoker's risk for heart disease is about the same as that of a lifelong nonsmoker.

In summary, prevention of chronic diseases is effective and does save lives. It can improve health outcomes for patients and address common risk factors. Disease prevention is also far less costly than waiting until a person is diagnosed with a chronic disease.

Causes of Infectious Chronic Diseases

Microbes, or microscopic organisms, including bacteria, viruses, fungi, and parasites, cause *infectious chronic diseases* (see Chapter 2). These microbes go through the body's barriers (e.g., skin, mouth, or nose) and multiply, creating signs and symptoms that range from mild to deadly. Once the microbes enter the body, they are known as germs or pathogens.

Bacteria are living single-cell organisms that grow and reproduce outside the human body. *Viruses* are biological agents that, unlike bacteria, are not complete cells; they are simply a combination of nucleic acid and proteins. They cannot reproduce themselves. Viruses can also infect bacteria by taking over a cell's structure and parts, often killing the bacteria in the process. Various kinds of bacteria and viruses infect humans.

Fungal diseases are caused by *fungi*, which are common in the environment They live outdoors in soil and on plants and trees as well as on many indoor surfaces and on human skin. Most fungi are not dangerous, but some types, such as ringworm, can be harmful to health.

Humans can also get an infectious chronic disease from protozoa. *Protozoa* are animal parasites that can live in the body. Roundworms, pinworms, tapeworms, and hookworms are the most common parasites that cause human infection.

Infectious diseases spread in a number of ways. They can come from another person (*communicable*) or from nonhuman sources (*noncommunicable*). They can spread from person to person directly via bodily fluids, or indirectly by way of air, foods, liquids, or surfaces. They can also spread by a *vector*, which is an infected animal or insect that bites a person.

Common ways in which people get infected are through skin contact, breathing in germs, eating or drinking contaminated foods or liquids, bites from vectors such as ticks, and sexual contact with an infected person. A person can also become infected through contact with fomites. *Fomites* are nonliving objects such as cups, doorknobs, or utensils that have infected water droplets on their surface. Mothers can give an infection to their unborn children through the birth canal and placenta.

Progress has been made in controlling many chronic infectious diseases. However, there is still a risk for new and reappearing germs. When germs undergo biological changes, new, potentially dangerous infections can arise. In addition, some germs can evolve and become more resistant to treatment—for example, new strains of bacteria that are resistant to antibiotics. Factors such as overcrowding and easy, effortless travel also make people increasingly vulnerable to the spread of infectious diseases.

Common Infectious Chronic Diseases

Most of the infectious chronic diseases are transmitted (spread) through sexual contact and are referred to as *sexually transmitted infections or diseases (STIs/STDs)*. The germs that cause these infections thrive in warm, dark, moist environments, which means that the body's reproductive organs are perfect environments for these germs.

According to the Infectious Diseases Society of America (2015), the most common STIs/STDs are chlamydia, followed by gonorrhea, syphilis, and AIDS. All of these diseases are preventable. The bacterial STIs/STDs—chlamydia, gonorrhea, and syphilis—can be cured if treated. If untreated, they create chronic health problems. The viral diseases, such as acquired immune deficiency syndrome (AIDS), can be treated but not cured. Each of the aforementioned STIs/STDs presents its own concerns:

- The bacteria that cause chlamydia can damage a woman's reproductive organs.

- The bacteria that cause gonorrhea grow and multiply easily in the reproductive tract of women and men. These bacteria can also grow in the mouth, throat, eyes, and anus. In addition, people with gonorrhea can more easily get HIV, the virus that causes AIDS.

- Bacteria cause syphilis. Many infected people do not have any symptoms for years. In the late stages of syphilis, the disease can damage internal organs, including the brain, nerves, eyes, heart, blood vessels, liver, bones, and joints.

• The human immunodeficiency virus (HIV) is the virus that can lead to AIDS. HIV damages a person's body by destroying specific blood cells that are crucial to helping the body fight diseases. If not treated early, HIV infection is linked to many chronic diseases including cardiovascular disease, kidney disease, liver disease, and cancer. AIDS is the late stage of HIV infection, when a person's immune system is damaged and has difficulty fighting diseases and certain cancers.

Controlling Infectious Diseases

As noted in Chapter 2, *epidemiologists* are scientists who work in the field of *epidemiology*. One of their jobs is to control the chain of infection that causes infectious diseases. The term *chain of infection* describes how an infectious disease is transmitted from one person to the next (Turnock, 2011). There are six links to the chain of infection (see Figure 3.1):

Pathogen or germ The virus, bacteria, fungi, or parasite that causes the infection.

Reservoir Any place where germs live and multiply. Some germs, such as the flu, spread directly from one human to another and have no reservoir. However, other germs first infect a nonhuman, such as a tick (reservoir), then spread from the reservoir to humans. Hosts that do not show any signs or symptoms of a disease but are still capable of transmitting the disease are known as *carriers*.

Place of exit Escape route for the germs from the reservoir. Examples of places of exit are respiratory droplets (sneeze), saliva, skin cuts, and blood exposure.

Method of transmission The germs' means of getting from one host to another. *Transmission* occurs through direct or indirect contact. For example, a method of transmission for syphilis is direct contact (sexual), and a method of transmission for Lyme disease is indirect (ticks).

Place of entry The route through which the germs enter the new host. These routes include the respiratory system (breathing), gastrointestinal system (eating or drinking), urinary and reproductive tracts (sexual contact), and skin cuts.

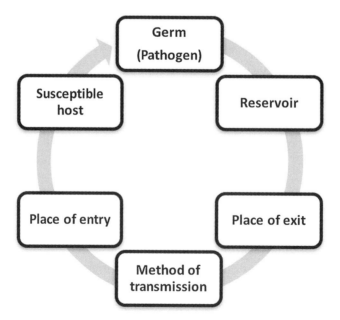

Figure 3.1 Chain of Infection

Susceptible host The organism that accepts the germs. Even if the germs gain entry, a person may not get the disease because he or she has immunity (through previous exposure to the germs) or is resistant to the germs due to having a strong immune system.

The way to control the transmission of an infectious disease is to interrupt the chain of infection at the various links. For example, the germs can be killed with medicines, such as antibiotics to kill bacteria. Another way is to get rid of the reservoir. For example, mosquito control reduces the chances of people getting malaria. Still another way to control an infectious disease is to block the passing of the germs—for example, by using condoms or by drinking clean water. Hand washing is another effective way to block the passing of germs from one host to another.

Vaccines increase the resistance of a host. They are the best defense we have against serious, preventable, and sometimes deadly infectious diseases. Vaccines are among the safest medical treatments available, but like any other medical treatment, there may be risks. Correct information about vaccines and their possible side effects helps people make informed decisions.

Understanding the differences among the terms *vaccine, vaccination,* and *immunization* can be tricky. A *vaccine* is a substance that produces *immunity* from an infectious disease and is given through needle injection, by mouth, or by aerosol spray. A *vaccination* is the injection of a vaccine that produces immunity in the body against a specific infectious disease. An *immunization* is the point at which a person becomes protected from a disease. Vaccines cause immunization.

Economic Costs of Chronic Diseases

The rising number of people who have chronic diseases is at the root of increasing US health care costs. According to the National Center for Chronic Disease Prevention and Health Promotion (2015), more than 86% of what Americans spend each year on health care is spent on chronic diseases. Those with multiple chronic diseases are the heaviest users of hospitalizations, office visits, home health care, prescription drugs, and other forms of health care.

Chronic diseases exact a huge toll on Americans today, but the future is even more troubling. According to the Robert Wood Johnson Foundation's report (McClellan & Riurin, 2009), over the next 15 years, the number of persons with chronic diseases in the United States will rise. Cases of cancer, diabetes, and mental disorders are expected to rise the most dramatically, up to 60% per condition. And according to the National Center for Chronic Disease Prevention and Health Promotion (2015), obesity is also a concern because the number of obese Americans is projected to increase. More than one third of children and adolescents are overweight or obese. Obese adolescents are more likely to become obese adults. Obese male youths have been found to be 18 times more likely to become obese adults, and obese female youths have been found to be 49 times more likely to become obese adults. Obesity-related diseases include heart disease, stroke, type 2 diabetes, and certain types of cancer.

Chronic diseases require ongoing management over years if not decades. However, most health care systems are not set up to provide this kind of care. According to the Robert Wood Johnson Foundation (2010), rushed health care providers often fail to coordinate patient care. Patients do not get the information they need to take more responsibility for their own health. Too often, there is no follow-up to make sure patients keep to their treatment plans.

We also know that people with chronic diseases receive conflicting advice and differing diagnoses from different physicians. Patients with chronic diseases are receiving services, but those services are not necessarily coordinated with one another, and they are not always the services needed (Lin et al., 2005). These gaps in care lead to increasing costs in health care as well as thousands of avoidable deaths each year (DeVol et al., 2007).

The United States in the 21st century faces a new reality: More and more people with chronic diseases need costly health care in a system that is too overburdened to respond (McClellan & Riurin, 2009). There is a dynamic created when so many Americans suffer from one or more chronic diseases and a health care system that does not respond adequately. This dynamic results in preventable illnesses and deaths, lifelong disability, compromised quality of life, and growing health care costs.

The Chronic Care Model

In response to the overburdened US health care system, Edward H. Wagner and colleagues in the 1990s developed the *Chronic Care Model (CCM)* (Wagner, 1998). The mission of the CCM is shown in Figure 3.2.

The CCM includes the following goals for chronic care patients:

- Regular visits with health care providers
- Prevention of complications or multiple diseases
- Emphasis on self-management
- Access to services proven to be effective
- Follow-up with patient done by health care provider

The CCM was developed as a response to the failures of the traditional care model, which involves expensive services, treatment only of signs and symptoms, multiple prescriptions, short education time, quick appointments, and little patient follow-up (Wagner, 1998). As the basis of the current US health care system, the traditional model has played a major role in the continuing increase in health care costs.

In contrast to the traditional care model, the CCM builds a health care system in which informed, proactive patients interact with health care teams. That is, the focus of health care is to contain the disease, slow its progress, manage its symptoms, and improve the quality of life for patients. One advantage of the CCM is that it can apply to most patients' chronic care issues. Still another advantage of the model is its emphasis on health care providers' working as a team and developing a relationship with their patients. For most chronic diseases, such as diabetes and asthma, self-care on the part of the patient is a crucial requirement of treatment. For treatment to be effective, there needs to be a strong relationship between the health care team and the patient.

As illustrated in Figure 3.3, there are six parts to Wagner's Chronic Care Model.

1. *Community resources and policies* need to meet patients' needs. For example, community resources need to focus on strategies, programs, and policies that improve patient care.

2. *Health care systems* need to be organized around goals that promote safe, high-quality care. Health care providers need to work as a team to create a comprehensive and inclusive system that coordinates and supports patient care.

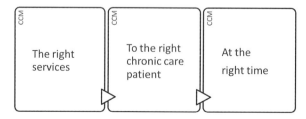

Figure 3.2 Mission of the Chronic Care Model (CCM)

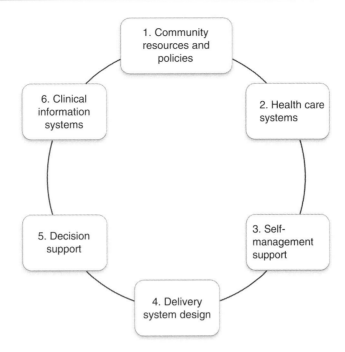

Figure 3.3 The Six Parts of the Chronic Care Model (CCM)

3. *Self-management support* reflects patients' needs as they manage as much of their disease as possible. Self-management support empowers and prepares patients to play a central role in their health care.

4. *Delivery system design* ensures effective, efficient health care and patient self-management support. Good design addresses the need for health care services that patients understand and that fit their culture.

5. *Decision support* increases the ability of health care provider teams to promote patient engagement and provide care that shares decisions with patients.

6. *Clinical information systems* use data to inform health care providers. Data systems monitor the quality of health care and help coordinate care among patients and their providers.

The model focuses on patient-centered prevention, treatment, and management of chronic diseases. It is an innovative model that puts patients first, and rewards health care providers who offer patient education and engagement, follow-up care, provider interaction, and information systems designed to improve the health of the patient and the quality of services.

Types of Palliative Care

As more people in the United States live longer lives, many will have life-threatening chronic diseases. People with these diseases want to live with dignity, receive quality health care, and be comfortable until the end of their lives. According to the National Hospice and Palliative Care Organization (2015), *palliative care* is the medical specialty that meets the needs of those living with a life-threatening chronic disease. The goal of palliative care is to provide the best possible quality of life for patients with life-threatening diseases (see Figure 3.4).

Palliative care is not a one-size-fits-all approach, however. A key benefit of palliative care is that it customizes treatment to meet the needs of each patient. The different approaches identified by the National Hospice and Palliative Care Organization (2015) include the following:

- Provides relief from such symptoms as pain, shortness of breath, loss of appetite, and difficulty sleeping. It can be used early in the illness, with other therapies that prolong life, such as chemotherapy or radiation therapy.

- Combines psychological and spiritual aspects of patient care.

- Improves the patient's quality of life and ability to tolerate treatments.

- Helps the patient gain strength to carry on with daily activities and to live as actively as possible until death.

- Can positively influence the course of a disease.

- Neither quickens nor postpones death.

- Uses a team approach to help patients better understand their choices for care.

- Offers a support system to help loved ones and family cope during the patient's illness and death.

Originally introduced in the 1960s, palliative care was limited to people who were dying of cancer. As a result, it was defined as health care given to people who no longer received treatment. It has since been realized that palliative care does help in the earlier course of a disease and that it can be provided alongside treatment.

Palliative care is provided by an interdisciplinary health care team that includes physicians, nurses, and social workers, and may include chaplains, massage therapists, nutritionists, and others. These teams specialize in the management of pain and other symptoms; intensive patient-physician communication; setting goals of care; and coordination of care across multiple settings.

Many people unfortunately believe that palliative care is only for people who are dying. Some patients refuse palliative care believing that to accept it will mean that they are going to die. They may

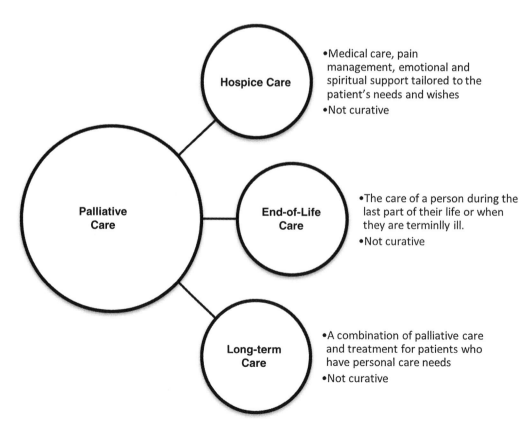

Figure 3.4 Types of Palliative Care

also believe that they will no longer receive any curative or healing treatments. Because of this misbelief, it is difficult to offer palliative care to patients early in their treatment.

Hospice care is one part of palliative care. It involves a team approach to health care with pain management and emotional and spiritual support tailored to the patient's needs and wishes. This support is extended to the patient's loved ones and family. Hospice care staff members have special training to address all types of physical or psychological symptoms that cause discomfort and pain. A patient who is dying can receive hospice care for an indefinite time as long as the patient's physician certifies that he or she has a life expectancy of 6 months or less.

Hospice care is the model for end-of-life care because it offers quality, compassionate care. At the center of hospice care is the belief that each of us should be able to die pain-free with dignity, and that our loved ones and families should receive the necessary support to allow us to do so. The focus is on caring, not curing.

Currently hospice programs serve more than 1.2 million patients, their loved ones, and their families each year (National Hospice and Palliative Care Organization, 2015). Hospice care is provided in centers known as hospices, in hospitals, in nursing homes, and also as a "hospice at home" service.

End-of-life care is available during the last part of a person's life, beginning from the point when it is clear that he or she is in a progressive state of decline. It is mainly health care providers who use the term *end of life*, whereas patients and their loved ones and families are more likely to use the term *terminal illness*.

Whether you call it end of life or terminal illness, how do you know when someone is dying? The reality is that no one ever knows exactly when someone is going to die. Some medical organizations define being terminally ill or at the end of life as when there is a short period of time, perhaps a few days or weeks, or at most a month or two, before a person is expected to die.

When patients are terminally ill, they may be cared for in a hospital, they may be at home with home-based care, or they may spend some time in hospice care. For most people, death comes after a long medical struggle with an incurable disease, such as advanced cancer or the bodily decline of old age. In all these cases, death is certain, but the "when" is unknown.

According to the National Hospice and Palliative Care Organization (2015), to receive quality end-of-life care, we all need to make a plan before a medical crisis arises by

1. Having a discussion about our wishes with loved ones and family—and our health care providers.

2. Writing down or videotaping how we want to be cared for at the end of life. We need to answer these questions: Do I want to have CPR (cardiopulmonary resuscitation) if my heart stops? Do I want aggressive treatments, such as being fed by a tube if I can't eat or being put on a breathing machine if I can't breathe on my own? Do I want antibiotics if I get an infection?

Despite medical advances, too many of us still die alone or in pain. Too many of us are subjected to costly and ineffective treatments. And too many of us at the end of life receive hospice care too late, or not at all. The National Hospice and Palliative Care Organization (2015) estimates that for every hospice patient, there are two more who could benefit from this care. For those living with life-threatening chronic diseases, palliative care needs to be offered more often and integrated across health care.

Long-term care (LTC) is a combination of palliative care and medical treatment, offering a range of medical, personal, and community services and supports needed to meet patients' personal care needs. Most LTC helps the patient with activities of daily living, such as taking medicines, bathing, dressing, eating, and using the toilet. It is available to those patients who have progressive chronic diseases, including dementia, multiple sclerosis, and Lou Gehrig's disease (ALS). Services can be in the person's home, in a community day care center, in an assisted living facility, or in a nursing home.

Chapter Summary

- Chronic diseases generally begin slowly and can last for the rest of a person's life. These diseases are not cured but are not immediately fatal. In other words, a chronic disease has an extended time span, does not go away quickly, and rarely is completely cured.

- Forty-five percent of all Americans live with a chronic disease, such as type 2 diabetes, depression, or cancer. By 2030, that percentage is expected to grow to more than 50%.

- Four lifestyle risk factors are the leading causes of many chronic diseases. These risk factors are lack of physical activity, poor dietary choices, tobacco use, and excessive alcohol use.

- The chain of infection identifies how an infectious disease is transmitted from one person to the next.

- The Chronic Care Model (CCM) builds a health care system in which informed, proactive patients interact with health care teams.

- Palliative care is the medical specialty that meets the needs of people with life-threatening chronic diseases. There are three types of palliative care: hospice care, end-of-life care, and long-term care.

REVIEW QUESTIONS

1. What are the most common noninfectious chronic diseases?

2. What are the differences between morbidity and mortality?

3. Identify ways to prevent infectious chronic diseases.

4. What are four causes of infectious diseases?

5. What are the four leading lifestyle factors linked to noninfectious chronic diseases?

6. Explain the chain of infection and its six links.

7. Summarize the differences among *vaccine, vaccination,* and *immunization.*

8. Explain the Chronic Care Model (CCM) and identify its six parts.

9. Describe the types of palliative care: hospice care, end-of-life care, and long-term care.

10. To receive quality end-of-life care, we all need to make a plan before a medical crisis arises. What questions should this plan answer?

KEY TERMS

Bacteria: Living single-cell organisms that grow and reproduce outside the human body

Carriers: Hosts that do not show any outward signs or symptoms of a disease but are still capable of transmitting the disease

Chain of infection: A term used to describe how an infectious disease is transmitted from one person to the next

Chronic Care Model (CCM): A model that builds a health care system in which informed, proactive patients interact with health care teams

Chronic disease or chronic condition: A disease or condition that begins slowly and lasts anywhere from 3 months to a year or longer, has no cure, limits what a person can do, and requires ongoing care

Communicable (chronic disease): An infectious chronic disease that is passed directly from one person to another through bodily fluids

Disease management: Multidisciplinary efforts to improve the quality and cost-effectiveness of care for patients suffering from chronic diseases

Early detection: Screening efforts to detect a chronic disease in its early stages when it is easier to treat

End-of-life care: Part of palliative care—care for a person in the last stages of his or her life

Epidemiologist: A scientist who works in the field of epidemiology

Epidemiology: The study of the distribution of deaths, diseases, and other health problems in a population

Fomites: Nonliving objects, such as cups, doorknobs, or utensils, that can carry germs or pathogens

Fungal diseases: Diseases often caused by fungi that are common in the environment

Fungi: Organisms found living outdoors in soil and on plants and trees as well as on many indoor surfaces and on human skin; some types can be harmful to health

Hospice care: A team approach to health care for patients with life-threatening illnesses

Immunity: Protection against diseases

Immunization: Provides protection from a disease; vaccines cause immunization

Infectious chronic disease: An infectious disease that limits what a person can do, requires ongoing care, and lasts anywhere from 3 months to a year or longer

Long-term care (LTC): A combination of services that help people who have chronic care needs

Method of transmission: The way a pathogen or germ travels from one host to another, or from a reservoir to a new host

Morbidity: Illness

Mortality: Death

Noninfectious chronic disease: A chronic disease that is not infectious and limits what a person can do, requires ongoing care, and lasts anywhere from 3 months to a year or longer

Palliative care: Medical treatment that meets the needs of people with life-threatening diseases

Pathogen or germ: The virus, bacterium, or parasite that has entered the body and causes a infectious disease

Place of entry: Route through which a pathogen enters the new host

Place of exit: Escape route for the pathogen from the reservoir

Protozoa: Single-celled parasites that can live in the body

Reservoir: Any place where a pathogen lives and multiplies

Screening: A method of checking a patient's body for cancer or other medical conditions before he or she has signs or symptoms

Sexually transmitted infections or diseases (STIs/STDs): A variety of infections and diseases that are caused and transmitted through sexual contact

Susceptible host: The organism that accepts germs, regardless of whether that organism contracts an illness or is resistant or immune

Terminal illness: An illness that ultimately results in death

Transmission: The means by which an infectious disease is spread

Vaccination: The injection of a killed or weakened microorganism that produces immunity in the body against that organism

Vaccine: A substance that produces immunity from a disease and can be given through needle injections, by mouth, or by aerosol

Vector: An animal or insect that is a carrier and transmits bacteria or a virus to a person

Viruses: Biological agents that, unlike bacteria, are not complete cells and cannot reproduce themselves

CHAPTER ACTIVITIES

1. The leading causes of many chronic diseases are four lifestyle risk factors: lack of physical activity, poor dietary choices, tobacco use, and excessive alcohol use. Brainstorm a list of chronic diseases that are caused by one or more of these lifestyle risk factors. Go to the CDC's website for more information: http://www.cdc.gov/chronicdisease/index.htm.

2. In small groups, discuss what type of patient would be best served by each of the following types of care: palliative care, hospice care, end-of-life care, and long-term care.

3. Select a way that a disease can be transmitted (kissing, sneezing, shaking hands, sexual contact, touching blood/bodily fluids, coughing, animal/insect bites, drinking water, food, not washing hands, etc.) and then describe the transmission. Use an actual disease to describe, such as the seasonal flu, chlamydia, or Lyme disease. What are examples of primary, secondary, and tertiary disease prevention strategies?

4. In teams of two, brainstorm the kinds of barriers and challenges to successful management of chronic diseases (for example, taking medicines, transportation, sick time). What are solutions to overcoming these barriers and challenges? Once each team has completed its task, join another team. With the other team, compare and combine your lists for class presentation and discussion.

5. Identify the six parts to the Chronic Care Model (CCM). Give two strategies for each of the six parts.

Bibliography and Works Cited

Anderson, G. (2007). *Chronic conditions: Making the case for ongoing care.* Baltimore, MD: Partnership for Solutions, Robert Wood Johnson Foundation.

Anderson, G. (2010). *Chronic care: Making the case for ongoing care.* Princeton, NJ: Robert Wood Johnson Foundation. Retrieved from http://www.rwjf.org/files/research/50968chronic.care.chartbook.pdf

Anderson, K., Anderson, L., & Glanze, W. (2012). *Mosby's medical, nursing, & allied health dictionary.* St. Louis, MO: Mosby.

DeVol R., Bedroussian, A., Charuworn, A., Chatterjee, A., Kim, I. K., Kim, S., & Klowden, K. (2007). *An unhealthy America: The economic burden of chronic disease.* Santa Monica, CA: Milken Institute. Retrieved from www.chronicdiseaseimpact.com

Faxon, D. P., Schwamm, L. H., Pasternak, R. C., Peterson, E. D., McNeil, B. J., Bufalino, V., & Shine, K. (2004). Improving quality of care through disease management: Principles and recommendations from the American Heart Association's expert panel on disease management. *Circulation, 21,* 2651–2654. Retrieved from http://www.ncbi.nlm.nih.gov/pubmed/15173048

Infectious Diseases Society of America. (2015). *Facts about infectious diseases.* Retrieved from http://www.idsociety.org/Facts_About_ID/

Lawrence, R. S. (2002). Health maintenance. In L. Breslow (Ed.), *Encyclopedia of public health* (p. 538) New York, NY: Macmillan Reference.

Lin, M., Marsteller, J., Shortell, S., Mendel, P., Pearson, M., . . . Rosen, M. (2005). Motivation to change chronic illness care: Results from a national evaluation of quality improvement collaboratives. *Health Care Management Review, 2,* 139–156.

McClellan, M., & Riurin, A. M. (Co-Chairs). (2009). *Beyond health care: New directions to a healthier America: Recommendations from the Robert Wood Johnson Foundation commission to build a healthier America.* Princeton, NJ: Robert Wood Johnson Foundation.

National Center for Chronic Disease Prevention and Health Promotion. (2009). *Power of prevention: Chronic disease . . . The public health challenge of the 21st century.* Retrieved from http://www.cdc.gov/chronic-disease/pdf/2009-power-of-prevention.pdf

National Center for Chronic Disease Prevention and Health Promotion. (2015). *Chronic diseases: The leading causes of death and disability in the United States.* Retrieved from http://www.cdc.gov/chronicdisease/overview/index.html

National Center for Chronic Disease Prevention and Health Promotion. (2016). Chronic disease overview. Retrieved from http://www.cdc.gov/chronicdisease/overview/index.htm

National Center for Health Statistics. (2013). Summary Health Statistics for the U.S. Population: National Health Interview Survey, 2012. Retrieved from http://www.cdc.gov/nchs/data/series/sr_10/sr10_259.pdf

National Center for Health Statistics. (2015). Health, United States, 2015. Retrieved from https://www.cdc.gov/nchs/hus/index.htm

National Health Council. (2014). About chronic diseases. Retrieved from http://www.nationalhealthcouncil.org/sites/default/files/NHC_Files/Pdf_Files/AboutChronicDisease.pdf

National Hospice and Palliative Care Organization. (2015). What is hospice and palliative care? Retrieved from http://www.nhpco.org/about/hospice-care

Robert Wood Johnson Foundation. (2010). *Chronic Care Model.* Improving Chronic Illness Care (ICIC). Retrieved from http://www.improvingchroniccare.org

Schrijvers, G. (2009, Jan.-Mar.). Disease management: A proposal for a new definition. *International Journal of Integrated Care*, p. 6. Retrieved from http://www.ncbi.nlm.nih.gov/pmc/articles/PMC2663707

Turnock, B. J. (2011). *Essentials of public health* (2nd ed.) Sudbury: MA: Jones and Bartlett.

Wagner, E. H. (1998). Chronic disease management: What will it take to improve care for chronic illness? *Effective Clinical Practice*, 2–4. Retrieved from http://www.improvingchroniccare.org/change/model/components.html

Wylie-Rosett, J., & Karanja, N. (2009). American Heart Association's behavioral roundtable for preventable disparities. *Prevention of Chronic Diseases, 2.* Retrieved from http://www.cdc.gov/pcd/issues/2009

CHAPTER 4

FUNDAMENTALS OF CULTURALLY COMPETENT HEALTH CARE

CHAPTER OBJECTIVES

- Summarize factors that cause racial and ethnic disparities in the United States.

- Define race, ethnicity, culture, and diversity.

- Explain cultural competency and identify four levels of culturally competent health care.

- Describe three approaches to culturally competent health care.

- State the merits of patient-centered care.

- Compare traditional medical practices of diverse populations in the United States.

The US population is highly diverse, and its racial and ethnic profile continues to change. Unfortunately, however, racial and ethnic minorities often receive lower quality health care than non-Hispanic Whites. Culturally competent health care has the potential to reduce these racial and ethnic health care disparities.

This chapter introduces key elements of culturally competent health care. Cultural competence is the ability of health care providers and settings to respond to the needs of diverse populations.

Culturally Competent Health Care

Health care providers work with increasing numbers of patients from racially and ethnically diverse populations. Nearly 1 in 5 Americans (32 million people) speaks a language other than English in the home, and 12% of the people in the United States are foreign-born (Centers for Disease Control and Prevention [CDC], 2013). The US Census Bureau predicts that within a few short decades, we will be a country of "minority majority"; that is, racial and ethnic minorities will exceed non-Hispanic Whites as the majority population (Berthold, Miller, & Avila-Esparza, 2009).

For purposes of this chapter, *race* refers to a population that differs from other populations of the same species on the basis of biological traits that are passed from ancestors. *Ethnicity* refers to a group's shared common and distinct racial, national, religious, linguistic, or cultural heritage. *Culture* comprises patterns of human behavior that include the language, thoughts, actions, customs, beliefs, and institutions of racial, ethnic, social, or religious groups. *Diversity* refers to differences from one another because of distinct characteristics, qualities, backgrounds, and beliefs (Office of Minority Health, 2015).

Racial and ethnic minorities, groups that have little representation or power in society, are underserved by our health care system. Despite improvement in overall health for most Americans, these minorities have higher rates of disease, disability, and death. And, as noted, they tend to receive lower quality of health care than non-Hispanic Whites. For example, according to the CDC's 2013 *Health Disparities and Inequalities Report,* African Americans have the highest death rate from colon and rectal cancer of any ethnic group in the United States. Native Americans are two to three times more likely to have type 2 diabetes than the general population. They also have higher mortality rates for heart disease, suicide, pneumonia, influenza, homicide, and alcoholism than the general population.

African Americans, Hispanics, Native Americans, Alaska Natives, and Native Hawaiians/Pacific Islanders are twice as likely to have and to die from certain diseases than non-Hispanic Whites. These differences in health outcomes between majority and minority populations are called *racial or ethnic health disparities* (see Table 4.1).

Health disparities exist because the relationship of illness to race, ethnicity, and culture is complex, dynamic, and interactive. It is complex because once people have received a diagnosis, there are many decisions as to how best to manage their disease. Often these decisions are based not just on what their provider tells them but also on their cultural beliefs and health practices. It is dynamic because patients have to balance their values and beliefs with the care they receive. It is interactive because they may have had negative experiences with and limited access to health care institutions due to racism, cultural issues, or poverty. Consequently, cultural values, beliefs, knowledge, and practices can be primary influences on patients' behaviors and create barriers to health care (see Figure 4.1).

There are many factors that lead to health disparities, including the following:

- Genetic makeup
- Socioeconomic status
- Lifestyle choices
- Immigration status
- Environmental conditions
- Family relationships
- Communication barriers or lack of bilingual staff
- Traditional health practices
- Lack of trust in health care providers and services

According to the Institute of Medicine (Smedley, Stith, & Nelson, 2003; Ulmer, McFadden, & Nerenz, 2009), there are four challenges related to racial or ethnic health care disparities:

1. Patients are more likely to refuse services, not stick to treatment plans, and delay seeking care.
2. Our health care system places time pressures on providers, making it difficult to make a diagnosis.
3. Time pressures increase shortcuts by providers because they are forced to make decisions without enough information, particularly when there are cultural or language barriers.
4. If a patient experiences discrimination, he or she will develop mistrust, which leads to less treatment.

Cultural competency in health care refers to a set of skills that allow providers to increase their understanding and appreciation of the racial, ethnic, cultural, and language differences of their patients (Brach & Fraser, 2000; CDC, 2015; Goode & Dunne, 2004; Oxendine, Goode, & Dunne, 2004). It is the

Table 4.1 General Health Profile of Racial and Ethnic Populations in the United States

	White (Non-Hispanic)	Black/African American (Non-Hispanic)	Hispanic/Latino/Latina Americans	Asian and Pacific Islander Americans (Non-Hispanic)	Native American Indians and Alaska Natives (Non-Hispanic)
Percent US Population	65	12	15	33	0.8
Median age	41	31	28	33	29
Countries of origin	European countries	Many African countries, West Indies, Dominican Republic, Haiti, Jamaica, and others	Mexico, Latin American countries, South American countries, Cuba, Puerto Rico, and others	India, Cambodia, Philippines, China, Japan, Vietnam, Korea, Hawaii, Samoa, Indonesia, and others	Americas, Nations of Cherokee, Chippewa, Choctaw, Navajo, Sioux, Mohawk, Algonquin, and 545 others
Leading causes of death (ages 18+)	Cardiovascular disease	Cardiovascular disease	Cardiovascular disease	Cardiovascular disease	Cardiovascular disease
	Cancer	Cancer	Cancer	Cancer	Cancer
	COPD[a]	Stroke	Stroke	Stroke	Accidents
	Accidents	Diabetes	Accidents	Accidents	Diabetes
	Stroke	Accidents	Diabetes	Diabetes	COPD[a]
	Alzheimer's disease	Kidney disease	COPD[a]	Influenza and pneumonia	Stroke
	Diabetes	COPD[a]	Chronic liver disease and cirrhosis	COPD[a]	Chronic liver disease and cirrhosis
	Influenza and pneumonia	Septicemia (blood poisoning)	Alzheimer's disease	Kidney disease	Kidney disease
	Kidney disease	Assaults (homicide)	Influenza and pneumonia	Alzheimer's disease	Influenza and pneumonia
	Suicide	Alzheimer' disease	Kidney disease	Suicide	Suicide

Note. Data from *Health Disparities and Inequalities Report—United States, 2013,* by Centers for Disease Control and Prevention, 2013, retrieved from http://www.cdc.gov/mmwr/preview/mmwrhtml/su6203a2.htm?s_cid=su6203a2_w; *Healthy People 2020: Disparities,* by Office of Disease Prevention and Health Promotion, 2015, retrieved from http://www.healthypeople.gov/2020/about/foundation-health-measures/Disparities

[a]COPD = Chronic Obstructive Pulmonary Disease

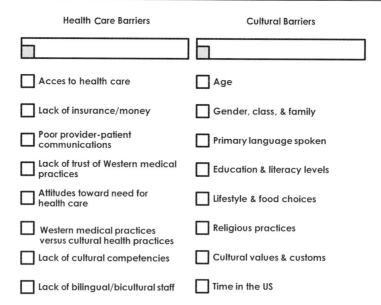

Figure 4.1 Examples of Cultural Barriers to Health Care

ability to interact and provide care to patients with diverse values, beliefs, and behaviors. Because the provider and the patient each bring his or her own culture to the health care experience, culturally competent care benefits providers as well as patients. There are four levels of culturally competent health care:

Cultural humility requires providers to self-evaluate and question assumptions, seek out resources and information on the cultural groups they serve, and ask patients to share their experiences, knowledge, resources, and needs.

Cultural knowledge requires providers to have information on different racial and ethnic groups as well as diseases and biological differences specific to these groups. It is more than being able to speak the same language and involves an understanding and acceptance of cultural practices.

Cultural skills require providers both to have cultural information on the patient's health issues and practices and to conduct a culturally based interaction. A culturally based interaction means that the provider combines Western medical practices with the patient's traditional medical practices. The provider needs to be aware of traditional medical beliefs and practices in the patient's community, know whether the patient uses these practices, and know how to negotiate with the patient between the traditional and Western medical practices.

Cultural encounter requires providers to know that their patients have their own health beliefs about their disease. Cultural encounter includes open communication about health beliefs that impact the patient's satisfaction with his or her diagnosis and treatment.

There are different models for providers to use when providing culturally competent health care. An example is Arthur Kleinman's explanatory model (1980, 1989). This model considers how a patient understands the causes and progress of his disease and how he thinks it should be treated. This model helps providers improve communications with patients, particularly those from ethnic and racial minorities. According to the explanatory model, providers who ask their patients the following questions will have a better understanding of their patients' health beliefs:

- What do you call your problem? What name does it have?
- What do you think caused your problem?

- Why do you think it started when it did?

- What does your sickness do to you? How does it work?

- How severe is it? Will it last a short or long time?

- What do you fear most about your illness?

- What are the chief problems that your illness has caused for you?

- What kind of treatment do you think you should receive?

- What are the most important results you hope to receive from the treatment?

Power Differences in Health Care

Recognizing power differences between health care providers and patients is key to culturally competent health care (Anderson et al., 2003; Goode & Dunne, 2004; Management Science for Health, 2010; Oxendine et al., 2004). Providers have an important role in the power differences—they hold knowledge, skills, and access to care. If patients believe that their providers have all the power, then interactions will be limited. When patients feel a lack of power, then they will be less engaged in their treatment (Berthold et al., 2009).

To have a balance of power, providers need to examine their beliefs and behaviors as the "person with power" with encouraging patient participation (Committee on Quality of Health Care in America, 2001; Health Resources and Services Administration, 2015). Health care settings also need to meet the needs of diverse populations.

To have a balance of power, culturally competent health care requires three approaches (Borkan & Fraser, 2000; Office of Minority Health, 2015). The *fact-centered approach* deals with cultural information about specific ethnic groups. The *attitude approach* supports cultural humility. The *skill-centered approach* involves communication skills that improve provider-patient interactions. These three approaches respect the patient and keep him or her as the center of the interaction (see Table 4.2).

Table 4.2 Culturally Competent Health Care Framework

	Culturally Incompetent	**Culturally Sensitive**	**Culturally Competent**
Fact-centered approach	Unaware	Aware	Knowledgeable
Attitude approach	Apathetic	Sympathetic	Committed to change
Skill-centered approach	Unskilled	Some skills	Highly skilled
Overall effect	**Destructive**	**Neutral**	**Constructive**

National Standards for Culturally Competent Health Care

As the United States becomes increasingly diverse, health care settings struggle to reduce health disparities. As already noted, almost 35 million US residents are foreign-born, and about 55 million people speak a language other than English at home. More than 24 million people who understand, speak, and write English still have *limited English proficiency (LEP)* (Office of Minority Health, 2015).

Federal law mandates that all health care settings receiving federal funding must meet standards of cultural competence. These standards—the National Standards for Culturally and Linguistically Appropriate Services in Health and Health Care (the National CLAS Standards) (Office of Minority Health, 2015; Smedley et al., 2003; Ulmer et al., 2009)—state that health care settings must:

- Offer and provide language assistance services, including bilingual staff and interpreter services, at no cost to each patient with limited English proficiency (LEP) at all points of contact and in a timely manner during all hours of operation.

- Provide to patients in their preferred language both verbal and written notices informing them of their right to receive language assistance services.

- Ensure the competence of language assistance provided to LEP patients by interpreters and bilingual staff. Loved ones and family members should not be used to provide interpretation services (except on request by the patient).

- Make available easily understood patient-related materials and post signs in the languages of the groups represented in their service area.

According to the National CLAS Standards, culturally competent health care results in improved communication, more effective use of time with patients, and fewer diagnostic errors. It also helps with negotiating differences and has positive effects on treatment outcomes. Unfortunately, the National CLAS Standards do not include federal funding, meaning that the costs of language services are the responsibility of health care settings. Trained interpreter services are costly, so the lack of funding results in many health care settings not meeting the National CLAS Standards.

Some health care settings use untrained interpreters, such as patients' family members. This can result in problems due to confidentiality issues and the untrained interpreter's lack of knowledge of medical terminology. In contrast, a trained medical interpreter provides to patients, family members, and their loved ones the following services:

- Obtaining the patient's medical history
- Explaining the treatment and procedures
- Discussion of discharge planning
- Obtaining consent for medical procedures
- Providing patient education

Patient-Centered Care

Health care settings that emphasize culturally competent services provide patient-centered care. *Patient-centered care* is a partnership among health care settings, providers, patients, and their loved ones and families (see Figure 4.2). It seeks patients' involvement in their own care (Committee on Quality of Health Care in America, 2001; Office of Disease Prevention and Health Promotion, 2015; Smedley et al., 2003; Ulmer et al., 2009). Patient-centered care is supported by a style of communication through which the patients' needs and goals are recognized and addressed by their provider. Patients can also understand and participate in their own care. Patient-centered care benefits every patient, not just those belonging to diverse populations. The principles of patient-centered care include the following:

- Treat everyone with dignity
- Strengthen patients' sense of control
- Share unbiased information and collaborate with patients and their family members and loved ones
- Identify community resources for patient support

Overview of Traditional Medical Practices

It is not possible for this overview to discuss all traditional medical practices. Further, I do not want to stereotype or suggest that all members of a particular race or culture follow certain health beliefs and

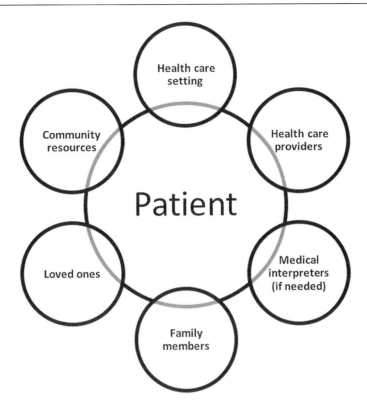

Figure 4.2 Patient-Centered Care

practices. Although information about a specific race or culture can help in understanding a patient, this can sometimes lead to stereotyping that patient. One must always remember to take into account the whole person and to see that a person can have different health beliefs and practices that are unique and not necessarily associated with his or her race or culture. It is also important to remember that there are factors beyond race and culture that influence a patient's health beliefs and practices, such as socioeconomic status, education, age, and environment.

According to the World Health Organization (WHO) (2015), *traditional medicine or traditional medical practices* are the knowledge, skills, and practices based on the theories, beliefs, and experiences of indigenous or native cultures. Traditional medicine maintains health as well as prevents and treats diseases.

Traditional medicine adopted by other populations (outside the native culture) is often called complementary, alternative, or integrative medicine. *Complementary medicine* is a combination of traditional medicine with Western medicine, such as using acupuncture along with medication to help manage pain. *Alternative medicine* is traditional medicine instead of Western medicine. *Integrative medicine or integrated medicine* is complementary medicine for which there is research evidence of safety and effectiveness (see Figure 4.3).

Following are descriptions that highlight traditional medical practices of select cultures (Goode & Dunne, 2004; Management Science for Health, 2010; Oxendine et al., 2004; University of Washington Health Services, 2015). These descriptions are limited and serve only as an overview of select healing beliefs and practices for each culture.

Asian Americans

Chinese medical practices have existed for over 5,000 years and are used to treat physical and mental health problems. The *traditional Chinese medicine (TCM)* approach to health and disease focuses on the dynamic balance between body, mind, and spirit, commonly expressed as yin and yang. Yin and yang symbolize the principle that for every action there is an equal and opposite reaction. Balancing yin

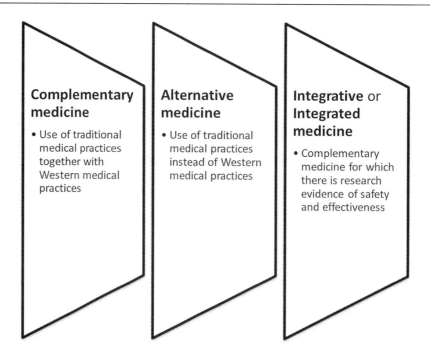

Complementary medicine

• Use of traditional medical practices together with Western medical practices

Alternative medicine

• Use of traditional medical practices instead of Western medical practices

Integrative or Integrated medicine

• Complementary medicine for which there is research evidence of safety and effectiveness

Figure 4.3 Traditional Medical Practices Adopted by Other Populations

and yang includes balancing aspects of our lives: cold and hot, wet and dry, inner and outer, body and mind. Because one cannot exist without the other, imbalance results in a disease. If there is an imbalance in a person's life, then there is a lack of harmony. It is important to have harmony because it means good health, good weather, and good fortune.

According to TCM, the body has three parts: *qi* (pronounced "chee"), moisture, and blood. *Qi* is the life force that gives us energy. Moisture is the liquid in our bodies that is necessary for life. Blood is the material from which all parts of our body are created—the building block. These three parts interact with each other in harmony so that the body exists in a state of health.

Diagnostic procedures in TCM identify the location and nature of energy imbalances in the body's organs. Treatment involves bringing more qi to organs that need it and drawing it away from organs with too much.

Qi is believed to travel throughout the body. It connects organs by meridians accessible at specific points on the body. To treat signs and symptoms, a practitioner treats the points to access the body's qi. Each point can have multiple functions, and different points can be used at the same time as part of treatment.

Two main practices associated with qi treatment are acupuncture and acupressure. In *acupuncture*, fine needles are inserted just below the skin on the body points. *Acupressure* uses the same points, but practitioners massage them one or two at a time. Acupressure usually has milder effects than acupuncture.

For many Asian Americans, eating certain foods can also cause a disease. Dietary treatment includes having a diet balanced in the five traditional flavors (sour, bitter, sweet, pungent, and salty). Because both food and illness can be classified as "hot" (yang) or "cold" (yin), to restore balance, a *yang* illness such as a fever is usually treated with *yin* foods, and vice versa.

It is important to note that for many Asian Americans, a disease can also be caused by fate or by ancestors from the spirit world who seek revenge. If this is believed to be the cause of a disease, then offerings and prayers are made to ward off harm.

Herbal medicines are among the oldest TCM treatments and can contain not only herbs but also parts of other plants, animals, or minerals. Traditional herbal medicines come in different forms, including pills or teas.

TCM strongly emphasizes prevention and determining the root cause of a disease once it develops. Many Asian cultures believe that good health is promoted through exercise, eating a balanced diet, and maintaining harmony with loved ones and family, both living and deceased.

Some Asian cultures rely on family as the first and sometimes only source of health care and make decisions based on what is best for the family rather than for individual family members. Others from Asian cultures may use traditional home remedies for minor illnesses such as colds, but seek care from Western health care providers for more serious diseases, such as lung diseases. Asian Americans may wish to consult only physicians of their own ethnic background, and women may prefer same-sex providers.

*   *   *

Ayurveda is a *traditional Indian medicine (TIM)* practice that has its roots in India and dates back thousands of years. It is based on the traditional customs, beliefs, and practices of the Hindu culture. Ayurveda has a focus on living a true and naturally balanced life. The treatment of a disease is grounded in bringing life back into balance.

Ayurveda offers a holistic approach with the understanding that there is no single cause for a disease. It brings together the knowledge, nature, and divinity within us. Health is defined as soundness of body (*shira*), mind (*manas*), and self (*atman*). Each of these must be nurtured if a person wants to be healthy.

A person needs to balance three forces called *doshas* to be healthy. No two people are alike because each is a unique combination of these forces. Those with a *pitta* makeup have different symptoms from those with a *vata* or *kapha* makeup:

1. Vata is the force compared to air.
2. Pitta is the force compared to fire.
3. Kapha is the force compared to mucus and water.

When these doshas are in balance, the functions of digestion, absorption, and elimination (physical and mental) create health. When there is an imbalance of the doshas, then a person becomes ill. As each dosha is responsible for specific areas of body and mind, the symptoms of imbalance indicate which of the doshas is weak or too strong. For example, too much vata causes arthritis, and too much pitta causes ulcers and liver disorders. The imbalance of doshas is caused by such factors as eating too much of certain foods, problems with relationships, or toxic environments.

Practicing Ayurveda puts balance in all things. Too much or too little of any one thing upsets the balance of the body and mind. Once a person knows what increases or decreases each of the doshas and understands the symptoms associated with each, he or she can apply Ayurvedic treatment to restore balance. Ayurvedic treatment removes the cause of imbalance in the doshas and includes natural medicines made of medicated oils, plants, and minerals. Yoga and meditation also create balance and help a person deepen his awareness of who he is and how he lives.

*   *   *

Traditional healers in some Southeast Asian countries such as Vietnam and Cambodia are revered and trusted. Many common illnesses—for example, bruises, flus, colds, and stomach pain—are treated with mentholated balms. Ginseng is considered a prevention and cure-all tonic. Traditional healers provide spiritual cleansing through *coining* (lightly scraping the skin with a coin or a spoon) or *cupping* (creating suction through heat on the skin with a cup) to rid the body of illness. Before coining or cupping, balms and other ointments are massaged in the area to prevent the skin from becoming red.

Hispanic/Latino/Latina Americans

For many Hispanic/Latino/Latina Americans, good health means that a person behaves according to God's will. They also follow the customs of their church, family, and local community. A disease is a result of many causes. Some causes are emotional states such as envy, anger, anxiety, family problems, and improper behavior. Other causes are environmental, such as air pollution, germs, bad food, or poverty. Supernatural causes such as evil spirits, bad luck, witchcraft, and vengeful enemies can also be responsible for a disease.

There are differences in traditional medical practices among subgroups. Mexican American traditional medical practice is *curanderismo,* derived from the Spanish verb *curar,* which means "to heal." Many Mexican American patients believe they are a victim of evil forces or suffer from soul loss. In addition, there are unique illnesses that are reported by Mexican Americans. *Susto* is sometimes called magical fright or soul loss and happens when a ghost or a frightening event causes the soul to leave the body. Symptoms include sleepiness, loss of appetite, and depression. *Bilis* is the result of excessive bile in the body. A person becomes ill with bilis if he or she is angry or frightened. *Empacho* is an illness caused by food that sticks to the stomach lining. This happens when a person eats a "hot" food instead of a "cold" food, or vice versa. Symptoms include stomach pain, diarrhea, vomiting, and fever. *Envidia,* or envy, is an illness caused when a person is envious of another. *Mal aire,* or bad air, is an illness caused by an evil wind, and can range from a cold or flu to joint pain.

Curanderismo is a combination of South American native traditions, Catholicism, European witchcraft, and traditions of other cultures. A *curandero* is the healer in the community and can be either gender. He or she may either be a generalist or have a specialty, such as midwifery, massage, or herbs. Curanderos treat physical and emotional illnesses, which include natural ones and those that are hexes brought on by witches and witchcraft. The curandero develops skills by apprenticing to an existing curandero, or he or she may have a spiritual experience and become aware of his or her calling to be a curandero. Skills are often passed down through generations within the same family.

Curanderos heal by using plants, rituals, prayers, charms, and magical spells. They locate the cause to treat the problem. These causes might be a magical bag placed in the hexed person's home or powder scattered near the hexed person. Catholicism is part of the healing, so some of the rituals and tools used might include prayers to and pictures of Jesus, crucifixes, or altars. The curandero deals with all aspects of a patient's life—the material, the spiritual, and the emotional—to cure. Treatment is most often a combination of herbs with ritual and counseling.

Puerto Ricans have a medical religious system called *Espiritismo,* which is a belief in one eternal good God. Espiritismo emphasizes the spiritual over the material, and everyone is believed to have a guardian spirit. An Espiritismo healer, or *espiritista,* believes in the spirit world of help and protection against harm and danger. The espiritista is a medium and usually a woman. To help patients with emotional, physical, and social problems, an espiritista gets rid of evil spirits as well as connects with good spirits.

Many Cuban Americans believe in *Santeria,* or Way of the Saints. It is a blending of African healing traditions with Catholicism. Santeria is practiced for well-being and for solving problems in the here and now. When its followers have a disease, they will ask not only how it happened but also why. Frequently, this is done by relating sickness to the ill person's social relations and lifestyle, and to the Santeria world of spirits and saints. For the followers of Santeria, illness is avoided and health achieved through rituals, offerings, and sacrifices to the Santeria saints. In this way, followers are empowered in their daily life and protected against supernatural forces.

According to Santeria practices, a person goes to a priest to be healed. The priest changes life's events in the person's favor by connecting with the evil spirits that are causing the disease. Some Cuban Americans believe that priests can undo evil spells.

African Americans

The traditional medical practices of African Americans are a blend from many cultures. The term African American is often used to identify Black populations who have diverse ethnic and cultural backgrounds. Many of the populations seen as African American identify themselves as Haitian, British, Brazilian, Jamaican, or other cultural/ethnic populations. New immigrants who are seen as African American may not identify with American-born Blacks or with those who are descended from slaves. Because of this complexity in racial and ethnic identity, the description here is limited to the practices of those African Americans who came to the United States with the slave trade from Africa in the 15th through 19th centuries. These African slaves brought with them many traditional health practices, which included local tribal traditions and Islamic medical practices.

African slaves who were brought to the Caribbean Islands practiced Santeria along with voodoo. *Voodoo* is also a blend of African tribal religion and Catholicism. A small number of African American communities practice voodoo, whose name comes from a West Indies god, Vodu. Traditional voodoo is combined with Catholic beliefs so that today's ceremonies include the healing powers of saints and relics. Voodoo health treatments include the use of *gris-gris,* which are good and bad oils and powders, as well as lighting candles for positive or negative hexes and spells.

Slaves in the United States took what they knew of healing from their African traditional beliefs and practices, combined it with what they could find in their new world, and developed their own type of healing practice. Healers were called *root workers* or *conjurers.*

Sadly, there is not much information on the root workers' medicines and other healing traditions of African slaves. Much of what they believed and practiced in their lands of origin was lost, as slaves were forced to adopt the religion and practices of their owners.

The blending of African traditional medical practices with religion is still present in many African American communities, where illness may be viewed as being caused by evil spirits such as the devil or by sinful actions. Healing comes from God through the power of prayer and the "laying on of hands."

Religion is an integral part of many African American communities, with prayer as a common practice of healing. For some African Americans, Jesus is necessary for healing powers. It is common for members of an African American church to pray together for the recovery of a fellow parishioner, with the preacher serving as a positive life force in the health of community members.

Some Africa Americans as well as other cultural groups, such as Indonesians, are practicing Muslims. Muslims are followers of Islam, a religion based on the teachings of Muhammad. The Islamic holy book, the Quran, teaches that all must live according to the laws of Allah. These laws instruct on respect for Allah, for self, for family, for others, and for the environment. If there is an interruption in glorifying and praising Allah and Allah's laws, then there is illness. Illness can be moral or physical or a combination of both. If patients are suffering from a moral illness, they must turn to the Quran as the guide to healing. If patients are suffering from a physical illness, they go to a physician who is a practicing Muslim.

Islamic and Western medical practices share similarities in their historical roots and training of physicians. The differences lie in the perceived therapeutic role of the physician. Western-trained physicians generally do not believe that they are agents of God. In contrast, Islamic-trained physicians believe that they are agents of God and that the act of healing is not entirely up to them. They may prescribe treatment, but Allah is the ultimate healer.

Native Americans and Alaska Natives

Native Americans and Alaska Natives comprise many different tribes that share both similar and different beliefs, languages, and traditions. The following description provides an overview of traditional medical practices among Native Americans and Alaska Natives. This overview is limited and is only a guideline in understanding tribal beliefs about illness and disease. Because there are many different traditional health beliefs and practices among the numerous groups of Native Americans and Alaska Natives, it is critical to develop awareness and sensitivity to this diversity.

Native American and Alaska Native cultures for centuries have understood health to mean the balance of all things physical, spiritual, emotional, and social. Illness occurs because something is out of balance. The belief that all people are part of the web of life means that what each person does to others, that person also does to himself or herself. The interrelatedness between people and the environment and the inclusion of a greater spirit is a common thread in the concept of wellness.

Many Native Americans and Alaska Natives believe that a disease is a consequence of a past, present, or future act. The cause can be either natural or unnatural. For example, a natural cause is a natural consequence of eating the wrong foods or having an accident.

Unnatural causes are the result of evil forces such as witchcraft, demons, and angry gods or ancestors. A disease is a form of punishment for violating certain customs. Evil forces enter the body and bring diseases with them. *Shamans* are special healers who remove the unnatural causes. For example, it might be necessary to call for a shaman to stop seizures caused by an evil force.

The special healers within most Native American and Alaska Native tribes go by different names, such as medicine man or woman and shaman. However, they are not the same—each has special powers. A medicine man or woman is not a true shaman. Shamans have the ability to journey in a meditative state to another world that is filled with objects, individuals, and various kinds of spirits. A shaman is a healer whose primary practice is treating diseases associated with unnatural causes. Medicine men and women, in contrast, are religious leaders as much as healers, treating spiritual and physical illness at the same time. They treat diseases caused by both natural and unnatural causes.

The sweat lodge ceremony is part of Native American traditional medical practices. This ceremony is one of physical and spiritual purification practiced to treat a disease. It is a communal affair. Participants know the person who is sick, and, through their participation, help the person heal.

Before the colonization of North America, many Native American tribes had their own remedies using plants and herbs. *Herbalists* are those within the community who heal by using herbal medicines. Unfortunately, forced tribal relocations, racist practices, and genocide resulted in the loss of knowledge of herbal remedies. However, a few herbal remedies did survive and are still practiced by some Native Americans.

Native Hawaiians and Other Pacific Islanders

The majority of Native Hawaiian and other Pacific Islanders in the United States live in Hawaii and the states of California, Washington, and Utah. Known as Pacific Islanders, the grouping clusters people by common heritage and by cultural beliefs and practices. However, the collective term Pacific Islander in no way implies that these populations are the same in nature.

Their homeland is Moananui—the islands and the ocean seas that surround them in the Pacific Ocean. They are referred to as Polynesians and Micronesians and are a highly diverse population with different historical backgrounds, cultural traditions, and more than 20 living traditional languages. They are Carolinians, Chamorros, Chuukese or Trukese, Hawaiians, Kosraeans, Marshallese, Palauans, Pohnpeians, Samoans, and Yapese, to name a few.

Traditional medical practices of Pacific Islanders have their basis in family, in nature, and in spiritual worlds that are interconnected and interdependent. A psychological unity binds the physical, mental, emotional, social, and spiritual being of the person with the universe. A person cannot be healthy unless the individual and the universe are in harmony. A feature of these islands' traditional medical practices is that people are integral to the balance of natural order.

The health of a Pacific Islander never is an individual matter but always is a collective concern. Among Pacific Islander cultures, the family is the basic unit of social structure, consisting of several nuclear families related by blood or marriage, as well as adopted members. The family as a whole is involved in both disease prevention and treatment. The extended family is headed by a chief who gives advice and approval on personal matters.

Obedience to the family is a primary responsibility of all its members. The family is the key to the "island way" and has structure, duties, and meaning that go beyond how the family is viewed in the West.

Common Threads in Traditional Medical Practices

This overview of traditional medical practices has identified common threads emphasizing the importance of body, mind, and spirit as well as harmony with nature in the healing process (Goode & Dunne, 2004; Kleinman, 1980, 1989; Management Science for Health, 2010; Oxendine et al., 2004). The holistic nature of healing is of prime importance and incorporates four factors:

1. *Patient.* The cause of a disease is the patient's responsibility. The patient has caused much of his or her illness through negative behaviors.

2. *Natural world.* This includes the natural aspects of a patient's environment. Common conditions include too much heat, cold, or wind. Natural causes also include outside organisms such as bacteria, viruses, and parasites.

3. *Social world.* Common causes of a disease can be witchcraft, spells, hexes, or voodoo. Other people also can give someone a disease.

4. *Supernatural world.* Unnatural forces such as evil spirits can cause a disease. These unnatural forces are brought on by moral or social misbehavior by the person. Repentance, prayer, and exorcism are needed to remove these supernatural forces.

Traditional medical practices see the causes of a disease as multidimensional and interdependent: The patient, the natural world, the social world, and the supernatural world influence each other.

Cultural Tips for Health Care Providers

The following is a list of tips for health care providers who work with patients from diverse racial and ethnic populations (Health Resources and Services Administration, 2015; Office of Minority Health, 2015; Smith et al., 2007):

- Avoid making judgments about the patient's beliefs and practices.
- Ask questions that help you learn about the patient's view of his or her disease.
- Find out what other treatments the patient is using.
- Ask the patient to bring to you any medications, herbs, and vitamins that he or she is taking.
- Explain procedures carefully, especially when they may be embarrassing for the patient. Tell the patient that you will make every attempt to maintain modesty.
- Ask the patient how much he or she wants to be informed and who he or she wants to involve in discussions about diagnoses, treatment, and prognoses.

Chapter Summary

- Nearly 1 in 5 Americans speaks a language other than English in the home, and 12% of the people in the United States are foreign-born.
- Despite improvement in overall health for most Americans, racial and ethnic minorities have higher rates of disease, disability, and death. They also tend to receive a lower quality of health care than non-Hispanic Whites.

- There are four levels of culturally competent care: cultural humility, cultural knowledge, cultural skills, and cultural encounters.

- The common theme in traditional medical practices is the importance of body, mind, spirit, and harmony with nature. These practices recognize the importance of the holistic nature of healing.

- According to traditional medical practices discussed in this chapter, the causes of a disease are multidimensional and interdependent.

REVIEW QUESTIONS

1. What is cultural competency in health care? Explain the four levels of and four approaches to culturally competent health care. What are the benefits of culturally competent health care?

2. What are the differences among race, ethnicity, culture, and diversity?

3. What are racial or ethnic health disparities?

4. What is patient-centered care?

5. Compare and contrast complementary, alternative, and integrated medical practices.

6. Why is it important to recognize power differences between patient and health care provider?

7. Compare and contrast three traditional medical practices.

8. Identify challenges related to racial and ethnic health care disparities.

9. Explain the importance of the National Standards for Culturally and Linguistically Appropriate Services in Health and Health Care (the National CLAS Standards).

10. What are some cultural tips for health care providers who work with racially and ethnically diverse patient populations?

KEY TERMS

Acupressure: Medical practice that uses the same points as acupuncture, but therapists massage the points one or two at a time

Acupuncture: Medical practice in which fine needles are inserted just below the skin on specific body points

Alternative medicine: Use of traditional medical practices instead of Western medical practices

Ayurveda: Indian medical practice based on the traditional customs, beliefs, and practices of the Hindu culture

Complementary medicine: Use of traditional medical practices together with Western medical practices

Cultural competency: Set of skills that allow a health care provider to increase his or her understanding and appreciation of the racial, ethnic, cultural, and language differences of his or her patients

Culture: Patterns of human behavior that include language, thoughts, actions, customs, beliefs, and institutions of racial, ethnic, social, or religious groups

Curanderismo: Healing practice that is a combination of South American native traditions, Catholicism, European witchcraft, and traditions from other cultures

Diversity: Differences from one another because of distinct characteristics, qualities, backgrounds, and beliefs

Doshas: In Ayurvedic practice, the three forces within a person's body

Espiritismo: Puerto Rican medical religious system, which is a belief in one eternal good God

Ethnicity: Shared common and distinct racial, national, religious, linguistic, or cultural heritage

Herbal medicine: Herbs, herbal preparations, and finished herbal products that contain parts of plants, animals, or mineral materials

Herbalist: Those who practice a specific form of healing, such as prescribing herbal medicines

Integrative medicine or integrated medicine: Combination of Western medical practices with complementary medicine for which there is research evidence of safety and effectiveness

Limited English proficiency (LEP): Skill level of people who understand, speak, and write English less than "very well"

Patient-centered care: Partnership among health care settings, providers, patients, and their families which ensures that decisions respect patients

Qi: Life force that gives us energy

Race: A population that differs from other populations of the same species by biological traits that are passed from ancestors

Racial or ethnic health disparities: Differences in health outcomes between majority and minority populations

Santeria: A healing practice that blends African healing traditions with Catholicism, in which a person goes to a priest instead of a medium or healer

Shamans: Special healers who are called on to remove the unnatural causes of illness

Traditional medical practices/traditional medicine: Knowledge, skills, and practices based on the theories, beliefs, and experiences of indigenous (native) or different cultures

Voodoo: A healing practice that combines African tribal religion and Catholicism

CHAPTER ACTIVITIES

1. A good way to avoid stereotyping is to start with a close look at your own culture. To identify how your culture influenced you, explore your childhood memories. Answer the following questions in two to three written paragraphs:

    a. *Health definitions.* What health beliefs did you learn from your family that have influenced your health behaviors? For example, what was a general assumption in your family if someone got sick from a cold or the flu? What was your family's assumption if someone was always "healthy"? What was the advice given to you on how to stay "healthy"?

    b. *Disease prevention.* What were your family's beliefs about the cause and prevention of a disease? For example, were you given vitamins or taken for yearly health physicals?

    c. *Illness treatment.* What happened when you became ill as a child? Did someone call your physician right away, or were home remedies tried first?

2. Refer to Arthur Kleinman's interview questions on the patient's health beliefs. Find a partner to practice asking and answering the questions. For confidentiality reasons, the answers can be for a real or an imagined disease. After completing this exercise, reflect on how it felt to be asked and to answer the questions.

3. Give examples of the three approaches in the culturally competent health care framework: culturally incompetent, culturally sensitive, and culturally competent. Be prepared to share your examples in class.

4. Work in groups of two or three and explain the principles of patient-centered care on one sheet of paper. Use fewer words and more visuals to emphasize points.

5. Select a racial or ethnic group whose traditional medical practices are of interest to you. Explain to class members through a PowerPoint presentation how the natural world, social world, and supernatural world are part of that practice.

Bibliography and Works Cited

Anderson, L., Scrimshaw, S., Fullilove, M., Fielding, J., Normand, J., & the Task Force on Community Prevention. (2003). Culturally competent healthcare systems: A systematic review. *American Journal of Preventive Medicine, 24*(3S), 68–79.

Berthold, T., Miller, J., & Avila-Esparza, A. (2009). *Foundations for community health workers.* San Francisco, CA: Jossey-Bass.

Borkan, J., & Neher, J. (1991). A developmental model of ethnosensitivity in family practice training. *Family Medicine, 23,* 212–217.

Brach, C., & Fraser, I. (2000). Can cultural competency reduce racial and ethnic health disparities? A review and conceptual model. *Medical Care Research and Review, 57*(1), 121–181.

Centers for Disease Control and Prevention. (2013). *Health disparities and inequalities report—United States, 2013.* Retrieved from http://www.cdc.gov/mmwr/preview/mmwrhtml/su6203a2.htm?s_cid=su6203a2_w

Committee on Quality of Health Care in America. (2001). *Crossing the quality chasm: A new health system for the 21st century.* Washington, DC: National Academies Press. Retrieved from http://www.nap.edu

Goode, T. D., & Dunne, C. (2004). *Cultural self-assessment. From the curricula enhancement module series.* Washington, DC: National Center for Cultural Competence, Georgetown University Center for Child and Human Development. Retrieved from http://ncccurricula.info/

Health Resources and Services Administration. (2015). Culture, language and health literacy. Retrieved from http://www.hrsa.gov/culturalcompetence/index.html

Kleinman, A. (1980). *Patients and healers in the context of culture: An exploration of the borderland between anthropology, medicine, and psychiatry.* Berkeley: University of California Press.

Kleinman, A. (1989). *The illness narratives: Suffering, healing, and the human condition.* New York, NY: Basic Books.

Management Science for Health. (2010). *The provider's guide to quality and culture.* Retrieved from http://erc .msh.org/mainpage.cfm?file=1.0.htm&module=provider&language=English&ggroup=&mgroup=

National Institutes of Health. (2016). Cultural respect: What is cultural respect? Retrieved from https://www .nih.gov/institutes-nih/nih-office-director/office-communications-public-liaison/clear-communication /cultural-respect

Office of Disease Prevention and Health Promotion. (2015). Disparities. *HealthyPeople.gov.* Retrieved from http://www.healthypeople.gov/2020/about/foundation-health-measures/Disparities

Office of Minority Health. (2015). *A physician's practical guide to culturally competent care.* Retrieved from https://cccm.thinkculturalhealth.hhs.gov/

Oxendine, J., Goode, T., & Dunne, C. (2004). *Public health in a multicultural environment: From the curricula enhancement module series.* Washington, DC: National Center for Cultural Competence, Georgetown University Center for Child and Human Development. Retrieved from http://ncccurricula.info

Smedley, B., Stith, A. Y., & Nelson, A. R. (Eds.). (2003). *Unequal treatment: Confronting racial and ethnic disparities in health care.* Washington, DC: National Academies Press. Retrieved from http://iom .nationalacademies.org/Reports/2002/Unequal-Treatment-Confronting-Racial-and-Ethnic-Disparities-in -Health-Care.aspx

Smith, W., Betancourt, J., Wynia, M., Bussey-Jones, J., Stone, V., Phillips, C., . . . Bowles, J. (2007). Recommendations for teaching about racial and ethnic disparities in health and health care. *Annals of Internal Medicine*, *147*, 654–665.

Ulmer, C., McFadden, B., & Nerenz, D. R. (Eds.). (2009). *Race, ethnicity, and language data: Standardization for health care quality improvement*. Washington, DC: National Academies Press. Retrieved from http://www .nap.edu/catalog/12696/race-ethnicity-and-language-data-standardization-for-health-care-quality

University of Washington Health Services. (2016). *EthnoMed*. Retrieved from https://ethnomed.org

World Health Organization. (2015). Traditional medicine: Definitions. Retrieved from http://www.who.int /medicines/areas/traditional/definitions/en/

CHAPTER 5

HEALTH BEHAVIOR AND PATIENT SELF-MANAGEMENT

CHAPTER OBJECTIVES

- Discuss differences between a theory and a model.

- Identify benefits of using theories and models in patient care.

- Compare and contrast theories and models discussed in this chapter.

- Explain the role of patient self-management education and support in health outcomes.

- Summarize the importance of patient empowerment in the delivery of health care.

Health care providers use health behavior theories and models as a way to improve the health of their patients. Theories and models guide changes in health behavior. This chapter explains four health behavior theories and models.

Health behavior theories and models lay the framework for disease management. The goal of disease management is to support patient education and self-advocacy. To meet this goal, health care providers offer strategies and programs that help patients manage their disease and improve health outcomes.

Differences Between Theory and Model

Many theories on health behavior have existed over the past 50 years. Health care providers use theories and models to answer the "why," "what," and "how" questions of health problems. That is, theories and models guide health care providers in understanding why patients do or do not engage in certain health behaviors (Glanz & Rimer, 1999; McKenzie, Pinger, & Kotecki, 2011).

A *theory* is an explanation of why events or situations happen. Theories are tools for understanding, explaining, and making predictions. The ideas of a theory are known as *concepts*. When a concept is used with a specific theory, it is known as a construct. *Constructs* are key ideas of a specific theory.

A *model* draws on a number of theories to explain a specific problem. Models provide a way to understand theories by breaking them down to their simplest form (see Figure 5.1).

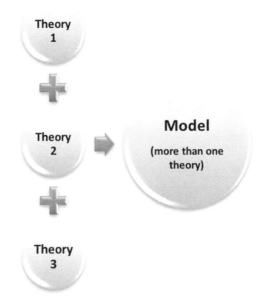

Figure 5.1 Difference Between Theory and Model

Benefits of Theories and Models

Health behavior theories and models exist for a reason. For example, a theory or model explains why a patient eats or does not eat a healthy diet. Health behavior theories and models:

- Explain why patients do or do not follow medical advice
- Identify information needed for an intervention
- Help in the design of educational strategies

Theories and models not only explain a health behavior but also identify ways to influence and change that behavior. Developing a theory about why a person chooses to smoke cigarettes is one step toward smoking cessation, but a well-explained model that is easy to follow gives a step-by-step guide on how a person can stop smoking.

To prevent disease, disability, and death, it is often necessary to change unhealthy behaviors. That is why it is important for health care providers to understand the health behaviors of their patients. A *health behavior* is any action that is related to disease prevention, health maintenance, and health improvement. Health behaviors are either *voluntary* or *involuntary.* These behaviors are performed for health reasons or because of a law or a requirement. An example of a voluntary health behavior is eating a healthy diet. Wearing a seat belt when driving is an example of an involuntary health behavior because it is one required by law.

Some health behaviors are engaged in daily, like brushing your teeth; others are done only once in a while, like getting a flu shot. Some of these behaviors a person does for himself or herself, like putting on sunscreen; some also affect others, like not drinking and driving. There are both short-term (e.g., losing 20 pounds in 3 months) and lifetime health behaviors (e.g., washing one's hands before eating). These long-term and regular patterns are known as *healthy lifestyle behaviors* (Glanz & Maddock, 2002; Glanz & Rimer, 1999; Green & Kreuter, 2005).

Most people do not practice healthy lifestyle behaviors all the time: Some might exercise every day of the week, but binge-drink several nights in a row; some might quit smoking, only to eat candy as a substitute. Ideally, the person who practices a variety of behaviors that improve his or her health is living a healthy lifestyle. Most people, however, practice some of these behaviors, some of the time.

Health behaviors are complex. It is not fully understood why some people engage in health behaviors and others do not. Researchers from the disciplines of psychology, education, sociology, epidemiology, and anthropology continue to explore the complex nature and causes of health behaviors (Green & Kreuter, 2005; McKenzie et al., 2011). Based on the work in these disciplines, theories and models exist to explain not only health behaviors but also their social and psychological influences.

Theories and models that explain health behaviors are classified as (a) individual, (b) interpersonal, and (c) community organization (Glanz & Rimer, 1999). Unfortunately, because health problems, populations, cultures, and environments are so varied and multilayered, there is no single theory or model that explains all health behaviors.

In summary, health behavior theories and models serve as a guide for health care providers to better understand health behaviors, develop interventions, and provide strategies for self-care. Health behavior theories and models guide health care providers to answer such key questions as:

* Why does a health problem exist in a patient?

* What is the best way to reach a patient to make a behavior change?

* Which strategies cause behavior change?

Overview of Four Theories and Models

We behave differently when we are feeling good as compared to when we are ill, and many theories and models explain why. In fact, there are college courses devoted to reviewing health behavior theories and models. This chapter provides an overview that looks at the importance of using theories and models as guides in changing health behaviors. The overview is limited to four commonly used theories and models that have been shown to positively affect health behaviors and to improve patient care:

1. Health belief model

2. Stages of change model

3. Social cognitive theory

4. Community organization

Health Belief Model

The *health belief model* (HBM), developed in the 1950s, was one of the first models to explain health behaviors. It is still one of the most common models used today by health care providers (Glanz & Rimer, 1999; McKenzie et al., 2011).

The HBM is an individual, psychological model that explains and predicts health behaviors. Its focus is on the attitudes and beliefs of individuals. The HBM is based on two main points: (a) the individual's view of the threat of a health problem and (2) the individual's view of the behavior needed for preventing this problem. This model has four constructs that explain and predict health behaviors (Glanz & Rimer, 1999) (see Table 5.1):

1. *Perceived susceptibility*—the person's belief in the chances of getting a certain disease

2. *Perceived severity*—the person's opinion of how serious this disease is in terms of pain, economic costs, or other costs

3. *Perceived benefits*—the person's opinion of the strategies to reduce the risk of the disease

4. *Perceived barriers*—the person's opinion of the physical and psychological costs of the strategies

Table 5.1 Health Belief Model Explained

Model	Description	What Does This Mean for the Health Care Provider?
Perceived susceptibility	Risk of getting a disease (low/high)	If patients think that there is low risk of getting a disease, then they are less likely to make behavior changes than if they think there is high risk of getting a disease. Example strategy: Make sure that the patient understands the risks of getting a disease.
Perceived severity	How serious a disease is and how serious its consequences	Patients are more likely to make changes in their behavior if they believe the disease is serious. Example strategy: Make sure that the patient has up-to-date information related to the disease.
Perceived benefits	Belief in the benefits of the treatment plan to reduce the seriousness of signs and symptoms	If patients are confident that the recommended treatment works, then they are more likely to make behavior changes, because they expect some benefit. Example strategy: Help the patient identify ways that the treatment plan is beneficial.
Perceived barriers	The physical and psychological downside of the advised treatment plan	A positive attitude with high hopes for the treatment plan is more likely to lead to behavior change. Example strategy: Help the patient identify barriers from an outside source (e.g., not having money or transportation) or within herself (e.g., making excuses or lacking motivation).
Cues to action	Events that stimulate readiness to change	If patients are worried about getting a serious disease, then they are more likely to engage in healthy behaviors. Example strategy: Help the patient identify ways that he can change the behavior(s) that put him at risk for a serious disease.
Self-efficacy	Confidence in one's ability to take action	The patient is ready to change and knows what to do—now it's time to take action. Example strategy: Reinforce and promote the patient's sense of self-efficacy.

There are two additional constructs of the HBM. The first is known as *cues to action*. These are events that stimulate an individual's readiness to act. An example of a cue to action is when the health care provider educates a patient at risk for heart disease on how to lower his blood pressure. The second construct is self-efficacy, or a person's confidence in his ability to successfully perform an action. An example of self-efficacy is confidence on the part of the patient at risk for heart disease that he can lower his blood pressure.

As a way to understand how the HBM works, let's explore condom use as an example. The HBM is based on the understanding that a person will take a health-related action (i.e., use condoms) if that person:

1. Feels that a negative health condition like HIV infection can be avoided

2. Has a positive expectation that by following a recommended strategy (using condoms), he will avoid a negative health condition

3. Believes that he can successfully follow the recommended strategy of using condoms correctly

The HBM not only explains health behaviors but also why these behaviors happen, and identifies points for possible change. The HBM is used to develop strategies that persuade a patient to make a healthy decision (Glanz & Rimer, 1999; Rosenstock, Strecher, & Becker, 1988; Strecher & Rosenstock, 1997). In summary, the health belief model (HBM) hypothesizes that a person makes health behavior changes if three factors exist at the same time:

1. The person is sufficiently concerned about a health problem.

2. The person believes that she is at risk for this health problem.

3. The person believes that if she uses specific strategies, she can reduce the health problem, and at a reasonable cost to her.

As helpful as the HBM is in working with patients, it does have limitations (Glanz & Rimer, 1999). One is that it is an individual, psychological model that does not consider environmental, social, or economic factors, which can also influence health behaviors.

Stages of Change Model

The *stages of change model* (SCM) or transtheoretical model, like the health belief model, focuses on the individual, psychological reasons why a person changes his or her behaviors (Prochaska & DiClemente, 1986; Prochaska & Velicer, 1997). The SCM, however, puts more emphasis than the HBM on how a person makes decisions. Making decisions is a process that involves the person's emotions, thoughts, and behaviors. According to the SCM, a person's motivation to change a health behavior is divided into three parts: the person's views, his or her behaviors, and the possibility of an action (Glanz & Rimer, 1999; Prochaska & DiClemente, 1986; Prochaska & Velicer, 1997).

According to the SCM, behavior change is a process that unfolds over time and is not a single event (Glanz & Rimer, 1999; McKenzie et al., 2011; Prochaska & DiClemente, 1986; Prochaska & Velicer, 1997). People are at different levels of motivation or readiness to change at different times in their lives. Further, the stages are not linear; instead, they are part of a cyclical process that varies for each person. The six stages of change are as follows:

1. *Precontemplation.* The person has a health problem (whether she knows it or not), and she does not change her behaviors—she is not ready to act.

2. *Contemplation.* The person knows she has a health problem and admits to it. She is seriously thinking about changing her behaviors in the near future—she is getting ready to act.

3. *Preparation.* The person recognizes that she has a health problem and intends to change her behaviors sometime in the near future; she makes some positive behavior changes, but not on a regular basis.

4. *Action.* The person develops an action plan, she makes regular behavior changes, and her actions are obvious.

5. *Maintenance.* The person adopts and keeps to her new behaviors for 6 months to 5 years; this means that the positive change in behaviors is kept to over time.

6. *Termination.* The person has no desire to go back to old behaviors, and continues with positive behaviors and resists relapse.

How a person passes through these stages varies, depending on the behaviors. For example, someone who is trying to give up his or her addiction to heroin can experience the stages differently than someone who wants to lose 20 pounds.

We are always at different points in the process of change, so there is a need for diverse strategies to motivate us. The strategies that work best are those that match our stage. By seeing health behavior change in stages, health care providers can tailor strategies to a patient's stage—for example, offering

Table 5.2   Stages of Change Model Explained

Model	Description	What Does This Mean for the Health Care Provider?
1. Precontemplation	The person has a health problem (whether he knows it or not), but he is not ready to act.	The patient has a health problem, but is not ready to change his behavior because it has little or no impact on his daily life. Example strategy: Explain to the patient the benefits and rewards of healthy behavior.
2. Contemplation	The person knows he has a health problem and admits to it. He is seriously thinking about changing his behaviors in the near future—he is getting ready to act.	The patient starts to get information on ways to manage his health problem, but has not changed his behavior. Example strategy: Make sure that the patient has the correct and most up-to-date information and knows how to change his behavior.
3. Preparation	The person recognizes that he has a health problem and intends to change his behaviors sometime in the near future; he makes some positive behavior changes, but not on a regular basis.	The patient recognizes the need to change health behaviors and has made some progress, but not on a regular basis. Example strategy: Explain to the patient the benefits and rewards of changing his behavior on a regular basis.
4. Action	The person develops an action plan, he makes regular behavior changes, and his actions are obvious.	The patient has a positive attitude about behavior change. He keeps to a regular schedule of changing his behavior. The patient starts to see and experience the benefits and rewards of behavior change. Example strategy: Provide positive feedback and support for behavior change.
5. Maintenance	The person adopts and keeps to his new behaviors for 6 months to 5 years; this means that the positive change in behaviors is kept to over time.	The patient has made a positive change in his health behavior over a period of time. Example strategy: Provide positive feedback for behavior change. Brainstorm with the patient on how he can keep to the behavior change over time and not relapse.
6. Termination	The person has no desire to go back to old behaviors, and continues with positive behaviors and resists relapse.	The patient feels better and realizes that his behavior change has been beneficial to his improved health. Example strategy: Discuss with the patient how he can keep the behavior change as part of his lifestyle over long periods of time.

education and feedback in the beginning stages, and reinforcement and support during the following stages. When patients know their stage, they can set realistic goals for themselves.

Relapse happens when a person goes back to an earlier stage. People generally do not simply move from one stage to the next, easily "graduating" from one set of behaviors to the next. Instead, they may enter at any stage, relapse to an earlier stage, and begin the process again. The person may cycle through this process often, or he or she can just give up, and the process stops at any point. In summary, according to the SCM, a person must feel threatened by the disease and believe that taking action is more beneficial than not taking action (see Table 5.2).

The SCM is useful, but has limitations (Glanz & Rimer, 1999). Like the health beliefs model, the SCM focuses on the individual without considering environmental, social, or economic factors that can also influence health behaviors. For example, a person may want to stop smoking cigarettes, but if his or her peers, loved ones, and family members smoke cigarettes, stopping is more difficult.

Social Cognitive Theory

Social cognitive theory (SCT) is a theory frequently used by health care providers. It is a complicated interpersonal theory with many constructs; therefore, this overview of SCT is limited to the key constructs. Albert Bandura and his researchers developed SCT in the early 1960s. SCT, also known as the social learning theory or social influence theory, examines how behaviors are learned, maintained, and changed over time (Bandura, 1986, 1989, 1997). The focus is on a person's *cognition*—his or her thinking, emotions, and behavior.

SCT describes an interactive, dynamic, and ongoing three-way process:

1. Personal factors, such as knowledge, emotions, and biological makeup

2. Environmental factors, including social influences, such as loved ones and family, and physical influences, such as pollution and housing

3. Human behavior factors, such as personal lifestyle choices

These three factors continually interact with each other. Changes in any one of the factors causes changes to the other two. This three-way process is known as *reciprocal determinism* (Bandura, 1986, 1989, 1997; Glanz & Rimer, 1999; McKenzie et al., 2011).

According to SCT, a person can change his or her health behavior with three elements (Bandura, 1986, 1989, 1997; Glanz & Rimer, 1999):

1. Behavioral capability

2. Self-efficacy

3. Outcome expectations

Behavioral capability is the ability to change a health behavior: The person knows what to do and how to do it. It is the knowledge and skills needed to perform a specific health behavior. Knowledge of health risks and benefits is the signal for change; however, if the person lacks this knowledge, there is little motivation to develop skills for change.

Self-efficacy is the sense of confidence in one's ability to successfully change behaviors. It is central to changing a behavior, the foundation for action. If a person has a low level of self-efficacy, then he or she will not be motivated to change. However, with a high level of self-efficacy, a person can change health behaviors even when faced with barriers.

A person's level of self-efficacy is dependent on the particular health behavior. For example, someone can have a strong sense of self-efficacy when exercising, but perceive a low level when trying to control smoking cigarettes. Regardless of the health behavior, a person can always increase his or her level of self-efficacy through:

• Skills development

• Observing behaviors of others

• Feedback and encouragement from others

• Coping with the anxiety associated with the behavior change

Outcome expectations are what a person expects from engaging in certain health behaviors. There are three types of outcomes:

1. **Physical:** positive (pleasure) and negative (pain) outcomes

2. **Social:** reactions from others about the behavior (approval and disapproval)

3. **Self-evaluation:** positive and negative reactions the person has toward his or her health behaviors and status

Bandura and others (Bandura, 1986, 1989, 1997; Glanz & Rimer, 1999; McKenzie et al., 2011) recognized that many theories of health behavior overlooked an important construct: learning by observing the behavior (modeling) of others. Therefore, observational learning is an important construct of SCT. *Observational learning* is learning through the experiences of others, rather than just by one's own experiences. That is, a person watches the behaviors of another person and observes their positive outcomes, and then engages in that behavior with the intent of yielding the same positive outcomes (Bandura, 1986, 1989, 1997).

The environment is another key construct in SCT. The environment is where observational learning takes place: It provides opportunities for a person to watch the behavior of others and learn the consequences of those behaviors.

When a person does change his or her health behavior, *reinforcements* increase or decrease the chances of repeating that behavior (Bandura, 1986, 1989, 1997). Positive reinforcements or rewards increase a person's chances of repeating the behavior. Negative reinforcements or penalties may increase the chances of repeated behavior by a negative stimulus. For example, the beeping alarm in a car (a negative stimulus) reminds drivers to fasten their seat belt.

Reinforcements can also be internal or external. Internal reinforcements are things people do to reward themselves, such as buying new clothes when they have lost weight. External reinforcements such as praise, money, or gifts from others encourage people to continue changing their behavior.

SCT has specific strategies to change behavior (Bandura, 1986, 1989, 1997) (see Table 5.3). One strategy is the use of role models whose behavior gets good results, such as using celebrities as

Table 5.3   Social Cognitive Theory Explained

Model	Description	What Does This Mean for the Health Care Provider?
1. Reciprocal determinism	Dynamic interaction of the person with her behavior and her environment	Your patient's health behaviors are influenced by who she is, what she knows, her behaviors, and her social and physical environments. Example strategy: Help the patient identify how behaviors as well as social and physical environments influence health.
2. Behavioral capability	Knowledge and skills needed to perform a certain health behavior	The patient has the knowledge and skills necessary to perform a health behavior. Example strategy: Help the patient identify the knowledge and skills necessary to engage in a health behavior.
3. Outcome expectations	What the person expects to happen if he changes his health behavior	The patient has expectations for what will happen if there are changes in a health behavior. Example strategy: Help the patient identify realistic expectations for changing a health behavior.
4. Self-efficacy	The person's confidence in his or her ability to change health behavior	The patient has a positive attitude toward his or her ability to change a health behavior. Example strategy: Provide the patient with verbal support that builds self-efficacy.
5. Observational learning (modeling)	Engaging in and maintaining new health behaviors by watching the behaviors of others and their outcomes	The patient looks for support and encouragement from those who have successfully changed a health behavior. Example strategy: Provide the patient with a resource listing of support groups.
6. Reinforcements (rewards)	Responses to the person's change in health behavior that increases or decreases the chances of the behavior happening again	The patient receives positive feedback from peers, loved ones, and family members for changing a health behavior. Example strategy: Explain and reinforce to the patient that his or her change in a health behavior will have long-lasting positive results.

spokespeople for a weight-loss program. Other strategies include reinforcements that modify behavior, or tools, resources, and environmental changes that make new behaviors easier to perform. Using SCT, the patient can:

- Observe positive health behaviors modeled by others

- Increase knowledge, skills, and confidence to engage in positive health behaviors

- Gain support for new health behaviors from his or her social and physical environments

SCT is effective, but does have limitations (Glanz & Rimer, 1999). Because SCT is so general, it lacks a step-by-step approach. People are seen as so dynamic that it is difficult to use the theory in its entirety. Instead, most health care providers tend to focus on one or two constructs, such as self-efficacy or observational learning. Finally, the theory has limited value for some diseases, such as dementia, which has more to do with chemical imbalances in the brain than low self-efficacy. Health care providers need to be aware that although SCT helps many patients engage in positive health behaviors, it has limited value for those who suffer from certain diseases or who are not in control of their behavior.

$$* \quad * \quad *$$

The theories and models of health behavior discussed thus far in this chapter share some similarities:

Health behavior change is a process. One central construct to these theories and models is that behavior change is a process, not a one-time event. Changes in health behaviors happen in stages. For example, most obese people cannot change their unhealthy eating habits all at once. It takes time to change health behaviors because they are so complex.

Behavior change can be difficult to maintain over time. Even when there is a good first attempt to change health behaviors, relapse is common. For example, it is common practice for someone to start a low-fat diet, only to give up on it after a few months.

Making a behavior change and then keeping to that change requires different strategies at different levels of influence. For example, someone could quit smoking by going "cold turkey," but he or she will be tempted again, perhaps just by being around family members who smoke.

It's important to identify the barriers. Everyone experiences barriers when he or she wants to change health behaviors. These barriers exist when a person weighs the pros and cons of changing his or her behaviors; and, because changing a behavior can be so difficult, it has to be worth it.

Community Organization

Although health behavior theories and models are useful, relying only on them is often not practical. People find it difficult to make health behavior changes in the face of unhealthy social and physical environments. Community organization addresses this issue of unhealthy environments and is an important consideration when helping patients (Glanz & Rimer, 1999: McKenzie et al., 2011).

Community organization is a process whereby community members identify issues, set goals, and mobilize resources (Berthold, Miller, & Avila-Esparza, 2009; Glanz & Rimer, 1999; McKenzie et al., 2011). They then develop and implement strategies for resolving their issues or for reaching their goals. Community organization is dependent on *social action*—community members coming together for a cause, especially one that involves a group that is being affected by a particular issue. Examples of this are activists who work in the arenas of gay rights, gun control, or human rights.

Community organization goes beyond the idea that a community is a place or a geographic location. Community is defined in other ways. There are communities of people with shared interests, such as persons with disabilities or LGBT (lesbian, gay, bisexual, and transgender) individuals. There are also communities of shared cultural identity—for example, Jewish, Irish American, or Mexican American. It is critical for health care providers to learn about the community they are working with and to know the community's unique characteristics. This knowledge leads to the delivery of health care that is for patients—not for providers.

Long-lasting change in health behavior requires change in the community. Community organization can promote and support long-term behavior change. However, community organization theories and models require the strength of local leaders and the demands of community stakeholders to make these changes. *Community stakeholders* are people in the community who are affected, or could be affected, by a community issue. They are individuals, groups, organizations, government departments, businesses—anyone with a stake or an interest in a community issue and its outcome (Berthold et al., 2009; KU Work Group for Community Health and Development, 2016).

Although there is not one theory or model for community organization, there are several key elements (Berthold et al., 2009; Glanz & Rimer, 1999; McKenzie et al., 2011):

1. *Community development.* Stakeholders identify and resolve their community's issues. The goal of community development is to improve environmental, economic, and social conditions within the community. Active local leadership and engaged community stakeholders work together to achieve this goal. Community development strategies include community participation, goal setting, problem solving, planning, and capacity building.

2. *Community capacity building.* Community stakeholders develop working relationships with each other, joining together to identify community issues, mobilize, and take action to resolve those issues.

3. *Community assessment and planning.* Community stakeholders create goals and strategies to problem-solve, sometimes with "experts" who provide technical assistance. Community assessment is a strategy through which community stakeholders gather information to understand the causes and consequences of issues. Then, with community leaders, they get together to discuss the situation and develop a plan to resolve these issues.

4. *Community action and results.* Community leaders and stakeholders increase their ability to resolve community issues and to make changes. They use the action plan to address the issue. Once the issue is resolved, an additional action plan is put in place to make sure that the changes last over time.

Community organization can result in change that is effective and sustained over time (see Table 5.4). There are many examples of how community organization has a lasting positive impact on the health behaviors of community members, including organizing for more community parks or bike paths, for community gardens, and against gun violence.

Some of the limits of community organization include the difficulty in getting started, building and maintaining interest, and evaluating success. Community organization can be politically charged, and, at times, communities and their health issues can suddenly change because of a new health crisis, lack of resources, a downturn in the economy, or even a natural disaster.

Disease Management

Every day, patients make health decisions—for example, taking medicines or keeping medical appointments. Health care providers use theories and models to develop disease management

Table 5.4 Community Organization Explained

Key Elements	Description	Example
1. Community development	Concerned members in the community (stakeholders) identify and resolve its issues.	You and other community members have gotten together to address the adolescent substance use issue in your community.
2. Community assessment and planning	Community stakeholders gather information to understand the causes and consequences of issues. Then, with other stakeholders, they get together to make a plan to resolve these issues.	You and other community stakeholders have contacted other stakeholders, such as the local departments of public health, school, police, and adolescent substance abuse treatment programs, to determine how much of an issue adolescent substance use is in the community. You find out that your community has the highest rate of adolescent alcohol use in the state. Together, stakeholders work to develop a plan that resolves the adolescent alcohol use issue.
3. Community action and results	Community stakeholders identify and discuss an action plan to resolve the issue. Once the issue has been resolved, an additional action plan is put into place to make sure that the changes last for the long term.	Together, stakeholders take action to address adolescent alcohol use. A task force is formed of community stakeholders who represent youth, schools, police, parents, treatment programs, religious organizations, and others who are concerned about this issue. The task force makes a plan to reduce adolescent alcohol use. Once implemented, this plan does reduce adolescent alcohol use. The plan is funded for years by local tax dollars.

educational tools, strategies, and programs that help patients make those health decisions and manage their disease.

Disease management is a multidisciplinary approach that improves the quality and cost-effectiveness of health care, especially for patients who have chronic diseases. Health care providers who use a disease management approach with their patients provide individualized treatment plans and educational tools, along with professional support (Betancourt & Like, 2000). The goal of disease management is to identify persons at risk for one or more chronic diseases, promote patient self-management, and provide effective and efficient health care. Disease management helps patients:

• Understand day-to-day management of their disease

• Reduce signs, symptoms, and complications

• Access quality health care

Chronic care management is part of disease management; however, as its name implies, it is specific to chronic diseases. The focus on chronic diseases is necessary because most of these diseases, such as diabetes, asthma, and arthritis, require the patient to follow a long-term treatment plan. The goal of chronic care management is to contain the disease, manage its signs and symptoms, and improve the patient's quality of life over a long period of time.

Also part of disease management is what is known as *integrated care*, which is a broad term that describes a goal of comprehensive care for patients with either acute or chronic diseases. Integrated care includes preventive care, social care, and home care based in the community. This type of care recognizes that social environments influence health; it focuses on the patient's view of what is needed. It addresses the complex nature of patients' needs, such as social and economic support (Institute for Healthcare Improvement, 2015; Institute of Medicine [IOM], 2001). Integrated care is most often used with elderly patients or patients who have a mental health disorder.

Patient Self-Management

Patients with one or more chronic diseases must often manage complex treatment plans and undergo major disruptions in their lives. Managing one or more chronic diseases also can be complicated because these diseases can go to extremes, changing from simple to complex, minor to major, mild to severe—even when the patient follows the treatment plan. Having a chronic disease is not only upsetting and complicated but also time-consuming. Treating these diseases often entails repeating many daily actions, such as checking symptoms or taking multiple medications even when the benefits are unclear.

Providing care to patients with chronic diseases is challenging and often complex, particularly for those who have more than one disease. However, what is supported by research is that patients who can self-manage their diseases and receive education and support from their health care providers have the best health outcomes (Institute for Healthcare Improvement, 2015; IOM, 2001).

Patient self-management refers to the patient's making decisions and taking actions to live well with one or more chronic diseases. It emphasizes not only patients' active participation but also developing skills:

1. *Taking care of illness.* The patient manages medical responsibilities, such as taking medicines as prescribed and keeping follow-up appointments.

2. *Carrying out normal activities.* The patient manages responsibilities related to work or school, loved ones, family, and community.

3. *Emotional responsibility.* The patient manages the changing emotions he or she feels as well as the changes in relationships with others.

Self-management skills not only allow a patient to be proactive but also can lead to better health outcomes. The role of the health care provider is to use the following strategies that encourage patients to use self-management skills.

Patient Self-Management Education

Patient self-management education is like traditional patient education in that it supports patients in living the best possible quality of life. However, traditional patient education offers information and technical skills, whereas self-management education teaches problem-solving skills (see Figure 5.2). A central concept in self-management is self-efficacy, or confidence (Bodenheimer & Abramowitz, 2010; Institute for Healthcare Improvement, 2015; Lorig & Holman, 2003).

Both traditional patient education and patient self-management education are necessary and beneficial to patients (Bodenheimer & Abramowitz, 2010; Institute for Healthcare Improvement, 2015). Some aspects of traditional patient education work well; some do not. For example, information is necessary, but it alone does not create behavior change.

Patient Self-Management Support

Patient self-management support is a type of counseling based on the partnership between the health care provider and the patient. The goal of self-management support is to help patients live as normal a life as possible. The following is a description of techniques a health care provider can use to support patient self-management (Bodenheimer & Abramowitz, 2010; Institute for Healthcare Improvement, 2015):

Establish a focus Establishing a focus is a first step in patient self-management. This is an opportunity for the health care provider to learn about the patient's concerns, knowledge, and behaviors related to

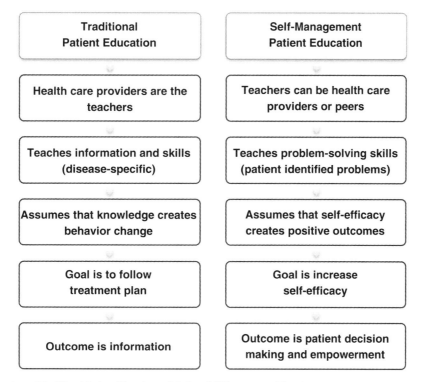

Figure 5.2 Comparison of Traditional Patient Education and Patient Self-Management Education

their chronic disease(s). By asking open-ended questions, the health care provider can learn about the patient's views and concerns and then help the patient focus on developing a realistic or doable action plan that is needed to manage his or her disease. The focus should not only be on identifying steps but also on what is realistic given the patient's personal circumstances.

Share information—advise and listen Health care providers need to share information about the disease(s) with the patient. However, the provider's emphasis should be on ensuring that he or she offers the information in a nonjudgmental manner and that the information addresses concerns raised by the patient. When advising, the providers should review behaviors to treat symptoms, such as taking medications. The patient's use of alternative and complementary medicine should also be part of sharing information.

Develop shared goals Shared goals incorporate both the health care provider's and the patient's views and concerns. The health care provider identifies not only the patient's views but also the barriers to reaching the patient's goals. For goals to be useful, they must be meaningful to the patient given his or her personal circumstances.

Develop an action plan The next step is to develop a realistic action plan that includes a discussion of the "how, what, when, and where" and the frequency of the new behaviors. It also includes a discussion of the barriers to success and some ways to overcome those barriers. An important aspect of developing an action plan is understanding the patient's level of self-efficacy as well as what are realistic steps given the patient's personal circumstances.

Use problem-solving techniques A follow-up plan solves any problems that might arise. It can be as simple as setting a specific date to check in. The key point is that the patient knows that the health care provider cares and will follow up.

Patient Empowerment

The patient—not the health care provider—has primary responsibility for his or her own health (Bodenheimer & Abramowitz, 2010; Institute for Healthcare Improvement, 2015; IOM, 2001; Lorig & Holman, 2003; Uldis, 2011). All of us self-manage when we get sick—sometimes for the better, sometimes for the worse. However, we do not always feel in control of our health or our health care. *Patient empowerment* refers to the patient's sense of being in control of his or her health and health care. The patient takes responsibility and feels empowered with the knowledge, attitudes, and skills that influence his or her health behavior. Health care providers are experts on diseases, but the patient is an expert on his or her own health.

There are actions that patients can take to empower themselves and improve their health (Bodenheimer & Abramowitz, 2010; Institute for Healthcare Improvement, 2015; IOM, 2001; Lorig & Holman, 2003; Schulman et al., 2012):

- Share current medical history with their health care provider(s)
- Write down questions before the medical visit
- Bring a loved one or family member to the medical visit to help understand the information given
- Ask questions on any piece of information they do not understood
- Write down instructions and take notes

Most patients want to play an active role in their health care. Many want to take control over their health and work in partnership with their health care providers. It is in the interest of health care providers to promote patient empowerment. When they do, their patients have better health outcomes (Institute for Healthcare Improvement, 2015; IOM, 2001).

In summary, everything that the health care provider does, such as perform blood tests or give physical exams, can improve care. However, almost everything that is a true health outcome—for example, symptom control or daily functioning—is dependent on the patient's actions. Self-management helps a patient feel more in control of his health because he makes decisions about it. For example, a patient, along with his health care provider, can set realistic treatment goals based on what is important to him.

Patient self-management has been associated not only with improved health outcomes but also with decreased use of health care services. The patient who understands his or her chronic disease(s), knows how to manage symptoms, and is able to get health care when needed will be less likely to require more expensive services (Institute for Healthcare Improvement, 2015; IOM, 2001).

Chapter Summary

- Health behavior theories and models explain why patients do or do not engage in certain health behaviors; they also identify information needed for a treatment plan and help in the design of educational strategies and professional support.

- Long-lasting change in health behavior requires change in the community. Community organization creates opportunities that promote and support long-term health behavior change.

- Disease management is a multidisciplinary approach that improves the quality and cost-effectiveness of health care, especially for patients who have one or more chronic diseases. Health care providers who use disease management with their patients provide individualized treatment plans and educational tools, along with professional support.

- The goal of disease management is to identify persons at risk for one or more chronic diseases, promote patient self-management, and provide effective and efficient health care.

- Health outcomes are dependent on patient actions. Everything that the health care provider does can improve the process of care. However, almost everything that is a true health outcome (e.g., symptom control or daily functioning) is dependent on the patient's actions.

- Patient self-management has been associated with improved health outcomes and decreased use of health care services.

REVIEW QUESTIONS

1. What is a health behavior? Distinguish between voluntary and involuntary health behaviors. List two to three examples for each.

2. Explain the differences between a theory and a model. What is a construct?

3. Compare and contrast the health belief model and social cognitive theory.

4. Explain key elements of community organization.

5. What is disease management? Compare and contrast chronic care management with integrated care.

6. Describe ways that a patient can increase his or her self-efficacy.

7. What are some of the differences between traditional patient education and patient self-management education?

8. Identify and list techniques a health care provider can use to promote patient self-management. What are some skills a patient needs to self-manage a chronic disease?

9. What is patient empowerment? Identify some actions a patient can take to feel empowered.

10. Identify two benefits of patient self-management.

KEY TERMS

Chronic care management: Care management focused on how to contain the disease and improve the patient's quality of life over a long period of time

Cognition: A person's way of thinking as well as his or her emotions and behaviors

Community action: Actions that try to resolve community issues and to result in long-lasting changes

Community assessment and planning: An element of community organization in which community stakeholders and leaders create tasks and goals to address a community issue

Community capacity building: The community's effort to develop and maintain strong working relationships among stakeholders and leaders

Community development: Community members' efforts to identify and resolve the community's issues

Community organization: Means by which community members identify issues, gather resources, and develop ways to resolve their issues

Community stakeholders: People in the community who are affected or could be affected by a community issue

Concept: An idea of a theory

Construct: A concept developed for use with a theory

Cues to action: Events that can stimulate an individual's readiness to act

Disease management: A multidisciplinary effort that improves the quality and cost-effectiveness of care for patients

Health behavior: Any action related to disease prevention, health maintenance, health improvement, or the rehabilitation of health

Health belief model (HBM): A model that explains and predicts health behaviors, with a focus on the attitudes and beliefs of individuals

Healthy lifestyle behavior: Long-term, regular pattern of health behaviors

Integrated care: Part of disease management and includes preventive care, social care, and home care

Model: A group of theories that help explain a specific problem

Observational learning: Learning through the experiences of others, rather than just through one's own experiences

Outcome expectations: What a person expects from engaging in certain health behaviors

Patient empowerment: The patient's feeling of being in control and able to make decisions about his or her health care

Patient self-management: Making decisions and taking actions to live well with one or more chronic diseases

Patient self-management education: Education that supports patients and teaches them problem-solving skills

Patient self-management support: Counseling technique that creates a partnership between the health care provider and the patient

Reinforcements: Consequences of a behavior that increase the chances that a person will repeat the behavior

Self-efficacy: A person's confidence in her or his ability to successfully perform an action

Social action: Action taken by community members joining together for a cause

Social cognitive theory (SCT): A theory that focuses on individual and psychological reasons why and how a person changes his or her behaviors

Stages of change model (SCM): A model that focuses on individual and psychological reasons why and how people change their behaviors

Theory: An explanation of why events or situations happen; an analytical tool for understanding, explaining, and making predictions

CHAPTER ACTIVITIES

1. In small groups, brainstorm examples of voluntary and involuntary health behaviors.

2. Interview two people: a health care provider and a person with a chronic disease. Use the following questions to conduct your interview. In small-group discussions, compare answers to the interview questions to identify differences in responses:

    a. Do you think that patients with chronic disease who are not doing well probably do not take their medications as prescribed?

    b. Do you think that chronic disease patients who only follow the health care provider's orders do better?

    c. Do you think that people with chronic diseases have caused their own illness?

    d. Do you think that most chronic diseases can be cured with proper attention and care?

    e. Do you think that pain, fatigue, emotional changes, and decreased physical activity are normally experienced by those living with chronic diseases?

    f. Do you think that health care providers are too busy to teach self-management skills to patients?

3.   In groups of three, review the health belief model, the stages of change model, and social cognitive theory (see Tables 5.1, 5.2, and 5.3). Each group member selects one of the tables and describes how a patient with a chronic disease, such as type 2 diabetes, heart disease, or alcoholism, would change his or her health behavior.

4.   Identify a health issue in your community. When the issue is identified, create a PowerPoint (no more than five slides) on how it can be addressed through key elements of community organization. Be prepared to present this PowerPoint in class for discussion.

5.   Brainstorm in groups of two to three people how to help a patient build self-efficacy. Identify barriers to self-management or reasons why some patients resist self-management. List ways that health care providers can help their patients overcome those barriers and/or resistance.

Bibliography and Works Cited

Bandura, A. (1986). *Social foundations of thought and action: A social cognitive theory.* Englewood Cliffs, NJ: Prentice Hall.

Bandura, A. (1989). Perceived self-efficacy in the exercise of control over AIDS infection. In V. M. Mayes, G. W. Albee, & S. F. Schneider (Eds.), *Primary prevention of AIDS: Psychological approaches* (pp. 128–141). London, England: Sage.

Bandura, A. (1997). *Self-efficacy: The exercise of control.* New York, NY: W. H. Freeman.

Berthold, T., Miller, J., & Avila-Esparza, A. (2009). *Foundations for community health workers.* San Francisco, CA: Jossey-Bass.

Betancourt, J., & Like, R. (2000, May 15). A new framework of care [Editorial]. *Patient care: The practical journal for primary care physicians. Special issue: Caring for Diverse Populations: Breaking Down Barriers, 34*(9), 10–12.

Bodenheimer, T., & Abramowitz, S. (2010). *Helping patients help themselves: How to implement self-management support.* Oakland: California HealthCare Foundation. Retrieved from http://www.chcf.org/~/media/MEDIA %20LIBRARY%20Files/PDF/H/PDF%20HelpingPtsHelpThemselvesImplementSelfMgtSupport.pdf

Bodenheimer, T., Lorig, K., Holman, H., & Grumbach, K. (2002). Patient self-management of chronic disease in primary care. *Journal of the American Medical Association, 288,* 2469–2475.

Corbin, J., & Strauss, A. (1988). *Unending work and care: Managing chronic illness at home.* San Francisco, CA: Jossey-Bass.

Glanz, K., & Maddock, J. (2002). Health-related behavior. In L. Breslow (Ed.), *Encyclopedia of public health* (Vol. 1, pp. 98–104). New York, NY: Macmillan Reference USA. Retrieved from http://go.galegroup.com/ps/i.do? id=GALE

Glanz, K., & Rimer, B. (1999). *Theory at a glance: A guide for health promotion practice.* Washington, DC: National Cancer Institute, US Department of Health and Human Services, and National Institutes of Health.

Green, L. W., & Kreuter, M. W. (2005). *Health promotion planning: An educational and ecological approach* (4th ed.) New York, NY: McGraw-Hill.

Institute for Healthcare Improvement. (2015). Partnering in self-management support: A toolkit for clinicians. Retrieved from http://www.ihi.org/resources/Pages/Tools/SelfManagementToolkitforClinicians.aspx

Institute of Medicine, the Committee on Quality of Health Care in America. (2001). *Crossing the quality chasm: A new health system for the 21st century.* Washington, DC: National Academies Press. Retrieved from http://www.nap.edu

KU Work Group for Community Health and Development. (2016). *Section 8. Identifying and analyzing stakeholders and their interests.* Lawrence: University of Kansas. Retrieved from the Community Tool Box: http://ctb.ku.edu/en/table-of-contents/participation/encouraging-involvement/identify-stakeholders /main

Lorig, K. R., & Holman, H. R. (2003). Self-management education: History, definition, outcomes and mechanisms. *Annals of Behavioral Medicine, 26*, 1–7.

Lorig, K. R., Sobel, D., Stewart, A., Brown, B., Bandura, A., Ritter, P., . . . Holman, H. (1999). Evidence suggesting that a chronic disease self-management program can improve health status while reducing hospitalization: A randomized trial. *Medical Care, 37*, 5–14.

Mattessich, P., & Monsey, B. (1997). *Community building: What makes it work: A review of factors influencing successful community building.* St. Paul, MN: Wilder Publishing Center.

McKenzie, J. F., Pinger, R. R., & Kotecki, J. E. (2011). *An introduction to community health* (7th ed.). Sudbury, MA: Jones & Bartlett.

McLeroy, K. R., Bibeau, D., Steckler, A., & Glanz, K. (1988). An ecological perspective on health promotion programs. *Health Education Quarterly, 15*, 351–377.

Prochaska, J. O., & DiClemente, C. C. (1986). Towards a comprehensive model of change. In U. Miller & N. Heather (Eds.), *Treating addictive behaviors* (pp. 3–27). New York, NY: Plenum Press.

Prochaska, J. O., & Velicer, W. F. (1997). The transtheoretical model of health behavior change. *American Journal of Health Promotion, 12*(1), 38–48.

Prochaska, J. O., Velicer, W. F., Rossi, J. S., Goldstein, M. G., Marcus, B. H., Rakowski, W., . . . Rossi, S. R. (1994). Stages of change and decisional balance for 12 problem behaviors. *Health Psychology, 13*(1), 39–46.

Rosenstock, I. M., Strecher, V. J., & Becker, M. H. (1988). Social learning theory and the health belief model. *Health Education Quarterly, 2*, 175–183.

Schulman-Green, D., Jaser, S., Martin, F., Alonzo, A., Grey, M., McCorkle, R., . . . Whittemore, R. (2012). Processes of self-management in chronic illness. *Journal of Nursing Scholarship, 44*, 136–144. doi:10.1111/j.1547-5069.2012.01444.x

Strecher, V. J., & Rosenstock, I. M. (1997). The health belief model. In K. Glanz, F. Lewis, & B. Rimer (Eds.), *Health behavior and health education: Theory, research, and practice* (pp. 41–60). San Francisco, CA: Jossey-Bass.

Udlis, K. A. (2011). Self-management in chronic illness: Concept and dimensional analysis. *Journal of Nursing & Healthcare of Chronic Illnesses, 3*, 130–139. doi:10.1111/j.1752-9824.2011.01085x

HEALTH LITERACY

CHAPTER OBJECTIVES

- Define health literacy.
- Identify and describe levels of health literacy.
- Explain causes and consequences of health literacy.
- Summarize why low health literacy is a problem in the United States.
- Outline strategies for improving low health literacy.
- Evaluate health information websites.

This chapter examines low health literacy and its impact on health care. It discusses in depth the causes and consequences of low health literacy. Health literacy strategies are identified and explained. Consideration is also given to the relationship between health literacy and access to quality health care.

Importance of Health Literacy

Seeking health information from multiple sources—television, websites, newspapers, radio, loved ones, family members, and neighbors—can be confusing and overwhelming for patients. It is not unusual for the media to tell us one thing one day and tell us something completely different the next. The following are some examples of just how confusing health information can be:

- Alcohol is bad for you, but drinking moderate amounts of wine can help prevent heart disease.
- Too much sun can cause skin cancer, but not enough sun can cause vitamin D deficiency.

- Too much stress is bad for you, but not all stress is bad.

- Birth control pills are effective against unwanted pregnancies, but not against sexually transmitted infections.

- Exercise is good, but too much exercise can lead to injuries.

- Too much caffeine is not good for you, but caffeine does have health benefits.

- Marijuana is an illegal drug in most states, but it can help relieve symptoms for some patients with chronic diseases.

As a health care provider, you may contribute to this confusion. But unlike other sources, health care providers have a responsibility to ensure that the information they share is understood and used by their patients. Fulfilling this responsibility is known as improving a patient's health literacy.

According to the American Medical Association's publication *Assessing the Nation's Health Literacy: Key Concepts and Findings of the National Assessment of Adult Literacy* (White, 2008), improving patients' health literacy—that is, the ability of individuals to read, understand, and act on health information and services—is critical to the health and safety of patients. Patients need to be health literate so that they can understand and act on the health information given and manage their disease(s).

Differences Between Literacy and Health Literacy

The 2003 National Assessment of Adult Literacy (NAAL) is a nationally representative assessment of English literacy among American adults age 16 and older. Sponsored by the National Center for Education Statistics (NCES), NAAL is the nation's most comprehensive measure of adult literacy since the 1992 National Adult Literacy Survey (NALS). Although the term *literacy* usually refers to the ability to read and write—to understand and communicate information—the NAAL has a more detailed definition for literacy that comprises two parts: skills and tasks. Literacy skills range from basic (such as recognizing words) to higher level (such as understanding what one has read in a book). Literacy tasks deal with a person's ability to read, write, speak, compute, and solve problems at levels necessary to:

- Function on the job and in society

- Achieve one's goals

- Develop one's knowledge and potential

Literacy helps us understand, communicate, and act on health information. When a person applies literacy skills and tasks to health, such as by eating a healthy diet, taking medication, or getting a flu shot, he or she is demonstrating *health literacy*. However, ordinary literacy is only one component of health literacy.

Health literacy goes beyond ordinary literacy because it requires knowledge of many areas, including the human body, medical terms, healthy behaviors, and how to access health care. It is also influenced by other factors, such as language, culture, age, socioeconomic status, education, and disabilities. For example, when anyone, regardless of literacy level, is feeling sick or in pain, it can be difficult to remember a health care provider's instructions. Health information provided in a stressful situation like a health care setting is unlikely to be remembered. It can also be difficult for an elderly person, regardless of literacy level, to remember how to correctly take multiple medications.

Levels of Health Literacy

To make the right health decisions and to act on them, patients must be at least somewhat health literate. The 2003 NAAL included a health literacy component. Each of the 19,000 participants was

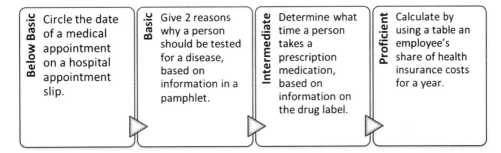

Figure 6.1 Examples of Skills at Each Level of Health Literacy
Note. From *The Health Literacy of America's Adults: Results from the 2003 National Assessment of Adult Literacy* (NCES Publication No. 2006-483), by M. Kutner, E. Greenberg, Y. Jin, and C. Paulsen, 2006, Washington, DC: US Department of Education.

asked to provide background information and to complete a set of tasks to measure his or her ability to read and understand text, interpret documents, and use and interpret numbers. The results were reported by dividing the health literacy skills of subjects into four levels: below basic, basic, intermediate, and proficient (see Figure 6.1).

Below Basic Level

Below basic is the lowest level of health literacy and includes such skills as being able to follow simple instructions or adding the amounts of medications. Adults also might be able to locate and circle the date of a medical appointment on a hospital appointment slip. An adult at this level might not know any English or not be able to read simple written instructions in his or her own language. About 14% of the US adult population has health literacy skills at the below basic level (White, 2008).

Basic Level

Adults at the basic level have the health literacy skills to perform simple tasks such as reading and understanding information in short, easy-to-read instructions. These individuals can understand an easy-to-read handout or brochure, and they might be able to state two reasons why a person should be tested for a disease, based on information in an easy-to-read handout. Patients need to be at the basic level of health literacy to access adequate services from health care providers. About 22% of the US adult population has health literacy skills at the basic level (White, 2008).

Intermediate Level

Adults at the intermediate level have the health literacy skills to perform slightly challenging tasks, such as summarizing written text, making simple connections, and identifying a specific location on a map. They also might be able to determine a healthy weight range for a person of a specified height, on the basis of a graph that relates height and weight. Most US adults (53%) fall into the intermediate category (White, 2008). They can apply information from moderately advanced text and make simple conclusions. Yet some types of health care information, such as insurance forms, consent forms, and medication instructions, are often complicated and can be overwhelming for most patients at this level.

Proficient Level

Adults at the proficient literacy level have the health literacy skills to perform complex activities. They can analyze many pieces of information, such as a table about blood pressure and physical activity. They also can find information about a medical term by searching through a credible website. Only about 12% of the US adult population has health literacy skills at the proficient level (White, 2008).

But even those who are most proficient at using text and numbers may be challenged in the understanding of health information when they are sick or in pain or feeling overwhelmed.

Core Skills of Health Literacy

As already noted, health literacy is more than the ability to read and write. It includes five core skills:

1. Reading
2. Writing
3. Math
4. Listening
5. Speaking

These five core skills enable patients to ask questions, follow a treatment plan, and discuss issues with their health care providers. Understanding a health care provider's instructions for self-care requires listening and speaking skills. Choosing between health plans or comparing prescription drug coverage requires reading and math skills to calculate premiums, copays, and deductibles. Signing medical waivers, writing down providers' instructions, and responding to providers' emails require reading and writing skills.

To be health literate, patients must not only have these five core skills but also know about the human body and diseases (Rudd, Anderson, Oppenheimer, & Nath, 2007). Even for those with advanced degrees, health literacy can be a challenge. To understand what patients go through to manage their health, think about the knowledge and skills required for the following tasks:

- Understanding a newspaper article about a recent Zika outbreak (reading and comprehension)
- Calculating the amount of calories in 1.5 servings of macaroni and cheese, based on a nutrition label (reading and math)
- Knowing that *glucose* is another word for sugar and choosing a product with less sugar over one with more sugar (reading and knowledge of nutrition and nutrition labels)
- Determining that "severe" is a more serious threat than "elevated," and deciding what to do with this information (knowledge and understanding risk)
- Giving medication to an elderly parent who lives at home and has diabetes, dementia, and high blood pressure (reading and math skills; knowledge of the human body, different diseases and their complications, and side effects of several medications)
- Negotiating a health claim with an insurance company claims manager (speaking, reading, and listening skills; understanding complex forms)

Understanding and accessing health information and services are overwhelming for most patients. To get a sense how overwhelming it can be, imagine yourself with a chronic disease such as type 2 diabetes. What are some of the daily skills needed to control your diabetes? You need to change your daily habits—the foods you eat, the activities you do; you must watch your symptoms on a regular basis; you take medicines and try to understand the directions about time, doses, and side effects; you access care when needed, complete medical and insurance forms, and make appointments for follow-up; when interacting with health care providers, you describe symptoms, report changes, ask questions, and try to follow instructions. You also need confidence, commitment, and will power in managing your diabetes over time.

Patients' health literacy has a direct impact on their ability to access health care, share personal information with health care providers, understand complicated information, and manage their disease(s). Health care providers have a responsibility to improve their patients' health literacy, because low health literacy increases the risk of harm. When patients receive accurate, easy-to-understand information, they are better able to manage their health, access services, and reduce harm.

Extent of the Problem of Low Health Literacy

Patient-centered care curbs rising health care costs because it allows patients to be active decision makers in their health care (Office of Disease Prevention and Health Promotion, 2011a, 2011b). To be active decision makers, however, patients need information that they can read, understand, and act on. Yet according to a landmark Institute of Medicine Committee report (Kohn, Corrigan, & Donaldson, 1999), two decades of research indicate that today's health information is not usable by the average adult. Nearly 9 out of 10 adults have difficulty using everyday health information that is available from health care providers, websites, media, and communities. Only 12% of US adults have the skills needed to manage their health and reduce harm.

The Institute of Medicine's 1999 findings suggest that most patients make decisions about their health care based on health information that they don't understand. Patients also make the majority of these decisions on their own—not with their health care providers in a face-to-face meeting. Most patients spend only a small amount of time with their health care providers, so they figure out by themselves how to make major health decisions, such as determining what type of health insurance they should have, how much medicine to take, or how to follow a treatment plan.

Reporting on the extent of the problem of low health literacy in the United States, the Institute of Medicine (Kohn et al., 1999) found that 25% of adults (50 million patients) are at some level of low health literacy. This means that they have trouble completing medical forms or understanding medical terms. Another 21% of adults (40 million patients) are functionally illiterate, meaning that they read at fifth-grade level or lower. They cannot perform the basic reading tasks required to access health care. Oral instructions are also difficult for them. Together, low health literacy and functional illiteracy account for at least 90 million adults; they lack the skills needed to prevent disease and protect their health. This represents between $50 billion to $73 billion a year in extra health care costs. Such statistics have sent an alarm to health care policymakers at the local, state, and national levels. Low health literacy is now recognized as a major problem in the United States, and remediating it is a priority, as stated in the Healthy People 2020 initiative, a project of the Centers for Disease Control and Prevention (CDC).

If measures are not taken to address low health literacy, the near future looks even bleaker. As the United States shifts toward a majority population of older adults, and with more people who have limited English proficiency (LEP), there will be even greater numbers of patients with low health literacy, creating a heavier economic burden on our already strained health care system (Centers for Disease Control and Prevention [CDC], 2016).

Causes of Low Health Literacy

Five factors can cause low health literacy (Office of Disease Prevention and Health Promotion, 2011a, 2011b). A patient with low health literacy may be dealing with one or more of these factors:

1. Functional difficulties
2. Physical disabilities
3. Cultural and language issues
4. Mental health disabilities
5. Computational or numerical difficulties

Patients with *functional* low health literacy lack ability to read and write. They also have trouble with spoken words of more than two syllables. But these patients are not stupid! They can figure out what you mean; however, they may miss things while struggling to understand what is said.

Physical disabilities, such as visual, hearing, and mobility impairments, can cause low health literacy. This also applies to patients who might be losing senses because of a certain disease or due to the aging process. For example, patients with multiple sclerosis may not be able to verbally respond to questions, or elderly patients may have hearing and vision loss.

Issues related to *culture* and *language* affect non-English-speaking populations and those with immigrant status; members of these groups may have *limited English proficiency (LEP).* Many people with LEP are literate in their own language; others are unable to read or write in their native language. Basic Western medicine practices—such as using a thermometer—may be completely unfamiliar to some patients with LEP. According to the Agency for Healthcare Research and Quality (2013), approximately 21 million people in the United States speak limited English, and there will be more in the years to come.

Patients with *mental health disabilities* will have difficulty understanding the status of their health care. They may interpret health information differently, and their judgment can be negatively affected. Sometimes patients with mental health disabilities are negative, paranoid, or passive when meeting with their health care providers. Consequently, they do not comprehend the information given or receive the care they need.

For patients with *computational or numerical difficulties,* the combined use of numbers and words is challenging. Yet much of health literacy entails following detailed directions that incorporate both numbers and words, and measuring medicines or food portions can be particularly difficult. For example, a diabetic patient can be challenged by the daily measuring of food portions and insulin injections.

Populations at Risk for Low Health Literacy

Persons with low health literacy are represented in every segment of society (see Figure 6.2). You, too, can be affected by low health literacy at some point in your life—regardless of your age, race, culture,

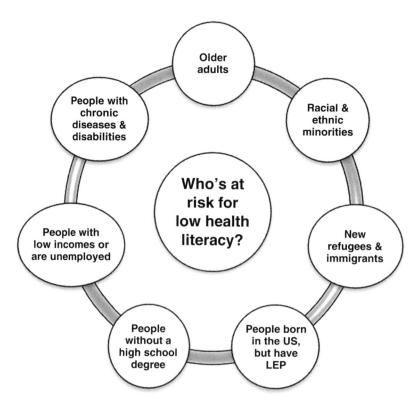

Figure 6.2 Populations at Risk for Low Health Literacy

income, or education. Nonetheless, low health literacy is much more common in certain US population groups. According to the Office of Disease Prevention and Health Promotion's *National Action Plan to Improve Health Literacy* (2010), although the majority of people with low health literacy skills in the United States are white and native-born, the people most at risk are those who

- Are over the age of 65
- Are members of racial and ethnic minority groups
- Are recent refugees and immigrants to the United States who do not speak English
- Were born in the United States but for whom English is a second language and who have LEP
- Did not graduate from high school
- Are working in low-income jobs or are unemployed
- Have chronic diseases and disabilities

Although patients who belong to these populations are known to be at higher risk for low health literacy, keep in mind that many do have the necessary skills. In other words, just because someone is a new immigrant or has a disability does not mean that he or she has low health literacy. It is also important to remember that many patients with low health literacy do not belong to an at-risk population. It is therefore important for health care providers to acknowledge the potential difficulty of identifying patients with low health literacy.

Shame and Low Health Literacy

Patients with low health literacy can feel shame about their lack of skills. As a result, they may hide reading, writing, or math difficulties from their health care providers to avoid embarrassment. This shame contributes to the "hidden" nature of health illiteracy. A landmark study on shame and low health literacy by Parikh, Parker, Nurss, Baker, and Williams (1996) found that 67% of patients with low health literacy never told their spouses, and 53% had never told their children of their literacy difficulties. Nineteen percent of these patients had never disclosed their difficulty reading to anyone.

Some patients may show signs of having low health literacy. If patients fill out their registration forms wrong or take their medications incorrectly, they may have done so because of low health literacy skills (Safeer & Keenan, 2005). Other signs of low health literacy are listed in Figure 6.3.

Because someone has low health literacy does not mean that he or she is stupid or can't function in everyday life. In fact, just the opposite is true for many of these patients, who function well without anyone knowing about their low literacy.

Consequences for Patients with Low Health Literacy

Low health literacy is linked to many health problems, such as greater risk of harm, limited access to care, and higher rates of hospitalization. According to the Office of Disease Prevention and Health Promotion (2010, 2011a, 2011b), the following are consequences for patients with low health literacy:

- They are less likely to receive preventive care, such as physicals, mammograms, and blood pressure screenings.
- They are less able to manage life-threatening diseases, such as heart disease, diabetes, and HIV/AIDS.
- They are more likely to miss medical appointments and to take medications incorrectly.
- They are more likely to lack skills needed for self-care.

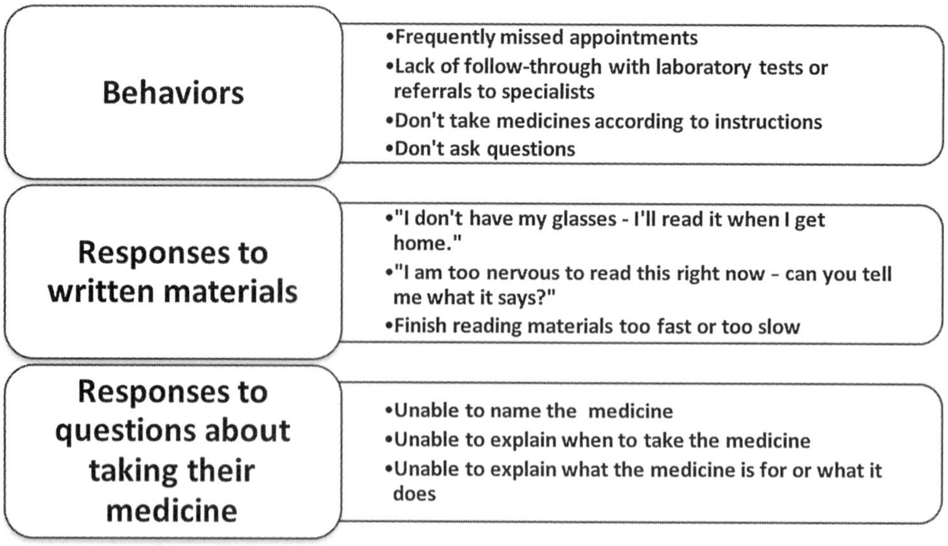

Behaviors	•Frequently missed appointments •Lack of follow-through with laboratory tests or referrals to specialists •Don't take medicines according to instructions •Don't ask questions
Responses to written materials	•"I don't have my glasses - I'll read it when I get home." •"I am too nervous to read this right now – can you tell me what it says?" •Finish reading materials too fast or too slow
Responses to questions about taking their medicine	•Unable to name the medicine •Unable to explain when to take the medicine •Unable to explain what the medicine is for or what it does

Figure 6.3 Signs of Low Health Literacy in Patients
Note. Adapted from *Health Literacy and Patient Safety: Help Patients Understand. Manual for Clinicians,* by B. D. Weiss, 2007, Chicago, IL: American Medical Association Foundation and American Medical Association.

- They are at higher risk of needing emergency services and hospitalization.

- They pay annual health care costs four times higher than those with higher levels of health literacy.

- They are more likely to report their health as poor and to have incomplete medical histories.

In summary, when patients with low health literacy interact with a complex health care system, the outcomes are often poor health, greater risk for harm, and higher medical costs.

Health Literacy and Health Care Providers

Factors that affect health literacy are complicated. They include not only patients' knowledge and skills but also health care providers' communication skills and the demands of the health care system.

Health literacy was once considered the responsibility of the individual, but now more attention is given to the role of health care providers because of the following (Safeer & Keenan, 2005):

Rising health care costs Providing health information and skills to patients decreases health care costs.

Managed care Managed care insurance plans want patients to be active decision makers in their health; low health literacy makes this difficult.

Complex treatment options Complex treatment options negatively affect a patient's ability to make informed health care decisions. Patients with low health literacy face significant challenges in following medicine instructions, preventing medical errors, and providing informed consent.

Aging population Aging is associated with decreased health literacy. Strategies to control costs and improve quality of care for older adults must include improving their health literacy.

Racial and ethnic diversity As the US population becomes more diverse, differences in language and cultural beliefs are barriers to communication between health care providers and patients.

As already noted, the main consequences for patients with low health literacy are poor health, greater risk for harm, and higher medical costs. One of the primary problems is that health care providers fail to speak to patients in easy-to-understand words, or *plain language*. They fail to make sure that patients understand what they are told, what they need to do, and why they need to do it. This lack of information spoken in plain language causes problems not only for patients and their health care providers but also for health care systems that are trying to control costs (Plain Language Action and Information Network, 2011).

The primary responsibility for improving patients' health literacy lies with health care providers and health care systems (Smedley, Stith, & Nelson, 2003). If they become better at communicating health information, the United States will be a health-literate society, leading to less harm to patients and lower health care costs.

Strategies That Improve Patients' Health Literacy

Low health literacy can affect anyone, regardless of age, race, education, gender, or income. It is sobering to know that low health literacy impacts nearly one in every three people living in the United States (CDC, 2016; Office of Disease Prevention and Health Promotion, 2010, 2011a, 2011b). It is a "condition" that can't be diagnosed by medical technology and is not visible to the eye, so health care providers need to have a certain awareness and develop certain skills to identify those patients who have low health literacy.

Health Care Providers

Health information needs to be spoken and written in easy-to-understand words—what's known as plain language. Plain language helps patients find what they need, understand what they find, and act on that understanding (Plain Language Action and Information Network, 2011).

Speaking plainly is just as important as writing plainly. Many of the same plain-language strategies for written messages apply to verbal messages. The plain-language strategies for health care providers listed in Table 6.1 improve patients' health literacy.

When working with patients, ask questions using the words "what" or "how" instead of those that can be answered with yes or no. For example, say, "Tell me about your problem. What may have caused it?"

Encourage patients to ask questions and to show you what they understand. A way to do this is by using the *teach-back method* to improve communication between health care providers and patients. The patient is asked to restate the information in his or her own words—not just repeat it—to make sure that the message is understood and remembered. When understanding is not correct, the health care provider repeats the information until the patient can understand and restate the information correctly.

When a patient has LEP, use a medically trained interpreter. Plain-language strategies do not necessarily help patients who have limited ability to speak or understand English. Health information for people with LEP needs to be communicated plainly in their primary language, using words and examples that fit the information into the context of their cultural norms and values.

Printed health information needs to be written in plain language and to be accessible to all audiences, including those with limited vision.

Determining the readability level of written materials is easy with Microsoft Word, which offers readability statistics in the spelling and grammar menu. The document is graded based on the Flesch-Kincaid Grade Level Formula. You should try to aim for the lowest level possible without losing the meaning of the information. To reach a general audience, a strategy is to keep your document at the fifth- or sixth-grade reading level (or lower) and never higher than eighth grade.

A word of caution: Readability tests give only a general idea of how difficult it will be to read the document, based on written words. They do not consider layout or design—or tell how well your

Table 6.1 Verbal Strategies for Health Care Providers

Before the Visit	During the Visit	Follow-Up
Know the languages and cultures of your patients.	Limit the amount of information provided at each visit.	Have staff schedule additional appointments to make sure that the patient knows when and where she is to go for her next appointment.
Determine what resources are needed by the patient (for example, a medical interpreter).	Use simple and familiar language.	Consider follow-up phone calls that repeat the important points you talked about during the visit.
Check the reading level of written materials that you give to patients; make sure the wording is not too advanced (fifth- to eighth-grade reading level, max.).	Start with the most important information first.	
	Speak slowly, take your time, and use repetition.	
	Use concrete examples that the patient can relate to.	
	Break complex information into smaller "chunks."	
	Give no more than one or two instructions at a time. Ask the patient questions to make sure that he understands instructions.	
	Avoid medical jargon or technical medical terms.	
	Use pictures or models to explain important ideas.	
	Invite a spouse or other family member into the room; this helps with comprehension and memory.	
	Use a quiet room with minimal distractions.	
	Consider color-coding medications or using some other visual aid (e.g., a sun to indicate taking them in the morning).	
	Use daily events as reminders—e.g., "Take these before breakfast" or "Check your sugar before you pick up the kids at school."	

audience understood your message. Pretesting with members of your target audience is the best way to judge the readability of your document.

Health information materials (see Table 6.2) should always take into account the target audience's culture and social context—race, ethnicity, language, nationality, religion, age, gender, sexual orientation, income level, disabilities, and occupation (Safeer & Keenan, 2005).

Table 6.2   Printed Materials Strategies (Including Brochures or Handouts)

Visuals	Layout	Writing Style
Whenever possible, use simple pictures, photos, line drawings, charts, and other visuals instead of text to make your points.	Use at least 12-point font.	Use simple language and simple writing style—avoid long sentences.
Use only visuals that help convey your message. (Don't just "decorate," as this will distract readers.)	Use headings and bullets to break up text.	Include no more than four main messages. Leave out information that is "nice to know" but not necessary.
Place visuals near to related text. Visuals need to include captions.	Avoid using all-capital letters, italics, and fancy script. Keep line length between 40 and 50 characters.	Organize similar information into several smaller groups.
Visuals need to be culturally appropriate and not complicated.	Highlight important points with color. Place the most important information at the beginning of the document and repeat it at the end.	Focus on changing behavior or on what needs to be done rather than trying to explain technical medical terms.
Make the cover of your document visually appealing to your target audience. The cover should include your main message.	Be sure to leave plenty of white space in the margins and between sections. Margins need to be at least one-half inch.	Review materials to make sure the literacy level is not above eighth grade.

Computer-Assisted Education

Computer-assisted education is an interactive way of teaching patients about the prevention and treatment of diseases. This is often more engaging than printed materials, especially for patients with low health literacy. It can be easily tailored to match their needs, and tailored messages can be easier to understand than one-size-fits-all presentations.

Many of the same health literacy strategies for verbal and written communication apply to computer-assisted education, including using plain language, large fonts, white space, and simple graphics. Accessibility also needs to be considered for persons with disabilities. Other specific strategies include the following:

- Use video and/or audio files, not just text
- Include interactive features such as quizzes
- Organize information to minimize searching and scrolling
- Give users the option to navigate from simple to more complex information
- Have a link with resources

Many federal, state, and local public health departments, universities, insurance plans, medical organizations, and health associations have websites that provide health information. These sites include the CDC (www.cdc.gov), Mayo Clinic (www.mayoclinic.org), MedlinePlus https://medlineplus (.gov/healthtopics.html), American Academy of Family Physicians (www.aafp.org), and others too numerous to list. Unfortunately, not all health information websites are at a reading level that is right for individuals with low health literacy; therefore, health care providers need to be careful about recommending websites to patients (Medical Library Association, 2015).

What health care providers can do to boost the general literacy skills of their patients is limited, but they can use strategies to improve health literacy. By ensuring that the health care setting is patient-friendly, communicating in plain language, using culturally appropriate materials, and using the teach-back method, health care providers can deliver effective care to all their patients.

Testing for Low Health Literacy

Health care providers can determine their patients' level of health literacy by using either the Test of Functional Health Literacy in Adults (TOFHLA) or the Rapid Estimate of Adult Literacy in Medicine (REALM) (Agency for Healthcare Research and Quality, 2009). The TOFHLA is available in English and Spanish. It uses health materials to evaluate reading comprehension and numeracy. The test has 50 questions and takes about 20 minutes to complete. A short version is available and takes around 7 minutes to complete. The REALM evaluates word recognition and pronunciation and takes about 5 minutes to complete.

These tests are usually administered in a research setting. Although health care providers can use these tests in a health care setting, doing so may be counterproductive: Having patients with low health literacy take a test when they go to see their health care provider may make it less likely for them to seek help, or it may leave them feeling ashamed.

Another approach suggested by the American Medical Association report (White, 2008) is to ask one or two simple questions that take less than a minute and are valid for English- and Spanish-speaking populations:

- "How often do you need to have someone help you when you read instructions, pamphlets, or other written material from your doctor or pharmacy?" (Answers indicating low health literacy are "sometimes," "often," or "always.")

- "How confident are you filling out medical forms by yourself?" (Answers indicating low health literacy are "somewhat," "a little bit," or "not at all.")

Patients

A specific strategy that patients can use when asking questions of their health care provider is *Ask Me 3*, developed by the CDC (2016). Ask Me 3 allows patients to get the information they need and in words that they understand. It is designed to promote communication between health care providers and patients. There are three simple questions that patients ask their health care providers at every visit and that health care providers should encourage their patients to ask (see Table 6.3):

1. What is my main problem? (diagnosis)
2. What do I need to do? (treatment)
3. Why is it important for me to do this? (context)

These three questions allow patients to know about their disease and medication, why the treatment is important, and steps to take to prevent a disease or to keep it under control.

The American Medical Association (Weiss, 2007) has developed a checklist for measuring patient understanding. This checklist has questions that a patient should be able to answer at the end of a visit.

What Health Care Systems Can Do to Improve Health Literacy

The following list shows steps that health care systems can take to improve health literacy. Please note that most of these steps would entail little or no expense, and if they were taken, the outcome would

Table 6.3 Checklist for Patients

At the end of each visit with your health care provider, you should be able to answer the following questions:

Ask-Me 3 Questions	Where Do I Go?	What Do I Do?	Next Steps
1. What is my main problem?	4. Where do I go for tests, medicine, and appointments?	5. How should I take my medicine? a. When do I take it? b. What will it do? c. How do I know if it is working? d. Whom do I call if I have questions, and when do I call?	7. When do I need to be seen again?
2. What do I need to do (about the problem)?			8. Do I have another appointment? If so, what is the date and time of the appointment?
3. Why is it important for me to do this?		6. Other instructions a. What to do? b. How to do it? c. When to do it?	9. Are there phone numbers to call?

Note. Adapted from *Health Literacy and Patient Safety: Help Patients Understand. Manual for Clinicians,* by B. D. Weiss, 2007, Chicago, IL: American Medical Association Foundation and American Medical Association.

result in better health for patients, less harm, and lower health care costs (Kohn et al., 1999; Nielsen-Bohlman, Pranzer, & Kindig, 2004).

- Change professional practice to emphasize health literacy improvement and shame-free environments
- At professional conferences and through the media, make the case for improving patients' health literacy
- Improve how patients with low health literacy use health services
- Improve how health forms and instructions are worded and used
- Improve access to the physical environment
- Improve access to culturally appropriate health information
- Create patient-centered environments that stress the use of plain language with patients in all interactions

Health Information Websites

Websites are one of the most widely used forms of communication. Millions of people search for health information on websites every day, whether for themselves or for a loved one. Sometimes when searching a website, a person can find correct information that is helpful. Other searches end badly because the information the person finds is out-of-date, incorrect, or even harmful.

All websites are not created equal. Anyone can set up a website and publish any kind of health information, so the problem becomes trying to figure out whether or not the information is correct. Patients need current, unbiased information from reliable sources to make decisions. Health care providers have a responsibility to guide their patients to the most helpful websites.

To assess a website's information, one needs to ask four questions (Medical Library Association, 2016): (a) Who or what is the source? (b) How accurate is the information? (c) Is the website trying to sell something? (d) If research results are used to support claims, how was the research conducted?

The first step in reviewing a website is to consider the source: Does the site use recognized experts, and who is responsible for the information? When you use a website, look for an "About Us" page. Check to see who runs the site. Is it a branch of the US federal government, a university, a nonprofit health organization, a hospital, a business, or an individual? There is a big difference between a site that states, "I developed this site after I was diagnosed with breast cancer" and one that states, "This page on breast cancer was developed by the American Cancer Society."

Some websites claim that their products have been "clinically tested." This type of claim gives the impression that the clinical testing proved the product's effectiveness. In truth, however, anyone can claim that the product has been clinically tested. The real question is, Have the clinical test results been published in a peer-reviewed professional journal? The safest solution is to choose sites created by the federal government or recognized institutions (public hospitals, universities, and nonprofit organizations). These sites exist only for public benefit and are not seeking to profit. They often contain comprehensive, up-to-date information and reliable advice based on peer-reviewed clinical tests.

Claims that a treatment works often are based only on animal testing. Studies that use animals as subjects are only the first steps in medical research. However, many drugs that show promising results in animals don't work in humans. Claims are stronger if they are based on research with human subjects. In general, the larger the number of people in a study, the more you can trust its results. Small studies may miss important differences because of the small sample size and are more at risk for finding things just by chance. When a site claims that the results were based on a study with only a handful of people, the value of the results is limited.

Does the website try to sell something with health claims that are too good to be true? Is the information written using obscure medical terms? A health information website should use plain language, not technical jargon.

Try to be aware of bias when reviewing a website. Who pays for the site? Check to see if the site is supported by public funds, donations, or by commercial advertising. A way to check is to look at a page on the site and see if it is clear who is providing the information. Advertisements should be labeled, saying "Advertisement" or "From Our Sponsor." For example, if a page about treatment of depression recommends one drug by name, try to determine whether the company that manufactures the drug sponsors the website. If it does, you should consult other sources to see what they say about the same drug.

Does the website promise quick, dramatic, miraculous results if you buy the product? Is this the only site making these claims? Beware of claims that one product will cure more than one disease, that it is a "breakthrough," or that it has a "secret ingredient." It is always better to get a second opinion and check more than one website. Also, use caution if the website uses a sensational writing style—for example, using lots of exclamation points.

Misinformation thrives on websites, so a focus on reliable and valid information is important. All websites should have a way to contact the organization. If the site provides no contact information, then the site is questionable at best. Does the site have an editorial board? Is the information reviewed before it is posted? This information is often on the "About Us" link of the website. See if the board members are experts in the subject of the site. For example, a site on injuries whose medical advisory board members are lawyers is not medically sound. Sometimes the site has information "about our contributors" or "about our authors" instead of an editorial board. Review this section to determine the level of expertise.

Is the information on the website current? Look for dates on the website to see when it was last updated. A site on coping with stress doesn't need to be as current as a site on the latest treatment of diabetes.

A person's health information is confidential, so a site should have a privacy policy. There should be a link saying "Privacy" or "Privacy Policy." Read the privacy policy to see if privacy is being protected. For example, if the site says, "We share information with companies that can provide you with useful products," then privacy is not protected.

Table 6.4 shows the Medical Library Association's 2016 list of the top most useful health information websites for patients.

Table 6.4 Medical Library Association's 2016 Most Useful Health Information Websites for Patients

Website	Description
Cancer.gov (http://www.cancer.gov/)	Official website for the National Cancer Institute (NCI). The NCI is the federal government's principal agency for cancer research and training. The NCI coordinates the National Cancer Program, which conducts and supports research, training, health information dissemination, and other cancer-related programs.
Centers for Disease Control and Prevention (CDC) (http://www.cdc.gov/)	An agency of the Department of Health and Human Services, the CDC is dedicated to promoting "health and quality of life by preventing and controlling disease, injury, and disability." Of special interest to patients are the resources about diseases, conditions, and other special topics arranged under "Health Topics A–Z" and "Travelers' Health," with health recommendations for travelers worldwide. Information is also available in Spanish.
Familydoctor.org (http://familydoctor.org/)	Operated by the American Academy of Family Physicians (AAFP), a national medical organization representing more than 93,700 family physicians, family practice residents, and medical students. All of the information on this site has been written and reviewed by physicians and patient education professionals at the AAFP.
Healthfinder® (http://www.healthfinder.gov/)	A gateway health information website whose goal is "to improve consumer access to selected health information from government agencies, their many partner organizations, and other reliable sources that serve the public interest." Menu lists on its home page provide links to online journals, medical dictionaries, minority health information, and information on prevention and self-care. The developer and sponsor of this site is the Office of Disease Prevention and Health Promotion, an office of the Department of Health and Human Services. Resources on the site are also available in Spanish.
HIV InSite (http://hivinsite.ucsf.edu/)	A project of the University of California San Francisco (UCSF) AIDS Research Institute. Designed as a gateway to in-depth information about particular aspects of HIV/AIDS, it provides numerous links to many authoritative sources. Information is also available in Spanish.
KidsHealth® (http://www.kidshealth.org/)	Provides doctor-approved health information about children, from before birth through adolescence. KidsHealth offers families useful, accurate, up-to-date, and jargon-free health information.
Mayo Clinic (http://www.mayoclinic.com/)	An extension of the Mayo Clinic's commitment to provide health education to patients and the general public. Editors of the site include more than 2,000 physicians, scientists, writers, and educators at the Mayo Clinic, a nonprofit institution with more than 100 years of experience in patient care, medical research, and education.
MedlinePlus (English/Spanish) (http://medlineplus.gov/)	A consumer-oriented website established by the National Library of Medicine, the world's largest biomedical library. An alphabetical "Health Topics" list of more than 300 diseases, conditions, and wellness issues. Additional resources include physician and hospital directories, several online medical dictionaries, and consumer drug information available by generic or brand name.
NIH SeniorHealth (https://nihseniorhealth.gov/)	Health and wellness information for older adults from the National Institutes of Health.
NetWellness (http://www.netwellness.org/)	Nonprofit consumer health website. Information is created and evaluated by medical and health professional faculty at the University of Cincinnati, Case Western Reserve University, and The Ohio State University.

Chapter Summary

- Health literacy is the ability of individuals to read, understand, and act on health information and services.

- As a health care provider, you have a responsibility to improve patients' health literacy.

- Five factors can cause low health literacy: functional difficulties, physical disabilities, cultural and language issues, mental health disabilities, and computational or numerical difficulties.

- There are about 90 million patients with low health literacy in the United States; they lack the skills needed to prevent disease and protect their health. These patients account for between $50 billion to $73 billion a year in extra health care costs.

- The main consequences for patients with low health literacy are poor health, greater risk of harm, and higher medical costs. One of the primary problems is that health care providers fail to speak to patients in easy-to-understand words (plain language). They fail to make sure that patients understand what they are told, what they are to do, and why they are to do it.

REVIEW QUESTIONS

1. What is health literacy?

2. What are the five core skills of health literacy?

3. Health literacy was once considered the responsibility of the individual, but now there is more attention given to the role of health care providers. Give three reasons why this statement is true.

4. What is the teach-back method?

5. What population(s) are most at risk for low health literacy?

6. What are the five causes of low health literacy?

7. List and discuss strategies a health care provider can use to improve the health literacy of his or her patients.

8. List and discuss strategies that a patient can use to improve his or her health literacy.

9. List and discuss strategies that a health care setting can use to improve patients' health literacy.

10. What are four questions to ask when reviewing a website?

KEY TERMS

Ask Me 3: Three questions that patients ask their health care providers at every visit, enabling patients to get the information they need and in words that they understand

Health literacy: The ability to read, understand, and act on health information and services

Limited English proficiency (LEP): Skill level of people who understand, speak, and write English less than "very well"

Literacy: The ability to read and write—to understand and communicate information

Plain language: Simple written and spoken language that makes health information easier to understand

Teach-back method: A method for ensuring that a message is understood and remembered, whereby the patient restates—not just repeats—the given information in his or her own words

CHAPTER ACTIVITIES

1. Make a brochure about a chronic disease of your choice. The brochure needs to be designed for a wide audience; it should use plain language and provide easy-to-understand health information. Follow the guidelines shown in Table 6.2, and include the following items:

   a. Easy to understand visuals that explain key ideas

   b. Action captions that clarify the point of the visual

   c. Interaction with the reader by posing questions

   d. Resources for more information

2. Identify and describe how a patient with a chronic disease would use the five core health literacy skills to manage his or her disease.

3. Role-play with a partner a scenario in which a health care provider is interacting with a patient who has a below basic or basic health literacy level. The below basic or basic health literacy level can be caused by functional difficulties, physical disabilities, cultural and language issues, mental health disabilities, or computational or numerical difficulties. The health care provider is trying to get the patient to understand what the problem is, what the patient needs to do, and why. Reverse roles after the first role play.

4. Create a list of 15 words related to management of such diseases as heart disease, diabetes, and breast cancer. The purpose of this word list is to help patients with low health literacy understand the terms necessary to manage their disease. Definitions in the word list need to be written in plain language and easy to understand.

5. Write a two- to three-page essay on strategies that help identify quality health information websites.

6. Develop a crossword puzzle of technical terms related to a chronic disease (20 words across, 20 words down). The clues need to be written in plain language and have a readability level of no higher than fifth grade.

7. The Medical Library Association lists its recommended health information websites at http://www.mlanet.org/p/cm /ld/fid=397. The websites are grouped into the following categories: General Health, Cancer, Breast Cancer, Diabetes, Eye Disease, Heart Disease, HIV/AIDS, and Stroke. For each category, identify three to four websites that you think are the most comprehensive for someone with low health literacy, and give reasons. Be prepared to write your responses in a two- to three-page paper.

Bibliography and Works Cited

Agency for Healthcare Research and Quality. (2004). Five steps to safer health care: Patient fact sheet. Retrieved from http://www.ahrq.gov/patients-consumers/care-planning/errors/5steps/index.html

Agency for Healthcare Research and Quality. (2009). Health literacy measurement tools. Retrieved from http://www.ahrq.gov/populations/sahlsatool.htm

Agency for Healthcare Research and Quality. (2012). Questions to ask your doctor. Retrieved from http://www.ahrq.gov/patients-consumers/patient-involvement/ask-your-doctor/index.html

Agency for Healthcare Research and Quality. (2013). 2013 national healthcare disparities report (NHDR), 1–277. Retrieved from http://www.ahrq.gov/research/findings/nhqrdr/nhdr13/2013nhdr.pdf

Centers for Disease Control and Prevention. (2016). Understanding health literacy. Retrieved from http://www.cdc.gov/healthliteracy/learn/understanding.html

Kohn, L.T.E., Corrigan, J.M.E., & Donaldson, M.S.E. (Eds.). (1999). To err is human: Building a safer health system. Retrieved from https://www.ncbi.nlm.nih.gov/pubmed/25077248

Kutner, M., Greenberg, E., Jin, Y., & Paulsen, C. (2006). The health literacy of America's adults: Results from the 2003 national assessment (NCES 2006-483). Retrieved from https://nces.ed.gov/pubsearch/pubsinfo.asp?pubid=2006483.

McLaughlin, G. H. (1969). SMOG grading: A new readability formula. *Journal of Reading, 12,* 639–646.

Medical Library Association. (2015). For health consumers and patients: Find good health information. Retrieved from http://www.mlanet.org/p/cm/ld/fid=398

Medical Library Association. (2016). For health consumers and patients: MLA top health websites. Retrieved from http://www.mlanet.org/p/cm/ld/fid=397

Nielsen-Bohlman, L., Panzer, A. M., & Kindig, D. A. (2004). *Health literacy: A prescription to end confusion.* Washington, DC: National Academies Press.

Office of Disease Prevention and Health Promotion. (2008). America's health literacy: Why we need accessible health information. Retrieved from http://www.health.gov/communication/literacy/issuebrief/

Office of Disease Prevention and Health Promotion. (2010). National action plan to improve health literacy. Retrieved from http://www.cdc.gov/healthliteracy/planact/index.html

Office of Disease Prevention and Health Promotion. (2011a). Health literacy improvement. Retrieved from http://www.health.gov/communication/literacy/

Office of Disease Prevention and Health Promotion. (2011b). Quick guide to health literacy. Retrieved from http://health.gov/communication/literacy/quickguide/

Parikh, N. S., Parker, R. M., Nurss, J. R., Baker, D. W., & Williams, M. V. (1996). Shame and health literacy: The unspoken connection. *Patient Education and Counseling, 27*(1), 33–39. Retrieved from http://www.sciencedirect.com/science/article/pii/0738399195007873

Plain Language Action and Information Network. (2011). Plain language: Improving communications from the federal government to the public. Retrieved from www.plainlanguage.gov.

Rudd, R. E., Anderson, J. E., Oppenheimer, S., & Nath, C. (2007). Health literacy: An update of public health and medical literature. In J. P. Comings, B. Garner, & C. Smith (Eds.), *Review of adult learning and literacy* (pp. 175–2014). Mahwah, NJ: Erlbaum.

Safeer, R. S., & Keenan, J. (2005). Health literacy: The gap between physicians and patients. *American Family Physician, 72,* 463–468. Retrieved from http://www.aafp.org/afp/2005/0801/p463.html

Schulz, P. J., & Nakamoto, K. (2013). Health literacy and patient empowerment in health communication: The importance of separating conjoined twins. *Patient Education and Counseling, 90*(1), 4–11.

Smedley, B. D., Stith, A. Y., & Nelson, A. R. (Eds.). (2003). *Unequal treatment: Confronting racial and ethnic disparities in health care.* Washington, DC: National Academies Press.

Weiss, B. D. (2007). *Health literacy and patient safety: Help patients understand. Manual for clinicians.* Chicago, IL: American Medical Association Foundation and American Medical Association.

White, S. (2008). *Assessing the nation's health literacy: Key concepts and findings of the National Assessment of Adult Literacy.* Atlanta, GA: American Medical Association.

White, S., & McCloskey, M. (2011). Framework: Definition of literacy (NCES 2005-531). Washington, DC: National Center for Education. Retrieved from http://nces.ed.gov/naal/fr_definition.asp

CHAPTER 7

COMMUNICATION SKILLS FOR HEALTH CARE PROVIDERS

CHAPTER OBJECTIVES

- Identify and explain types of communication skills for health care providers.

- Summarize the importance of effective communication skills for health care providers.

- Describe the five major emotions that patients experience.

- Describe difficult situations in the provider-patient relationship.

- Discuss special considerations for patients who are communication-vulnerable.

- Explain and defend the Patient's Bill of Rights.

This chapter explores the ways that effective health care provider communication can improve health outcomes for patients. Effective communication skills enable health care providers to understand not only the patient's health status but also his or her cultural healing beliefs. Communication skills also help providers identify and assist patients who have learning, physical, or mental health disabilities.

There are work situations where effective communication is crucial, particularly when medical errors and adverse events occur. In such situations, the patient should be informed not only of the error or event but also of his or her rights.

Communication Skills for the Health Care Provider

Communication is the process of relating to and interacting with other people. When communicating with someone, a person shares information that expresses ideas, emotions, and needs.

Effective communication includes listening and understanding, and expressing ideas, feelings, and information to others in a respectful, caring, and clear manner. Effective communication is a mutual process between two or more people. It can be both an art and a science, and it can be learned and mastered. That is, the more someone practices, the better at it he or she becomes.

The Joint Commission (2010), the leading accreditation agency for hospitals and other health care services, offers the following definition of effective communication

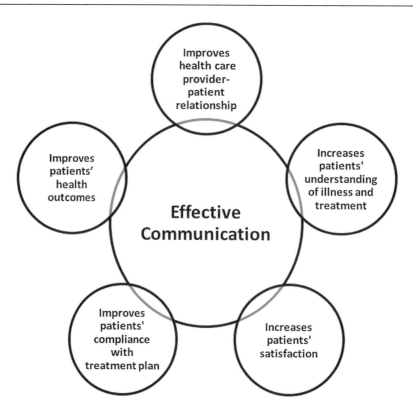

Figure 7.1 Benefits of Effective Communication

in its publication *Advancing Effective Communication, Cultural Competence, and Patient- and Family-Centered Care*:

> Patients and health care providers exchange information, enabling patients to participate actively in their care from admission through discharge, and ensuring that the responsibilities of both patients and providers are understood. To be truly effective, communication requires a two-way process (expressive and receptive) in which messages are negotiated until the information is correctly understood by both parties. Successful communication takes place only when providers understand and integrate the information gleaned from patients, and when patients comprehend accurate, timely, complete, and unambiguous messages from providers in a way that enables them to participate responsibly in their care. (p. 1)

See Figure 7.1 for a summary of the benefits of effective health care provider communication.

There are two main forms of communication that health care providers use with patients: verbal (talking) and nonverbal (body language). A provider who develops skills in these areas can improve the health outcomes of their patients. How a provider and a patient communicate with each other lays the foundation of care throughout the spectrum of health, illness, and recovery.

Verbal Communication

A provider communicates with patients differently than with friends, loved ones, or family members. Provider-patient communications are health focused and patient centered, with defined professional boundaries. There are three ingredients to communicating and engaging with patients: respect, genuineness, and empathy.

To communicate with *respect* means using statements that show understanding of the patient's experiences. After carefully listening to what a patient says, the provider can let the patient know that his or her feelings are understandable. Other ways that a health care provider can show respect are to

- Find something to praise in the patient's behavior, particularly when the patient is experiencing stress over his or her illness

- Be aware of the patient's personal space, which can vary among cultures

- Sit or stand at the patient's eye level to show that you are listening

- Invite the patient to tell his or her story by using open-ended questions like "How can I help you today?"

- Dressing professionally or in a way that is appropriate for the workplace

Communicating with *genuineness* means that the provider is "being real" and showing true interest in the patient. Genuineness means that it is okay to laugh with patients, to show concern, or, if a patient has experienced loss, to express sadness.

Often patients complain of not being understood by their health care providers. They want their providers to understand them and to support them; that is, they want providers to show *empathy*. Empathy is more than feeling sorry for the patient. It is an appreciation, understanding, and acceptance of the patient's emotional state, his or her experiences and perspectives (American Academy on Communication in Healthcare, 2011; O'Toole, 2008; Roter & Hall, 2006). Empathy is an active process that shows the patient that the provider has been listening and understands the patient's experiences. By expressing empathy, a provider can gather information as well as build trust. There are many different ways to communicate empathy. The challenge, however, is learning how to communicate empathy that is genuine.

Most providers already have basic skills in showing empathy, but the demands of providing health care often require more developed skills (Barnard, Hughes, & St. James, 2001; Chonchinov, 2007; Roter & Hall, 2006). Providers ask patients about personal issues, and patients often talk about things they tell no one else, such as sexual problems, addictions, and anxieties. It takes not only learning empathy skills but also practice and experience to comfortably listen to patients' most personal stories.

To show empathy requires listening, remaining silent, and letting the patient talk. Being comfortable with silence is a valuable skill for a provider. Silence allows the importance of a verbal message to sink in. When the patient is silent, it might indicate that a message from the health care provider was powerful enough to raise strong emotions (Chi & Verghese, 2013).

Some providers feel uncomfortable with a patient's silence. With experience, it becomes easier to know when words of comfort or even a touch is helpful during a patient's silence (Chi & Verghese, 2013; Finch, 2006). See Figure 7.2 for guidance on different ways of responding to a patient's silence, depending on the reason for it.

Nonverbal Communication

Patients often show their feelings and concerns not with words but through *nonverbal communication or body language.* This way of communicating requires providers to carefully assess what remains unspoken. There are five types of body language between provider and patient:

1. Body posture
2. Facial expressions and eye contact
3. Hand and arm gestures
4. Body space
5. Touch

Although providers need to understand the body language of their patients, they also must keep in mind that each culture has its own rules about body language (The Joint Commission,

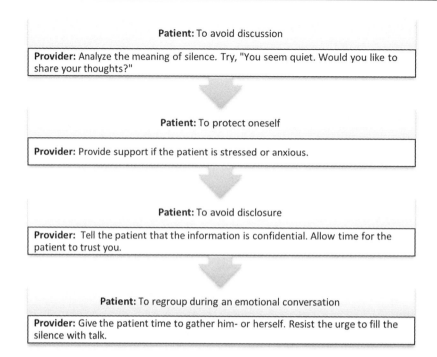

Figure 7.2   Health Care Provider Responses to a Patient's Silence

2010). In some cultures, for example, direct eye contact is considered disrespectful or even hostile. What may be acceptable body language in one culture can be offensive in another. If a provider is unsure about a patient's cultural background, then a simple approach is to just ask the patient.

Body posture shows how open a person feels toward another. A rigid posture by the provider shows reluctance to engage with the patient. The provider should appear interested in the patient and ready to listen, and use body posture that is engaging yet relaxed.

When a patient is receiving information, his or her *facial expressions* and *eye contact* express different emotional responses. The provider needs to observe whether these responses are appropriate to the information given to the patient. If the patient's responses are not in keeping with the information given, then the provider may need to change his or her words to ensure that the patient truly understands the information.

The patient's *hand and arm gestures* provide clues as to how the patient is feeling. Crossed arms and closed hands or laced fingers give the message that the patient might be reluctant to talk. He or she can feel angry or scared or threatened. Providers can also give messages to patients with their hand and arm gestures. Open hands and arms show patients openness, honesty, and willingness to engage with them.

Body space, sometimes referred to as personal space, has to do with what a person considers a comfortable distance from another. This distance varies not only by culture but also by the type of relationship. Social distance is considered to be about 4 to 12 feet between people and is used in conversations between friends or in the workplace.

Each patient is unique, however, and each has different body space requirements. An anxious patient might need more space to feel comfortable, whereas patients who are in pain might need the provider to be closer. Each provider-patient situation requires ongoing body space adjustment to make the patient feel safe and comfortable (The Joint Commission, 2010; Sheldon, 2009). See Figure 7.3 for an illustration of body space distances.

Touch is the universal language of caring. Providers use touch in a variety of ways to communicate different messages to patients, such as showing interest and expressing care.

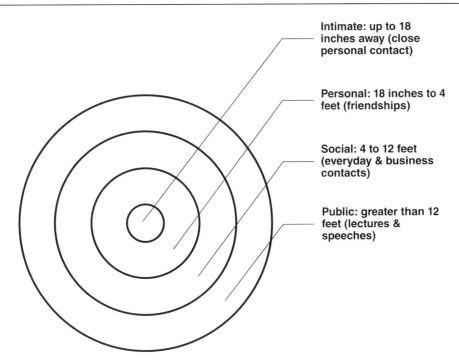

Figure 7.3 Body Space Distances

Touch is a powerful connecting tool, yet it can be easily misunderstood. A firm touch by a provider can be seen by the patient as controlling or hostile. It can also be seen as sexual by some patients. The meaning of the touch should be explained beforehand to avoid misunderstandings (Chi & Verghese, 2013; Finch, 2006; O'Toole, 2008; The Joint Commission, 2010). As a general rule, touching above the elbow, when not part of physical care, can be confusing to patients.

Active Listening

What a provider says should be consistent with his or her body language. Otherwise, the provider sends mixed messages. One way to prevent mixed messages is to use a technique known as active listening. *Active listening* is an interactive process between the provider and the patient: The provider involves the patient, hears and understands his or her message, and gives feedback about what was heard. Active listening requires the provider to observe the patient's verbal and nonverbal messages without judgment.

Instead of judging, the provider focuses on what the patient is saying and not saying. When providers use active listening, they get better information from their patients, save time, and solve problems. Table 7.1 describes ways that providers can use active listening.

Table 7.1 Active Listening for the Health Care Provider

Skill	Example
Concentrate and make an effort to focus on the patient speaking.	Listen without interrupting or offering explanations. Use body language that shows interest, such as nodding your head in agreement or eye contact.
Ask questions to be certain you understand the message correctly.	Summarize and paraphrase what you heard. Use the patient's words when you summarize. Ask for more details. Take notes; this helps with remembering what was said.
Help the patient feel at ease when speaking.	Use body language or words that encourage the patient to speak and contribute to the conversation.

There are barriers to active listening. Some are easily removed with a medical interpreter, but others are not so easily removed. Before starting a discussion, the provider needs to determine the patient's readiness to talk. If a patient has been recently diagnosed with cancer, for example, then talking about ways to get support services may be helpful. Talking about more complicated topics like long-term care should wait until later, when the patient is ready to hear detailed information. Offering information in chunks is better than bombarding the patient with information that he or she is not ready to hear.

A patient's anxiety can also create a barrier to active listening. The higher the patient's level of anxiety, the less information he or she can understand. The patient might try to use humor, silence, or sarcasm to avoid talking about subjects that make him or her anxious. Anxiety can also affect the provider's ability to engage in difficult conversations (Chi & Verghese, 2013; O'Toole, 2008; Sheldon, 2009). Although there may be no way to decrease anxiety in these situations, it is important to realize that listening can be inaccurate during these conversations. One solution is for providers to check in with one another to confirm what they believe they heard.

The Patient's Emotional Health

Being a patient is both a physical and emotional experience, one that continually demands adjustments to cope with the inherent stress of being a patient (Chapman, 2009: Chi & Verghese, 2013; Finch, 2006; O'Toole, 2008). The ability to recognize a patient's emotions and emotional health is an important part of a health care provider's communication skills, because understanding the patient's emotional state can lead to improved relationships and treatment outcomes (American Academy on Communications in Healthcare, 2011). For example, when a patient first hears his diagnosis, he might find it difficult to cope with the emotional stress. Struggling to cope with emotions can interfere with the patient's ability to understand or hear information. As a result, the patient becomes more upset and confused, and may not interact in ways that are helpful. This barrier to interaction is frustrating for both the patient and the health care provider.

Living with a disease causes a patient to experience and express emotions in new ways (Finch, 2006; The Joint Commission, 2010). As part of the provider-patient relationship, there needs to be the understanding that each patient has a unique way of expressing emotions. But regardless of the emotion, the health care provider needs to see the patient as a human being—not just as a product of his or her disease (Chonchinov, 2007).

One way to view an emotion is to see it as a flow of energy that changes a person's relationships with self and others (Tomm, 1995). With this view in mind, an emotion is seen as an energy field. For example, we can often feel someone else's anger or sadness. How we choose to release that emotional energy determines how we are in the world—that is, how we are seen and how we interact.

There are five basic emotions that are part of who we are and are always with us: fear, anger, sorrow, joy, and compassion. When we are a patient, we experience these emotions in unique ways and spend a lot of time expressing them. These emotions are not to be judged; there is no right or wrong emotion. They come and go like clouds in the sky, and just as the sky cannot control the clouds, we cannot control emotions (Tomm, 1995). However, we can control how we express emotions.

Fear helps us survive, and how a patient chooses to respond to a diagnosis is often based on a sense of survival. The fight-or-flight response is rooted in fear. If a patient decides to fight and thus to follow the treatment plan, such a decision is usually based on the expectation of a positive outcome. A patient is more likely to follow her treatment plan as long as she believes there is a chance of a positive outcome—no matter how small. Patients will fight back against their disease if there is a benefit to fighting (Tomm, 1995).

Fear is a healthy response to a diagnosis. However, when fear becomes the dominant emotion, it becomes *maladaptive fear* and can turn into *paranoia*, excessive suspicion of others. Sometimes a patient experiences intense fear of dying, of being sick, or of being disabled. The fear can be so strong that such a patient can worry himself or herself into sickness or death.

Anger is related to fear. It helps a patient move from self-blame to placing responsibility on the causes of the disease (Tomm, 1995). It can mobilize a patient to action and to change. When the cause is revealed and anger is expressed in healthy ways, then the patient is less likely to be depressed.

When anger is expressed in negative ways, it is *destructive anger* and can spiral out of control. For example, a patient might be so angry that she acts hostile toward her health care providers. This type of anger interferes with the patient's treatment. A patient can instead have *constructive anger*, behaving in ways that lead to positive action and change (Tomm, 1995). For example, a patient can use her anger to her advantage by being her own health advocate.

Sadness is the third emotion that patients commonly experience. Embracing sadness is accepting one's vulnerability. Sadness means opening up to loss. Once a patient opens up to his loss of health, he can be more open to himself and to others (Tomm, 1995).

Embracing sadness depends on support from others. A function of sadness is to be open to support and to offer support (Tomm, 1995). When patients actively seek support from others, they can support others in similar situations. For example, support groups for patients with chronic diseases are often an essential part of their treatment plan. Support groups help patients cope with the physical and emotional burdens of their chronic disease.

A patient also experiences *joy.* Joy enables a patient to see with new eyes after being released from fear, anger, or sadness. When a person sees herself with new eyes, she also can listen in new ways. She can listen to new possibilities rather than limit herself to the role of a patient (Tomm, 1995). For example, it is not unusual for some patients who recover from a life-threatening disease to make major changes in their life. With feelings of joy, the possibilities can be endless. Having joy does not mean that fear, anger, or sadness go away; instead, joy allows these emotions to exist in relation to each other. Each emotion has its own time for expression.

Compassion is a healing emotion. Feeling compassion for others and oneself can help in the healing process. However, to feel compassion, a person has to love and forgive all his strengths and weaknesses. He celebrates his talents and yet forgives himself when he experiences challenges and defeats. In other words, compassion is an acceptance of self.

Compassion depends on our ability to be, love, know, and see in ways that are empty of judgment. It means being open to ourselves and the world around us. The calmness that comes from compassion encourages social engagement (Tomm, 1995). For example, at an Alcoholics Anonymous (AA) meeting, people in recovery experience the compassion of others who are open, supportive, nonjudgmental, and accepting; those struggling with addiction receive kindness and support from others, and thus feel less alone.

Difficult Situations in the Provider-Patient Relationship

Communication can be challenging in health care settings. Typically, the provider and the patient are strangers, the situation is stressful, and the risks can be high. Provider-patient communications are often complex and need to be completed quickly. When the provider and the patient are unable to speak to, listen to, or understand each other, what begins as difficult can quickly become impossible (American Academy on Communications in Healthcare, 2011; Chapman, 2009).

When situations become difficult, providers tend to blame patients, and patients tend to blame providers (Platt & Gordon, 2004; Roter & Hall, 2006). Often, both can be correct. Whether it is the provider or the patient who contributes to the difficulty, it is the provider who has the most influence in improving the situation. It is better for the provider to focus on improving the situation instead of trying to change the patient (American Academy on Communications in Healthcare, 2011).

The first opportunity to manage a difficult situation arises when the provider interviews the patient. One strategy is to offer brief explanations as part of the interview, using such statements as "If I could know a little about your life, it would help me ask the right questions." In addition to gathering patient information, the provider can assess the patient's expectations of the provider and the services. The interview can also give clues as to the patient's willingness to comply with his or her treatment plan.

Working together as partners is more likely to succeed when the provider and the patient understand each other's expectations. To understand a patient's expectations, the provider can ask the following interview questions:

- "What do you think are realistic goals in managing your illness?"
- "What do you think of the treatment plan?"
- "Will you take your medicines as directed?"

Many types of difficult situations occur in health care settings. In this chapter, discussion of difficult situations is limited to delivering bad news, working with noncompliant patients, and working with patients who experience somatization. There is also a discussion of patients who are communication-vulnerable.

Delivering Bad News

Timing is important when delivering bad news to a patient. For purposes of this chapter, *bad news* is any medical news that drastically and negatively changes the patient's view of his or her future.

When the provider delivers bad news, the goal is to do so in a compassionate yet direct way that helps the patient. Before meeting with the patient, the provider needs to think about what to say and have all the necessary information available. There also needs to be enough time to communicate the information and for the patient to react.

The next step is for the provider to deliver the bad news with sensitivity and care. The information also needs to be:

- *Objective.* Do not jump to conclusions about how the patient will react.
- *Precise.* The information should be detailed, clear, to the point, and stated using simple language.
- *Accurate.* The information should be based on the most current research.

See Table 7.2 for examples of language to use when delivering bad news to a patient.

Not all patients react the same way when they hear bad news. Some will react as if they are in shock. Others will react in mixed ways: Anger, sorrow, denial, blame, disbelief, and guilt all are common

Table 7.2   The Language of Bad News

Delivering Bad News (Accurate)	Responding to Patient Reactions (Objective)	Dealing with the Prognosis (Precise)
"I'm afraid the news is not good. The biopsy showed you have colon cancer."	"I imagine this is difficult news."	"What are you expecting to happen?"
"Unfortunately, there is no question about the results. You have emphysema."	"I wish the news were different."	"What would you like to have happen?"
"I have the report, and it's not as we had hoped. It confirms that you have dementia."	"Is there anyone you'd like me to call?"	"How specific would you like me to be?"
"It looks like you have tested positive for HIV. I know this must be difficult for you to hear."	"Does this news frighten you?"	"What are your fears about what might happen?"

reactions. The provider should give the patient enough time and privacy to react. In follow-up conversations, the patient may want to talk again about the bad news and need additional support. When a patient receives bad news, the provider's support is important particularly if there is uncertainty about treatment (Chonchinov, 2007).

Noncompliant Patients

Providers expect patients to cooperate and follow their treatment plan. When patients do not cooperate and do not follow their treatment plan, then they are known as *noncompliant*. In truth, many patients do not comply with or follow their treatment plan. The average compliance to prescribed medications varies from 30% to 70% (Viswanathan et al., 2012). When providers advise patients on behavior changes, such as to stop smoking, they are even less successful with patients' compliance. Noncompliant patients not only put their own health at risk but also are a financial burden to our health care system. According to Viswanathan et al. (2012), the cost of noncompliance is between $100 billion and $289 billion annually in the United States.

There is no way to predict whether a particular patient will be compliant or noncompliant. Instead, the predictors have more to do with the quality of the provider-patient relationship (Viswanathan et al., 2012):

- Provider's failure to explain well
- Patient's failure to understand what the provider said
- Written materials that are beyond the patient's reading level
- Patient's lack of belief in his or her provider or treatment plan

One explanation for noncompliance is that many patients choose to follow their own treatment plan. In these cases, it is up to the provider to understand the patient's view of the diagnosis, its cause, and treatment. The provider should ask questions that lead to a better understanding of why the patient is noncompliant with the treatment plan. Once the provider begins the conversation on why there is noncompliance, then he or she can ask the patient about ways the two of them can work together for better results. The provider can try to address the noncompliance by changing the treatment plan with the patient's help, making sure that the patient understands by asking him or her to state the new agreed-on treatment plan (American Academy on Communication in Healthcare, 2011).

Somatization

Some patients have symptoms but do not have a diagnosis. Their physical examinations and laboratory tests do not show a cause for their symptoms. These patients are experiencing what is known as *somatization*. Patients with somatization believe that there is something wrong physically, and they keep coming back for more health care services. Meanwhile, the provider cannot find anything wrong. These patients may have a psychiatric disorder and express it as physical symptoms that drive them to seek more health care services. To summarize, the three characteristics of patients with somatization are (a) undiagnosed physical symptoms, (b) a psychiatric disorder that the patient does not recognize, and (c) high usage of health care services.

For both the provider and the patient, the central issue in somatization is the stress caused by lack of a diagnosis. The key in treating a patient with somatization is attention to and relief of his suffering, regardless of his diagnosis. The provider's efforts to understand the patient's suffering means better care for the patient. It is important to recognize and respect a patient's suffering even if there is no evidence to support a medical diagnosis.

Special Considerations for Patients Who Are Communication-Vulnerable

Patients have the right to know about the health care they receive, to make decisions about the care, and to be listened to by their providers. But sometimes providers find it difficult to inform certain patients, especially those who have difficulty with communication. *Communication-vulnerable* patients need assistance with communication (The Joint Commission, n.d.). Examples of communication-vulnerable patients are those who:

- Have a physical issue and have difficulty speaking, hearing, or seeing

- Have a psychiatric disorder such as schizophrenia or autism

- Are age 65 and older

- Are in an emergency situation and can't communicate

Providing health care to a patient who is communication-vulnerable can be a challenge. According to The Joint Commission (n.d.), communication-vulnerable patients are at risk for decreased access to medical care and higher rates of drug complications and hospitalization. They are also more likely to leave the hospital against medical advice (American Academy on Communication in Healthcare, 2011; Finke, Light, & Kitko, 2008).

Patients with Speech and Writing Difficulty

A patient's speech and writing difficulty can be caused by a disease, such as multiple sclerosis or cerebral palsy, an injury, or a surgical procedure. There are methods known as *augmentative and alternative communication* (AAC) that improve communication with such patients. AAC includes signing and gesture, picture or letter charts, electronic devices with speech output, and computer technology. These methods can help patients understand what is said and communicate with their provider.

Conversations with patients who have speech difficulties take longer, both because the provider needs to ask questions slowly and because the patient needs more time to answer. The provider needs to look at the patient directly to gain more information. If the provider does not understand what the patient is saying, the provider should ask the patient to repeat what he or she said or, if possible, to write it down. If all else fails, the provider needs to ask a relative or caregiver to interpret.

Sensory Impairments

Some communication-vulnerable patients have *sensory impairments*, such as hearing and/or vision loss. According to the National Center for Health Statistics (2010), sensory impairments are a substantial problem for older Americans: One out of four has impaired hearing, and one out of six has impaired vision. For those with hearing problems, 72% might benefit from a hearing aid, but do not use one. Over half of those with impaired vision could improve their eyesight by using glasses or by getting a corrected prescription. There are skills that make it easier to communicate with a patient who has hearing loss:

- Ask if the patient uses a hearing aid

- Talk slowly and clearly in a normal tone—do not shout or yell

- Face the person directly so that he or she can lip-read or pick up other visual clues

Visual impairments are limitations in one or more functions; the most common ones affect the sharpness of vision, the distance a person can see, and color. There are skills that make it easier to communicate with a patient who has visual impairments (Finke, Light, & Kitko, 2008):

+ Check to see if the patient has and wears eyeglasses

+ Make sure that handwritten instructions are clear

+ Ensure that any printed materials have large, easy-to-read type

+ Use pictures if the patient has trouble reading words

Cognitive Impairment

A person is said to have a *cognitive impairment* when he or she has difficulty concentrating, learning new things, making decisions, or remembering. Severe stress, medications, a mental health disorder, or a disability that affects cognition (e.g., dementia or autism) can cause cognitive impairment.

The following are the most common reasons why patients have cognitive impairments:

1. *Delirium*, a disorder of thinking and memory

2. *Dementia*, a loss of brain function that occurs with certain diseases and can affect memory, thinking, language, judgment, and behavior

3. Stroke, trauma, and congenital defects that produce brain defects

The challenge for providers in working with patients with cognitive impairment is that many of these patients do not know where they are and can't remember people, places, or events. Their stories are often confusing, leading to incomplete information, and they are often unable to follow treatment plans.

Patients with cognitive impairment also experience behavioral changes; for example, they may lose interest in previously enjoyable activities. They can be irritable and insensitive to other people's feelings. During more advanced stages of cognitive impairment, patients' behavior may change, and they may even kick, hit, or scream.

Some older patients may develop *mild cognitive impairment (MCI)*. People with MCI have ongoing memory problems, but do not have the confusion associated with dementia. Some patients' MCI may not progress, whereas others' MCI may progress to Alzheimer's disease. The following list outlines communication skills for providers to use with a cognitively impaired patient.

Provider Communication Skills for Cognitively Impaired Patients

Talk to the patient directly.

Get the patient's attention and keep eye contact.

Speak clearly at a natural speed—do not speak loudly or shout.

Use simple words when possible.

Say one question or statement at a time.

Explain who you are and what you will be doing.

If the patient hears you but does not understand you, reword your statements.

Have a family member or caregiver present if needed.

Show support and understanding to the patient.

Use a yes-or-no format for your questions.

Make it clear that you are not giving a "test"—you are searching for information to help the patient.

A health care provider can screen a patient for cognitive impairment. The most commonly used cognitive impairment screening test is the Mini-Mental State Examination (MMSE). A positive result suggests the need for referral to a neurologist or neuropsychologist for a more detailed diagnosis. There are limitations to any cognitive impairment screening test, however, because results may reflect the patient's education level instead of a health problem.

Patient's Bill of Rights

An important part of effective communication is for patients to know they have certain rights, guaranteed by federal laws. The US Advisory Commission on Consumer Protection and Quality in the Health Care Industry created the first nationally recognized Patient's Bill of Rights in 1998. In 2010, a new Patient's Bill of Rights was created along with the Affordable Care Act, and there are eight principle areas of rights and responsibilities (US Office of Personnel Management, n.d.):

1. Patients have the right to accurate and easily understood information about their health plan, health care providers, and health care settings. If a patient speaks another language, has a physical or mental disability, or just does not understand something, help should be given so that he or she can make informed health care decisions.

2. Patients have the right to choose health care providers who can give quality health care when needed.

3. If a patient has severe pain, an injury, or sudden illness that he believes puts his health in danger, he has the right to be screened and stabilized using emergency services. A patient should be able to use these services without needing to wait for authorization and without any financial penalty.

4. A patient has the right to know her treatment options and take part in decisions about her care. This right is known as *informed consent*.

5. Patients have a right to considerate, respectful care from their health care providers and to care that does not discriminate against the patient.

6. A patient has the right to confidentiality. *Confidentiality* is the principle that a patient must be able to talk privately with his health care providers and have his health care information protected. Patients also have the right to read and copy their own medical record. They have the right to ask that their physician change their record if it is not correct, relevant, or complete.

7. Patients have the right to a fair, fast, and objective review of any complaint they have against their health care provider and health plan.

8. In a health care system that protects patients' rights, patients are expected to take some responsibility to get well and/or stay well (for instance, by not using tobacco products). Patients are expected to treat health care providers and other patients with respect, try to pay their medical bills, and follow the rules and benefits of their health plan coverage.

Two areas in the 2010 Patient's Bill of Rights, informed consent and confidentiality, have legal importance for providers and their patients (American Cancer Society, 2011). Patients can give informed consent only when they understand how their disease will be treated, agree to the treatment plan, understand the risks, are aware of other treatment options available to them, and know what can happen if they refuse treatment.

After the provider informs the patient and the patient agrees to the treatment, the patient signs a legal agreement form stating that he or she understands and agrees to the treatment. In giving his or her informed consent, the patient expects that the provider's primary concern is the patient's health, well-being, and safety.

Providers have a legal responsibility to provide patients with all the information they need to make decisions (American Cancer Society, 2011). Providers are also legally required to give information about potential consequences the patient may experience by participating in the treatment.

The protection of a patient's confidentiality or personal information is also a legal right. Exposing a patient's confidential health information is a breach of his or her trust and violates professional standards established in the standards from the Health Insurance Portability and Accountability Act of 1996 (HIPAA). *HIPAA* requires most physicians, nurses, hospitals, nursing homes, and other health care providers to protect the privacy of a patient's confidential health information. Only information that is important to the patient's treatment is shared with other providers.

HIPAA forbids providers from disclosing a patient's confidential health information, except in specific situations. One type of situation arises when there could be harm to innocent people, including patient self-harm. These situations include instances of child or elder abuse, gunshot wounds, an admission of a crime, and communicable diseases. The provider is legally required to share this information with the appropriate authorities, such as police, protective services, and departments of public health.

Another legal exception for sharing patients' confidential health information is when the patient is unconscious or cannot give permission. The provider may share the health information of unconscious patients with family or others involved in their care. The provider can do this only if he or she believes that it is in the patient's best interest.

Medical Errors

As part of the Patient's Bill of Rights, health care providers need to protect their patients from medical errors. *Medical errors* occur when something that was planned doesn't work out or when the wrong plan was used in the first place. This might include an inaccurate diagnosis or treatment. Medical errors can occur in any health care setting as well as in a patient's home. Errors can involve medicines, surgery, diagnosis, equipment, or lab reports.

Medical errors are a serious problem in US health care settings. According to research conducted over a 10-year span by the Agency for Healthcare Research and Quality (2009), an estimated 48,000 to 100,000 patients die each year as a result of medical errors. According to researchers Makary and Daniel's (2016) study, deaths resulting from medical errors are the third leading cause of mortality in the United States, ranking just behind heart disease and cancer. Medical errors that can lead to death range from surgical problems that go undetected to wrong doses or types of medications that patients receive.

The best way for a provider to prevent errors and improve quality of patient care is to encourage patients to be active participants in their health care (Kohn, Corrigan, & Donaldson, 2000). When a medical error happens, patients need their providers to:

- *Admit to the error and be honest in describing its implications.* Patients have a legal right to full disclosure of errors. Providers, however, need to check with their employer's policy on disclosing medical errors. Admitting an error can lead to a lawsuit.

- *Apologize.* Patients want their providers to take responsibility for the error. An apology can go a long way toward addressing a patient's anger.

- *Give evidence* that steps are being taken to prevent such an error in the future.

There is a difference between injury or death caused by errors made by providers, on the one hand, and unfortunate results of treatment, on the other. Some allergic reactions to medications, for example, stem from physical differences among patients and not from prescribing the wrong drug to a patient. This type of negative outcome is referred to as an adverse event. *Adverse events* are not preventable. They are undesirable and unintentional, though not necessarily unexpected, results of medical treatment (Classen et al., 2011; Kohn et al., 2000).

In contrast, a medical error can be prevented given the current state of medical knowledge. A medical error happens when a provider chooses an incorrect method of care or chooses the right method of care but performs the method incorrectly.

Chapter Summary

- When working with patients, a health care provider needs skills in listening, hearing, speaking, nonverbal communication or body language, and behaving professionally at all times.

- Effective communication is an essential part of the provider-patient relationship. To be effective, communication is a two-way process in which messages are negotiated until both parties correctly understand.

- There are three essential ingredients in communicating with patients: respect, genuineness, and empathy.

- The more that patients are engaged in their health care, the better their health outcomes. It takes specific skills, however, to engage and communicate with certain patients.

- Part of effective communication is that patients know they have certain rights. Federal laws guarantee certain rights of patients.

- A medical error is one that could be prevented given the current state of medical knowledge. An adverse event is an undesirable and unintentional, though not necessarily unexpected, result from a medical treatment.

REVIEW QUESTIONS

1. Explain the five types of body language between provider and patient. What are some strategies a provider can use to improve nonverbal communications?

2. How can a provider communicate with respect, genuineness, and empathy during a provider-patient interaction?

3. Describe active listening.

4. Why is it important for a provider to know the emotional health of their patients? Explain the five basic emotions that a patient may experience.

5. What are examples of a health care provider's responses to a patient's silence?

6. What are the three characteristics of somatization?

7. Identify steps to take when delivering bad news.

8. What types of patients are communication-vulnerable?

9. What is the difference between maladaptive fear and paranoia? Between destructive anger and constructive anger?

10. What is the difference between a medical error and an adverse event?

KEY TERMS

Active listening: Listening through which the health care provider involves the patient, hears and understands his or her message, and gives feedback about what was heard

Adverse event: An undesirable and unintentional, though not necessarily unexpected, result of medical treatment

Augmentative and alternative communication: Communication aids or devices

Bad news: News that drastically and negatively changes the patient's view of his or her future

Cognitive impairment: In the case of patients, difficulty concentrating, learning new things, making decisions, or remembering, due to severe stress, cognitive disabilities, psychiatric disorders, or medications

Communication: The process of relating to and interacting with other people

Communication-vulnerable patients: Patients who need assistance in communication

Confidentiality: The principle that a patient must be able to talk privately with his health care providers and have his health care information protected

Constructive anger: Anger that stimulates the person to behave in ways that lead to positive action and change

Delirium: A disorder of thinking and memory

Dementia: A loss of brain function that happens with certain diseases and can affect memory, thinking, language, judgment, and behavior

Destructive anger: Anger that is expressed in negative ways

HIPAA: Government standards that require most physicians, nurses, hospitals, nursing homes, and other health care providers to protect the privacy of a patient's confidential health information

Informed consent: Patient's permission to be put on a treatment plan and to be given treatment, based on his or her knowledge and understanding of all relevant information, which is required by law to be supplied in writing

Maladaptive fear: Fear that becomes the main emotion a person experiences and that is no longer healthy

Medical error: Something planned as a part of health care services that doesn't work out, or use of the wrong plan

Mild cognitive impairment (MCI): Ongoing memory problems, but not the confusion associated with dementia

Noncompliant: Describes a patient who does not follow his or her treatment plan

Nonverbal communication or body language: Communication of information without using words

Paranoia: Excessive suspicion of others

Sensory impairments: Hearing loss and/or vision loss that affects communication

Somatization: A condition that exists when a patient has symptoms but does not have a diagnosis

CHAPTER ACTIVITIES

1. Form groups of three: One student is the provider, one is the patient, and the third is the observer/recorder. Using simple instructions, the provider will teach the patient a series of exercise routines or a daily activity, such as correctly brushing teeth. The patient requires special considerations as a communication-vulnerable person. The trio decides on the communication need. Once the 5–10-minute instruction begins, the observer/recorder writes down what he or she sees and hears. Upon completion of the activity, the observer/recorder gives feedback to the provider and patient.

2. This is an activity done with a partner. Choose one of the following role-playing situations. Each partner will choose whether he or she will use effective or poor listening skills. Act out the scenario. Discuss the scenario with each other.

    a. One of your coworkers is complaining about another coworker's always showing up late and being lazy on the job. Your coworker is concerned about having to work extra hard to prevent medical errors caused by the other coworker. He is very frustrated and angry, and wants to yell at the coworker for his or her lazy work habits.

    b. You are working with a diabetic patient who is not compliant with his or her treatment plan. Your task is to talk to the patient about ways to be more compliant with the treatment plan.

3. Health care providers encourage dialogue by asking open-ended questions that require more than simply a yes or no. These questions offer the patient an opportunity to disclose problems more freely. Examples of open-ended questions about a patient's health complaint are "What can you tell me about when you first noticed your symptoms?" "How are you feeling right now?" "What are your concerns about having this disease?" An example of a closed-ended question is "When did the symptoms start?" Many health care providers fear that asking open-ended questions takes too much time. However, when used correctly, these questions can save time and improve efficiency by uncovering important information early in the patient-provider relationship. Create a patient case study and the open-ended questions you would ask as their provider.

4. Brainstorm five different examples each of medical errors and adverse events.

5. In pairs, create a "problem tree" that identifies barriers to communicating with communication-vulnerable patients. On one side of the tree, identify the barriers; on the other side of the tree, identify possible strategies.

Bibliography and Works Cited

Agency for Healthcare Research and Quality. (2009). *Advancing patient safety: A decade of evidence, design, and implementation.* Retrieved from http://www.ahrq.gov/professionals/quality-patient-safety/patient-safety-resources/resources/advancing-patient-safety/advancing-patient-safety.pdf

American Academy on Communication in Healthcare. (2011). *Improving healthcare communications: Build the relationship.* Retrieved from http://www.aachonline.org

American Cancer Society. (2011). *Patient's bill of rights.* Retrieved from http://www.cancer.org/Treatment/FindingandPayingforTreatment/UnderstandingFinancialandLegalMatters/patients-bill-of-rights

Barnard, S. R., Hughes, K. T., & St. James, D. (2001). *Writing, speaking, and communication skills for health professionals.* New Haven, CT: Yale University Press.

Berthold, T., Miller, J., & Avila-Esparza, A. (2009). *Foundations for community health workers.* San Francisco, CA: Jossey-Bass.

Chapman, B.K.B. (2009). Improving communication among nurses, patients, and physicians. *American Journal of Nursing, 109*(11), 21–25.

Chi, J., & Verghese, A. (2013). Improving communication with patients: Learning by doing. *Journal of the American Medical Association, 310,* 2257–2258.

Chonchinov, H. (2007). Dignity and the essence of medicine: The A, B, C, and D of dignity conserving care. *British Medical Journal, 335*(7612), 184–187.

Classen, D. C., Resar, R., Griffin, F., Federico, F., Frankel, T., Kimmel, N., . . . James, B. C. (2011). "Global trigger tool" shows that adverse events in hospitals may be ten times greater than previously measured. *Health Affairs, 30,* 581–589. Retrieved from http://content.healthaffairs.org/content/30/4/581.short

Dillon, C. F., Gu, Q., Hoffman H., & Ko, C. W. (2010). Vision, hearing, balance, and sensory impairment in Americans aged 70 years and over: United States, 1999–2006. NCHS Data Brief No. 31. Hyattsville, MD: National Center for Health Statistics.

Finch, L. P. (2006). Patients' communication with nurses: Relational communication and preferred nurse behaviors. *International Journal for Human Caring.* Retrieved from http://search.ebscohost.com/login.aspx?direct=true&db=psyh&AN=2008-02723–003&login.asp&site=ehost-live\nlfinch@menphis.edu

Finke, E. H., Light, J., & Kitko, L. (2008). A systematic review of the effectiveness of nurse communication with patients with complex communication needs with a focus on the use of augmentative and alternative communication. *Journal of Clinical Nursing, 17,* 2102–2115.

The Joint Commission. (n.d.). Call to action: Improving care to communication vulnerable patients. Retrieved from http://www.patientprovidercommunication.org/files/CommunicationVulnerableWebinar.pdf

The Joint Commission. (2010). *Advancing effective communication, cultural competence, and patient- and family-centered care: A roadmap for hospitals.* Oakbrook Terrace, IL: Author.

Kleinsinger, F. (2010). Working with the noncompliant patient. *Permanente Journal, 14*(1), 54–60.

Kohn, L.T.E., Corrigan, J.M.E., & Donaldson, M.S.E. (Eds.). (1999). To err is human: Building a safer health system. Retrieved from https://www.ncbi.nlm.nih.gov/pubmed/25077248

Makary, M. A., & Daniel, M. (2016). Medical error—the third leading cause of death in the US. *BMJ, 353*, i2139. doi: http://dx.doi.org/10.1136/bmj.i2139

O'Toole, G. (2008). *Communication: Core interpersonal skills for health professionals.* Chatswood, NSW, Australia: Elsevier.

Pauker, S. G., Zane, E. M., & Salem, D. N. (2005). Creating a safer health care system: Finding the constraint. *Journal of the American Medical Association, 294*, 2906–2908. Retrieved from http://www.innoqare.com/wp-content/uploads/Publicatie+creating+a+safer+healthcare.pdf

Platt, F. W., & Gordon, G. H. (2004). *Field guide to the difficult patient interview.* Philadelphia, PA: Lippincott Willliams & Wilkins.

Roter, D. L., & Hall, J. A. (2006). *Doctors talking with patients/patients talking with doctors: Improving communication in medical visits* (2nd ed.). Westport, CT: Praeger.

Sheldon, L. K. (2009). *Communication for nurses* (2nd ed.). Sudbury, MA: Jones and Bartlett.

Tomm, W. (1995). *Bodied mindfulness: Women's spirits, bodies and places.* Waterloo, ON, Canada: Wilfrid Laurier University Press.

US Office of Personnel Management. (n.d.). Patients' bill of rights. Retrieved from https://www.opm.gov/healthcare-insurance/healthcare/reference-materials/#url=Bill-of-Rights

Viswanathan M., Golin, C. E., Jones, C. D., Ashok, M., Blalock, S. J., Wines, R. C., . . . Lohr, K. N. (2012, December). Interventions to improve adherence to self-administered medications for chronic diseases in the United States: A systematic review. *Annals of Internal Medicine, 157*, 785–795. doi:10.7326/0003-4819-157-11-201212040-00538

World Health Organization. (2005). What is a health system? Retrieved from http://www.who.int/features/qa/28/en/

CHAPTER 8

PATIENT NAVIGATORS AND PATIENT SELF-ADVOCACY

CHAPTER OBJECTIVES

- Identify the function and skills of patient navigators.

- Explain how patient navigators access quality health care.

- Discuss the importance for health care providers to set boundaries with patients.

- Compare and contrast complementary, alternative, and integrative medicine.

- Identify ways patients can self-advocate for quality health care.

- Explain advance directives and their importance to patient care.

This chapter covers two areas related to patient-centered health care: patient navigation and the role of patient navigators, and patient self-advocacy. It begins with an overview of patient navigation. There is a discussion of the functions and skills of patient navigators, as well as of how they improve health care services for patients. Also included in this section is an explanation of how patient navigators and other health care providers can set professional boundaries with patients.

The second part of the chapter identifies ways that patients can self-advocate for quality health care. It also includes a general overview of complementary, alternative, and integrative medicine because many patients use these practices as part of their treatment plan. Finally, the chapter discusses advance directives and their importance to patient autonomy.

What Are Patient Navigators?

In a perfect world, there are no barriers to health care. No patient goes untreated or experiences delays. But this is not a perfect world, and, unfortunately, barriers do prevent patients from getting the health care they need.

Table 8.1   Health Care Barriers

Types of Barriers	Specific Barriers to Care	Solutions to Barriers
Financial or economic	Lack or inadequate insurance Inability to afford medication or health care	Guide patients to sources of financial support Answer questions about financial forms and assistance
Education	Low level of health literacy Difficulty completing forms Anxiety about the patient's disease and health care	Help complete paperwork Explain the health care system Educate patients on diagnoses and medical procedures
Logistic	Child care or elder care responsibilities Conflicts between appointments and work schedules	Help with arranging child care or elder care
Transportation	Lack of access to public transportation Difficulty arranging transportation	Help patients find resources for transportation
Language and culture	Cultural beliefs about US health care Difficulty speaking or reading English	Help patients access culturally appropriate care Direct patients to language interpretation services
Health care system	Lack of coordination among services Unavailability of care information when needed	Coordinate appointments for diagnostic and treatment services Make sure that medical records arrive at scheduled appointments
Emotional	Mental health issues in dealing with their disease	Direct patients to support groups or counseling services

Health care barriers are any nonmedical situations that make getting a diagnosis or treatment difficult (Freeman, 2001; Freund, 2011; McGlynn et al., 2003). The following are examples of health care barriers:

Income Low-income populations have higher morbidity and mortality rates than those of higher-income populations.

Language difficulties or cultural differences Patients who have language difficulties or cultural differences are at higher risk for not getting health care they need.

Provider-centered health care Health care should be centered on the patient, not on health care providers. Unfortunately, many patients experience *provider-centered care*: Health care is offered at the convenience of providers. For example, when health care providers do not communicate with each other because it is inconvenient, patients can experience delays in treatment. In *patient-centered care*, patients receive emotional, administrative, and educational support in managing their disease. This type of care improves patients' health outcomes.

Geographic barriers Some places, such as rural and inner-city areas, have shortages of health care providers. These shortages result in limited options in accessing health care services.

For a more detailed explanation of types of health care barriers and possible solutions, see Table 8.1.

Health care barriers create problems because they cause patients to avoid care, delay treatment, and miss appointments. Delays in care make diseases more difficult to manage and lower a patient's chances of getting well. The Commonwealth Fund (Stremikis, Schoen, Fryer, & the Commonwealth Fund, 2011) found that more than half of adult patients experience poorly organized health care (see Figure 8.1).

There is a critical three-part time period to save lives from most chronic diseases: from the time when there is a positive finding, to getting the diagnosis, and then receiving the follow-up treatment.

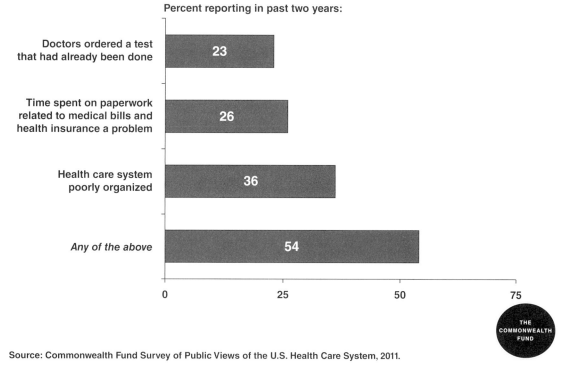

Figure 8.1   Potential Waste and Inefficiency in US Health Care

Note. From "A Call for Change: The 2011 Commonwealth Fund Survey of Public Views of the U.S. Health System," by K. Stremikis, C. Schoen, A. K. Fryer, and the Commonwealth Fund, 2011. Retrieved from http://www.commonwealthfund.org/~/media/Files/Publications/Issue%20Brief /2011/Apr/1492_Stremikis_public_views_2011_survey_ib.pdf

During this three-part time period, patients can experience barriers that cause a delay in their health care. As already noted, the delay can be dangerous for patients because it puts their chances of getting well at risk and makes their treatment difficult.

To address this problem of delay in health care, a new specialty has emerged: the patient navigator. *Patient navigators (PNs)* assist patients who are coping with chronic diseases, particularly those that require complex testing and treatment, as in the case of cancer. They navigate patients through the health care system, support them in the management of their disease, and help them overcome barriers to care. PNs help patients get what they need from a health care system that may otherwise make them feel powerless (Risendal, Valverde, Calhoun, Esparza, & Whitley, 2009).

Patient navigation is unique to the US health care system, and it is based on the concept that there is power in people helping people. With help from a PN, a patient is more likely to learn how to navigate and advocate for himself or herself. PNs build relationships, solve problems, advocate, and offer support to patients (University of Colorado Cancer Center, 2011). They also help patients understand the importance of timely diagnosis and treatment.

The Function of Patient Navigators

There are at least seven problems that patients encounter when seeking health care (Jansson, 2011; Risendal et al., 2009). Patients often:

1. Cannot afford their medical care

2. Receive medical care that does not meet best practices

3. Experience violations of their rights, including insufficient or inaccurate information

4. Receive medical care that is not culturally appropriate

5. Receive insufficient preventive care for specific chronic diseases or ones linked to environmental factors

6. Have high levels of anxiety, depression, and other mental health conditions that remain unaddressed

7. Receive health care that often fails to link them with health-related programs and services in their communities

Patients often experience a combination of two or more of these problems. Some patients advocate for themselves and seek second opinions or fight for medical insurance coverage. But others need assistance, for many reasons—for example, they don't know how to access resources, they have a language barrier, or they fear negative consequences if they ask too many questions.

PNs help patients at two levels. First, they help patients access services that otherwise are not given to them. Second, they advocate for changing policies in their institutions and communities that create barriers to health care.

PNs do more than just point the way for patients, however. According to the University of Colorado Cancer Center's Patient Navigator Training Program (2011), they perform a broad range of functions, including the following:

-   Work with health care teams to coordinate patient care

-   Maintain communication between patients and their health care team

-   Connect patients with culturally appropriate resources

-   Monitor progress and provide outreach to noncompliant patients

-   Access health care insurance coverage and other financial aid

-   Promote and protect patients' health through health education, screening services, and clinical trials information

-   Identify and use community services

-   Support and guide patients to self-navigate and self-advocate

-   Conduct ongoing outreach to populations that experience barriers

Figure 8.2 details the demands of a day in the life of a PN.

There are different models of patient navigation. Some models focus on services, others focus on addressing a specific type of barrier, and still others focus on both services and barriers. Service-focused PNs help chronic care patients arrange financial support, transportation, and/or counseling. Other service-focused models do community outreach. They also enroll patients in clinical trials or build partnerships with local agencies to which patients can be referred. Barrier-focused PNs identify and try to remove barriers in a particular community. Examples of these activities are outreach, screenings, and advocacy for quality health care.

The PN's functions can sometimes overlap with the job responsibilities of other health care providers, such as nurses, social workers, health educators, psychologists, counselors, and community health workers. There is no set educational requirement to be a PN; PNs can have a degree in social work, nursing, or health education, for example, or they might not have a degree. Regardless of education level, the function of a PN is to guide chronic care patients through a complex health care system and provide services that reduce barriers to quality health care.

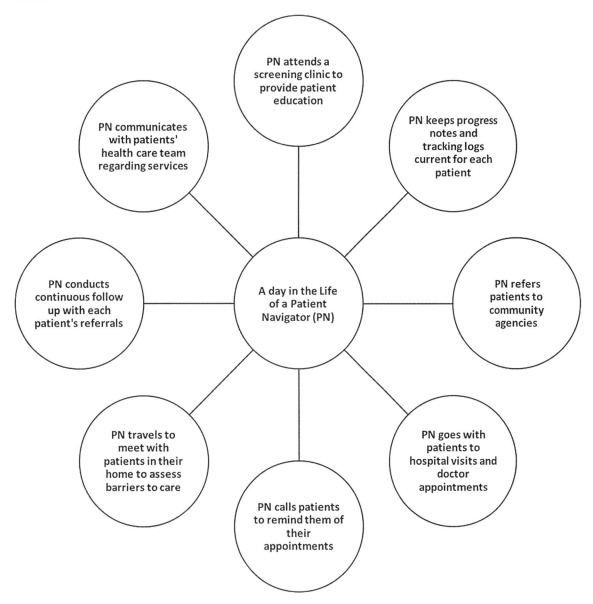

Figure 8.2 A Day in the Life of a Patient Navigator (PN)

Skills of Patient Navigators

Building trust with chronic care patients is critical to patient navigation. If patients do not trust their PN, they might not discuss concerns or accept help. There are three skills that PNs need to earn patients' trust (see Figure 8.3):

1. *Caring or empathy.* Coping with a chronic disease such as cancer can be a traumatic and overwhelming experience. It can also be complicated by a confusing health care system. PNs are trained to be caring, or to have empathy, which helps guide patients through a challenging time.

2. *Communication.* Building trust with patients requires effective communication, including being a good listener (see Chapter 7). A first step in establishing a patient's trust is to engage in a discussion that clearly explains the PN's functions and responsibilities, covers the topic of protection of the patient's privacy, and communicates the patient's expectations.

3. *Competence.* Being knowledgeable, prepared, and organized demonstrates that a PN is competent. To be more specific, PNs should have the following skills:

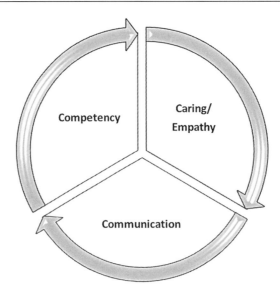

Figure 8.3 Patient Navigators and Patient's Trust

- Cultural competency with patients and the community where they live
- Knowledge of the system that patients must navigate
- Ability to connect with decision makers, especially insurance representatives
- Ability to maintain current chronic disease information for patients
- Ability to identify community resources

Patient Navigators and Health Care Teams

PNs work with health care teams to coordinate patients' care. Each team member has a unique role in diagnosing and treating the patient (see Figure 8.4). The following are some team members who work closely with chronic care patients:

- *Primary care physicians* oversee a patient's general health and his or her treatment.
- *Physician specialists* concentrate on diagnosing and treating specific diseases.
- *Nurses* are in charge of implementing the plan of care that the physician and the specialist have set up. They administer medications and monitor side effects.
- *Administrators,* such as clinic coordinators, case managers, and medical billing coordinators, coordinate and facilitate patient care.

PNs work with these team members and with those who offer additional support services to the patient, such as clergy, home health aides, psychologists, and social workers. PNs also work with individuals and community-based organizations. These can include transportation services, language translators, and insurance representatives.

Setting Professional Boundaries

PNs work closely with patients, develop their trust, and learn about their lives. This level of intimacy can lead to professional boundary issues. Patients may ask for help that is beyond the role of a PN. It then becomes necessary for the PN to set boundaries and clarify them for patients. *Professional boundaries* are ethical guidelines that a professional uses in relationships developed through work. The purpose of professional boundaries is to provide safety and structure for patients.

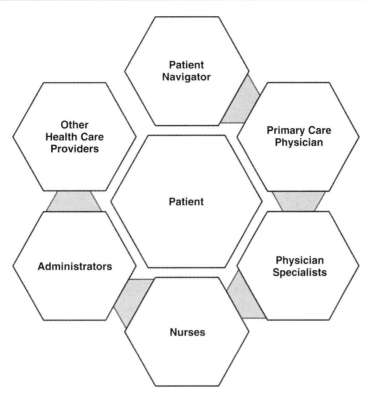

Figure 8.4 Patient Navigators and Health Care Team Members

As part of professional boundaries, a PN acts in the patient's best interests and respects his or her dignity. This means that a PN does not obtain personal gain at a patient's expense and does not have inappropriate involvement in a patient's life.

To set professional boundaries, a PN knows what the boundaries are and when they have been crossed. Setting professional boundaries and clarifying them with patients establish appropriate relationships.

Some PNs as well as other health care providers do violate boundaries. They use their power over patients to advance their own emotional, financial, sexual, or personal needs. Examples of danger zones in boundary violations are excessive personal disclosure, receiving gifts, inappropriate touch, and/or sexual relationships (HANYS Breast Cancer Demonstration Project, 2002; Risendal et al., 2009).

As a health care provider, the PN—not the patient—is ultimately responsible for managing boundary issues. The best time for a PN to set boundaries is at the beginning of the relationship with the patient. A way to determine if a boundary has been crossed with a patient is to review the following questions:

• Is what I am doing in the patient's best interest?

• How would this be viewed by the patient's family or loved ones?

• Am I taking advantage of the patient?

• Would I tell a coworker about my behavior?

Patient Autonomy

Once a person becomes ill and becomes a patient, his or her life changes. Being ill can feel strange, frightening, and out of control—the patient is in a crisis (Robert Wood Johnson Foundation, 2011; Walsh-Burke & Marcusen, 1999). Having an illness is a crisis on at least three levels (Freeman, 2001; Norcross, 2010). First, it is a biological crisis threatening the body, and can prevent a person from functioning. Second, it is a psychological crisis, stirring up strong feelings that challenge the patient emotionally and intellectually. Third, being ill is a social crisis because the person's identity is likely to be affected. That is, once the person is ill, family, friends, loved ones, and strangers treat him or her differently.

In the past, patients simply let their physicians make all their health decisions. However, the role of health care providers has shifted away from that of the expert who always knows best; providers now share the role of decision maker with their patients. This shift means that patients are educating themselves as best as they can about their disease and its treatment to make their own decisions, which is known as *patient autonomy*. Patient autonomy places patients' decisions at the heart of their health care.

Patient autonomy does have its challenges (Groopman, 2010; Norcross, 2010). With too much autonomy, patients can feel abandoned by their health care providers. They may be overwhelmed with the choices they need to make, and receive little guidance from their providers.

There is no one way to be a patient. Some patients want the more traditional approach: the provider explains little, chooses the treatment, and tells the patient what to do. Others want a provider who explains the disease, describes treatment options, answers questions, and then lets the patient make the decision. Still other patients want a partnership, working together with their provider as decisions are made throughout the treatment. Each patient needs to ask herself what she wants from her providers and what she wants to do. Does she as a patient want to choose by herself what is best, or does she want to share the responsibility with her provider?

Patient Self-Advocacy

Treatments for chronic diseases are complex and ongoing. Patients with chronic diseases can find it difficult to manage their treatment plans because there are different health care providers to work with, tests to take, and instructions to follow.

When a patient is receiving treatment, he needs to be proactive and to self-advocate. Self-advocacy is an ongoing process, from diagnosis through to treatment and finally to follow-up care. Being a self-advocate means that the patient takes an active role in his health care. The following are ways that health care providers can encourage self-advocacy in their patients:

- *Patients need to talk to their health care providers about what matters to them.* Patients should share what matters and the type of care they want. They should make a list of all the questions they want to ask, and write down the answers. If possible, they should take a friend, family member, or loved one with them to medical appointments. This person can listen, take notes, and help remember what was said. Patients also should consider seeking a second opinion about their diagnosis and treatment plan, which may help them feel more confident about their decisions.

- *Patients can learn about the best treatments for their disease.* Learning more helps in following the treatment plan and in knowing what questions to ask during appointments. Patients can learn more about chronic diseases from reliable websites, such as MedlinePlus and other government sites.

- *Patients need to take advantage of other services offered* at their physician's office, hospital, or clinic, such as counseling and support groups.

- *Patients need to make connections with others who are living with their chronic disease* and learn from the experiences of others.

- *If the patient has a physician whose communication style does not match theirs or they want a different approach for their care, they should find a new physician.* Regardless of whom the patient chooses, there should be one physician or health care provider to coordinate his or her treatment plan. With one physician or health care provider who knows about all of the treatment the patient is receiving, the patient is more likely to get what he or she needs and not receive unnecessary or harmful treatment.

- *Patients need to create lists of medical information.* Patients should list all medications that they take, including vitamins, herbal remedies, and over-the-counter drugs. They should also write down or record information during visits with their health care providers. Lists of their medical history, contact information, and insurance information also should be readily available.

- *Patients need to know the difference between more care and better care.* Sometimes, more care can do harm or create unnecessary risks.

See Table 8.2 for more examples of self-advocacy questions and tasks.

Self-advocacy doesn't have to be time-consuming or difficult; it can be as simple as just asking more questions. Being a self-advocate doesn't mean that the patient alone is responsible for his or her care. In fact, it commonly involves seeking additional support not only from others such as family and loved ones but also from nonprofit organizations and the federal government. For example, patients can access publicly available reports that provide consumer protection information on physicians, hospitals, and health plans. The federal government tracks and publishes information on the quality of hospitals, nursing homes, and physicians through www.healthcare.gov.

Complementary, Alternative, and Integrative Medicine

As part of exercising patient autonomy and self-advocacy, some patients seek a different kind of medical treatment from what is offered by their health care providers. Such medical treatments are not taught widely at US medical schools or are not generally available in US health care settings. These treatments are called *complementary and alternative medicine (CAM)*. Precisely defining CAM is difficult because the field is broad and constantly changing. The National Center for Complementary and Alternative Medicine (NCCAM, 2016) defines CAM as a group of diverse medical and health care systems, practices, and products that are not generally considered part of conventional medicine.

Conventional medicine (also called Western medicine) is medicine as practiced by MDs (medical doctors or physicians) and DOs (doctors of osteopathic medicine). It can also be practiced by other health care providers, such as physician assistants, psychologists, and registered nurses. *Complementary medicine* refers to use of CAM together with conventional medicine, such as using massage in addition to a physician's care to lessen back pain. *Alternative medicine* refers to use of CAM only and not using conventional medicine, such as using only massage to lessen back pain, without the care of a physician.

Integrative medicine combines treatments from conventional medicine and from CAM for which there is some scientific evidence of safety and effectiveness. An example of integrative medicine is drinking green tea because there is scientific evidence from laboratory studies that it may protect against the growth of certain cancers.

To understand the many different types of CAM practices, NCCAM (2016) has grouped them into broad categories: whole medical systems, natural products, mind and body medicine, energy fields, movement therapies, traditional healers, and manipulative and body-based practices (see Table 8.3). Keep in mind that the differences among practices aren't always clear, and some practices use techniques from more than one group.

Decisions about health care are important—including decisions about whether or not to use CAM health practices. The best way for a patient to self-advocate when choosing CAM health practices is to become informed—finding out and considering what scientific studies have been done on the safety

Table 8.2 Patients' Questions and Tasks for a Health Care Provider Appointment

Questions to Ask When Making the Appointment	Before the Appointment	During the Appointment	After the Appointment
What is the location of the office (including floor, room, or suite number)?	Write down your questions.	Speak up if you have questions or concerns; you have the right to question anyone involved in your care. Ask as many questions as you need in order to feel comfortable with the information. If you don't understand something, ask to have it explained again.	Try to keep all of your information in one place. Doing so will make it easier to find later.
Where should I park? (If you do not drive, ask about using public transportation.)	Have as much of your medical history written down as possible, including current medicines as well as diagnostic and treatment history.	Learn about your disease and treatment options by asking your health care provider and by using reliable sources.	Have one place in your home and/or office for those things you need regularly, such as prescription medications and contact information for providers, hospitals, and insurance companies.
What is the cancellation policy for appointments?	Bring someone with you. If you have permission, bring a tape recorder to tape the conversation between you and your health care provider(s).	When your physician or other health care provider writes you a prescription, make sure you can read and understand it. Make sure your physician or other health care provider knows about allergies and adverse reactions you have had to medicines. Ask for written information about the side effects your medicine could cause. Ask questions if you are not sure how to take your medicine.	When you pick up your medication from the pharmacy, ask: Is this the medicine that my physician or other health care provider prescribed?
What insurance plans does this office participate in?		Ask for educational material that might be available (books, pamphlets, tapes, and videos).	Keep copies of all insurance policies and refer to them by name and number in any communication with insurers. Keep a written record of conversations with insurance company representatives; include the date, name of the person you spoke with, and what was said.
As a new patient, do I need to arrive early to fill out forms?			If you have been diagnosed with a chronic disease that requires costly treatment, try to decide ahead of time how to adjust your budget to deal with loss of income or expenses that are not covered by insurance.
What does the physician or other health care provider expect me to bring when I come to my appointment?			
Can a family member or friend be present during the visit?			

Table 8.3   Examples of Complementary and Alternative Medicine (CAM) Practices

Whole Medical Systems	Natural Products	Mind and Body Medicine	Energy Fields	Movement Therapies	Traditional Healers	Manipulative and Body-Based Practices
Complete systems of healing theory and practice.	Herbal medicines, botanicals, vitamins, and other natural products.	Focus on the mind-body connection. The mind affects health.	Change energy fields to affect health.	Body movement improves health.	Healing methods based on cultural traditions.	Focus on the structures and systems of the body.
Chinese medicine, homeopathy	*Vitamin C, fish oil, green tea*	*Meditation, yoga*	*Healing touch, Reiki, qigong*	*Alexander Technique, Pilates*	*Medicine man or woman, shaman*	*Massage, spinal manipulation*

and effectiveness of the health practice in question. The following are other strategies patients can use in selecting a CAM health practice:

- Discuss the information with their health care providers before making a decision.

- Choose a complementary health care provider, such as an acupuncturist, as carefully as a conventional health care provider.

- Before using any dietary supplement or herbal product, find out about potential side effects with medications they may be taking.

- Only use treatments that have been proven safe and effective.

- Tell all their health care providers—CAM and conventional—about the health care services they use. For safety reasons, give all providers a full picture of what patients do to manage their health.

Advance Directives

Patients have rights regarding their medical care. The principle of *informed consent*, as discussed in Chapter 7, legally requires health care providers to supply in writing all the information patients need to make an informed decision about whether or not to participate in a particular treatment.

Patients also have the right to make decisions about their own care—about how much or how little treatment to receive. Some patients with a life-ending disease may decide to try every available and aggressive treatment, hoping that something will work. Other patients may decide to limit or completely avoid aggressive treatment. Whatever the patient decides, it is important to make the decisions known to others, particularly family and loved ones.

Informing others is crucial if the patient has a terminal disease or is in an irreversible condition. A *terminal disease* is an incurable condition that will produce death within 6 months, even with life-sustaining treatment; an *irreversible condition* is one that can be treated but never cured. It is fatal without life-sustaining treatment.

If a patient has a terminal disease or is in an irreversible condition, he or she often is unable to make decisions. Before a patient loses the capacity to make medical decisions, it is wise for him or her to consider and prepare an advance directive. *Advance directives* communicate to health care providers, family, and loved ones about the type of health care the patient wants when he or she can no longer make decisions. *Advance directive* is a broad term for any legal document dealing with health care decisions, such as a living will or who will be health care proxy (sometimes known as durable power of attorney).

A *living will* is a set of instructions that spell out what types of medical treatment the patient wants at the end of his or her life. It tells health care providers his or her wishes. A living will protects the patient's rights and removes the burden of making difficult decisions from family, loved ones, and health care providers.

There are different types of medical decisions to address when making a living will (Robert Wood Johnson Foundation, 2011), including the following:

- The use of life-sustaining equipment (dialysis machines, ventilators, and respirators)

- *Do-not-resuscitate (DNR)* orders (instructions not to use CPR if breathing or heartbeat stops)

- Artificial hydration and nutrition (tube feeding)

- Withholding of food and fluids

- Palliative or comfort care

- HIPAA authorization (allows the patient to identify others with whom health care providers can share his or her information)

- Organ and tissue donation

A decision not to receive aggressive medical treatment is not the same as deciding to withhold all medical treatment. A patient can still receive antibiotics, nutrition, pain medication, and other treatments when the goal becomes comfort rather than cure. This type of treatment is called *palliative care*, and its primary focus is on helping the patient remain as comfortable as possible. Patients can, however, change their minds at any time and ask for more aggressive treatment.

Health care proxy or durable power of attorney is another type of advance directive. It is a legal document that appoints someone as the health care proxy who makes the patient's health care decisions. The health care proxy makes decisions when the patient can't communicate on his or her own. The document goes into effect only when the patient's physician says that the patient can't understand and cannot make decisions about his or her health care. Unless that happens, no one can make decisions for the patient.

The role of the health care proxy is not only to make health care decisions for the patient but also to act as the patient's spokesperson and advocate in regard to a range of medical decisions. Therefore, the person appointed as health care proxy should know the patient well and be someone who can carry out the wishes as stated in the living will. The proxy should be able to do this regardless of personal feelings or influence from family and loved ones. Being someone's proxy is challenging because the proxy may have to make decisions even in circumstances where the patient's wishes are not generally known. It is therefore important for patients to choose their health care proxy wisely. The best person to have as a health proxy is someone who can:

- Understand your wishes and can speak out on your behalf if necessary

- Act on your wishes and separate his or her own feelings from yours

- Be your advocate

- Handle conflict among family, loved ones, and health care providers

- Travel to be at your side if needed

- Be available long into the future

Although a lawyer is not needed to complete advance directives, patients should be aware that each state has its own laws for creating advance directives, and take special care to follow the laws of the state where they live or where they are receiving health care. Forms for making advance directives can be obtained from health care providers, Offices on Aging, state health departments, and online from the US Department of Health and Human Services (DHHS). There are also private companies that offer online advance directive services.

Advance directives are important for all of us, because choices about end-of-life care are difficult even when we are well. If a person has a terminal disease or is in an irreversible condition, these decisions can seem overwhelming. Avoiding these decisions when we are well will only put a heavier burden on us, our family, and our loved ones later on. Communicating our wishes about end-of-life care ahead of time will ensure that if we become seriously ill, we can face the end of our lives with dignity.

Chapter Summary

- Patient navigators help patients who are coping with chronic diseases that require complex testing and treatment. They help patients enter and navigate the health care system, manage their disease, and overcome barriers to care.

- Patient navigators help patients at two levels: (a) they help specific patients obtain services and rights that would otherwise not be given to them; (b) they advocate to change dysfunctional policies in their institutions and communities.

- Patient navigators build working relationships to solve problems, direct patients to resources, and manage information.

- Patient navigators and other health care providers are most effective when they have examined their professional boundaries. They understand when, where, and with whom their boundaries have become blurred.

- Health care providers work as a team, but the most important team member is the patient. The more that patients participate in their own health care, the greater the likelihood that they will experience positive outcomes.

- Complementary and alternative medicine comprises diverse medical and health care systems, practices, and products that are not generally considered part of conventional or Western medicine.

- Advance directives communicate wishes about end-of-life care ahead of time. A living will and health proxy, as part of advance directives, ensure that if a person is seriously ill, he or she can face the end of his or her life with dignity.

REVIEW QUESTIONS

1. Define health care barriers and give some examples.

2. List and explain three functions of a patient navigator.

3. Compare and contrast two models of patient navigation.

4. What are some of the skills a patient navigator needs in order to be effective?

5. Identify some team members who work closely with patients with chronic disease.

6. List three examples of crossing professional boundaries.

7. What is the difference between patient autonomy and patient self-advocacy?

8. What are ways a patient can self-advocate?

9. Discuss the differences among complementary, alternative, and integrative medicine.

10. Why is it important to have an advance directive?

11. What is the difference between a living will and a health proxy?

KEY TERMS

Advance directive: A legal document dealing with health care decisions

Alternative medicine: Use of CAM only and not using conventional medicine

Complementary and alternative medicine (CAM): Diverse medical and health care systems, practices, and products that are not generally considered part of conventional or Western medicine

Complementary medicine: Use of CAM together with conventional medicine

Conventional medicine: Medicine as practiced by MDs and other health care providers trained in Western medicine

Do-not-resuscitate (DNR) orders: Instructions not to use CPR if breathing or heartbeat stops

Health care barrier: Any nonmedical situation that makes getting a diagnosis or treatment difficult

Health care proxy or durable power of attorney: Legal document that appoints someone (the health care proxy) to make health care decisions for the patient

Informed consent: Patient's permission to be put on a treatment plan and to be given treatment, based on his or her knowledge and understanding of all relevant information, which is required by law to be supplied in writing

Integrative medicine: Medical practices that combine treatments from conventional medicine and from CAM for which there is some scientific evidence of safety and effectiveness

Irreversible condition: A condition that can be treated but never cured and that is fatal without life-sustaining treatment

Living will: Document that states what types of medical treatment a person wants at the end of life if the person is unable to speak

Palliative care: Treatment whose primary focus is helping the patient remain as comfortable as possible

Patient autonomy: The ability of patients to educate themselves about their disease and its treatment, and make informed decisions

Patient-centered care: Health care that includes support to patients in managing their disease

Patient navigators (PNs): Individuals who assist patients with chronic diseases, particularly those that require complex testing and treatment

Professional boundaries: Ethical guidelines that a professional uses for relationships developed through work

Provider-centered care: Health care that is offered at the convenience of providers, not patients

Terminal disease: An incurable condition that will produce death within six months, even with life-sustaining treatment

CHAPTER ACTIVITIES

1. On one side of a piece of paper, list those things that frustrate you about health care in the United States; on the other side, list the ways in which receiving health care in the United States can be a positive experience. Pair off with someone in the class and compare your lists. Choose one shared frustration to focus on, and brainstorm specific behavior(s) that a person could follow to relieve some of the frustrations.

2. You are working as a patient navigator with a small group of new immigrants (approximately 10 adults) who are new to the US health care system. English is the second language of most members of the group, or they have low health literacy. Brainstorm some of the barriers to health care that the group members might experience and some ways to overcome those barriers.

3. Write a one-page information sheet on a complementary, alternative, or integrative medical practice of interest. Use visuals instead of text when appropriate. Remember to include resources and references as part of the information sheet.

4. You have been asked to present an educational workshop on the importance of advance directives. Your audience is made up of seniors who live in an assisted living community (approximately 20 people ages 65–85). Write three objectives or learning outcomes that you feel would be appropriate for this situation. In other words, what do you expect the participants to learn from attending this workshop? Select two strategies or methods that you feel might help you meet your objectives.

5. You are a patient navigator who is working with two African American women who have type 2 diabetes. Give examples of strategies that you will use to guide these women toward self-advocacy and patient autonomy.

Bibliography and Works Cited

Davis, K., & Guterman, S. (2011). Achieving Medicare and Medicaid savings: Cutting eligibility and benefits, trimming payments, or ensuring the right care? Retrieved from 2011\n http://www.commonwealthfund.org /Blog/2011/Jul/Achieving-Medicare-and-Medicaid-Savings.aspx#citation

Freeman, H. P. (2001). *Voices of a broken system: Real people, real problems.* Bethesda, MD: President's Cancer Panel. Retrieved from http://deainfo.nci.nih.gov/advisory/pcp/archive/pcp00-01rpt/PCPvideo/voices_files /PDFfiles/PCPbook.pdf

Freund, K. M. (2011). Patient navigation: The promise to reduce health disparities. *Journal of General Internal Medicine, 26,* 110–112. Retrieved from https://www.ncbi.nlm.nih.gov/pmc/articles/PMC3019331

Groopman, L. C. (2010). Letter to patients: On becoming the "good" patient and finding the "right" doctor. In T. Kushner (Ed.), *Surviving health care: A manual for patients and their families* (pp. 1–12). New York, NY: Cambridge University Press.

HANYS, Breast Cancer Demonstration Project. (2002). *Breast health patient navigator resource kit.* Rensselaer, NY: Healthcare Association of New York State. Retrieved from https://www.hanys.org/bcdp/resource_kits /upload/Complete-PNP-Kit-PDF.pdf

Jansson, B. S. (2011). *Improving health care through advocacy: A guide for the health and helping professions.* Hoboken, NJ: Wiley.

McGlynn, E. A., Asch, S. M., Adams, J., Keesey, J., Hicks, J., DeCristofaro, A., & Kerr, E. A. (2003). The quality of health care delivered to adults in the United States. *New England Journal of Medicine, 348,* 2635–2645. doi:10.1056/NEJMsa022615

National Center for Complementary and Alternative Medicine. (2016). What is complementary and alternative medicine? Retrieved from http://nccam.nih.gov/health/whatiscam/

Norcross, W. A., (2010). Becoming an active member of your health care team. In T. Kushner (Ed.), *Surviving health care: A manual for patients and their families* (pp. 13–25). New York, NY: Cambridge University Press.

Risendal, B., Valverde, P., Calhoun, E., Esparza, A., & Whitley, E. (2009). Patient navigator training and competencies [Abstract]. *Psycho-Oncology, 18,* S15. Retrieved from http://onlinelibrary.wiley.com/doi /10.1002/pon.1526/full

Robert Wood Johnson Foundation. (2011). Care about your care. Retrieved from http://www.rwjf.org/en/library /collections/cayc.html?cid=xdr_cayc

Stone, N. J. (2006). Clinical confidence and the three C's: Caring, communicating, and competence. *American Journal of Medicine, 119*(1), 1–2.

Stremikis, K., Schoen, C., Fryer, A. K., & the Commonwealth Fund. (2011). A call for change: The 2011 Commonwealth Fund survey of public views of the U.S. health system. Retrieved from http://www .commonwealthfund.org/~/media/Files/Publications/Issue%20Brief/2011/Apr/1492_Stremikis_public_views _2011_survey_ib.pdf

Taking charge of your care. (2015). *Cancer.Net.* Retrieved from http://www.cancer.net/navigating-cancer-care/managing-your-care/taking-charge-your-care

University of Colorado Cancer Center. (2011). Colorado patient navigator training program. Retrieved from http://www.patientnavigatortraining.org

Walsh-Burke, K., & Marcusen, C. (1999). Self-advocacy training for cancer survivors. The Cancer Survival Toolbox. *Cancer Practice, 7,* 297–301. Retrieved from http://www.ncbi.nlm.nih.gov/pubmed/10732527

BASICS OF DISEASE AND DIAGNOSIS

CHAPTER OBJECTIVES

- Identify major categories and types of diseases.

- Describe elements of a physical examination.

- Explain electronic health records and electronic prescriptions.

- Summarize types of screenings.

- Identify and describe common diagnostic tests and procedures.

- Review medical specialties.

Physical examinations can detect health problems before they start. They also can find health problems early, when treatment outcomes are better. By having regular physical examinations with the right screenings, diagnostic tests, and procedures, patients can improve their chances of living a longer, healthier life.

Disease Categories and Types

Diseases are what health care providers study. A *disease* is a biological condition that is a change from normal bodily functions or structures. There are many different categories and types of diseases. For the purposes of this textbook, the discussion of categories and types is limited to how a disease develops. There are five major categories based on how a disease develops (see Figure 9.1):

1. *Degenerative disease.* These diseases cause the function of tissues, organs, or body structure to decline over time.

2. *Genetic disease, or hereditary or inherited disease, and congenital disease.* These diseases are caused by defects in a person's genetic makeup. When these defects occur at birth, the condition is known as a congenital disease. Not all congenital diseases are genetic, however.

3. *Inflammatory disease.* This category comprises a large and diverse group of diseases. The body reacts to injuries or infection with *inflammation,* meaning that it becomes red, swollen, hot, and sometimes painful. The immune system is

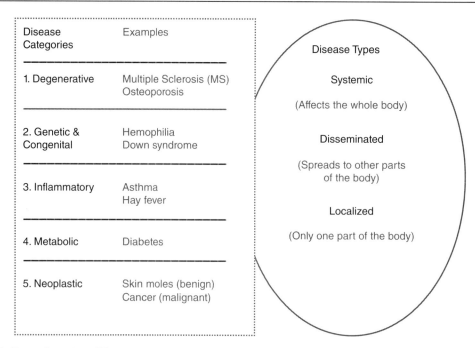

Figure 9.1 Disease Categories and Types

usually the cause of inflammation. However, some inflammatory diseases, such as certain cancers, are not caused by the immune system.

4. *Metabolic disease.* These are diseases caused by abnormal chemical reactions in the body that disrupt metabolism. *Metabolism* is a chemical process that takes place in the cells and the fluids of the body, enabling the body to get or produce energy from food.

5. *Neoplastic disease.* A tissue mass caused by an abnormal growth of cells is a *neoplasm*. A *tumor* is a neoplasm that has formed into a lump. Not all neoplasms form tumors. There are different types of neoplastic diseases: Some involve harmless neoplasms; others involve neoplasms that are harmful (cancers).

In addition to these categories, diseases are also grouped based on how they exist in the body. *Localized diseases* affect only one part of the body. *Disseminated diseases* spread to other parts of the body. *Systemic diseases* affect the entire body.

Physical Examination

Certain health care providers, such as physicians, nurse practitioners, and physician assistants, provide a diagnosis to a patient. A *diagnosis* identifies the nature and causes of a patient's disease. To give a diagnosis, these providers perform tests and procedures based on a patient's signs and symptoms. *Signs* are the evidence of a disease that can be observed or measured by medical tests and procedures; high blood pressure is an example of a sign. *Symptoms* are what the patient reports to have—for example, feeling tired; symptoms can't be measured or observed.

A *physical examination* is the first way to determine a diagnosis. During a physical examination, a provider studies a patient's body and performs the following actions (Llewelyn, Ang, Lewis, & Al-Abdullah, 2014):

Inspection The provider looks at a patient's body or at a body part.

Palpation The provider uses his or her fingers and hands to touch and feel a patient's body to examine the size, texture, location, and tenderness of an organ or body part.

Auscultation The provider, typically using a stethoscope, listens to a patient's lungs, heart, and intestines to evaluate the number and quality of sounds.

Percussion Using small instruments or his or her fingers or hands, the provider taps body parts to make a sound. The purpose is to evaluate the size, consistency, and borders of body organs as well as the presence or absence of fluid in body areas.

A complete physical examination includes checking the patient's height, weight, body temperature, pulse rate, respiratory rate, and blood pressure for signs. General appearance, skin, eyes, ears, nose, mouth, neck, lungs, heart, lymph nodes, back, legs, feet bones, joints, and reflexes are also checked.

The provider performs multiple tasks while conducting a physical examination. In addition to examining the patient's body, the provider takes a health history, orders diagnostic tests and procedures, suggests screenings, prescribes medicines, recommends a treatment plan, and gives a prognosis. A *prognosis* is the provider's opinion of how the patient's disease will develop—whether it will get better or worse. The following sections of this chapter explain the provider's tasks that are performed during and as a result of a physical examination.

Health History

During a physical examination, the provider asks the patient questions about his or her health. These questions relate to the patient's health or medical history, and the responses are crucial elements in the provider's diagnosis.

There are two parts to a patient's health history. The first part is a record of the patient's personal health, such as past diseases, allergies, and drug sensitivities as well as a history of medical care. The second part is information on the patient's family health history. Many diseases can run in families. If one generation of a family has high blood pressure, for example, it is not unusual for the next generation also to have high blood pressure. Putting together a family health history and learning how genes, the environment, and lifestyle interact lead to a better understanding of how and why a patient has a disease. It can also help the provider predict diseases for which the patient may be at risk.

Health Records

There are two types of health records. The first is a health history record that the patient keeps. The second is the record that a provider keeps on the patient's health history.

It is recommended that patients keep track of their health history. The patient's health record includes personal information on medications taken, allergies, test results, illnesses, surgeries, and family health history (see list). By keeping a health record, a patient can avoid undergoing duplicate procedures and tests. These records also help providers get the information they need to treat a patient in an emergency.

Personal Health Record Information

Personal information (name, birth date, and address)

Names and phone numbers of contact people

Names, addresses, and phone numbers of health care providers

Health insurance information

Current medications and dosages

Allergies

Important diseases in family health history

A list and dates of important diseases and surgeries

Information from recent health care provider visits

Important tests results

Over-the-counter and herbal medicines

Mental health services

The health record that providers keep includes the patient's health history and the results of physical examinations. Each time a patient visits his or her provider and receives treatment, somebody makes a note of it in the patient's health record. These health records contain the basics (e.g., name and date of birth) as well as the information a patient tells his or her provider during a physical examination.

Providers often ask questions during a physical examination that relate to the patient's health. All of the patient's answers go into his or her health record, along with the results of any physical examinations, test and procedure findings, treatments, medications, and notes providers make about the patient's health. These health records include not only the patient's physical health care but also his or her mental health care. Each medical specialist who treats a patient keeps his or her own file, and each of these is part of a patient's health record.

Providers usually store their patients' health records online as *electronic health records* (EHRs). EHRs let providers share up-to-date information about a patient's diseases, treatments, tests, procedures, and prescriptions. If a provider uses EHRs, he or she can join a network to securely share a patient's records with other providers. EHRs cut down on medical errors and prevent patients from receiving duplicate services.

Patients should know what's in their health records, how to access them, who else sees them, and what laws are in place to keep them private. In the United States, patients have the right to see, get copies of, and sometimes even change their health records. If a patient notices a mistake in his health records, he has the right to request a correction from his provider.

Most health care providers protect their patients' privacy. Patient information can, however, be legally used and shared with the following people or groups when needed:

- Other health care providers who provide the patient with treatment.

- Insurance companies and other groups responsible for paying the patient's health care costs.

- Public health agencies as needed to protect the public's health.

- Law enforcement agencies.

- Family, relatives, friends, or others in a patient's life—but only if the patient gives permission. Parents have access to their child's health records up to age 18.

Not only are there electronic health records, but there are also electronic prescriptions. The following are benefits of *electronic prescriptions* for patients and providers:

- Patients do not need to drop off the prescription and wait for the pharmacist to fill it.

- Providers can easily check which drugs the patient's insurance covers.

- Providers have secure access to the patient's prescription history, so they can know about drug interactions, allergies, and other warnings.

- Prescriptions are easier for the pharmacist to read than handwritten ones, resulting in fewer mistakes.

Diagnostic Tests and Procedures

The health care provider orders diagnostic tests and procedures during the physical examination. A *diagnostic test* is an analysis of a specimen removed from a patient. A *diagnostic procedure* is the moving around of the patient's body that goes beyond what is done during a normal physical examination.

Diagnostic tests and procedures are either invasive or noninvasive. *Invasive* means that the test or procedure "invades" the patient's body and can cause pain. A *noninvasive* test or procedure causes little or no pain.

Most diagnostic tests and procedures carry a degree of risk. The risk is greater when tests and procedures are invasive; however, even the noninvasive can present problems. For example, having many X-rays can expose a patient to unhealthy levels of radiation.

It is the legal responsibility of providers to advise their patients about the risks and benefits of a diagnostic test or procedure. Only when patients understand the risks and benefits of a test or procedure can they give their informed consent. It often is a challenge, however, for providers to explain a specific test or procedure to a patient. Many tests and procedures are complex, technically advanced, and difficult to understand.

Providers order diagnostic tests or procedures for five main reasons:

- To establish a diagnosis
- To provide prognosis information
- To screen for a disease in asymptomatic patients
- To monitor treatment
- To prove that a patient is free from a disease

There are hundreds of diagnostic tests and procedures. This chapter discusses the most common categories (see Figure 9.2).

Clinical Laboratory Tests

A *clinical laboratory test* checks a sample of blood, urine, tissue, or other substances in the body for health problems. An example of a clinical laboratory test is the *complete blood count (CBC)*. A CBC measures the levels of different types of blood cells and can detect diseases or signs of infection.

A *urinalysis* is the physical, chemical, and microscopic examination of urine. It involves a number of tests that detect and measure compounds that pass through the urine. A patient's urine sample is examined for color, appearance, microscopic parts, and chemical content.

Many factors, such as sex, age, race, and health history, affect clinical laboratory test results. For example, how closely the patient follows pretest instructions can affect test results, as can drugs the patient is taking. Specific foods affect test results, which is why a patient may be asked not to eat or drink for several hours before a test.

Cytologic and Histologic Exams

A *cytologic test* is the laboratory examination of cells to see what the cells look like and how they form and function. A cytologic test is usually done to look for cancers and infections. The Pap smear is a common cytologic test that looks at cells from the cervix. There are multiple locations for cytologic materials, such as urine, mucus from the lungs, vaginal smears, abdominal and chest cavity fluids, and fluid removed during a biopsy. A *biopsy* is removal of a small sample of tissue for examination and diagnosis. A biopsy can be performed in the following ways:

- A needle withdraws tissue or fluid.
- An endoscope looks at areas inside the body and removes cells or tissues (Figure 9.4).
- Part or all of the tissue is surgically removed.

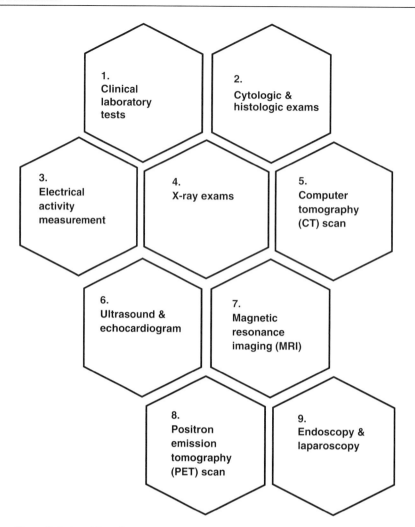

Figure 9.2 Common Diagnostic Tests and Procedures

Diseased tissue removed during a biopsy is sent to a pathology laboratory, where the pathologist does a *histologic test*. This test examines tissue cells and structure for health problems.

Measurement of Electrical Activity

The *electrocardiogram (ECG)* is a painless procedure that measures and records electrical activity of the heart. Electrical currents within the heart control its pumping. An ECG measures those currents and identifies changes in heart rate or heart rhythm. It can also provide clues about other diseases. Twelve metal discs with thin wires called electrode patches are attached to the patient's skin on the legs, arms, and chest, and voltage differences are recorded.

A similar procedure that measures electrical activity is the *electroencephalogram (EEG)*. Electrode patches are placed on the scalp and then the EEG measures the electrical activity of brain waves. An EEG detects abnormal patterns in the brain waves. Diseases such as brain tumors and strokes as well as brain injuries can change brain wave patterns.

X-Ray Exam

The basic principle of X-rays is the use of electromagnetic radiation to make images. X-rays pass through the part of the body to be examined. The image is then recorded on a film called a *radiograph*. X-rays can detect broken bones, cavities in the teeth, and other health problems.

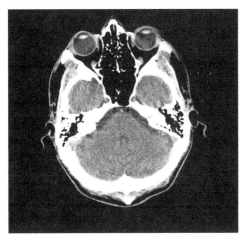 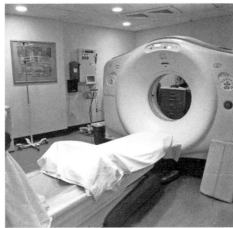

Figure 9.3 CT/CAT Scan of the Head and CT/CAT Scan Machine

Note. Head scan from Andrew Ciscel (Flickr) [CC BY-SA 2.0 (http://creativecommons.org/licenses/by-sa/2.0)], via Wikimedia Commons, https://commons.wikimedia.org/wiki/File%3AHead_CT_scan.jpg

Machine photo from NithinRao (Own work) [Public domain], via Wikimedia Commons, https://commons.wikimedia.org/wiki/File%3ACt-scan.jpg

Having an X-ray is painless, and the amount of radiation from a single X-ray is too small to cause any harm. Some providers are concerned, however, that multiple X-rays may expose patients to harmful amounts of radiation. If a patient is pregnant, she should talk to her provider about having X-rays, because radiation may be harmful to a fetus (US National Library of Medicine, 2016).

Computed Tomography Scan

A *scan* is an advanced X-ray that uses a computer to make pictures of the inside of the body. A *computed tomography scan (CT/CAT scan)* uses special X-ray technology and computers to create cross-sectional pictures of parts of the body. A CT/CAT scan beams X-rays through a patient's body part at multiple angles to capture data. The data are then fed to a computer and made into a three-dimensional (3-D) picture projected onto a screen.

CT/CAT scans show internal organs impossible to see with X-rays. X-rays look all the way through a body, but can't tell how deep anything is. A CT/CAT scan, in contrast, tells not only whether something abnormal is present but also roughly how deep it is in the body. CT/CAT scans are used to analyze major parts of the body, including the abdomen, back, and head (see Figure 9.3). Other uses of CT/CAT scans include looking for broken bones, tumors, blood clots, and internal bleeding.

The patient lies still on a table when having a CT/CAT scan. The table passes through the center of a large machine. Some scans require the patient to be given a contrast dye. The dye improves the visibility of certain tissues or blood vessels.

CT/CAT scans release more radiation into the patient than do regular X-rays, but the amount is still too small to cause harm unless the patient is pregnant (Porter, Kaplan, & Albert, 2011). As with X-rays, some providers are concerned that multiple CT/CAT scans may expose patients to harmful amounts of radiation (US National Library of Medicine, 2016).

Ultrasound and Echocardiogram

An *ultrasound, or sonogram,* uses high-frequency sound waves that humans cannot hear. It is painless and, unlike X-rays or CT/CAT scans, does not involve radiation exposure.

For an ultrasound, special jelly is applied to the skin, and a handheld device that sends out sound waves is moved over the skin. The sound waves bounce off organs in the body, and the handheld device captures the sound waves that bounce back. These sound waves create pictures of the patient's organs, which are projected on a screen (see Figure 9.4).

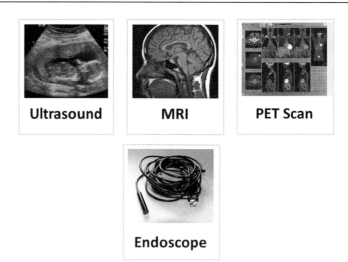

Figure 9.4 Images Related to an Ultrasound, MRI, PET Scan, and Endoscopy
Note. Images are from the following sources:

1. Ultrasound image: Wikimedia Commons
   Retrieved from https://upload.wikimedia.org/wikipedia/commons/thumb/f/f7/Praenatal.png/673px-Praenatal.png. Permission to upload is given by the physician and the mother.
2. MRI image: Wikimedia Commons
   Retrieved from https://commons.wikimedia.org/w/index.php?title=Magnetic_resonance_imaging&redirect=no#/media/File:MRI_head_side.jpg
3. PET scan image: Wikimedia Commons
   By OpenStax College [CC BY 3.0 (http://creativecommons.org/licenses/by/3.0)], via Wikimedia Commons. Retrieved from https://commons.wikimedia.org/wiki/File%3A205_Multi-image_Panel_of_PET_Scan-01.jpg
4. Endoscope image: Wikimedia Commons
   By Finn Årup Nielsen (Own work) [CC BY-SA 4.0 (http://creativecommons.org/licenses/by-sa/4.0)], via Wikimedia Commons. Retrieved from https://commons.wikimedia.org/wiki/File%3AEndoscope%2C_USB%2C_2015-05-30.jpg

Although usually associated with fetal examination, ultrasounds are used for different diagnoses. For example, ultrasound is used to look at the heart, brain, kidneys, and liver. Ultrasound detects tumors and can guide surgeons in performing a biopsy.

An *echocardiogram* is an ultrasound of the heart. It aids in examining heart valves and in determining the heart's size and functioning. This test estimates how forcefully the heart is pumping blood. It can also spot areas of the heart wall that have been injured by a previous heart attack or some other cause.

Magnetic Resonance Imaging (MRI)

Magnetic resonance imaging (MRI) uses a large magnet and radio waves to make images of body organs and structures. Tissues in organs emit a signal based on their chemical makeup. During the scan, an electric current is passed through wires to create a temporary magnetic field in a patient's body. Radio waves are sent from and received by a transmitter/receiver in the machine, and these signals are used to make 3-D images of the scanned area of the body. These images help pinpoint problems in the body. A typical MRI scan last from 20 to 90 minutes, depending on the part of the body being imaged (see Figure 9.4).

MRI is used to detect a variety of diseases, including problems of the brain, spinal cord, joints, ligaments, heart, abdomen, eyes, and heart. It can also identify infections, inflammatory diseases, and tumors. In some cases, an MRI can provide images of body parts that can't be seen as well with an X-ray, CT/CAT scan, or ultrasound.

During the scan, the patient lies on a table that slides inside a tunnel-shaped machine. The patient may be given a dye to highlight certain organs or structures so that problem areas can be seen in detail.

An MRI is a more sensitive scan for showing soft tissues, whereas CT/CAT scans are better at imaging bones.

Positron Emission Tomography (PET) Scan

A *positron emission tomography (PET) scan* uses a radioactive substance that can show how tissues, organs, and structures are changing (see Figure 9.4). A PET scan requires the patient to ingest a *tracer*, a small amount of radioactive materials mixed with sugar. After receiving the tracer, the patient lies still while the radioactive sugar circulates through the blood and collects in organs and tissues. If a tumor is present, the tracer will concentrate in the tumor.

The patient then lies on a table, which slides into a tunnel-shaped PET scanner. The scanner detects signals from the tracer, and a computer records the results as 3-D images.

The combination of a CT/CAT scan with PET images improves the ability to distinguish normal from abnormal tissues. However, PET scans are more accurate in showing large and more aggressive tumors than they are in locating tumors that are small or less aggressive. The good news is that they can detect cancer when other imaging techniques show normal results.

Endoscopy and Laparoscopy

Endoscopy is a procedure used to look inside a patient's body. It is an invasive procedure that uses an instrument called an *endoscope* (see Figure 9.4). An endoscope has a tiny camera attached to a long, thin tube. It is inserted through a body opening to see inside an organ and, if necessary, perform surgery.

This procedure is done in the hospital or outpatient surgical center under general anesthesia, which means that the patient is unconscious and pain-free. A small cut is made in the abdominal area below the belly button and a needle is inserted. Carbon dioxide gas is passed into the area to help move the abdominal wall and any organs out of the way, creating a larger space to work in. The tube of the endoscope is then placed through the cut. A tiny video camera goes through this tube and is used to see the inside of the pelvis and abdomen.

A common endoscopic procedure is the *laparoscopy*. A laparoscopy is a surgery performed on the abdomen and pelvis areas, including the reproductive organs, stomach, appendix, liver, and gallbladder. Many types of abdominal surgery can be done with a laparoscopy, including diagnosis and treatment of infertility or pelvic pain, and removal of the gallbladder or appendix.

There are many different kinds of endoscopy procedures. The following are the names of some of them and where they look:

- Arthroscopy: joints
- Bronchoscopy: lungs
- Colonoscopy and sigmoidoscopy: large intestine
- Cystoscopy: urinary system
- Upper gastrointestinal endoscopy: esophagus and stomach

Health Screenings

Health screenings are tests and procedures that are essential to *preventive medicine*, which are medical actions that a person can take to prevent a disease. The benefits of screenings are that they detect health problems early and sometimes even prevent a disease. Many diseases are *asymptomatic*, meaning that they have no symptoms, so the patient feels fine. But a screening tries to find a disease before the patient has symptoms. According to the Centers for Disease Control and Prevention (2015), there are other benefits to screenings in that patients can:

Table 9.1   US Preventive Services Task Force 2016 Recommendations for Health Screenings by Age Group

Screening Tests for Newborns and Infants	Screening Tests for Children (Ages 2–12)	Screening Tests for Teens (Ages 13–18)
Congenital disorders	Obesity	Obesity
Infectious diseases	*If at risk:*	*If at risk:*
Genetic (inherited) disorders	Diabetes	Cervical cancer
If at risk:	Cholesterol	Chlamydia and gonorrhea
Iron deficiency	Lead poisoning	Diabetes
Lead poisoning	Tuberculosis	Cholesterol
Tuberculosis		HIV
		Tuberculosis

Screening Tests for Young Adults (Ages 19–29)	Screening Tests for Adults (Ages 30–49)	Screening Tests for Older Adults (Ages 50 and Up)
Breast cancer	Breast cancer	Breast cancer
Hypertension	Diabetes	Diabetes
Cervical cancer	Hypertension	Hypertension
Chlamydia and gonorrhea	Cervical cancer	Cervical cancer
Cholesterol	Cholesterol	Colorectal cancer
HIV	HIV	Cholesterol
Obesity	Obesity	HIV
If at risk:	Thyroid dysfunction	Obesity
Diabetes	*If at risk:*	Osteoporosis
Tuberculosis	Chlamydia and gonorrhea	Thyroid dysfunction
Colon cancer	Colorectal cancer	Prostate cancer
	Osteoporosis	*If at risk:*
	Prostate cancer	Chlamydia and gonorrhea
	Tuberculosis	Tuberculosis
		Lung cancer

Note. Adapted from *Published Recommendations,* by US Preventive Services Task Force, 2016. Retrieved from https://www.uspreventiveservicestaskforce.org/BrowseRec/Index

- Take steps to reduce the risk of developing a disease
- Take better care of their health when a screening shows a risk for a disease
- Detect a disease early so that easier and more effective treatment can be provided

The need for particular screenings depends on age, gender, race and ethnicity, family history, and risk factors for certain diseases. Knowing what screenings are necessary and when to have them can be confusing. Table 9.1 summarizes health screenings that are recommended by the US Preventive Services Task Force (2016) for people in different age groups. Please keep in mind that for many of these screenings, there is no national agreement on recommendations. Recommendations differ based on the patient's health history, family health history, and lifestyle, as well as on the experiences of the health care provider (Centers for Disease Control and Prevention, 2015). The patient and his or her provider need to work together to develop an individualized health screening plan.

This section of the chapter is limited to discussion of seven common health screenings:

1. Screenings for cancer

2. Self-examinations

3. Blood screening tests

4. Bone mineral density (BMD) test

5. Eye examinations

6. Dental examinations

7. Genetic testing and counseling

Screenings for Cancer

As part of women's routine health care, a pelvic exam and a Pap smear test detect infection, inflammation, and cancer (see Figure 9.5). The provider performs a *pelvic exam* to feel for lumps and for changes in the shape of a woman's uterus, ovaries, and cervix. During the exam, the woman lies on her back on an examination table with her feet in stirrups and legs apart. The provider uses a *speculum*, a device for opening the vagina. Once the vagina is open, the provider examines the cervix for health problems or takes cell samples for a Pap smear test. These samples of cells are examined in a clinical laboratory.

The *Pap smear test* checks for cervical cancer and other abnormal cells. This test can also detect infections or inflammation. Women should start getting regular Pap smear tests at age 21 or within 3 years of the first time of having sex—whichever occurs first (US Preventive Services Task Force, 2016).

A Pap smear test is one of the most reliable and effective cervical cancer screening tests available. The *human papillomavirus (HPV)* is the virus that causes most cervical cancers and is tested as part of the Pap smear test. The Pap smear test does not screen for ovarian, uterine, vaginal, or vulvar cancers.

If a patient is 30 years old or older and her screening tests are normal, her chances of getting cervical cancer in the next few years are low. For that reason, she may not need another screening test

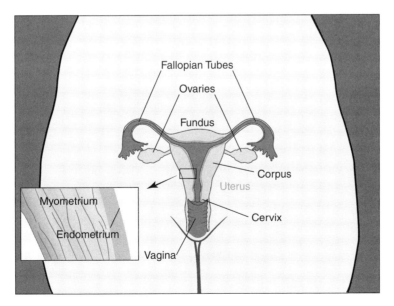

Figure 9.5 Female Reproductive System

Note. Adapted from the National Cancer Institute, Visuals Online, n.d., unknown illustrator. This image is in the public domain and can be freely reused. Retrieved from https://visualsonline.cancer.gov/details.cfm?imageid=1783

for up to 3 years (US Preventive Services Task Force, 2016). If a woman is older than 65 and has had normal Pap test results for several years, or if she has had her cervix removed (during an operation called a *hysterectomy*, which also removes the uterus), she may stop getting regular Pap smear tests (US Preventive Services Task Force, 2016).

Breast cancer is the second most common type of cancer in women. The older a woman is, the greater her risk. Most women who develop breast cancer have no special risk factors for the disease.

There are two screenings that a health care provider can use to help detect breast cancer in a patient. The first screening is a *clinical breast exam* (CBE). A provider checks the patient's breasts and underarms for any lumps, nipple discharge, or other changes.

The *mammogram* is a screening that uses an X-ray picture of the breast to look for early signs of breast cancer. Regular mammograms are the best tests to find breast cancer early, sometimes up to 3 years before it can be felt.

A stool test is used for early detection of colorectal cancer. Colorectal cancer affects the large intestine and the rectum. An example of a stool test is the *fecal occult blood test* (FOBT). To perform a FOBT, tiny stool samples are put on a special card or cloth and sent to a clinical laboratory for testing. With some FOBT kits, patients can do the testing themselves at home.

The FOBT checks for blood in the stool because blood may be a sign of colorectal cancer; however, not all bloody stools are caused by cancer. Other diseases, such as ulcers or Crohn's disease, can also cause bloody stools.

Everyone should have his first colonoscopy after he turns 50 because it helps in preventing colorectal cancer. A *colonoscopy* is an outpatient procedure in which the colon and rectum are examined (see Figure 9.6). The colon is the lower part of the intestinal tract that ends at the rectum and anus.

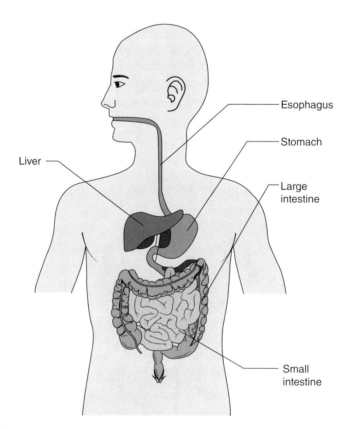

Figure 9.6 Colon and Rectum
Note. Adapted from National Institute of Diabetes and Digestive and Kidney Diseases, 2014. This information is not copyrighted. The NIDDK encourages people to share this content freely. Retrieved from https://www.niddk.nih.gov/health-information/health-topics/digestive-diseases /microscopic-colitis/Pages/facts.aspx

A colonoscopy shows inflamed tissue, abnormal growths, ulcers, bleeding, and muscle spasms. If abnormal tissue growths known as polyps are detected during the colonoscopy, they are removed before they produce symptoms. That polyp tissue is then sent to a clinical laboratory for testing.

The patient lies on his or her left side on the examining table when having a colonoscopy. Pain medication and a mild sedative are given to keep the patient comfortable during the procedure. A long, flexible, lighted tube called a *colonoscope* is inserted into the rectum and then guided into the colon. The colonoscope transmits an image of the inside of the colon onto a computer screen, so that the lining of the colon can be examined.

The *virtual colonoscopy* is another type of colonoscopy. It is done with an X-ray machine instead of a colonoscope. When a virtual colonoscopy is being performed, the patient has to lie on a table while a technician inserts a thin tube through the patient's anus and into the rectum. The tube inflates the large intestine with air for a better view. The table slides into a tunnel-shaped device, where the technician takes the X-ray images. The patient may have to hold his or her breath several times during the procedure to steady the images.

A procedure similar to the colonoscopy is the *flexible sigmoidoscopy*. The colon has three main parts: the ascending colon, the transverse colon, and the sigmoid colon. The flexible sigmoidoscopy sees inside the sigmoid colon and rectum and is used to look for early signs of cancer. It can detect inflamed tissue, abnormal growths, and ulcers. A flexible sigmoidoscopy allows for the viewing of only the sigmoid colon, whereas the colonoscopy allows the entire colon to be viewed. If polyps are found during a flexible sigmoidoscopy, then the rest of the colon is examined with a colonoscopy.

The National Institute of Diabetes and Digestive and Kidney Diseases (2015) recommends that men talk to their provider about the benefits, risks, and limitations of prostate cancer screening before deciding whether to be tested. For most men at average risk, discussions about screening are started at age 50. However, some providers recommend that men at higher risk of prostate cancer—African American men or men with a family history of prostate cancer—start screening earlier.

A *digital rectal exam (DRE)* is a physical examination of the prostate. It is often part of a physical examination in men age 50 or older, whether or not the man has urinary problems (see Figure 9.7).

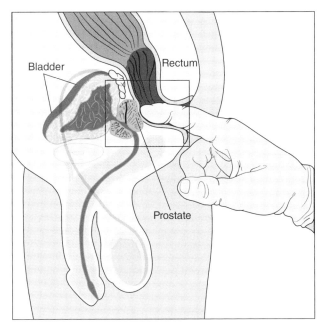

Figure 9.7 Digital Rectal Exam in Men

Note. Adapted from the National Cancer Institute, Visuals Online, n.d. This image is in the public domain and can be freely reused. Retrieved from https://visualsonline.cancer.gov/details.cfm?imageid=7136

A DRE is done to examine the prostate gland for enlargement or cancer. When conducting a DRE, the provider asks the patient to bend over a table or lie on his side while holding his knees close to the chest. The provider then slides a gloved, lubricated finger into the rectum and feels the part of the prostate that lies next to it. This exam reveals whether the prostate has any abnormal changes. A DRE can also be part of a routine pelvic examination in women and is done to find causes of pelvic pain and rectal bleeding.

Prostate problems tend to be more common as men age. *Prostate-specific antigen (PSA)* is a protein made by the cells of the prostate gland. The *PSA blood test* measures the level of PSA in the blood. It is normal for men to have low levels of PSA in their blood, but prostate cancer often raises PSA levels. A PSA blood test can detect prostate cancer; however, an elevated PSA level does not always mean that the person has prostate cancer.

Many providers use the PSA blood test along with a DRE to help detect prostate cancer in men ages 50 and older. Yet there is ongoing debate about how to interpret a PSA blood test. Detection of prostate cancer does not necessarily save men's lives. A PSA blood test may detect a small, slow-growing cancer that will never become life threatening. Most prostate cancers are slow growing and can exist for decades before causing health problems. In addition, a PSA test may not help if it detects a fast-growing cancer that has already spread to other body parts. To add to the debate, the PSA test is known to have high false-positive rates. Providers and patients should weigh the benefits of PSA blood testing against the risks of follow-up procedures (US National Library of Medicine, 2016). Some of the follow-up procedures used to diagnose prostate cancer may cause significant side effects, including bleeding and infection.

Self-Exams

Self-exams are done by people at home to check for abnormal changes in their body. The most commonly recommended include breast self-exam for women, testicular self-exam for men, and self-exam for skin cancer.

Many women check their own breasts for changes or problems by doing a breast self-exam (BSE). Although not recommended as part of breast cancer screening, a BSE does help women become familiar with the way their breasts normally look and feel, so that if they find a lump, they will know to call their provider (US National Library of Medicine, 2016). Breast self-exams should include visual inspection to see any changes in contour or texture. There should also be manual inspection in standing and reclining positions to feel for lumps or thicknesses.

A testicular self-exam involves the male reproductive organs (see Figure 9.8). The testicles are located in the scrotum under the penis. Males who have reached puberty or are over 15 should examine their testicles at least once a month to check for testicular cancer. Testicular cancer affects mostly young men between the ages 20 and 39 (US National Library of Medicine, 2016). If a male notices any lumps or changes in the size of his testicle, he needs to contact his provider. It could be just an infection, but it also could be the first sign of testicular cancer.

Sometimes men experience no symptoms of testicular cancer until it reaches an advanced stage, yet most testicular cancers are treatable. Men 40 and older should perform a testicular self-exam every month if they have a family history of testicular cancer, an undescended testicle, or a past testicular cancer.

US Preventive Services Task Force (2016) recommends that if you are over 20 years old, it's important to check your own skin at least once a month for skin cancer. This advice is most important to the person who has frequent exposure to the sun or bad sunburns early in life or who has fair skin, moles, or a history of skin cancer. Many skin cancers can be cured when detected and treated early.

A skin self-exam is best done in front of a full-length mirror. A handheld mirror can help with looking at areas that are hard to see. Special attention needs to be given to skin areas that are often

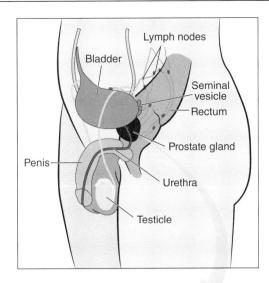

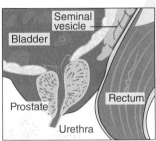

Figure 9.8 Male Reproductive System

Note. Adapted from the National Institute of Diabetes and Digestive and Kidney Diseases, 2014. This information is not copyrighted. The NIDDK encourages people to share this content freely. Retrieved from https://www.niddk.nih.gov/health-information/health-topics/diagnostic-tests /Medical%20tests-prostate-problems/Pages/medical-tests-prostate-problems.aspx

exposed to the sun, such as the hands, arms, chest, and head. If moles, blemishes, freckles, and other marks on the skin do not change over time, there is no need for concern.

Blood Screening Tests

Some screening tests use a blood sample taken from the patient's arm. This section describes blood screening tests for three widespread diseases: heart disease, diabetes, and HIV infection.

A diet high in cholesterol can lead to premature heart disease. To test for cholesterol levels, a sample of blood is taken from the patient's arm and sent to a laboratory for analysis. This test gives information about the patient's cholesterol elements: total cholesterol, LDL (harmful) cholesterol, HDL (good) cholesterol, and triglycerides, which are fats that store energy. If you are 20 years of age and older, it is recommended that you have your cholesterol tested at least once every 5 years and every 2 years if you have a family history of heart disease, high cholesterol, or diabetes (US Preventive Services Task Force, 2016).

There are three blood tests that measure the level of glucose in the blood or blood sugar and are used to diagnose type 2 diabetes. The *fasting plasma glucose test* measures the level of glucose in the blood. This test is recommended for everyone starting at age 20. The *oral glucose tolerance test* measures the body's ability to use glucose. The *A1C test* is a blood test that provides information about a person's average levels of blood glucose over the previous 3 months. The A1C test is the primary test used for diabetes management.

It is recommended by the US Preventive Services Task Force (2016) that adolescents and adults between the ages of 13 and 64 be screened for HIV (human immunodeficiency virus) infection. This screening is recommended because HIV can be detected and diagnosed early. Patients who are infected with HIV gain years of healthy living if they receive treatment early. For pregnant women, an HIV screening can detect infection and prevent transmission to the fetus. A blood sample or a saliva sample taken from a person's gums with a swab can be used for an HIV test.

Bone Mineral Density (BMD) Test

A *bone mineral density (BMD) test* measures calcium and other minerals in the bone. This test predicts a patient's risk for bone fractures and for osteoporosis. *Osteoporosis* is the thinning of bone tissue and loss of bone density. The BMD uses a low-dose X-ray scan and is painless.

Patients should have a bone density screening if they are at risk for osteoporosis (US Preventive Services Task Force, 2016). People are more likely to get osteoporosis if they are a woman over 65 or a man over age 70. Women under age 65 and men ages 50–70 are at increased risk for osteoporosis if they have a family history of osteoporosis, rheumatoid arthritis, eating disorders, early menopause, or a history of smoking or alcoholism.

Eye Examinations

A routine eye exam is a series of tests that check the vision and the health of a patient's eyes. The *refraction test* measures whether a person needs a prescription for eyeglasses or contact lenses. For this test, the patient looks through a special device called a refractor and focuses on an eye chart 20 feet away. The patient is asked if the chart appears more or less clear when different lenses are in place.

People age 40 and older tend to have more vision problems than younger people. By age 65, patients should have eye exams every year (US Preventive Services Task Force, 2016). Those at higher risk for eye diseases need to be examined more often—for example, those patients with a damaged optic nerve, glaucoma, or diabetes, or who have a family history of eye diseases.

Dental Examinations

For a person to have good oral health, his or her whole mouth, not just the teeth, needs care. The word *oral* refers to the mouth, which includes teeth, gums, jawbone, and supporting tissues. The health of the mouth is a sign of the body's health. Many diseases, such as diabetes, HIV infection, and cancer can cause oral health problems.

During a routine dental exam, the dentist does a complete examination of the soft tissue in the mouth and throat to look for signs of cancer. This exam includes an inspection of the tongue and salivary glands as well as of the face, head, and neck areas to look for abnormal changes in the lymph nodes.

Next, the dentist or dental hygienist uses a metal probe to measure how deep the gum tissue is around each tooth. This is done to identify gum disease in the early stages, when treatment is most effective. The dentist also notes any cavities, fillings, and crowns, and the condition of each tooth. X-rays of the teeth are ordered periodically to detect decay, bone loss, or abscesses.

Adults should see their dentist for a checkup and cleaning every 6 months. More frequent visits may be needed if the patient is pregnant, has type 2 diabetes, has HIV infection, smokes, uses chewing tobacco, drinks alcohol excessively, or has gum disease.

Genetic Tests and Counseling

Genetic tests find genetic diseases by identifying changes in chromosomes, genes, or proteins. The results of a genetic test can confirm or rule out a suspected genetic disease. These tests can also help determine a person's chance of developing or passing on a genetic disease. More than 1,000 genetic tests are currently in use, and more are being developed (Genetics Home Reference, 2016).

When a gene is abnormal, it is called a *genetic mutation*. Genetic mutations may run in families or just happen by chance. Those mutations that run in families are inherited or hereditary genetic diseases. A mutated gene is passed down through a family, and each generation of children can inherit the disease caused by the mutated gene. By reviewing a patient's family health history, a provider can tell if his or her patient is likely to inherit a genetic mutation.

People from certain ethnic groups can also get hereditary diseases. For example, sickle-cell disease occurs primarily in the children of African American parents who carry the gene mutation. Other genetic diseases are not inherited but instead are due to problems with the number of chromosomes. In Down syndrome, for example, there is an extra copy of a chromosome.

A sample of blood or skin is usually needed for genetic testing. If a patient has a positive test result, she may be more likely to get a certain disease than most people, but it doesn't mean that she will definitely get it. A negative test result shows that the patient doesn't have that particular gene mutation and that it doesn't run in her family. A negative result doesn't mean that the patient won't get that disease; it only means that she is not more likely to get the disease than other people.

Patients have their reasons for being tested or not tested for a genetic disease. For many, it is important to know whether a disease can be prevented or treated if a gene mutation is found. For some genetic diseases, however, there is no treatment. Nevertheless, test results might help a patient make life decisions, such as career choice or family planning. For example, a pregnant woman can have genetic tests to determine the health of both herself and her baby and be proactive in family planning.

Many health care providers recommend genetic counseling to patients considering genetic testing. *Genetic counseling* provides information and support to people who have or are at risk for a genetic disease. A genetic counselor provides education, guidance, and support to patients so that they can make informed decisions.

Some diseases have a genetic feature but are not considered to be primarily a genetic disease. For example, some cancers are caused by gene mutations. These mutations occur randomly or because of exposure to toxins in the environment, such as cigarette smoke.

Medical Specialties

Many physicians are trained in a medical specialty that helps in the diagnosis and treatment of diseases (see Table 9.2.). Medical specialties are organized into three groups. *Surgical specialties* focus on operative techniques to treat disease. *Medical specialties* focus on the diagnosis and nonsurgical treatment of disease. *Diagnostic specialties* focus primarily on the diagnosis of diseases.

Table 9.2 Examples of Medical Specialties

Specialty	Type	Focus
Allergy and immunology	Medical/diagnostic	Allergies, asthma, immune system
Anesthesiology	Surgical	Control of the anesthesia the patient receives during surgery
Cardiology	Medical	Heart
Dermatology	Medical	Skin
Emergency medicine	Medical	First treatment in an emergency medical situation
Endocrinology	Medical	Diabetes and hormonal problems
Family medicine	Medical	Primary care for adults and their families
Gastroenterology	Medicine	GI tract

(continued)

Table 9.2 *Continued*

Specialty	Type	Focus
General surgery	Surgical	Variety of surgeries
Geriatrics	Medical	Older adults
Hematology	Diagnostic	Blood
Infectious diseases	Medical	Infectious biological agents
Intensive care medicine	Medical	Life support and critical care
Internal medicine	Medical	Primary care for adults
Medical genetics	Medical	Heredity
Neurology	Medical	Brain and nervous system disorders
Obstetrics and gynecology	Medical and surgical	Female reproductive health, oncology, childbirth
Oncology	Medical	Cancer
Ophthalmology	Medical and surgical	Eyes
Orthopedic surgery	Surgical	Muscles, bones, and joints
Otolaryngology (ENT)	Medical and surgical	Ear, nose, and throat
Palliative care	Medical	Pain relief for terminally ill patients
Pediatrics	Medical	Infants, children, and adolescents
Physical medicine and rehabilitation	Medical	Function after an injury or because of a disease
Plastic surgery	Surgery	Cosmetic and reconstructive surgery
Preventive medicine	Medical	Public health
Proctology	Medical	Rectum, anus, and colon
Psychiatry	Medical and diagnostic	Mental and emotional problems
Pulmonology	Medical	Lungs
Radiology	Diagnostic	Medical imaging
Rheumatology	Medical	Arthritis and other connective tissue disorders
Urology	Surgical	Urinary tract of males and females; male reproductive system

Note. Adapted from *ABMS Guide to Medical Specialties,* by American Board of Medical Specialties, 2016a, Maryland Heights, MO: Elsevier; and *Specialty and Subspecialty Certificates,* by American Board of Medical Specialties, 2016b. Retrieved from http://www.who.int/hrh/statistics/Health_workers_classification; see references

Chapter Summary

- Diseases are classified into five major categories: degenerative, genetic and congenital, inflammatory, metabolic, and neoplastic.

- There are four elements to a physical examination: inspection, palpation, auscultation, and percussion.

- Screenings are essential to preventive medicine. Preventive medicine comprises medical actions that a person can take to prevent a disease.

- Screening recommendations differ depending on the patient's health history, family health history, and lifestyle, as well as on their provider's experiences.

- Many diseases have a genetic feature. For example, some cancers are caused by gene mutations. These mutations can occur randomly or because of an environmental exposure.

- Most diagnostic tests and procedures have a degree of risk. The risk is greater when tests and procedures are invasive; however, even the noninvasive can present problems.

- Physicians can be trained in different medical specialties that help in the diagnosis and treatment of diseases.

REVIEW QUESTIONS

1. List and describe three types of diseases based on how they exist in the body.

2. Explain the four elements of a physical examination.

3. Who can have access to a patient's health records?

4. Describe a self-exam for a woman and a self-exam for a man.

5. What are the benefits of electronic health records and electronic prescriptions?

6. What is the difference between an ECG and an EEG?

7. Identify and explain two screenings for cancer.

8. What is genetic counseling?

9. What are the benefits and limitations of the following scans: CT/CAT, PET, and MRI?

10. Identify and explain three medical specialties.

KEY TERMS

A1C test: Blood test that provides information about a person's average levels of blood glucose over the previous 3 months

Asymptomatic: Term that describes diseases that have no symptoms

Auscultation: Procedure in which the health care provider listens to a patient's lungs, heart, and intestines to evaluate the number and quality of sounds

Biopsy: Abnormal tissue removed during surgery for examination

Bone mineral density (BMD) test: Test that measures calcium and other minerals in the bone

Clinical breast exam (CBE): Breast exam performed by a health care provider

Clinical laboratory test: Test that checks a sample of blood or other substances in the body for certain diseases

Colonoscope: A tube with a scope that is inserted into the rectum and the colon

Colonoscopy: Outpatient procedure in which the large intestine is examined to detect polyps (and, if any are found, to remove them)

Complete blood count (CBC): Clinical laboratory test that measures the levels of different types of blood cells and can detect diseases or signs of infection

Computed tomography scan (CT/CAT scan): X-ray technology that creates cross-sectional pictures of parts of the body

Congenital disease: Disease caused by a genetic defect and that occurs at birth

Cytologic test: Laboratory examination of cells to see what the cells look like and how they form and function

Degenerative disease: Disease that causes a progressive decline in the function of tissues, organs, or body structure

Diagnosis: Identification of the nature and causes of a disease

Diagnostic procedure: Moving around of the patient's body that goes beyond what is done during a normal physical examination

Diagnostic test: Analysis of a specimen removed from a patient

Digital rectal exam (DRE): Physical exam of the prostate

Disease: Biological condition that is a change from normal bodily functions or structures

Disseminated disease: A disease that spreads to other parts of the body

Echocardiogram: Ultrasound of the heart

Electrocardiogram (ECG): Test that measures the electrical activity of the heart

Electroencephalogram (EEG): Test that measures the electrical activity of the brain

Electronic health record (EHR): Confidential patient health record that providers or a hospital keeps on a computer

Electronic prescriptions: Prescriptions that are written up on a computer and sent directly to the pharmacy

Endoscope: A device that looks at areas inside the body and removes cells or tissues

Endoscopy: Invasive procedure that lets a health care provider look inside a patient's body

Fasting plasma glucose test: Test that measures the level of sugar in the blood

Fecal occult blood test (FOBT): Test that checks for blood in the stool

Flexible sigmoidoscopy: Procedure that sees inside the sigmoid colon and rectum

Genetic counseling: Information and support for people who have or are at risk for a genetic disease

Genetic disease, or hereditary or inherited disease: Disease caused by a defect or defects in a person's genetic makeup brought about by genetic mutations that run in families

Genetic mutation: An abnormal gene

Genetic tests: Tests done on blood and other tissue to find genetic diseases

Health screening: Test or procedure that is essential to preventive medicine

Histologic test: Test that examines tissue cells and structure for health problems

Human papillomavirus (HPV): Virus that causes most cervical cancers

Hysterectomy: Surgery that removes the uterus and cervix

Inflammation: A reaction in the body that causes the affected area to become sore, red, or swollen

Inflammatory disease: A disease caused by a body's reaction to injuries or infection with inflammation, meaning that the affected area becomes sore, red, or swollen

Inspection: The provider's visual review of a patient's body or body part

Invasive: Characteristic of a test or procedure that invades the patient's body and can cause pain

Laparoscopy: Procedure that allows a surgeon to see and operate on the abdomen and pelvis areas

Localized disease: A disease that affects only one part of the body

Magnetic resonance imaging (MRI): Magnetic field and radio waves that make images of body organs and structures

Mammogram: X-ray picture of the breast

Metabolic disease: Abnormality in the body's metabolism

Metabolism: Chemical process that takes place in the cells and the fluids of the body, enabling the body to get or produce energy from food

Neoplasm: An abnormal tissue mass caused by an abnormal growth of cells

Neoplastic disease: Disease involving neoplasms that can be harmless or that can be malignant and cause cancer

Noninvasive: Characteristic of a test or procedure that causes little or no pain for the patient

Oral glucose tolerance test: Test that measures the body's ability to use glucose

Osteoporosis: Thinning of bone tissue and loss of bone density over time

Palpation: Procedure in which the health care provider uses his or her fingers and hands to touch and feel the patient's body to examine an organ or body part

Pap smear test: Test for cervical cancer and abnormal cells

Pelvic exam: Examination of a woman's reproductive organs

Percussion: Method of tapping body parts with fingers, hands, or small instruments

Physical examination: The examination of a patient's body to see whether there are health problems

Positron emission tomography (PET) scan: Scan that uses a radioactive substance to show changes in tissues, organs, and structures

Preventive medicine: Medical actions that a person can take to prevent a disease

Prognosis: A health care provider's opinion of how the patient's disease will develop

Prostate-specific antigen (PSA): Protein produced by the cells of the prostate gland

PSA blood test: Test that measures the level of PSA in the blood

Radiograph: X-ray image that is recorded on a film

Refraction test: Eye exam that measures whether a person needs a prescription for eyeglasses or contact lenses

Scan: X-ray taken with a machine that uses a computer to make detailed pictures of the inside of the body

Sign: Evidence of a disease that can be observed during a physical examination

Speculum: Device that opens the vagina

Symptom: What the patient reports to be experiencing and that cannot be measured by medical tests and procedures

Systemic disease: A disease that affects the entire body

Tracer: Radioactive material mixed with sugar

Tumor: A neoplasm that has formed into a lump

Ultrasound, or sonogram: Procedure in which sound waves create pictures of the patient's organs, which are projected on a screen

Urinalysis: Physical, chemical, and microscopic examination of urine

Virtual colonoscopy: Colonoscopy that is done with an X-ray machine

CHAPTER ACTIVITIES

1. Your class will identify and invite a health care provider from the community to speak to the class about diagnostic tests and procedures that he or she performs. Prepare one to three questions to ask the health care provider about a specific diagnostic tool.

2. You have been recently hired by a public health department located in a seaside resort. Your job responsibility is to develop a community-wide skin cancer health awareness campaign. Brainstorm in small groups five strategies that promote skin cancer prevention. The strategies can target the individual, family, school/workplace, and community.

3. Identify three phone and/or iPad apps that explain diagnostic tests and procedures. Compare and contrast the qualities of each app (e.g., cost, ease of use and readability, visuals, source) from a patient's perspective.

4. With a partner, write a script for a short YouTube clip or commercial recommending dental exams for adults and children. As part of the script, discuss the benefits of daily brushing and flossing of teeth in preventing cavities and gum disease.

5. There is debate in the medical community concerning the recommendations for certain cancer screenings, such as PSA tests and mammograms. Select a screening and write a two- to three-page paper on its pros and cons. On the basis of your research, what are your recommendations about the screening? Be prepared to present your findings and recommendation in class discussions.

Bibliography and Works Cited

Ackley, B. J., & Ladwig, G. B. (2014). *Nursing diagnosis handbook: An evidence-based guide to planning care* (10th ed.) Maryland Heights, MO: Elsevier.

American Association for Clinical Chemistry. (2015). Understanding your tests. *Lab Tests Online.* Retrieved from https://labtestsonline.org/understanding/

American Board of Medical Specialties. (2016a). *ABMS guide to medical specialties.* Maryland Heights, MO: Elsevier. Retrieved from https://www.abmsdirectory.com/pdf/Resources_guide_physicians.pdf

American Board of Medical Specialties. (2016b). Specialty and subspecialty certificates. Retrieved from http://www.abms.org/member-boards/specialty-subspecialty-certificates/

American Cancer Society. (2015). American Cancer Society guidelines for the early detection of cancer. Retrieved from http://www.cancer.org/healthy/findcancerearly/cancerscreeningguidelines/american-cancer-society-guidelines-for-the-early-detection-of-cancer

Centers for Disease Control and Prevention. (2015). CDC prevention checklist: Preventive care: Everyone needs an ounce of prevention. Retrieved from http://www.cdc.gov/prevention/

Llewelyn, H., Ang, H. A., Lewis, K. E., & Al-Abdullah, A. (2014). *Oxford handbook of clinical diagnosis* (3rd ed.) Oxford, England: Oxford University Press.

National Cancer Institute. (2011). How to check your skin for skin cancer. Retrieved from https://www.cancer.gov/types/skin/self-exam

National Cancer Institute. (2015). Colorectal cancer screening (PDQ®)–Patient version. Retrieved from https://www.cancer.gov/types/colorectal/patient/colorectal-screening-pdq#section/_13

National Heart, Lung and Blood Institute. (2012). What are blood tests? Retrieved from http://www.nhlbi.nih.gov/health/health-topics/topics/bdt/

National Institute of Diabetes and Digestive and Kidney Diseases. (2014). Medical tests for prostate problems. Retrieved from https://www.niddk.nih.gov/health-information/health-topics/diagnostic-tests/Medical%20tests-prostate-problems/Pages/medical-tests-prostate-problems.aspx

Nemours Foundation. (2016). Medical tests and exams. *KidsHealth.* Retrieved from https://kidshealth.org/en/parents/system/medical?ref=search

Nicoll, D., Lu, C. M., Pignone, M., & McPhee, S. J. (2012). *Pocket guide to diagnostic tests.* Columbus, OH: McGraw-Hill Education.

Porter, R. S., Kaplan, J. L., & Albert, R. K. (2011). *The Merck manual of diagnosis and therapy* (19th ed.). Whitehouse Station, NJ: Merck Sharp & Dohme.

Thompson, M. J., & Van den Bruel, A. (2011). *Diagnostic tests toolkit* (EBM toolkit series). Oxford, England: Wiley-Blackwell. doi:10.1002/9781119951827

US National Library of Medicine. (2016a). Diagnostic tests. *MedlinePlus.* Retrieved from https://www.nlm.nih .gov/medlineplus/diagnostictests.html

US National Library of Medicine. (2016b). What is genetic testing? *Genetics home reference.* Retrieved from https://ghr.nlm.nih.gov/primer/testing/genetictesting

US Preventive Services Task Force. (2016). *Published recommendations.* Retrieved from https://www .uspreventiveservicestaskforce.org/BrowseRec/Index

WebMD. (2016). Annual physical examinations. Retrieved from http://www.webmd.com/a-to-z-guides/annual -physical-examinations#1-2

PART 2

HUMAN DISEASES FROM A SYSTEMIC APPROACH

IMMUNE SYSTEM AND RELATED DISEASES

CHAPTER OBJECTIVES

- Define and explain antigens and antibodies.

- Describe the structure and function of the immune system.

- Identify types and functions of selected immune cells.

- Compare and contrast natural, active, and passive immunity.

- Review causes, signs, and symptoms as well as treatment of selected immune deficiency and autoimmune diseases.

- Review causes, signs, and symptoms as well as treatment of select allergies.

The immune system is the body's major defense against foreign microorganisms and other harmful substances. The immune system's job is to keep out these "invaders" or, failing that, to seek out and destroy them. In most cases, the immune system does a skillful job of keeping people healthy and preventing diseases. But sometimes problems with the immune system lead to a group of illnesses referred to as immunological diseases.

Immune System Function

The human body protects itself against disease-causing microorganisms, called pathogens. *Pathogens,* or germs, are infectious agents: bacteria, viruses, fungi, and parasites. The *immune system,* a network of specific organs, tissues, vessels, and cells, is the body's way of protecting itself. This network works to defend the body against pathogens and other harmful substances, such as poisons, and foreign objects, for example a splinter lodged in the skin. The network's job is to keep out these invaders or, failing that, to seek out and destroy them itself.

The immune system is complex. It can recognize and remember millions of different pathogens, as well as release *secretions*, or fluids, and cells to wipe them out. The system owes its success to its communication network. Millions of cells,

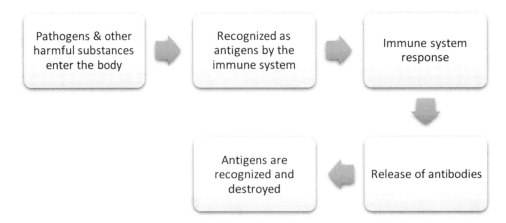

Figure 10.1 The Immune Response

organized into groups and subgroups, gather and pass information back and forth in response to any changes in the body. Once immune cells receive the alarm, they make chemicals. These chemicals enable the immune cells to regulate their own growth and behavior, enlist other immune cells, and direct the new recruits to infected areas.

The immune system protects the body by recognizing and destroying antigens. *Antigens* are any substance recognized as foreign by the immune system. When the immune system defends itself against antigens, the defense is known as an *immune response*. In an immune response, antibodies are released to attack the antigens. Antibodies, or immunoglobulins, are proteins naturally present in the body (see Figure 10.1).

The most common antigens are bacteria, viruses, and parasites. Each antigen uses different tactics to infect a person and each requires a unique immune response. Most bacteria live in the spaces between cells. Viruses, along with a few types of bacteria and parasites, must enter cells to survive, whereas parasites live either inside or outside cells.

Immune System Structure

Antigens that try to get into the body must first move past the body's external barriers, which are the skin and the cells that line the body's internal passageways. The skin, an important part of the immune system, is tough and sealed off to antigens except when it is cut, burned, or scratched. The skin also secretes antibacterial substances that destroy most antigens that land on it.

The respiratory and digestive systems also protect against antigens. Antigens that enter the nose meet up with protective mucus. In addition, attempts to enter the nose or lungs trigger a sneeze or cough that forces antigens out of the respiratory passageways. The stomach contains a strong acid that destroys antigens that are swallowed with food.

If antigens survive the body's frontline defenses, they still have to find a way through the walls of the digestive, respiratory, genital, or urological passageways to the underlying cells. These passageways are lined with cells covered in mucus that block antigens from getting into deeper cell layers.

Once an antigen does make it inside the body, it has to fight with the immune system. The immune system has its own circulatory system, called the *lymphatic system*. The lymphatic system is a network of organs, vessels, tissues, and cells that keeps away infection and balances the body's fluids. It is supported in its tasks by being inter-connected with the cardiovascular system via the flow of blood in and out of arteries, into the veins, and through the lymphatic system. The following are the organs of the lymphatic system (see Figure 10.2):

Bone marrow Soft tissue in the hollow center of bones. It is the ultimate source of all blood cells, including the immune cells.

Tonsils Clumps of tissue that are located in the back of the mouth. They recognize antigens that enter the body via air or food.

Thymus A gland that lies in the lower part of the neck, between the breastbone and your heart. It is responsible for making immune cells.

Spleen An organ at the left of the abdomen, near the stomach. It's the largest of the lymphoid organs and has chambers where immune cells gather and confront antigens. It filters the blood, looking for antigens; makes white blood cells; stores blood cells; and destroys old blood cells.

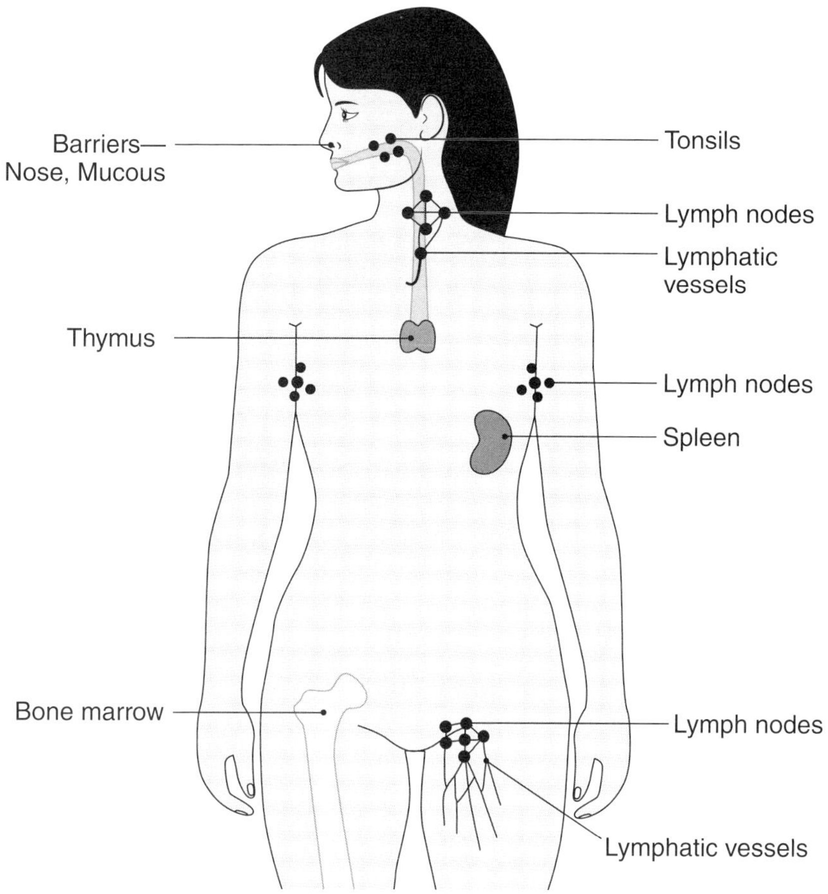

Lymph nodes Small, bean-shaped glands, lymph nodes cluster in the neck, armpits, and groin, and inside the chest and abdomen. There are more than 100 lymph nodes in the body, and they contain filtering tissue along with a large number of immune cells. Like the spleen, these nodes are where immune cells fight antigens. Swelling or inflammation of these nodes is a response to antigens.

Figure 10.2 Organs of the Immune System

Note. Reproduced with permission from the National Institute on Aging and the National Institute of Allergy and Infectious Diseases, 2015.

Retrieved from https://www.nia.nih.gov/health/publication/biology-aging/immune-system-can-your-immune-system-still-defend-you-you-age

The lymph nodes filter *lymph*, a clear fluid that contains white blood cells as well as proteins and fats that defend against antigens. Lymph seeps outside the blood vessels into body tissues then passes through the lymph nodes before being put back into the blood via a large vein just below the neck.

The organs of the immune system are connected with one another and with other organs by a network of lymphatic vessels, which are thin tubes that carry lymph. The immune cells travel through the lymphatic vessels, which run along the body's circulatory system. Lymphatic vessels are present wherever there are blood vessels. Cells and fluids are exchanged between blood and lymphatic vessels, allowing the lymphatic system to monitor the body for antigens. Lymphatic vessels carry lymph without the "pumping" action of the circulatory system; instead, fluids ooze into the lymph system and get pushed by normal body and muscle motion to the lymph nodes.

Lymphatic tissue is scattered throughout the body and is home to immune cells. Immune cells are packed into tissue clusters in the walls of parts of the body that are often exposed to antigens. These sites include the gastrointestinal system as well as the tonsils, adenoids, and appendix. In addition to these sites, clumps of lymphatic tissue are found in the lungs.

Cells of the Immune System

The immune system has different ways of fighting antigens. One way is to stockpile a huge number of immune cells. A *cell* is the smallest unit of life and is the basis of all plant, animal, and human tissue.

Blood cells, including immune cells, are made in the bone marrow. Bone marrow is like a factory, mass-producing red and white blood cells. The marrow makes blood cells from *stem cells*, so named because they can branch off and become many different types of cells.

Some of the immune cells attack all antigens; others are designed for specific targets. When there are no antigens, the immune system stores just a few of each type of immune cell. If an antigen does appear, the few immune cells that respond to it mushroom into an army of cells. After their job is done, most of the immune cells fade away, leaving a few cells behind to watch for future attacks.

It is *leukocytes*, or white blood cells, that are key to the immune system. Leukocytes are not like normal cells in the body because they are independent, living single-cell organisms and can move and capture antigens on their own. They behave like a moving blob and swallow up other cells.

There are different types of leukocytes, and they work together to destroy antigens. The most common are presented in the following list:

Types of Leukocytes

    Lymphocytes

    B-cells

    T-cells

    Killer T-cells

    Helper T-cells

    Regulatory T-cells

    Phagocytes

    Neutrophils

    Complements

Each type of leukocyte has a special role in the immune system. Regardless of the type, however, communication among them becomes critical. Sometimes leukocytes communicate by physical contact, and sometimes they communicate by chemical signals. The following description gives an overview of leukocytes and how they protect the body from antigens.

Lymphocytes have multiple functions, such as making antibodies that recognize and remember previous antigens (e.g., bacteria, viruses, and toxins) and then destroy them. They also destroy the body's own cells that have themselves been taken over by antigens or become cancerous. Lymphocytes travel throughout the body via the circulatory and lymphatic systems, patrolling everywhere for antigens. As lymphocytes develop, they learn to tell the difference between body tissues and those antigens not normally found in the body.

There are two types of lymphocytes, *B-cells* and *T-cells*. Lymphocytes start out in bone marrow, and they either stay there and mature into B-cells or migrate through the bloodstream to the thymus and mature there, becoming T-cells (*T* stands for "thymus"). When mature, T-cells leave the thymus and travel to other tissues.

B-cells and T-cells are found in the bloodstream, but tend to concentrate in some of the lymphatic organs and tissues, such as the lymph nodes, thymus, spleen, bone marrow, and lymphatic vessels. They are also found in the digestive system. Once B-cells and T-cells are formed, a few of those cells multiply and provide "memory" for the immune system. This enables the immune system to respond faster and more efficiently the next time the body is exposed to the same antigen.

B-cells and T-cells have different functions. Each specific B-cell is tuned in to a specific antigen, and when that antigen is in the body, the B-cell clones itself and produces millions of antibodies designed to eliminate that antigen.

T-cells contribute to immune defenses in two major ways. First, they direct and regulate immune responses; second, they directly attack and kill antigens. A way to think about the difference between B-cells and T-cells is that B-cells are like the body's spy system, seeking out their targets and sending defenses to lock onto them. T-cells are like the soldiers, destroying the antigens that the B-cell spies on.

There are three kinds of T-cells: killer, helper, and regulatory:

Killer T-cells help rid the body of antigens. They directly attack and kill antigens on contact using lethal chemicals. These cells are also responsible for the rejection of tissue and organ grafts.

Helper T-cells coordinate immune responses by communicating with and activating other cells, including B-cells and other T-cells.

Regulatory T-cells tell the B-cells and other T-cells when the body is healthy again and they can stop attacking antigens.

B-cells, when stimulated, mature into *plasma cells*—these are the cells that make antibodies. An *antibody, or immunoglobulin*, is a blood protein made by the body's immune system that helps fight a specific antigen.

As noted, each B-cell makes one specific antibody. For example, one B-cell makes an antibody that blocks a cold virus; another makes an antibody that attacks bacteria that cause pneumonia. Each type of antibody is unique and defends the body against one specific type of antigen.

Antibodies are Y-shaped proteins. They have a special section (at the tips of the two branches of the Y) that is sensitive to a specific antigen and locks on to it. Antibodies mill around a lymph node, then lock on antigens circulating in the bloodstream. They are not capable of destroying antigens without help, however—that's the job of T-cells. Antibodies can also cancel out the negative effects of poisons and other damaging substances made by different organisms. Lastly, antibodies can activate a group of proteins called the complement (discussed later in this section), which is also part of the immune system. There are five categories of antibodies; each has specific functions:

- Immunoglobulin A (IgA)—in bodily fluids; guards the entrances to the body
- Immunoglobulin D (IgD)—helps start early B-cell responses and regulates the cell's activation
- Immunoglobulin E (IgE)—normally present in only small amounts; protects against parasites and is responsible for allergy symptoms
- Immunoglobulin G (IgG)—travels in the blood to coat antigens
- Immunoglobulin M (IgM)—kills bacteria and protects blood from infection

Another type of leukocyte is the phagocyte. *Phagocytes* swallow and digest antigens as well as send signals to other phagocytes. Some phagocytes circulate in the blood; others migrate into tissues. Specialized types of phagocytes are found in many organs, including the lungs, kidneys, brain, and liver.

There are different cells that are considered phagocytes. The most common is a *neutrophil*. The bone marrow makes trillions of neutrophils every day and releases them into the bloodstream, but their life span is short—generally less than a day.

Neutrophils are attracted to inflammation and bacteria. They circulate in the blood, but move into the site of infection in large numbers and release chemicals. At a site of serious infection, where lots of bacteria have reproduced in the area, pus will form. *Pus, or purulent,* is simply dead neutrophils and other cellular debris. Sometimes it forms into a *pustule,* known as a blister or pimple, filled with pus.

The last protector is the complement. The *complement* is a cluster of about 25 proteins working together to protect against antigens. The complement cluster floats freely in blood and works with antibodies and phagocytes to help get rid of antigens faster.

Complements are manufactured in the liver. When the first protein in the complement cluster is activated, it sets an attack in motion. Complements cause bursting of cells and signal to phagocytes that a cell needs to be removed. Complement proteins, which cause blood vessels to become dilated and then leaky, contribute to the redness, warmth, swelling, pain, and loss of function that characterize an *inflammatory response.*

In summary, the basic cells in the immune system are antibodies (immunoglobulins) made in B-cells, three kinds of T-cells (killer, helper, and regulatory/suppressor), phagocytes (e.g., neutrophils), and complements.

For an example of how these immune cells communicate and work together, consider what happens when a virus enters a person's body. If a virus gets past the first barriers of the immune system (e.g., the mouth or nose), then the body responds by activating an immune response. First, the body recognizes the virus as an antigen and pushes it, via the respiratory and circulatory systems, into the lymphatic system, where a phagocyte ingests but does not kill it. Then the phagocyte displays the antigens on its own exterior. The antigens chemically alert a helper T-cell. Next, the helper T-cell chemically sounds an alarm for more immune cells to respond. A B-cell responds (with antibodies for a virus) to this alarm and comes to read the antigen. This B-cell then is activated and makes millions of antibodies that are specific to the antigen. The antibodies attach to the virus and hold on tight. The antibodies then send an alarm to other phagocytes and T-cells to come and kill the virus.

The last stage of the immune response is the responsibility of the regulatory T-cells. Once the number of antigens has dropped significantly and the virus is killed, regulatory T-cells signal other immune cells to rest. This is an important step because extended activity of an immune response could lead to the damage of healthy cells (see Figure 10.3).

Self and Non-Self Immune Response

A healthy immune system has the ability to tell the difference between the body's own cells, known as "self," and foreign antigens known as "non-self." There is a peaceful coexistence among cells that carry "self" markers. But when these cells meet up with antigens carrying markers that say "non-self," they quickly launch an immune response and attack.

How do immune cells know what to attack and what to leave alone? Each of the cells in the body has *human leukocyte antigen* (HLA) that marks the cell as self, and each person bears a slightly unique set. The immune system learns to see these body cells as normal and usually does not react against them. Anything that the immune system finds that does not have these markings is definitely non-self and is therefore fair game for an attack.

In the case of what are known as *autoimmune diseases,* the immune system mistakes self for non-self and attacks the body's own cells. In other cases, the immune cells respond to a seemingly harmless foreign antigen, such as ragweed pollen, and launches a full attack. The result is an allergy, and this kind of antigen is called an *allergen.* Cells from another person (except an identical twin) also carry non-self markers and act as antigens.

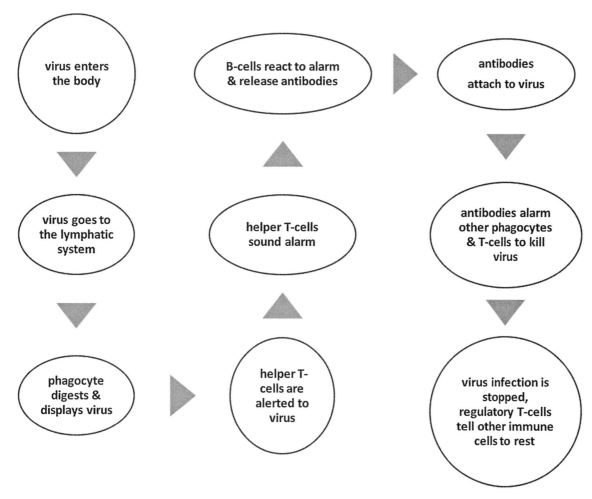

Figure 10.3 Immune Response to Virus Infection

Immunity and Immunizations

Antibodies create *immunity*, or protection against diseases. Antibodies are disease specific; for example, a measles antibody protects a person from measles, but not mumps.

Immunity can be strong or weak, short lived or long lasting, depending on several factors: the type and amount of antigen, how the antigen enters the body, and an individual's genetic makeup. When faced with the same antigen, some patients' response is strong, others' is weak, and some is nonexistent.

Because everyone's immune system is different, some people never seem to get infections, whereas others seem to be sick all the time. As people age, they usually become immune to more antigens because they have come into contact with more of them over the years. That's why adults tend to get fewer colds than children: Their bodies have learned to recognize and immediately attack many of the viruses that cause colds.

Three Types of Immunity

There are three types of immunity: natural, active, and passive (see Figure 10.4).

Everyone is born with *natural immunity*, a general protection. Natural immunity involves barriers that keep antigens from entering the body. These barriers—cough, tears, mucus, skin, and stomach acid—form the first defense in the immune response.

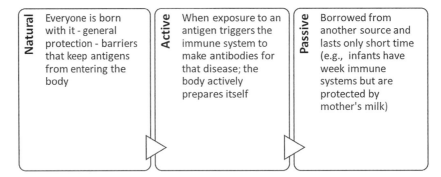

Figure 10.4 Three Types of Immunity

The second kind of protection is *active immunity*, which develops over time as people are exposed to diseases or are immunized or vaccinated against diseases; the body's immune system "actively" prepares itself for future challenges. As discussed earlier, exposure to an antigen triggers the immune system to make antibodies targeted to that disease. If an immune person comes into contact with that disease in the future, his or her immune system recognizes it and will immediately make the antibodies needed to fight it. Active immunity can be lifelong.

As part of active immunity, an *immunization, or vaccination*, gives the body a disease-specific antigen that doesn't make the person sick but allows the body to make antibodies. These antibodies protect against future attacks from that specific disease. A vaccination is a weakened form of a disease—that is, either a killed form of the disease or a similar but less potent strain. Once the vaccination is inside the body, the immune system starts to attack, but because the disease is different or weaker, there are few or no symptoms. Now, when the real disease invades the body, the immune system is able to get rid of it immediately (see Figure 10.5). For example, a polio vaccine does not give a person polio, but it allows the body to make antibodies that will protect that person from future exposure to polio.

Immunizations are one of the best ways to prevent infectious diseases, and vaccines have an excellent safety record. The Centers for Disease Control and Prevention (CDC, 2014b) recommend immunizations throughout the life span; however, immunizations work best at specific ages. Although some parents are against childhood immunizations, there is scientific evidence supporting the benefits of vaccinating children in particular. According to the CDC (2014b):

- If an unvaccinated child is exposed to a disease, the child's body may not be strong enough to fight it. Before vaccines, many children died from diseases that vaccines now prevent, such as whooping cough, measles, and polio. Those same germs exist today, but because babies are protected by vaccines, we don't see these diseases nearly as often.

- Immunizing individual children also helps protect the health of our community, especially those people who cannot be immunized, such as children who are too young to be vaccinated or the people who don't respond to a particular vaccine.

- Vaccine-preventable diseases are costly; they result in physician visits, hospitalizations, and premature deaths. Sick children can also cause parents to lose time from work.

Passive immunity is immunity "borrowed" from another source, and it usually lasts only a few weeks or months. For example, infants are born with weak immune systems, but are protected for the first few months of life by antibodies in their mother's breast milk. These antibodies protect a baby's digestive tract and help defend the baby against infection for up to 12 months. This is passive immunity

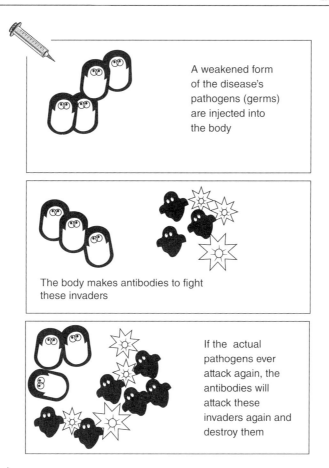

Figure 10.5 How Vaccines Work

Note. Adapted from "Vaccines & Immunizations," by Centers for Disease Control and Prevention, n.d., http://www.cdc.gov/vaccines/vac-gen
/howvpd.htm

because the infant who is protected does not make antibodies but borrows them from his or her mother.

Stress and the Immune System

Smoking, obesity, surgery, infections, and trauma all put stress on the body and weaken the immune system. With stress exposure, the nervous system activates immune responses that help the body maintain balance. However, when stress is excessive and long lasting, it negatively impacts the immune response and leaves the body vulnerable to diseases. The quality, intensity, and length of a stressful experience determine the effect that stress has on the immune system.

Age and the Immune System

A healthy young person's body is like a T-cell factory, able to fight off an antigen with a powerful immune response. As mentioned earlier, the immune response is not as powerful in older adults because they make fewer T-cells and fewer antibodies. Immune cells also lose some of their ability to communicate with each other.

A weakened immune response makes older adults less responsive to immunizations. Even though immunizations may not work as well, however, immunizations against influenza, pneumonia, hepatitis B, tuberculosis, diphtheria, and tetanus still can decrease death rates in older adults. There are ongoing research efforts to develop other immunizations that respond to age-related changes in the immune system.

As people age, they tend to have mild, chronic inflammation, which is associated with an increased risk for heart disease, arthritis, type 2 diabetes, physical disability, and dementia. Understanding the underlying risks for and causes of chronic inflammation in older adults—and why some older adults do not have this problem—will help health care providers find better ways to treat its associated diseases.

Age-related negative changes to the immune system are known as *immunosenescence*. A lifetime of stress on our bodies is thought to contribute to immunosenescence. Radiation, chemical exposure, and exposure to certain diseases also speed up the deterioration of the immune system. Research is still needed to better understand immunosenescence and to determine which areas of the immune system are most vulnerable to aging (National Institute on Aging, 2015).

Immunological Diseases

Immunological diseases, or diseases of the immune system, fall into five main categories (see Figure 10.6):

1. *Immune deficiency diseases:* Resistance to diseases becomes dangerously low.

2. *Autoimmune diseases:* The body's immune system attacks its own cells and tissues by mistake.

3. *Allergies or hypersensitivities:* Immune responses overreact to substances that are usually harmless.

4. *Cancers of the immune system:* Cells of the immune system grow out of control.

5. *Graft-versus-host disease:* The immune system rejects an organ transplant and causes a life-threatening reaction.

The next sections discuss each of these five categories.

Immune Deficiency Diseases

The importance of the immune system is evident in patients born with an immune system that is inadequate or that doesn't work at all. These patients are infected easily, and the consequences can be

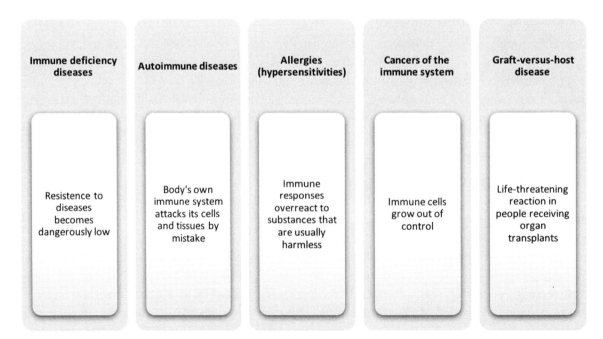

Figure 10.6 Five Main Categories of Immune System Diseases

fatal. When the immune system is missing one or more of its parts, the result is an *immune deficiency disease, or immunodeficiency disease.*

Sometimes a person is born with an immune deficiency, although symptoms might not appear until later in life. Immune deficiency can also be caused by an infection or occur as a side effect of drugs. Organ transplants, chemotherapy, blood transfusions, surgery, malnutrition, smoking, and stress can also cause an immune deficiency. Some patients can have temporary immune deficiency caused by virus infections, including influenza, infectious mononucleosis, and measles. The severity of immune deficiency disease symptoms depends on the type of cells affected. These diseases can range from a manageable chronic infection to a life-threatening condition. The following are two examples of immune deficiency diseases.

IgA Deficiency

IgA is an immunoglobulin found primarily in saliva and other body fluids, and it helps guard the entrances to the body. If the body doesn't make enough IgA, the deficiency causes food and other allergies, or an increased number of respiratory infections. *IgA deficiency* is the most common immune deficiency disease, but the condition is usually not severe. There is no cure or prevention for IgA deficiency, although some patients can suddenly begin to make IgA. Those patients with IgA deficiency need to avoid infections, eat healthy diets, get adequate rest, and have regular follow-up care.

Human Immunodeficiency Virus Infection (HIV)/ Acquired Immunodeficiency Syndrome (AIDS)

The *human immunodeficiency virus (HIV)* is a virus that wipes out vital helper T-cells. Without helper T-cells, the immune system is unable to defend the body against normally harmless organisms. These organisms can cause life-threatening infections in people with HIV and *acquired immunodeficiency syndrome (AIDS).* Patients with HIV have symptoms similar to those born without immune systems. As HIV weakens the immune system, a person develops AIDS and has unusual, often life-threatening infections and rare cancers.

People become infected with HIV by having unprotected sexual intercourse with an infected person or from sharing contaminated needles. Newborns can get HIV infection from their infected mothers while in the uterus, during the birth process, or during breastfeeding.

Some patients develop signs and symptoms within days of the infection; others may not have any signs or symptoms for up to 10 years. The long period without signs and symptoms increases the risk of spreading the disease to others because a person might not know he or she has the disease. Some of the symptoms of HIV infection are swollen glands, weight loss, fatigue, flu-like symptoms, and night sweats.

HIV/AIDS is caused by a retrovirus (a type of virus), and the medications to treat this retrovirus are called antiretroviral. These medications control the virus and slow the progression of HIV infection, but they do not cure it.

Autoimmune Diseases

With an *autoimmune disease*, the immune system mistakenly attacks the body's healthy organs, tissues, and cells as though they were antigens. At the core of the immune system is the ability to tell the difference between what's you and what's foreign (or, as discussed earlier, self and non-self). Sometimes, the body is unable to tell the difference, and when this happens, the body makes *autoantibodies* that attack normal cells by mistake. At the same time, T-cells fail to do their job of keeping the immune system healthy. The result is a misguided attack on the body. Healthy organs, tissues, and cells are destroyed, which leaves the body unable to perform important daily functions.

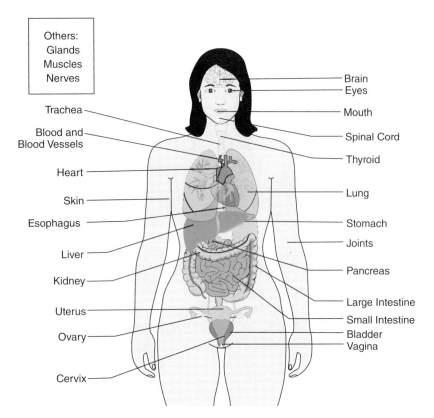

Others:
Glands
Muscles
Nerves

Trachea
Blood and Blood Vessels
Heart
Skin
Esophagus
Liver
Kidney
Uterus
Ovary
Cervix

Brain
Eyes
Mouth
Spinal Cord
Thyroid
Lung
Stomach
Joints
Pancreas
Large Intestine
Small Intestine
Bladder
Vagina

Figure 10.7 Body Parts Affected by Autoimmune Diseases

Autoimmune diseases are serious and chronic, and affect almost all the parts of the body (see Figure 10.7). There are more than 80 known types, and some have similar symptoms. Although each disease is unique, many share the first warnings of illness, such as fatigue, dizziness, muscle aches, and fever. This makes it hard for providers to diagnose these diseases, which can be frustrating and stressful for patients.

Autoimmune diseases are common, affecting more than 23.5 million Americans, and are a leading cause of death and disability. It is unknown what causes an autoimmune disease, but many factors are involved, including the following:

Gender More women than men have autoimmune diseases, which often start during their childbearing years.

Family history Some autoimmune diseases run in families, so inheriting certain genes makes it more likely to get an autoimmune disease.

Environmental exposure Certain environmental exposures may cause or worsen some autoimmune diseases. Sunlight, chemicals, and infections are linked to many autoimmune diseases.

Race or ethnic background Some autoimmune diseases are more common and more severe in certain racial and ethnic groups than in others.

For many autoimmune diseases, symptoms can come and go and can vary in severity at different times. When symptoms go away for a while or disappear, the patient is said to be in *remission*. The diseases may also have *flares*, or sudden and severe symptoms. Autoimmune diseases are chronic and do not usually go away, but symptoms can be treated. Some autoimmune diseases are described elsewhere in this book, but an overview of the following common autoimmune diseases is in this section:

- Alopecia areata
- Celiac disease
- Type 1 diabetes
- Guillain-Barre syndrome
- Multiple sclerosis (MS)
- Myasthenia gravis (MG)
- Rheumatoid arthritis (RA)
- Juvenile rheumatoid arthritis (JRA)
- Scleroderma
- Lupus

Alopecia areata is caused by the immune system attacking hair follicles (the structures from which hair grows). It usually is not serious; however, it can affect the way a person looks. In most cases, hair falls out in small, round patches the size of a quarter. Some patients do lose more hair, but rarely is there total loss of hair on the head or on other parts of the body.

Anyone can have alopecia, and it often starts in childhood. There is a slight increase of risk of having the disease if a family member has it. Unfortunately, there is no cure for alopecia, and there are no medications approved to treat it. Health care providers may use medications approved for other diseases to help the hair grow back.

Celiac disease is a genetic disease that limits the body's ability to break down certain foods that contain gluten. Gluten is found mainly in wheat, rye, and barley and in some prepared foods, but can also be found in other products, such as in some medications. With celiac disease, the immune system responds abnormally or overreacts to ingested gluten. The immune system's abnormal response can cause damage to the linings of the small intestine. Because the small intestine is responsible for absorbing the nutrients in food, damage to the lining interferes with absorption. Celiac disease affects each person differently, and symptoms can occur in the digestive system or in other parts of the body. For example, one patient might have diarrhea and stomach pain; another might be anxious or depressed. Other symptoms are constipation, weight loss or gain, fatigue, skin rash, missed menstrual periods, and infertility. Some patients have no symptoms. Blood tests as well as a small piece of tissue, or biopsy, from the small intestine can help diagnose the disease. Although celiac disease cannot be cured, avoiding gluten usually stops the damage and associated symptoms.

Type 1 diabetes is a disease caused by the immune system attacking the cells in the pancreas that make insulin, a hormone that is needed to control glucose (sugar) levels in the blood. When the cells that make insulin are attacked, then the pancreas cannot make insulin. Without insulin, there is too much glucose that stays in the blood. Too much glucose can hurt the eyes, kidneys, nerves, gums, and teeth, but the most serious problem caused by type 1 diabetes is heart disease.

A blood test detects type 1 diabetes; if the test is positive, then the patient needs to take insulin for the rest of his or her life. Type 1 diabetes occurs most often in children and young adults, but it can appear at any age. The following are some of the symptoms of type 1 diabetes (National Institute of Arthritis and Musculoskeletal and Skin Diseases, 2016):

- Extreme thirst
- Frequent urination
- Extreme hunger or fatigue
- Unintended weight loss
- Sores that heal slowly
- Dry, itchy skin
- Loss of feeling (numbness) in the feet
- Blurry vision

Guillain-Barre syndrome causes the immune system to attack the nerves that connect the brain and spinal cord with the rest of the body. Damage to the nerves makes it hard for them to transmit signals, causing muscles to have trouble responding to the brain. The cause of this syndrome is unknown. Sometimes it is triggered by an infection, surgery, or a vaccination. The first symptom is usually weakness or a tingling feeling in the legs, which can spread to the upper body. Symptoms usually worsen over a period of weeks, then stabilize. In severe cases, Guillain-Barre syndrome can cause paralysis and be life threatening; some patients need a respirator to breathe.

Most patients do recover, however; recovery can take a few weeks to a few years. Treatment options include medications or a procedure called plasma exchange. In *plasma exchange*, whole blood is withdrawn from the person, the plasma is removed from the blood and replaced, and then the blood is transfused back into the person.

The causes of *multiple sclerosis (MS)* are unknown. MS is a disease in which the immune system attacks and damages the coating around the nerves called the myelin sheath. This damage affects the brain and spinal cord, blocking or slowing down messages between the brain and the body. MS affects women more than men and it usually begins between the ages of 20 and 40. The disease is often mild, but some patients lose the ability to write, speak, or walk. There is no cure for MS, but medications can slow it down and help control symptoms. Physical and occupational therapy can also help. Symptoms depend on the location and extent of each attack, but they often include the following (Office of Women's Health, 2011):

- Problems with vision and speech
- Muscle weakness, causing trouble with coordination and balance
- Numbness and tingling
- Thinking and memory issues
- Tremors
- Paralysis

Myasthenia gravis (MG) is a disease where the immune system makes abnormal antibodies that block or change the nerve signals to the muscles. The blocked signals create a communication problem between nerves and muscles. Common symptoms are weak muscles, difficult motor coordination, and drooping head. A patient can also experience trouble with vision, facial expression, talking, and swallowing. The MG weakness gets worse with activity but better with rest.

There are medications that keep the body from making abnormal antibodies and help strengthen muscles. Treatments can also filter abnormal antibodies from the blood or add healthy antibodies from donated blood. Sometimes surgery to remove the thymus gland can also help.

If patients with MG follow their treatment plan, they can expect a normal life, or close to it. MG can also go into temporary or permanent remission, during which time patients do not need treatments.

Rheumatoid arthritis (RA) occurs when the immune system attacks joint tissues and causes inflammation. As RA progresses, the surrounding muscles, ligaments, and tendons that support and stabilize joints become weak and unable to work. RA can affect any joint tissue, but it is common in the wrist and fingers. RA can also affect other body parts besides joint tissue, such as the eyes, mouth, and lungs. More women than men get RA, and it often starts between ages 25 and 55. The disease can last for only a short time, or symptoms might come and go. The severe form of RA can last a lifetime.

The cause of RA is unknown, but genes, environment, and hormones might contribute. Treatments include medications, lifestyle changes, and surgery that can slow or stop joint damage and reduce pain and swelling. The following are some of the symptoms of RA:

- Painful, stiff, swollen, and deformed joints
- Reduced motion
- Eye inflammation
- Lumps of tissue under the skin, often at the elbows
- Anemia

Juvenile rheumatoid arthritis (JRA) is a type of arthritis that occurs in children age 16 or younger. The signs and symptoms are similar to the adult form of RA, such as joint inflammation and reduced motion. It can affect any joint tissue and, in some cases, internal organs. JRA causes growth problems in some children.

Symptoms can come and go. An early sign of JRA is limping in the morning. Some children have just one or two flares; others have symptoms that never go away.

It is uncertain what causes JRA, but whatever the cause, there are two components. First, something in a child's genetic makeup gives him or her a tendency to develop JRA; then an environmental factor, such as a virus, triggers the disease. Medications and physical therapy can help maintain movement and reduce swelling and pain.

Although it is often referred to as if it were a single disease, *scleroderma* is really a symptom of a group of diseases that involve abnormal growth of connective tissue. The word *scleroderma* means "hard skin." In localized scleroderma, hard, tight skin is the extent of the problem. In systemic scleroderma, however, the problem goes much deeper, affecting blood vessels and internal organs, such as the heart, lungs, and kidneys. Symptoms of scleroderma include calcium deposits in connective tissues; swelling of the esophagus; thick, tight skin on the fingers; and red spots on the hands and face (National Institute of Arthritis and Musculoskeletal and Skin Diseases, 2016).

It is unknown what causes scleroderma. It is more common in women than men, especially those between 30 and 50 years of age. It can be mild or severe and can be life threatening. There is no cure, but various treatments, including physical therapy, can help relieve symptoms.

Some patients with scleroderma may experience *Raynaud's phenomenon*, in which blood vessels narrow, and blood can't get to the surface of the skin. The affected areas, usually the fingers and toes, turn white and blue. A patient may also feel cold and numb from lack of blood flow. When the blood flow returns, the skin turns red and throbs or tingles. Raynaud's phenomenon usually occurs when a person is cold or feeling stressed. Women are more likely than men to have it, and it is more common in people who live in colder climates.

Treatment of Raynaud's depends on its severity and whether the patient has other health conditions. For most people, Raynaud's isn't disabling, but can affect quality of life.

Lupus disease occurs when something goes wrong with the immune system, causing it to create autoantibodies that attack healthy cells and tissue anywhere in the body—joints, skin, blood vessels, and organs—leading to inflammation, pain, and damage. There are many kinds of lupus, but the most common type is systemic lupus erythematosus (SLE), which affects many parts of the body. Anyone can get lupus, but young women in their 30s and 40s are most at risk. Lupus is also more common in African American, Hispanic, Asian, and Native American women. The cause of lupus is unknown, but genetic, environmental, and hormonal factors may contribute. Lupus is a mild disease for some patients; for others, it causes severe signs and symptoms. Some common signs and symptoms of lupus are joint and muscle pain with swelling, fever, red rashes, hair loss, weight loss, and memory problems (Lupus Foundation of America, 2015).

There is no one test to diagnose lupus, and it may take years to make the diagnosis. There is no cure for lupus, but anti-inflammatory medications and lifestyle changes such as stress management can help control signs and symptoms. Lupus is a serious disease that needs constant monitoring and treatment because it can damage organs and be life threatening if left untreated.

Allergies

Allergies, or hypersensitivities, are an overreaction of the immune system to antigens in the environment. The most common types of allergies occur when the immune system responds to a false alarm. For example, in an allergic person, a normally harmless substance such as grass pollen or mold is mistaken for a threat and is attacked. The substances that provoke such attacks are called allergens, and a possibly endless variety of allergens exist. Dust mites, seasonal allergies, drug allergies, food allergies, animal hair allergies, and allergies to toxins are the most common. A patient can have several types of allergies, because those with allergies often are sensitive to more than one allergen.

The immune response to allergens causes such symptoms as swelling, watery eyes, rashes, difficulty breathing, and sneezing. The part of the body the allergen comes into contact with affects the symptoms (US National Library of Medicine, 2016b):

- Allergens that you inhale (breathe in) may cause stuffy nose, itchy throat, thick mucus, cough, or wheezing.

- Allergens that touch the eyes may cause itchy, watery, red, swollen eyes.

- Eating something you are allergic to may cause nausea, vomiting, cramping, diarrhea, or a life-threatening reaction.

- Allergens that touch the skin may cause a skin rash, hives, itching, blisters, or peeling skin.

- Drug allergies usually involve the whole body and can cause many different of symptoms.

A life-threatening response to an allergen is called *anaphylactic shock*, in which the person experiences severe respiratory distress and a fall in blood pressure. When a person goes into shock, immediate medical treatment is necessary. The best treatment is a prompt intramuscular injection of *epinephrine*, or adrenalin. Some people with allergies must carry epinephrine at all times in an EpiPen™, which can be self-injected in an emergency.

Medications called antihistamines relieve most symptoms of allergies. Antihistamines can reduce symptoms, but the best method is avoidance of antigens. A process called desensitization holds the most promise in treating allergies. In desensitization, a patient is exposed to small amounts of the identified allergen until he or she no longer has a reaction. Sometimes a change in residence is needed when all else fails to control allergies.

Both genes and the environment have something to do with why people get allergies. A specific allergy is not usually inherited, but if both parents have allergies, then their children are at risk. If only the mother has allergies, the risk is greater for the child than if it is only the father who has allergies.

Cancers of the Immune System

Cancer is uncontrolled growth of cells, and this can occur with the cells of the immune system. *Lymphoma* involves the lymphoid tissues and is a common childhood cancer. *Leukemia*, which involves abnormal overgrowth of leukocytes, is the most common childhood cancer. With current medications and treatment, most cases of both types of cancer in children and adolescents are curable.

Graft-Versus-Host Disease

Graft-versus-host disease (GVHD) is a complication that can happen after a bone marrow or stem cell transplant. As noted earlier in this chapter, the bone marrow is the soft tissue inside bones that helps form immune cells. Stem cells are normally found inside bone marrow.

Because only identical twins have identical tissue types, a donor's bone marrow is normally a close, but not perfect, match to the recipient's tissues. The differences between the donor's cells and recipient's tissues often cause T-cells from the donor to recognize the recipient's body tissues as foreign. When this happens, the newly transplanted cells attack the transplant recipient's body.

Rates of GVHD vary from between 30% to 40% among related donors and recipients to 60% to 80% between unrelated donors and recipients (US National Library of Medicine, 2016b). The greater the mismatch between donor and recipient, the greater the risk of GVHD. After a transplant, the recipient usually takes medications that suppress the immune system, which helps reduce the chances or severity of GVHD. With GVHD, the patient is very vulnerable to infections. Common symptoms include abdominal pain, fever, skin rashes, hair loss, and lung and digestive tract disorders.

The goal of treatment is to suppress the immune response without damaging the new cells. GVHD can be treated successfully, but that does not guarantee that the transplant itself will succeed in treating the original disease or condition. Some cases of GVHD can lead to death.

Chapter Summary

- Immunity is the body's ability to defend itself against pathogens and other harmful substances.

- Antigens are pathogens that trigger an immune response.

- The most common antigens are bacteria, viruses, and parasites. Each antigen uses different tactics to infect a person, and each requires a unique immune response.

- The lymphatic system is the immune system's own circulatory system. The lymphatic system is a network of organs, vessels, tissues, and cells that keeps away infection and balances the body's fluids.

- Diseases of the immune system fall into five main categories: immune deficiency or immuno-deficiency diseases, autoimmune diseases, allergies (hypersensitivities), cancers, and graft-versus-host disease.

- Immunizations are one of the best ways to prevent infectious diseases, and vaccines have an excellent safety record. Although some parents are against childhood immunizations, there is scientific evidence supporting the importance of vaccination for children in particular.

REVIEW QUESTIONS

1.   What is the term for a substance that triggers an immune response?

2.   What causes cancers of the immune system?

3.   Describe the lymphatic system and give reasons why it is important to the immune system.

4.   What type of immunity do infants receive from their mothers?

5.   Identify and describe the following: B-cells, T-cells, and phagocytes.

6.   What is the human leukocyte antigen (HLA), and how does it help in defending the body against infection?

7.   What are immunoglobulins, and how do they function?

8.   Why is it important for children to receive the recommended childhood immunizations?

9.   How do stress and age affect the immune system?

10. Explain why identical twins are ideal for stem cell transplants.

KEY TERMS

Acquired immunodeficiency syndrome (AIDS): The final stage of HIV infection, in which the immune system is so damaged that it is unable to fight off infections or cancers

Active immunity: Immunity that develops when exposure to an antigen triggers the immune system to make antibodies to that disease

Allergen: Harmless antigen that the immune cells attack

Allergy: Condition in which the immune cells respond to an otherwise harmless foreign antigen and launch an attack

Alopecia areata: Disease in which the immune system attacks the structures from which hair grows (hair follicles)

Anaphylactic shock: A life-threatening response to an allergen, causing severe respiratory distress and a fall in blood pressure

Antibodies, or immunoglobulins: Blood proteins that attack antigens

Antigens: Any substance recognized as foreign by the immune system and that can cause an immune response

Autoantibodies: Antibodies that attack normal cells by mistake

Autoimmune diseases: Diseases in which the immune system attacks healthy cells by mistake, while at the same time, T-cells fail to keep the immune system healthy

B-cells and T-cells: Lymphocytes that are created in bone marrow

Celiac disease: Genetic disease caused by the affected person's inability to tolerate gluten

Cell: Smallest unit of life and the basis of all plant, animal, and human tissue

Complement: A cluster of proteins working together to protect the body from antigens

Epinephrine: Adrenalin

Flares: Sudden and severe symptoms

Graft-versus-host disease (GVHD): Mature T-cells' reaction that causes complications after a bone marrow or stem cell transplant

Guillain-Barre syndrome: A syndrome in which the immune system attacks the nerves that connect the brain and spinal cord with the rest of the body

Helper T-cells: Immune cells that coordinate immune responses

Human leukocyte antigen (HLA): A system built into all body cells that marks them as "self"

Human immunodeficiency virus (HIV): Virus that wipes out vital helper T-cells, leaving the immune system unable to defend the body against normally harmless organisms

IgA deficiency: The most common immune deficiency disease, caused by the body's failure to produce enough of the antibody IgA

Immune deficiency diseases, or immunodeficiency diseases: Diseases that prevent a person's body from fighting back against infections and other diseases

Immune response: The immune system's defense against antigens

Immune system: Network of specific organs, tissues, vessels, and cells that work together to defend the body against harmful substances

Immunity: Protection against diseases

Immunization/vaccination: Procedure that gives the body a disease-specific antigen that allows the body to make antibodies to protect from future attacks from that specific disease

Immunological diseases: Diseases of the immune system

Immunosenescence: Age-related negative changes to the immune system

Inflammatory response: Redness, warmth, swelling, pain, and loss of function

Juvenile rheumatoid arthritis (JRA): Type of arthritis that occurs in children age 16 or younger

Killer T-cells: Immune cells that help rid the body of antigens

Leukemia: Childhood cancer that involves abnormal growth of leukocytes

Leukocyte: White blood cell

Lupus disease: Disease in which the immune system damages healthy connective tissue anywhere in the body

Lymph: Body fluid that carries and stores immune cells

Lymphatic system: The immune system's own circulatory system

Lymphocyte: A type of leukocyte that has many functions

Lymphoma: Childhood cancer that involves the lymphoid tissues

Multiple sclerosis (MS): Condition in which the immune system attacks the protective coating around the nerves

Myasthenia gravis (MG): Disease that occurs when the immune system makes antibodies that block or change the nerve signals to muscles

Natural immunity: General protection that everyone is born with

Neutrophil: Phagocyte that is attracted to inflammation and bacteria

Passive immunity: Immunity borrowed from another source

Pathogens: Disease-causing microorganisms such as bacteria, viruses, fungi, and parasites

Phagocyte: A type of leukocyte that attacks and ingests antigens

Plasma cell: Cell that makes antibodies

Plasma exchange: A process in which whole blood is withdrawn from a person, plasma is removed from the blood and replaced, and then the blood is transfused back into the person

Pus, or purulent: Dead neutrophils and other cellular debris

Pustule: A blister or pimple filled with pus

Raynaud's phenomenon: Condition that occurs when blood can't get to the surface of the skin, and the affected areas turn white and blue

Regulatory T-cells: Immune cells that tell B-cells and other T-cells when the body is better

Remission: Body state in which all signs and symptoms of a disease have gone away for a while or have disappeared

Rheumatoid arthritis (RA): Condition in which the immune system attacks the connective tissue of the joints throughout the body

Scleroderma: Disease that affects collagen and causes abnormal growth of connective tissue

Secretions: Fluids released by the immune system

Stem cell: Blood cell made in the bone marrow

Type 1 diabetes: Disease in which the immune system attacks cells that make insulin

CHAPTER ACTIVITIES

1.   Autoimmune diseases are a group of more than 80 chronic diseases that involve almost every human organ system. In small groups, identify as many autoimmune diseases for each organ system as you can. The group that has correctly identified the most diseases for every organ system wins the challenge.

2. You have been hired as a community health worker for adolescent HIV/AIDS prevention. Your target population is from the LGBTQ (lesbian, gay, bisexual, transgender, and queer) community. Identify five health promotion strategies specific to this target population. Develop three health promotion messages that encourage testing for this target population.

3. You are a patient advocate who works with pediatric patients. A patient's parents are reluctant to give their child immunizations as recommended by the CDC. In pairs, role-play how you would talk with these parents about the importance of childhood immunizations.

4. Create a one-page handout on how immune system cells attack antigens. This handout is for a low-health-literacy target population (e.g., the elderly, people with limited English proficiency, or those with low literacy). Use graphics or pictures instead of words when possible. Figure 10.5 can be used as model for this activity.

5. In groups of four, each member chooses one or two cells in the immune system. Through individual research, each group member learns about the function of his or her chosen cell(s). Following the research activity, each member shows his or her understanding by answering specific questions about his or her cell(s) from group members and/or the class as a whole.

Bibliography and Works Cited

AIDS.gov. (2011). Immune system 101. Retrieved from https://www.aids.gov/hiv-aids-basics/just-diagnosed-with-hiv-aids/hiv-in-your-body/immune-system-101/

American Academy of Allergy Asthma & Immunology. (2015). Conditions & treatments. Retrieved from http://www.aaaai.org/conditions-and-treatments.aspx

Arthritis Foundation. (2015). Understanding arthritis. Retrieved from http://www.arthritis.org/about-arthritis/understanding-arthritis/

Centers for Disease Control and Prevention. (2014a). Immunity types. Retrieved from http://www.cdc.gov/vaccines/vac-gen/immunity-types.htm

Centers for Disease Control and Prevention. (2014b). Why are childhood vaccines so important? Retrieved from http://www.cdc.gov/vaccines/vac-gen/howvpd.htm

Lupus Foundation of America. (2015). Get answers: I have lupus. Retrieved from http://www.lupus.org/answers/topic/i-have-lupus

Mineo, T. C. (2015). *Novel challenges in myasthenia gravis*. New York, NY: Nova Biomedical.

National Institute of Aging. (2015). Immune system: Can your immune system still defend you as you age? Retrieved from https://www.nia.nih.gov/health/publication/biology-aging/immune-system-can-your-immune-system-still-defend-you-you-age

National Institute of Allergy and Infectious Diseases. (2013). Overview of the immune system. Retrieved from https://www.niaid.nih.gov/research/immune-system-overview

National Institute of Allergy and Infectious Diseases. (2015). Diseases & conditions. Retrieved from https://www.niaid.nih.gov/diseases-conditions/all

National Institute of Arthritis and Musculoskeletal and Skin Diseases. (2016). Understanding autoimmune diseases. Retrieved from http://www.niams.nih.gov/Health_Info/Autoimmune/default.asp

Nemours Foundation. (2015). The immune system. *KidsHealth*. Retrieved from http://kidshealth.org/parent/general/body_basics/immune.html

Office of Women's Health. (2011). *A lifetime of good health: Your guide to staying healthy*. Retrieved from http://www.womenshealth.gov/publications/our-publications/lifetime-good-health/

Paul, W. E. (2008). The immune system. In W. E. Paul (Ed.), *Fundamental immunology* (6th ed., pp. 2–25). Philadelphia, PA: Lippincott Williams & Wilkins.

Sompayrac, L. (2003). *How the immune system works* (2nd ed.). Malden, MA: Blackwell.

US National Library of Medicine. (2016a). Autoimmune diseases. *MedlinePlus.* Retrieved from https://www.nlm .nih.gov/medlineplus/autoimmunediseases.html

US National Library of Medicine. (2016b). Immune system and disorders. *MedlinePlus.* Retrieved from https:// www.nlm.nih.gov/medlineplus/immunesystemanddisorders.html

CHAPTER 11

ENDOCRINE SYSTEM AND RELATED DISEASES

CHAPTER OBJECTIVES

- List and summarize major glands and organs in the endocrine system.

- Discuss how the endocrine system hormones influence body functions.

- Explain the role of the pancreas.

- Describe how aging, illness, the environment, and stress affect the endocrine system.

- Identify and discuss endocrine system diseases.

- Review treatment plans for endocrine system diseases.

The endocrine system is made up of glands located throughout the body. These glands secrete hormones directly into the bloodstream. Hormones are essential to metabolic function, such as energy use, growth and development, muscle and fat distribution, sexual development, and water balance. The most common endocrine diseases occur when one or more of the glands and organs of the endocrine system are either overactive or underactive; that is, glands secrete hormones in amounts that are either too much or not enough for the body to work normally.

Function of the Endocrine System

The *endocrine system* is a control station that communicates, influences, and coordinates the body's work from head to toe. It affects almost every cell, organ, and function of the body. In general, this system controls those functions that are performed slowly, such as body growth. Faster functions, such as breathing and body movement, are controlled by the nervous system. Like the nervous system, the endocrine system is one of the body's main communicators; and even though the endocrine system and nervous system are separate, they often work together to help the body maintain homeostasis. *Homeostasis* is the state of balance and stability of the body's internal organs and functions. In addition to helping maintain homeostasis, the endocrine system is responsible for or affects the following (Crowley, 2012):

- Metabolism—digestion, elimination, breathing, blood circulation, and maintaining body temperature

- Tissue function

- Reproduction and sexual function

- Growth and development

- Mood
- Responses to stress

These various functions are performed and controlled by a network of glands and organs that make, store, and secrete hormones directly into the bloodstream. *Hormones* are the body's chemical messengers that regulate the activities of cells and organs. They are either proteins or steroids and are released into the bloodstream and then transported to cells and organs throughout the body.

Hormones send chemical information and instructions from one set of cells to another to coordinate bodily functions. Although different hormones circulate throughout the bloodstream, each one affects only the cells that are targeted to receive its message. When the hormone reaches its target cell, it transmits chemical information and instructions to the cell.

The environment, stress, and infection influence hormone levels in the body. The levels are also influenced by changes in the balance of fluid and minerals in the blood. When hormone levels reach a normal amount, any further secretion is "turned off" to maintain homeostasis. This turnoff process is called the *negative feedback system* because information about the hormone's level is fed back to the gland that makes it, which then responds by decreasing or increasing production.

Influences on Endocrine System Function

Everyone's body goes through changes that affect the functioning of the endocrine system. Some of these changes are related to aging, disease, stress, and the environment.

Aging

Aging affects nearly every gland in the endocrine system. The system's response time becomes slower, especially in people who might be at risk for a particular disease. The changes during aging are either impaired secretion or inability to respond to the body's internal environment.

Aging in particular affects the endocrine functions related to women's ovaries and that cause menopause. With *menopause*, the production of the ovarian hormones estrogen and progesterone slows down and then stops. Without these hormones, a woman is unable to become pregnant. Menopause usually occurs when women are between the ages of 40 to 58 years old. Given that the average life expectancy for US women today is 84 years, many women spend almost half their adult life as either a menopausal or postmenopausal woman.

Women can experience menopause at a younger age if they smoked, never had a baby, were exposed to toxic chemicals, had heart disease, or used certain medications. Hormone therapy and other medications are helpful in dealing with menopause symptoms.

Disease

A disease can affect the endocrine system in several ways. For example, one of the functions of the liver and kidneys is to clear hormones from the body. If a person has chronic liver or kidney disease that impairs the function of these organs, the hormone clearing is slowed down and causes complications.

Stress

Many factors can start a stress response in the endocrine system, but physical stress has the most impact. For the body to respond to physical stress, the adrenal glands need to make more of the hormone *cortisol*. The following are examples of physical stress that causes the endocrine system to release cortisol (National Institute of Diabetes and Digestive and Kidney Diseases [NIDDK], 2014):

- Injuries
- Surgery

- Allergic reactions

- Intense heat or cold

- Life-threatening diseases or severe infections

Environment

An *environmental endocrine disruptor (EED)* is a chemical outside the body that causes negative effects on the endocrine system. There are currently more than 84,000 chemicals used internationally for commercial purposes, and at least 30,000 have been in the US environment since 1979 (Endocrine Society, 2016c; National Institute of Diabetes and Digestive and Kidney Diseases, 2014; STEERS Institute, 2016). Research has over time increased scientists' understanding of how a broad range of these chemicals negatively affect the endocrine system. There is research-based evidence at the local, national, and international levels that strongly suggests that prolonged exposure to EEDs negatively impacts the endocrine system in a number of ways, including delayed sexual development and decreased fertility (Endocrine Society, 2016c; NIDDK, 2014; STEERS Institute, 2016).

Structure of the Endocrine System

The endocrine system is made up of glands scattered throughout the body. A *gland* is a group of cells that function like a factory to make, store, and release hormones into the bloodstream. Glands release more than 20 major hormones that influence almost every cell, organ, and function of the body. Keep in mind that although the endocrine glands are the body's main hormone makers, some non-endocrine organs, such as the brain, heart, lungs, and liver, also make and release hormones.

There are eight major glands in the endocrine system: the hypothalamus, and the pituitary, thyroid, parathyroid, adrenal, pineal, and reproductive glands. The pancreas is also part of this system; however, it is also part of the digestive system because it makes and secretes digestive enzymes. What follows is an overview of each endocrine gland (National Cancer Institute, 2016):

Hypothalamus This gland lies in the lower part of the brain, just above the pituitary gland, and is the primary link between the endocrine and nervous systems (see Figure 11.1). The *hypothalamus* controls the part of the nervous system that is responsible for breathing, sleep, hunger, and maintaining body temperature. It also controls the pituitary gland by either increasing or decreasing the gland's hormone secretions.

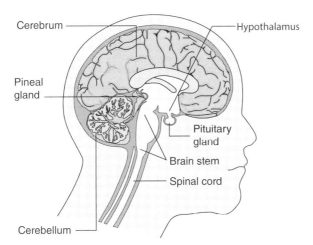

Figure 11.1 Hypothalamus, Pituitary Gland, and Pineal Glands

Note. Adapted from the National Cancer Institute, Visuals Online, 2001. This image is in the public domain. Retrieved from https://visualsonline.cancer.gov/details.cfm?imageid=2717

Pituitary gland The *pituitary gland* makes hormones that influence other endocrine glands; it also regulates homeostasis. It is located at the base of the brain just beneath the hypothalamus (see Figure 11.1). Although no bigger than a pea, this gland is the most important part of the endocrine system and is sometimes called the "master gland" for this reason. The secretion of pituitary hormones is influenced by such factors as emotions, stress, and the environment. These factors first affect the hypothalamus. Then the hypothalamus sends information to the pituitary, which then secretes hormones that affect the following body functions:

- Growth of body tissues
- Making of sex hormones
- Regulating the body's water balance
- Reducing sensitivity to pain
- Controlling the menstrual cycle
- Contractions of the uterus during labor

Pineal gland The size of a grain of rice with a pinecone shape (see Figure 11.1), the *pineal gland* is located in the middle of the brain. This gland secretes melatonin, a hormone that may help regulate the daily wake-and-sleep cycle, in response to light.

Thyroid gland Located in the front part of the lower neck, the *thyroid gland* is shaped like a butterfly and makes thyroid hormones (see Figure 11.2). Thyroid hormones control the rate at which cells burn fuels from food to make energy. These hormones also play a key role in bone growth and brain development and in the nervous system in children.

Parathyroid glands The four *parathyroid glands* are attached to the thyroid and are each about the size of a grain of rice (see Figure 11.2). These glands function together to release parathyroid hormone, which regulates calcium levels in blood and bones.

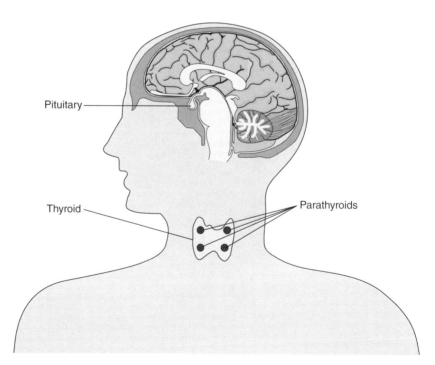

Figure 11.2   Pituitary, Thyroid, and Parathyroid Glands

Note. Adapted from the NIDDK Image Library, National Institute of Diabetes and Digestive and Kidney Diseases, 2012. Retrieved from https://catalog.niddk.nih.gov/Catalog/imagelibrary/detail.cfm?id=1073

Adrenal glands The body has two triangular *adrenal glands,* one on top of each kidney. The glands have two sections; each makes hormones with different functions. The outer section makes hormones that influence salt and water balance and the body's response to stress. These hormones also influence metabolism, the immune system, and sexual development and function. The inner section makes hormones such as epinephrine. Epinephrine, or adrenaline, increases blood pressure and heart rate when the body experiences stress.

Reproductive glands (gonads) The *reproductive glands (gonads)* secrete sex hormones that influence female and male characteristics. Males have twin reproductive glands called *testes,* which make *testosterone,* a hormone associated with sexual development. During puberty, testosterone influences the growth of the penis and testes, growth of facial and pubic hair, deepening of the voice, and increasing muscle mass and height. Throughout adult life, testosterone helps maintain male sex drive, sperm production, hair patterns, muscle mass, and bone mass.

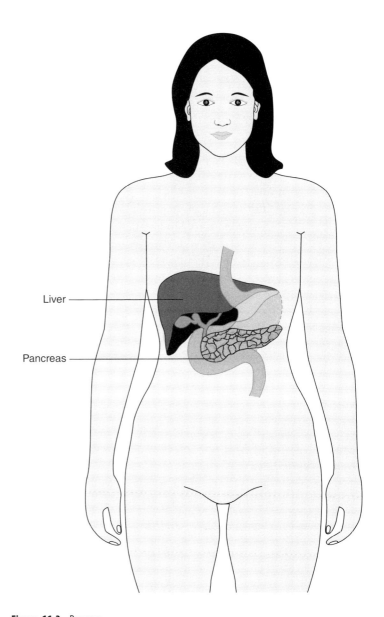

Ovaries are the female reproductive glands and are located in the pelvis. They make eggs and secrete the female hormones estrogen and progesterone. *Estrogen* helps in the development of female sexual features, such as breast growth, the buildup of body fat, and the growth spurt that occurs during puberty. Both estrogen and *progesterone* are also involved in pregnancy and the regulation of the menstrual cycle.

Pancreas The *pancreas* is a large gland behind the stomach that helps maintain healthy glucose levels (see Figure 11.3). It secretes the hormone *insulin,* which controls the use of glucose by the body. Insulin helps glucose move from the blood into the cells, where it is used for energy. The pancreas also secretes the hormone *glucagon* when glucose is low. These two hormones work together to keep a steady level of glucose in the blood and to keep the body supplied with fuel for energy.

Diseases of the Endocrine System

Over- or underactivity of one or more of the endocrine system's glands and organs leads to what is known as a hormone imbalance, which is the cause of most endocrine diseases. The body also can have difficulty controlling hormone levels because of difficulty in removing hormones from the blood.

Endocrinology is the branch of medicine concerned with endocrine glands, organs, and hormones. Patients with an endocrine disease often see a medical specialist called an *endocrinologist,* who is a physician specifically trained to diagnose and treat endocrine diseases. In the case of these diseases, making a diagnosis entails correctly

Figure 11.3 Pancreas

Note. Adapted from the National Institute of Diabetes and Digestive and Kidney Diseases, 2014. Retrieved from https://www.niddk.nih.gov/health-information/diabetes/delaying-preventing-type -2-diabetes

matching the patient's signs and symptoms with a specific hormone dysfunction. It also requires lab results that confirm overproduction or underproduction of a particular hormone or hormones. Two common lab blood tests that detect hormone levels are *radioimmunoassay (RIA)* and 24-hour urine tests.

Signs and symptoms of an endocrine disease depend on age, sex of the patient, and the level of hormone secretion. For example, if the pituitary gland over- or underproduces growth hormone, then children's height can be seriously affected.

Glands of the endocrine system are the basis for discussion of diseases in this chapter. The diseases of the pancreas include prediabetes, diabetes mellitus (type 1 and type 2), gestational diabetes, hypoglycemia, and metabolic syndrome. The diseases of the pituitary gland include gigantism and acromegaly. The diseases of the thyroid include Graves disease, hyperthyroidism, hypothyroidism, Hashimoto's disease, and thyroid cancer. The diseases of the reproductive glands (gonads) include precocious puberty and hypogonadism.

Diabetes and Associated Diseases

Diabetes can affect anyone, but some population groups have a higher risk for developing the disease than others. Diabetes is more common in African Americans, Latinos, Native Americans, and Asian Americans/Pacific Islanders. In some groups, such as certain Native American tribes, as many as 40% of the adult population have type 2 diabetes.

The high rate of diabetes in certain populations means that many others are at increased risk for prediabetes. Patients with prediabetes can prevent type 2 diabetes by making changes in their diet and increasing physical activity. They may even be able to return their glucose levels to a normal range. According to the American Diabetes Association (2016), diet and physical activity work better than medications to delay the development of diabetes. Just 30 minutes a day of moderate physical activity, coupled with a 5–10% reduction in body weight, causes a 58% reduction in risk of diabetes.

Diabetes Mellitus

A major disease of the pancreas is *diabetes mellitus*. It is caused by the failure of the pancreas to secrete enough insulin or by the body's inability to use insulin correctly. *Insulin* is the hormone needed to convert sugar, starches, and other carbohydrates into *blood glucose* (blood sugar). Glucose is an important source of energy for body cells. Carbohydrates, such as bread, the sugar found in milk, and fruits are the main food source of glucose. After a meal, glucose is absorbed into the bloodstream and carried to the body's cells. Insulin takes the glucose from the blood, puts it into the cells, and helps the cells use glucose for energy. If a person takes in more glucose than the body needs, then the body stores the extra glucose in the liver and muscles as *glycogen*. The body uses glycogen for energy between meals. Extra glucose can also be changed into fat and stored in fat cells.

When diabetes leads to buildup of glucose in the blood, it can cause two major problems. One problem is that the cells become starved for energy; the second is that high blood glucose levels over time can damage eyes, kidneys, nerves, and heart. When there is a high level of blood glucose, the condition is called *hyperglycemia*.

Diabetes mellitus is divided into two types, depending on the cause of the disease. If the diabetes is caused by insulin deficiency, it is type 1 diabetes. If there is an inadequate response to insulin, then it is type 2 diabetes (see Figure 11.4).

In the past, type 1 diabetes was called juvenile-onset diabetes because it had to do with insulin problems that happened in young children and adolescents. Type 2 diabetes was called adult-onset diabetes because it was far more common in adults. Now, however, the two types of diabetes are no

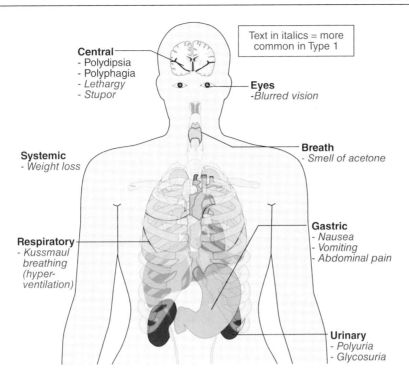

Figure 11.4 Main Symptoms of Diabetes

Note. Adapted from Mikael Häggström, "Medical gallery of Mikael Häggström 2014," by Mikael Häggström, Wikiversity Journal of Medicine 1 (2). doi:10.15347/wjm/2014.008. ISSN 20018762. (All used images are in public domain.) [Public domain], via Wikimedia Commons. Retrieved from https://commons.wikimedia.org/wiki/File%3AMain_symptoms_of_diabetes.png

longer limited to particular age groups. The terms juvenile-onset diabetes and adult-onset diabetes are used less frequently because young children and adolescents are increasingly being diagnosed with type 2 diabetes. Approximately 30 million children and adults have diabetes in the United States. Of that number, nearly 95% have type 2 diabetes (American Heart Association, 2015; Centers for Disease Control and Prevention, 2015).

Type 1 Diabetes Mellitus   *Type 1 diabetes mellitus*, in which the body does not make insulin, is usually diagnosed in children and young adults. Only 5% of patients with diabetes mellitus have this form of the disease (American Diabetes Association, 2016). With the help of insulin therapy and other treatments, patients with type 1 diabetes learn to manage their disease and can live long, healthy lives.

Usually patients need to inherit risk factors from both parents to have type 1 diabetes. These factors are more common in those of European descent. However, according to the American Diabetes Association (2016), most people who are at risk do not get type 1 diabetes. Because inherited risk factors are difficult to identify, research into this disease has shifted focus to identify environmental triggers. One trigger might be cold weather, because it develops more often in winter than summer and is more common in cold climates. Another trigger might be viruses. Perhaps a virus that has only mild effects on most people triggers type 1 diabetes in others. Early diet may also play a role because type 1 diabetes is less common in those who were breastfed and first ate solid foods at later ages. Regardless of how a patient gets type 1 diabetes, this disease takes many years to develop. Once patients have it, they are likely to develop *diabetic ketosis*, which is abnormal fat metabolism caused by a lack of insulin.

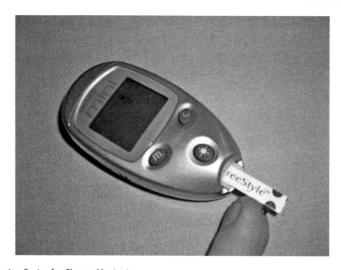

Figure 11.5   Automatic Lancing Device for Glucose Monitoring

Note. From "Glucose Test.JPG," by Erik1980, 2007, via Wikimedia Commons. Retrieved from https://commons.wikimedia.org/wiki/File:Glucose_test.JPG

Treatment for diabetes requires a diet that controls carbohydrate intake. Type 1 diabetes patients also need insulin, with doses adjusted to their individual glucose needs. Most type 1 diabetic patients need several insulin injections throughout the day in order to maintain a normal level of glucose. The most common way to check glucose levels is to gather a blood sample by pricking a fingertip with an automatic lancing device and then use a glucose meter to measure the blood's glucose level (American Diabetes Association, 2016) (see Figure 11.5).

Insulin pumps are used by type 1 diabetic patients who need frequent insulin shots or injections. An insulin pump is a small device that is attached to the patient's clothing. From the pump, a short tube with a needle is inserted into the skin near the abdomen wall and kept in place with tape. The pump gives dosages of insulin just as a healthy pancreas would.

Type 2 Diabetes Mellitus   In *type 2 diabetes mellitus*, the pancreas secretes normal amounts of insulin, but then tissues are insensitive to the insulin and respond the wrong way. The reason for the incorrect response to insulin is not completely understood, but it seems to be related to obesity. Type 2 diabetes develops most often in older overweight and obese adults. With weight reduction there is an improvement in tissue response to insulin. The American Diabetes Association (2016) has shown through numerous studies that overweight or obese people can delay or prevent type 2 diabetes by exercising and losing weight.

Type 2 diabetes has a strong link to family health history and lifestyle factors. Obesity tends to run in families, and families tend to have similar eating and physical activity habits. If a patient has a family history of type 2 diabetes, it may be difficult to figure out whether his or her diabetes is caused by lifestyle factors or genetics. Most likely it is due to both.

Type 2 diabetic patients often manage their disease through behavior changes in diet, weight control, and physical activity. If these behavior changes are not enough to maintain a healthy level of blood glucose, then the patient is prescribed diabetes medications. If diet, weight control, physical activity, and medications don't work, then insulin is given in the same way as for type 1 diabetics.

Gestational Diabetes

Some women develop *gestational diabetes* when pregnant. It usually occurs in late pregnancy when the fetus's body has already been formed but while it is still growing. A diagnosis of gestational diabetes doesn't mean that the patient had diabetes before pregnancy or that she will have diabetes after giving birth.

About 18% of all pregnancies are affected by gestational diabetes (Centers for Disease Control and Prevention, 2015; March of Dimes, 2016). It is not known what causes it, but there are clues. The placenta secretes hormones that help the baby develop, but they also block the action of the mother's insulin, causing insulin resistance. *Insulin resistance* makes it hard for the mother's body to properly make and use the insulin it needs during pregnancy. Without enough insulin, blood glucose builds up to high levels, causing hyperglycemia, which is harmful to the fetus.

Gestational diabetes is treated by dietary changes or with insulin medication. Although glucose levels return to normal after delivery, a woman who has had gestational diabetes is at risk for developing diabetes later in life.

Poorly controlled gestational diabetes can cause the fetus to have high glucose levels, which in turn cause the pancreas of the fetus to make more insulin to get rid of the glucose. Because the fetus is getting more glucose than it needs, the extra is stored as fat, causing fetal macrosomia. *Fetal macrosomia* is a term used to describe newborn babies who are significantly larger than average. A baby diagnosed with fetal macrosomia has a birth weight of more than 8 pounds, 13 ounces, regardless of whether the baby's delivery is preterm (born before 37 weeks of pregnancy), term (born after 37 weeks of pregnancy), or postterm (born after 42 weeks of pregnancy). Fetal macrosomia is often difficult to detect and diagnose during pregnancy, but it can both complicate vaginal delivery and put the baby at risk of injury during birth. It also puts the baby at increased risk for health problems later in life, including childhood obesity, heart disease, breathing difficulties, and diabetes (Mayo Clinic, 2016).

Hypoglycemia

Hypoglycemia occurs when blood glucose (blood sugar), the body's main source of energy, drops below normal levels. A blood glucose level below 70 mg/dl is considered hypoglycemia (American Diabetes Association, 2016). In a healthy person, when glucose levels drop, the liver breaks down glycogen and releases it into the bloodstream, causing blood glucose to rise to a normal level. For patients with diabetes, however, this response to hypoglycemia doesn't work as quickly, causing blood glucose levels to remain low.

Hypoglycemia isn't a disease itself; instead, it's an indicator of a health problem. Although it can come on suddenly, hypoglycemia is usually mild and can be treated quickly by eating or drinking glucose-rich foods (carbohydrates), such as rice, potatoes, bread, tortillas, milk, fruit, and sweets. If left untreated, however, hypoglycemia gets worse and causes confusion, sweating, dizziness, or fainting. Severe hypoglycemia can lead to seizures, coma, and even death (American Diabetes Association, 2016).

Diabetes medications or treatments are the most common cause of hypoglycemia. In patients on diabetes medication, low blood glucose can be caused by meals that are too small or skipped, increased physical activity, and alcoholic beverages. Diabetes treatment plans are specifically designed to match the dose and timing of medication to a patient's usual schedule of meals and activities. Mismatches, such as taking a dose of insulin and then skipping a meal, can result in hypoglycemia.

When a diabetic patient thinks his blood glucose level is too low, he needs to check it with a blood sample and use a blood glucose meter. If the level is below 70 mg/dl, he should eat or drink quick-fix foods or liquids right away to raise the glucose level. A quick fix can be three or four glucose tablets, a half cup of any fruit juice, or a tablespoon of sugar or honey. The next step is to recheck blood glucose in 15 minutes to make sure it is at 70 mg/dl or above. If it's still too low, the patient should eat another serving of a quick-fix food. He repeats these steps until the blood glucose level is 70 mg/dl or above.

According to the American Diabetes Association (2016), patients with diabetes should be prepared to prevent low blood glucose by

- Learning what can trigger changes in the glucose level
- Always having several quick-fix foods or drinks handy
- Telling family members, loved ones, and coworkers about hypoglycemia and how they can help if needed
- Having a blood glucose meter readily available for frequent testing
- Wearing a medical identification bracelet or necklace

As already noted, severe hypoglycemia causes a patient to pass out, and it can even be life threatening. Another person can help by giving an injection of prescribed glucagon to the patient. Glucagon rapidly brings the glucose level back to normal and helps the patient regain consciousness. Family, friends, or coworkers of the diabetic patient can be trained on how to give a glucagon injection and when to call 911 for medical help.

Hypoglycemia unawareness occurs in some diabetic patients: They do not experience early warning signs of low blood glucose. This unawareness develops when frequent episodes of hypoglycemia cause changes in how the body reacts to low glucose levels. The body stops releasing stress hormones when glucose drops too low. The condition occurs most often in those with type 1 diabetes; these patients may need to check their glucose level often to prevent hypoglycemia.

Metabolic Syndrome

The term *metabolic* refers to the biochemical processes involved in the body's normal functioning. When these biochemical processes are not working correctly, the person is at risk for health problems, such as heart disease, diabetes, stroke, and obesity; this condition is referred to as *metabolic syndrome*. Metabolic syndrome is basically a clustering of often interconnected metabolic problems. One example of interconnectedness is the way that *abdominal obesity*, or a larger than normal waistline, contributes to high blood pressure, high blood cholesterol, and high blood glucose levels.

Insulin resistance, the body's inability to make and use insulin properly, increases the risk for metabolic syndrome. Some people inherit a tendency toward insulin resistance. For these people, factors such as obesity and lack of physical activity can trigger insulin resistance.

Metabolic syndrome has become much more common in the United States due to the rise in obesity. About 20% to 25% of adult Americans are estimated to have metabolic syndrome (American Heart Association, 2014; National Institute of Diabetes and Digestive and Kidney Disease, 2015a). In the future, metabolic syndrome may overtake smoking as a leading risk factor for heart disease. It is possible to delay or control metabolic syndrome, but it requires a lifelong commitment to healthy lifestyle choices, such as weight control and regular physical activity.

Diseases of the Thyroid

The thyroid releases hormones that control many bodily activities, including heart rate and how fast a person burns calories. Diseases of the thyroid happen when the thyroid either over- or underproduces thyroid hormones. Women are more likely than men to have thyroid diseases, especially after pregnancy and after menopause.

Graves Disease

Graves disease is the most common cause of hyperthyroidism in the United States. *Hyperthyroidism* occurs when the thyroid gland makes more of thyroid hormones than the body needs. As noted earlier, thyroid hormones affect a number of body functions, such as metabolism, breathing, heart rate, and control of body temperature; they also affect weight and cholesterol levels. Hyperthyroidism causes these body functions to speed up.

Patients with Graves disease may have some of the symptoms of hyperthyroidism, such as nervousness or irritability, heat intolerance, rapid heartbeat, hair loss and weight loss (Endocrine Society, 2016b) (see Figure 11.6). They may also develop a *goiter*, which is an enlarged thyroid that is painless but causes the neck to look swollen. In addition, the eyes of patients with Graves appear enlarged because the eyelids are pulled back and the eyes bulge out from the eye sockets. This eye condition is called *Graves ophthalmopathy*; it can last for a couple of years, but it often improves on its own.

It is not known why some people develop Graves disease, but age, sex, heredity, and stress factors are involved. Graves usually occurs in people younger than age 40 and is up to eight times more common in women than in men. Patients with autoimmune diseases

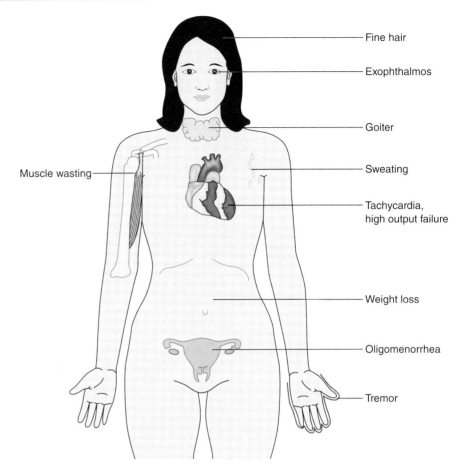

Figure 11.6 Signs and Symptoms of Graves Disease

Note. Adapted from "HyperaldosteronismSymptoms.jpeg," by Madhero88 at English Wikipedia [CC BY 3.0 (http://creativecommons.org/licenses/by/3.0)], via Wikimedia Commons. Retrieved from https://commons.wikimedia.org/wiki/File%3AHyperaldosteronismSymptoms.jpeg

such as rheumatoid arthritis have an increased chance of developing Graves, as do those with a family health history of the disease. Given that some of the signs and symptoms of Graves disease are visible, such as hair loss and a goiter, it can sometimes be easily diagnosed based only on a physical examination and a family health history. Laboratory tests or a thyroid scan can confirm the diagnosis.

There are three treatment options for Graves disease: radioiodine therapy, antithyroid medications, and thyroid surgery. Graves is most often treated with radioactive iodine (radioiodine) therapy, which destroys the cells of the thyroid gland. Almost everyone who receives radioiodine treatment eventually develops *hypothyroidism*, meaning that the thyroid does not make enough thyroid hormones for the needs of the body. Patients with hypothyroidism must take synthetic thyroid hormone.

Health care providers sometimes prescribe antithyroid medications as the first or only treatment for Graves disease. Antithyroid medications, however, require frequent monitoring by a provider and do not usually have permanent results.

Surgery is another treatment for Graves disease, but it is usually limited to patients with thyroid cancer, pregnant women who cannot tolerate drugs, or those who fail other forms of treatment. When surgery is used, usually the entire thyroid is removed. If the entire thyroid is removed, lifelong thyroid hormone replacement is necessary.

Hashimoto's Disease

In *Hashimoto's disease*, the immune system attacks the thyroid gland. This chronic inflammation damages the thyroid gland, leading to hypothyroidism. Hashimoto's disease is the most common cause of hypothyroidism in the United States; however, not everyone with this disease develops hypothyroidism.

Many patients with Hashimoto's disease have no symptoms at first, but over time, the thyroid enlarges and causes a goiter. Other symptoms can be mild or severe and include fatigue, weight gain, cold intolerance, and a slowed heart rate.

Hashimoto's disease is about seven times more common in women than in men, and it more commonly appears between 40 and 60 years of age. Hashimoto's tends to run in families, but there are also possible environmental factors, such as pesticides, excessive iodine consumption, and certain medications. Viral infections may also cause this disease. Patients with other autoimmune diseases are more likely to develop Hashimoto's disease, and vice versa; for example, patients with Hashimoto's are more likely to develop rheumatoid arthritis, and those with rheumatoid arthritis are more likely to develop Hashimoto's.

Diagnosis begins with a physical examination and health history. An endocrinologist will do RIA blood tests along with an ultrasound or CT scan to confirm the diagnosis.

Treatment depends on whether or not the thyroid is damaged enough to cause hypothyroidism. If there is hypothyroidism, then synthetic thyroid hormone treatment is required to return hormone levels up to normal. If there is no hypothyroidism, then the focus of treatment is on trying to reduce the size of the goiter. Hashimoto's disease may not always need treatment, and an option is to simply monitor the progress of the disease.

Thyroid Cancer

As the term implies, thyroid cancer is a cancer of the thyroid gland tissues. This cancer is the ninth most common cancer in the United States, with yearly estimates of nearly 63,000 Americans being diagnosed and nearly 1,900 deaths (National Cancer Institute, 2015). The number of thyroid cancer diagnoses is increasing more rapidly than that of any other cancer in the United States. This increase has been seen in all racial and ethnic population groups and in both males and females. The incidence of thyroid cancer is nearly three times higher in women than in men and nearly twice as high in Whites as in African Americans.

Thyroid cancer can occur in any age group, although it is most common in people over age 30, and it is significantly more aggressive in older patients. Risk factors for thyroid cancer include the following:

- Being female and between the ages of 25 and 65
- Being exposed to radiation as a child
- Having had a goiter
- Having a family health history of thyroid disease or thyroid cancer

There are usually no early signs or symptoms of thyroid cancer. They may arise as the tumor gets bigger. When they do eventually appear, signs and symptoms include a lump in the neck, hoarseness, and trouble breathing and swallowing. Diagnostic tests include ultrasound examination, CAT scan, and surgical biopsy.

Treatment for thyroid cancer can be a combination of surgery, radiation therapy, chemotherapy, thyroid hormone therapy, and targeted therapy. Targeted cancer therapies, sometimes called "precision medicines," are drugs or other substances that block the growth and spread of cancer.

The treatment and prognosis for thyroid cancer depend on the age of the patient and his or her general health, the type and stage of the cancer, and whether the patient has had thyroid cancer in the past.

Growth Hormone Disorders

The pituitary is the small gland in the brain that makes *growth hormone* (GH). GH is responsible for body growth and development during childhood and adolescence; and maintenance of a normal level of GH is also important for adults. Almost all body tissues are affected by GH.

Acromegaly

Acromegaly is a result of too much GH and is caused by a noncancerous tumor in the pituitary gland. Although symptoms can appear at any age, acromegaly is most often diagnosed in middle-aged adults. One of its most common symptoms is abnormal bone growth in the hands and feet. Similar bone changes can also change facial features: The brow and lower jaw stick out, the nasal bone grows, the facial features enlarge, and the teeth space out. Other symptoms include joint aches, breast discharge in women, and erectile dysfunction in men.

Acromegaly is first diagnosed through an RIA blood test, then an MRI of the pituitary is used to locate and detect the size of the tumor.

The first line of treatment is usually surgical removal of the tumor, but medication or radiation may be used instead of surgery. Treatment options depend on the patient's health status and the size of the tumor. Even if treatment is effective, a patient needs long-term monitoring of GH levels. The most serious health consequences of acromegaly are type 2 diabetes, high blood pressure, increased risk of cardiovascular disease, and arthritis. If not treated, acromegaly can lead to serious illness and even premature death.

About 60 out of every million people suffer from this disease at any given time, but the actual number of people with this disease is not known. Because of its slow onset (start), acromegaly is often not diagnosed early, or it is diagnosed incorrectly.

When pituitary gland tumors cause overproduction of GH in childhood, then the disease is called gigantism rather than acromegaly. A pediatrician should be consulted if a child's growth rate suddenly increases beyond what would be predicted before puberty and by how tall the child's parents are.

Sex Hormone Disorders

The *gonads*, or ovaries and testes, are endocrine glands that make and secrete sex hormones. Precocious puberty and hypogonadism are examples of diseases caused by problems with how the gonads produce and secrete sex hormones.

Precocious Puberty

Puberty is the stage during which children develop physically and emotionally into young men and women. The onset of puberty is normally triggered by the hypothalamus. It signals the pituitary gland to release hormones that stimulate the ovaries or testicles to make sex hormones. Puberty starts no earlier than about 8 years of age for girls and 9 years of age for boys.

When a child begins showing signs of puberty before age 8 in girls and age 9 in boys, the condition is known as *precocious puberty, or hypergonadism*. It can be physically and emotionally difficult for children and can be a sign of other health problems. Most cases of precocious puberty have no known cause, but some possible causes are thought to be obesity as well as social and environmental factors. There is some research evidence which suggests that chemicals in the environment and certain processed foods may negatively affect puberty. In addition, radiation received from childhood cancer treatments can lead to early puberty.

For the majority of girls, there's no medical problem at fault; they simply start puberty too early for an unknown reason. The signs and symptoms of precocious puberty in girls include the following (Eunice Kennedy Shriver National Institute of Child Health and Human Development, 2013):

- Breast development
- Rapid increase in height
- Acne
- Growth of pubic and underarm hair
- Menstruation
- Body odor

Precocious puberty is less common for boys and more likely to be related to another medical problem. The signs and symptoms in boys include the following (Eunice Kennedy Shriver National Institute of Child Health and Human Development, 2013):

- Enlarged testicles or penis
- Rapid increase in height
- Acne
- Growth of pubic, underarm, or facial hair
- Deepening voice
- Body odor

When skeletons mature and bone growth stops at an early age, then children with precocious puberty don't achieve their full adult height. Their early growth spurt may make them tall when compared with their peers, but they stop growing too soon and end up at a shorter height than they would have otherwise.

The physical changes that boys and girls undergo during puberty can be observed through a physical examination. To confirm a diagnosis of precocious puberty, RIA and urine tests can detect higher levels of sex hormones. X-rays of a child's wrist and hand show whether the bones are maturing too fast. A CT scan, MRI scan, and ultrasound can also help with diagnosis.

The treatment goal for precocious puberty is to stop sexual development and rapid bone growth. Lowering levels of sex hormones with synthetic hormone therapy is one way to stop precocious puberty. With hormone therapy, a girl's breast size decreases or stops growing. In a boy, the penis and testicles shrink back to the size expected for his age. Growth in height will also slow down to a rate expected for children before puberty.

Hypogonadism

Hypogonadism occurs when the gonads do not make enough of the sex hormone testosterone. Testosterone is found in both males and females, although it is commonly called the male hormone because it plays a key role in male growth and development. Hypogonadism usually affects males, but it can also affect females and often happens during puberty.

There are two types of hypogonadism: Primary hypogonadism occurs because the gonads are not making enough testosterone; in secondary hypogonadism, the brain's hypothalamus and pituitary glands aren't working properly and can't control gonad function.

Hypogonadism can be caused by an injury, other diseases, tumors, or treatment for certain diseases, such as cancer. It can also be the result of a history of steroid abuse, even if the patient no longer uses steroids.

Signs and symptoms of hypogonadism includes growth problems, hair loss, genital underdevelopment, sexual dysfunction, infertility, decrease in muscle and bone mass, increase in fat mass, enlarged male breasts, loss of cognitive function, and depression (Endocrine Society, 2016a). Males and females can experience similar signs and symptoms. If hypogonadism begins during fetal development, a baby may be born with abnormal sex organs. If it develops before puberty, hypogonadism may impair penis and testicle growth.

A physical examination can determine if a patient's sexual development is at an age-appropriate level. RIA blood tests to check testosterone level as well as pituitary hormone level help diagnosis hypogonadism. Hormone-based medications and injections are available for men and for women. For some patients, surgery and radiation therapy may be needed. If hypogonadism is treated, the prognosis is generally positive.

Chapter Summary

- A gland is a group of cells that make and release hormones.

- Endocrine glands are scattered throughout the body; they secrete hormones that regulate many bodily functions.

- Endocrine glands release more than 20 major hormones into the bloodstream, and these hormones influence almost every cell, organ, and function of our bodies.

- The pituitary gland is sometimes called the "master gland" because it regulates growth and metabolism.

- Endocrine diseases are caused by an abnormal over- or undersecretion of hormones. They can also be caused when the body has difficulty in removing hormones from the blood.

- Aging, disease, stress, and the environment can affect how the endocrine system works.

- Endocrinology is the medical field that specializes in endocrine diseases. An endocrinologist is a physician with specialized training in endocrinology.

- Insulin is secreted when the blood glucose level rises. Insulin helps blood glucose enter cells. Without insulin, glucose cannot enter the cells, which leads to an increase in the blood glucose (blood sugar) level.

REVIEW QUESTIONS

1. What is the difference between type 1 and type 2 diabetes?

2. What is the negative feedback system, and how does it control hormones?

3. Name the hormones that cause the development of female and male sex characteristics.

4. Define *metabolic* and identify the risks factors for metabolic syndrome.

5. Describe the differences between Graves disease and Hashimoto's disease.

6. What is a goiter? What diseases cause a goiter?

7. Describe the difference between acromegaly and gigantism.

8. Identify the signs of precocious puberty and explain why it is a concern.

9. What are three strategies a patient with diabetes can do to prevent low blood glucose?

10. List some of the causes of hypogonadism.

KEY TERMS

Abdominal obesity: Larger waistline than normal

Acromegaly: Condition caused by excessive growth hormone, commonly leading to abnormal bone growth of hands and feet

Adrenal glands: Two glands, one on top of each kidney, that secrete hormones that influence the body's response to stress, metabolism, blood chemicals, and body characteristics such as sexual development

Blood glucose: A source of energy for body cells

Cortisol: Hormone that helps the body respond to physical stress

Diabetes mellitus: Disease caused by the failure of the pancreas to secrete enough insulin or by the body's inability to use insulin correctly

Diabetic ketosis: Abnormal fat metabolism caused by a lack of insulin

Endocrine system: System made up of glands, located throughout the body, that secrete hormones essential to metabolic function

Endocrinologist: Specially trained physician who diagnoses and treats diseases of the endocrine system

Endocrinology: Branch of medicine concerned with the endocrine system

Environmental endocrine disruptor (EED): A chemical outside the body that has negative effects on the endocrine system

Estrogen: Female hormone

Fetal macrosomia: Condition caused by poorly controlled gestational diabetes, which leads to excessive blood glucose in babies

Gestational diabetes: Diabetes that develops during pregnancy

Gigantism: Overproduction of the growth hormone

Gland: Group of cells that make and release chemicals

Glucagon: Hormone that is released by the pancreas when blood glucose is low

Glycogen: Extra glucose that is stored in the liver and muscles and used for energy during meals

Goiter: Enlarged thyroid gland

Gonads: Ovaries and testes

Graves disease: Disease affecting a number of body functions, including metabolism, heart rate, weight, and breathing; the most common cause of hyperthyroidism in the United States

Graves ophthalmopathy: Disease condition in which the eyes of patients with Graves disease appear enlarged because the eyelids are pulled back and the eyes bulge out from the eye sockets

Growth hormone (GH): A hormone responsible for body growth and development

Hashimoto's disease: Chronic inflammation of the thyroid gland, often causing hypothyroidism

Homeostasis: State in which internal organs and functions are balanced and stable

Hormones: Chemical messengers that regulate the activities of cells and organs

Hyperglycemia: Condition in which glucose builds up to high levels in the blood

Hyperthyroidism: Condition in which the thyroid gland produces more thyroid hormones than the body needs and causes certain body functions to speed up

Hypoglycemia: Condition in which blood glucose drops below normal levels

Hypoglycemia unawareness: State in which diabetic patients do not experience early warning signs of low blood glucose

Hypogonadism: Condition that occurs when the gonads under-produce sex hormones

Hypothalamus: Gland that lies in the lower part of the brain and is the primary link between the endocrine and nervous systems

Hypothyroidism: Condition in which the thyroid gland does not produce enough hormones for the needs of the body.

Insulin: Hormone that helps convert sugar, starches, and other carbohydrates into glucose for energy

Insulin resistance: In the context of gestational diabetes, a state in which the mother's body has difficulty producing and using all the insulin it needs for pregnancy; more generally, difficulty using insulin effectively, resulting in an elevated blood glucose level

Menopause: Age-related changes to the ovaries

Metabolic: Concerning biochemical processes involved in the body's normal functioning

Metabolic syndrome: Group of metabolic risk factors that exist in a person

Negative feedback system: A feedback loop in which information about a hormone's level is fed back to the gland that makes it and that then responds.

Ovaries: Female reproductive glands that produce estrogen and progesterone

Pancreas: Gland that helps the body maintain healthy blood glucose levels

Parathyroid glands: A group of four glands, attached to the thyroid, that release parathyroid hormone.

Pineal gland: Gland that is located in the middle of the brain and that is involved with daily and seasonal sleep-and-waking cycles.

Pituitary gland: Gland that regulates homeostasis and produces hormones that influence other endocrine glands

Precocious puberty, or hypergonadism: Signs of puberty that begin abnormally early, before age 8 in girls and age 9 in boys

Progesterone: Female hormone

Puberty: Stage in which children develop physically and emotionally into young men and women

Radioimmunoassay (RIA): Blood test that detects hormone levels

Reproductive glands (gonads): The ovaries in women and the testes in men

Testes: Male reproductive glands that produce testosterone

Testosterone: Male hormone

Thyroid gland: Gland that is located in the front part of the neck and makes thyroid hormones.

Type 1 diabetes mellitus: Diabetes mellitus caused by insufficient insulin

Type 2 diabetes mellitus: Diabetes mellitus caused by an inadequate response to insulin

CHAPTER ACTIVITIES

1. Managing a chronic disease such as type 2 diabetes can be a challenge for newly diagnosed patients. To understand these challenges, imagine yourself as someone who has been recently diagnosed with type 2 diabetes. Create a "5 A's list" for self-care, using the American Diabetes Association website (www.diabetes.org) as a resource. Present the list on a current one-month calendar daily planner. Each section of the 5 A's list has a name:

    a. *Arrange.* What do you do now that you know you have type 2 diabetes? What are your appointments, medicines, phone calls, and emails or letters? [Use your imagination and refer to your own relationship with your health care provider.]

    b. *Advise.* What information do you need to tell your health care provider and care team? They need to know the foods you eat and drink, the exercise you do, and all medicines you take and their side effects. What information do you need to know from them?

    c. *Assist.* Name the problem that stops you from taking care of yourself—for example, you don't understand your health care provider, medicines cost too much, or family does not help. Then identify someone who can help you with that problem. If there is no one who can help you, write how can you help yourself.

    d. *Agree.* What are the goals that you and your health care provider have identified? For each goal, identify what, when, and how you will meet it.

    e. *Act.* What are the blocks to those goals you and your health care provider have identified? How will you overcome those blocks? Who can help you with your goals?

    Once you have completed this activity, write a one- to two-page reflection paper identifying some of the difficulties or barriers in managing type 2 diabetes as a patient with low health literacy.

2. In small groups, make a health bingo game. The target audience is made up of residents who live either in an urban assisted living facility or in public housing. The topic is type 2 diabetes awareness. Create 24 questions, and write the answers on the bingo card (with one free space). Questions are based on prevention concepts related to diabetes. To win, a player needs to get five correct answers in a row, column, or diagonal line.

3. Answer the following questions in two to three pages and be prepared to discuss answers in class: For people with type 1 diabetes, what problem is there with insulin? How do people get the disease? How do they manage it? For people with type 2 diabetes, what problem exists with insulin? How do people get the disease? How do they manage it? Do you know anyone with diabetes? Have you noticed things he or she does to manage the disease? What steps can you take as a health educator to help those with type 1 and type 2 diabetes?

4. You are working as a patient advocate with those who have thyroid diseases. As part of your job, you will make a poster board with pictures that show how low-health-literacy patients with a thyroid disease can protect their health. Use those pictures that best illustrate points and minimize wording.

5. Your instructor will fill a container with slips of paper printed with descriptive statements related to endocrine diseases. The statements do not identify the disease but do describe a feature. Select one slip. You will have a few minutes to think about what disease the statement describes and then you will read your statement and identify the disease.

Bibliography and Works Cited

American Diabetes Association. (2016). National diabetes education program. Retrieved from http://www.diabetes.org/diabetes-basics/?loc=GlobalNavDB

American Heart Association. (2014). *Metabolic syndrome.* Retrieved from http://www.heart.org/HEARTORG/Conditions/More/MetabolicSyndrome/Metabolic-Syndrome_UCM_002080_SubHomePage.jsp

American Heart Association. (2015). About diabetes. Retrieved from http://www.heart.org/HEARTORG/Conditions/Diabetes/AboutDiabetes/About-Diabetes_UCM_002032_Article.jsp#.Vo2wsLYrLtQ

American Medical Association. (2015). *Prevent diabetes STAT: Screen/test/act today.* Retrieved from http://www.ama-assn.org/sub/prevent-diabetes-stat/index.html

Centers for Disease Control and Prevention. (2015). Diabetes home. Retrieved from http://www.cdc.gov/diabetes/home/index.html

Crowley, L. V. (2012). *Introduction to human disease* (9th ed.). Boston, MA: Jones and Bartlett.

Endocrine Society. (2016a). *Hypogonadism.* Retrieved from http://www.hormone.org/diseases-and-conditions/mens-health/hypogonadism

Endocrine Society. (2016b). *Thyroid disorders.* Retrieved from http://www.hormone.org/diseases-and-conditions/thyroid

Endocrine Society. (2016c). *What are hormones, and what do they do?* Retrieved from http://www.hormone.org/hormones-and-health/what-do-hormones-do

Eunice Kennedy Shriver National Institute of Child Health and Human Development. (2013). Puberty and precocious puberty: Condition information. Retrieved from https://www.nichd.nih.gov/health/topics/puberty/conditioninfo/Pages/default.aspx

March of Dimes. (2016). *Gestational diabetes.* Retrieved from http://www.marchofdimes.org/complications/gestational-diabetes.aspx

Mayo Clinic. (2016). Fetal macrosomia. Retrieved from http://www.mayoclinic.org/diseases-conditions/fetal-macrosomia/basics/definition/CON-20035423?p=1

National Cancer Institute. (2015). Thyroid cancer—patient version. Retrieved from http://www.cancer.gov/types/thyroid

National Cancer Institute. (2016). SEER training modules: Endocrine system. Retrieved from https://training.seer.cancer.gov/anatomy/endocrine/

National Institute of Diabetes and Digestive and Kidney Diseases. (2014). *Causes of diabetes.* Retrieved from http://www.niddk.nih.gov/health-information/health-topics/Diabetes/causes-diabetes/Pages/index.aspx

National Institute of Diabetes and Digestive and Kidney Diseases. (2015a). Endocrine diseases. Retrieved from http://www.niddk.nih.gov/health-information/health-topics/endocrine/Pages/default.aspx

National Institute of Diabetes and Digestive and Kidney Diseases. (2015b). National diabetes education program. Retrieved from http://www.niddk.nih.gov/health-information/health-communication-programs/ndep/pages/index.aspx

US National Library of Medicine. (2014). Diabetes (diabetes mellitus). *PubMed Health.* Retrieved from http://www.ncbi.nlm.nih.gov/pubmedhealth/PMHT0024704/

US National Library of Medicine. (2016). Endocrine system. *MedlinePlus.* Retrieved from https://medlineplus.gov/endocrinesystem.html#topics

CHAPTER 12

NERVOUS SYSTEM, SENSORY SYSTEM, AND RELATED DISEASES

CHAPTER OBJECTIVES

- Identify three functions of the nervous system.

- Compare and contrast the central nervous system and the peripheral nervous system.

- Review and explain common infectious and degenerative neurological diseases discussed in this chapter.

- Review and explain brain and spinal cord tumors discussed in this chapter.

- Review and explain common brain and spinal cord injuries discussed in this chapter.

- Review and explain sensory diseases discussed in this chapter.

The nervous system is among the smallest body systems in terms of weight, yet it is the most complex. What is the nervous system? What does it do? How does it work? The first two questions are easy to answer, but the third is much more difficult. Neuroscientists can explain what the nervous system is and what it does, but because there are so many complex levels of understanding, the ability to explain how it works is more challenging. Described as the final frontier of biology, neuroscience is beginning to reveal some of the mysteries of the nervous system.

Function of the Nervous System

The body's systems do not function separately. All have to work together as one unit to maintain homeostasis, or internal balance. The function of the nervous system is to help the body's systems communicate with each other. It does this by using both electrical and chemical impulses that send and receive messages.

A way to explain what the nervous system does is to describe its three main functions. Millions of *neurons*, or nerve cells, in the body detect *stimuli*, or things that cause physiological changes in a cell, tissue, or organ. Neurons detect stimuli outside the body, such as changes in pressure, oxygen, and water balance. Neurons also detect stimuli inside the body, such as temperature, light, and sound. The gathering of all this information that is perceived by the senses (smell, sight, touch, taste, and hearing), otherwise known as *sensory input*, is the first function of the nervous system.

Sensory input is processed and then made into electrical signals, or *nerve impulses*, that are transmitted to the brain. There the nerve impulses create sensations, thoughts, emotions, and memory. The process of making decisions each moment based on sensory input is called *integration*, which is the second function of the nervous system.

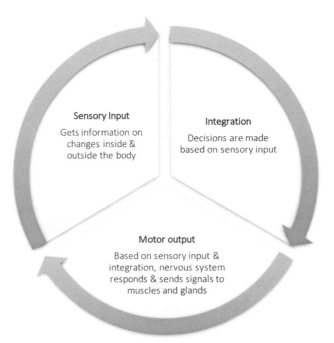

Figure 12.1   Three Functions of the Nervous System

In response to sensory input and integration, the nervous system sends signals to muscles, causing them to contract or relax, and also to glands, causing them to secrete hormones. This activity is called *motor output*, the third function of the nervous system.

Together these three functions keep us in touch with what is going on inside and outside our body, maintain homeostasis, and explain our mental state (see Figure 12.1).

Control of the body's billions of cells is the responsibility of two communication systems: the nervous system and the endocrine system. Both systems send messages from one part of the body to another, but they do it in different ways. The nervous system sends messages fast, using nerve impulses. The endocrine system sends messages slowly, using hormones secreted by glands into the bloodstream. Nerve impulses and hormones communicate information to body structures, increasing and decreasing their activities as needed to maintain a healthy body.

Structure of the Nervous System

The organs of the nervous system include the brain, spinal cord, nerves, and *ganglia*, which are masses of nerve tissue outside the brain or spinal cord. As previously noted, the nervous system depends on tiny nerve cells called neurons. Neurons send information about any changes inside and outside the body. They send information through a complex electrical and chemical process, making connections that affect the way we think, learn, move, feel, and act.

There are about 20 billion neurons in the body. Each receives information from 100,000 different sources, and each has a special job to do. For example, sensory neurons take information from the eyes, ears, nose, tongue, and skin to the brain. Motor neurons carry messages away from the brain and out to the rest of the body for movement.

Neurons have features that make them different from other body cells; for example, they are shaped differently depending on what role they play. But all neurons have the same three parts (see Figure 12.2):

•   The central body

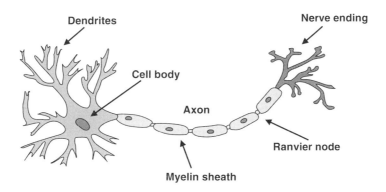

Figure 12.2 Neuron

Note. Adapted from "Derived Neuron Schema With no Labels.svg," by Dhp1080, svg adaptation by Actam (Image:Neuron.svg) [CC BY-SA 3.0 (http://creativecommons.org/licenses/by-sa/3.0) or GFDL (http://www.gnu.org/copyleft/fdl.html)], via Wikimedia Commons. Retrieved from https://commons.wikimedia.org/wiki/File%3ADerived_Neuron_schema_with_no_labels.svg

- *Dendrites*, which are finger-like projections that carry impulses into the neuron
- The *axon*, which is made up of long fibers that carry impulses out of the neuron

The axon has a fatty protective coating called a *myelin sheath*. The myelin sheath wraps around the axon and creates a number of bumps on it (see Figure 12.2). The space or gap between each bump is called a *node of ranvier*, which exposes the neuron membrane to the external environment. Messages jump off the node from one neuron to the next, using special chemicals called *neurotransmitters*.

We are born with all the neurons that we will ever have, but many of the neurons are not connected to each other. As we grow and learn, messages travel from one neuron to another over and over, creating *neural pathways*, or connections in the brain. This is why some physical tasks like riding a bike can be difficult to learn at first, but then become easy because the pathway is established. Unlike other cells in the body, if a neuron is damaged by disease or injury, it is not repaired or replaced.

Another type of cell in the nervous system is a *neuroglia*. These cells do not send messages as neurons do but instead support, nourish, and protect neurons. They are a special type of "connective tissue" for the nervous system.

There is only one nervous system, but each part of the system is also called a nervous system, which can be confusing. All subsystems belong to one nervous system, and each has a structure and function that make it different from the others. The nervous system is divided into two major subsystems: the central nervous system (CNS) and the peripheral nervous system (PNS). The PNS has two subsystems, the somatic and the automatic. The automatic system has its own subsystems, the sympathetic and the parasympathetic. Use Figure 12.3 as a visual guide as you read about the various subsystems in the next sections.

Central Nervous System

The brain and spinal cord are organs of the *central nervous system (CNS)*. The brain is protected by the bones of the skull; the spinal cord is protected by round bones called *vertebrae*. In addition to bones, there are *meninges*, or membranes, as well as a special fluid called *cerebrospinal fluid* that provide protection.

The spinal cord, in the spinal column, is an extension of the brain and is the network that sends messages through nerves. *Nerves* are bundles of nerve fibers. The nerves within the spinal cord go up to and down from the brain carrying messages to and from muscles, organs, and glands.

The spinal cord is about 18 inches long and $\frac{1}{4}$-inch thick, and goes from the lower part of the brain down through the spine. Along the way, many nerves branch out to the entire body, particularly into the arms, torso, and legs.

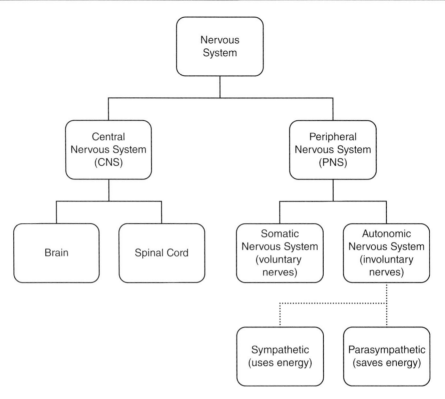

Figure 12.3 The Nervous System and Subsystems

The brain is the control center of the nervous system and is at the top of the spinal cord. This soft organ has the most neurons of the nervous system. Because it controls just about everything, when something is wrong with the brain, the problem is often serious and can affect different parts of the body. The adult brain weighs about 2 to 3 pounds and is compact, with many folds and grooves. It is divided into three major parts: the *cerebrum, cerebellum,* and *brain stem* (see Figure 12.4). The cerebrum is the largest part of the brain and is located in the front part of the skull. It performs motor, sensory, and higher mental functions, such as thought, reason, emotion, and memory. The cerebellum is located at the back of the skull. It coordinates and controls muscle activity, balance, and equilibrium. The brain stem is located below the cerebellum. It controls the flow of messages between the brain and

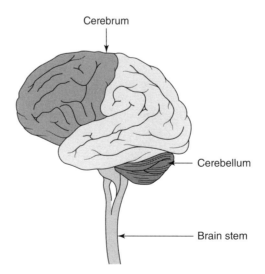

Figure 12.4 Parts of the Brain

the rest of the body, and is also responsible for basic vital life functions, such as breathing, heart rate, and blood pressure.

When the brain receives a message from anywhere in the body, the brain tells the body what to do. For example, if you touch a hot stove, the nerves in your skin shoot a message of pain to the brain. The brain then sends a message back telling the hand muscles to pull away.

In children, the brain is particularly flexible; in fact, when one part of a child's brain is injured, another part can often learn to take over some of the lost function. But as we age, the brain works harder, making it challenging sometimes to master new tasks or change behavior. However, throughout adulthood, the brain can reorganize itself and allow neurons to respond in ways that lessen the consequences of injury and disease. It can also adjust neural activity in response to new situations or to changes in the environment.

Peripheral Nervous System

The *peripheral nervous system (PNS)* comprises the nerves outside the CNS, starting with 12 pairs of cranial nerves and 31 pairs of spinal nerves. The PNS has nerves that run throughout the body like strings, making connections with the brain, other parts of the body, and often with each other (see Figure 12.5). The nerves are wrapped with myelin sheath, which speeds up the transmission of nerve impulses.

The PNS nerves are the communication network between the CNS and the arms, legs, eyes, ears, and other organs. These nerves carry signals from the CNS to a specific part of the body to perform an action. That part of the body then keeps the CNS informed of what is going on inside and outside the body.

The PNS is subdivided into the somatic nervous system and the autonomic nervous system. The *somatic nervous system*, or voluntary nervous system, is made up of nerves that go to the skin and muscles. The somatic nervous system controls skeletal muscles that allow us to voluntarily move and to receive information from our senses.

The *autonomic nervous system*, or the involuntary nervous system, is made up of nerves that connect the CNS to organs, such as the heart and stomach. It is also helps control involuntary functions like breathing, digesting, and sweating.

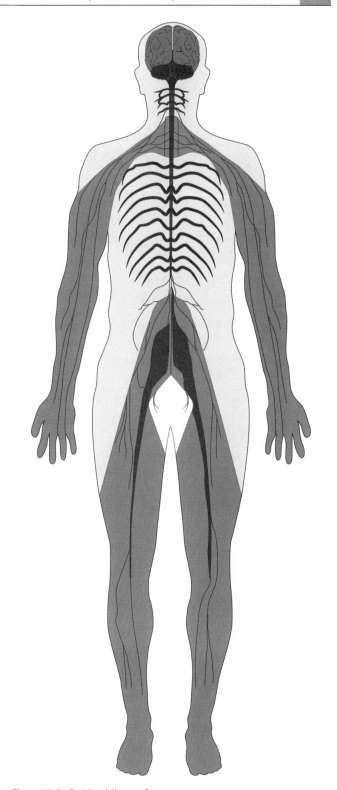

Figure 12.5 Peripheral Nervous System
Shaded areas showing the location of the peripheral nerves. Peripheral nerves go from the spinal cord to arms, hands, legs, and feet.

The autonomic nervous system is further divided into the *sympathetic nervous system* and the *parasympathetic nervous system*. These two nervous systems work together, but act on the body in opposite ways. The sympathetic increases the actions of the body, whereas the parasympathetic decreases them.

The sympathetic nervous system's main function is to prepare the body for emergency situations. In emergency situations, this system causes the adrenal glands to release the hormone adrenaline, which gives extra power to the muscles for a quick getaway. (This is what's commonly known as the "fight-or-flight" response.) The parasympathetic nervous system's function is to prepare the body for rest by slowing the heart rate and breathing. It also calms down systems and saves energy.

Diseases of the Nervous System

Neurology is the medical specialty concerned with the nervous system. A *neurologist* is a physician who specializes in neurology and is trained in the diagnosis, treatment, and management of neurological diseases. Many neurologists also have additional training in specific areas of neurology, such as stroke and epilepsy.

Headaches

According to the American Migraine Foundation (2016), *tension headaches* are the most common type of headache for adults. These headaches are from tight muscles in the shoulders, neck, scalp, and jaw. They are often related to stress, depression, or anxiety. Tension headaches are more likely to happen when a person is overworking, not getting enough sleep, missing meals, or using alcohol. Sensitivity to light or sound may also be a cause.

These headaches happen infrequently and can last minutes to days. The pain is usually on both sides of the head, accompanied by a tightening feeling. Tension headaches do not worsen with physical activity and may not cause disability.

The cause of a tension headache determines the treatment. If there is no medical cause for the headache, the use of aspirin, acetaminophen, muscle relaxants, anti-inflammatory medications, massage, acupuncture, and meditation provide temporary relief from pain.

Migraine headaches are less common than tension headaches (American Migraine Foundation, 2016). A migraine is a repeating headache that lasts from 4 to 72 hours and often causes moderate to intense pain on one side of the face, nausea, and sensitivity to sound and light. Migraine pain is made worse by physical activity and causes disability. Some migraines sufferers can tell when they are about to have a migraine because they see flashing lights or zigzag lines, or they temporarily can't see.

The cause of migraines may be related to genes. Medications can help prevent migraine attacks or help relieve symptoms. For many patients, stress management can also help. A migraine can be diagnosed through a review of the patient's health history of repeating, severe headaches; a CT or MRI scan; and an EEG. Treatment includes bed rest, staying in a dark room, and aspirin or anti-inflammatory medications. For others, pain relievers as well as biofeedback, relaxation techniques, massage, and acupuncture can help relieve symptoms.

Cluster headaches are the most painful of headaches (American Migraine Foundation, 2016). They are repeated periods of intense pain on one side of the head around the eye, and they cause high blood pressure. Severe pain can last up to 3 hours and occur once every other day or up to eight times in one day. The pain can last for 4 to 6 weeks, then entirely disappear for up to a year. Correct diagnosis of cluster headaches requires the health care provider to know that the patient has suffered short-lasting headaches with red eye, tearing, runny nose, and other related symptoms that occur on one side of the head over weeks.

Infectious Diseases

Infection of the nervous system can involve the brain or the meninges or both. These infections can be either acute or chronic. They pose a challenge to health care providers due both to the high potential for morbidity (illness) and mortality (death) and to difficulties in treatment (Parikh, Tucci, & Galwankar, 2012). There are four main causes of neurological infection: fungal, bacterial, parasitic, or viral. The infectious diseases discussed in this section are meningitis, encephalitis, West Nile virus, and shingles.

Meningitis

Meningitis is a swelling of the meninges, the membranes that surround the brain and spinal cord, and is usually due to an infection. This swelling causes severe headache, fever, confusion, vomiting, and a stiff neck, which develop over several hours or over a couple of days.

The usual cause of meningitis is viral, but bacterial and fungal infections can also cause it. Depending on the cause, meningitis can either resolve on its own in a couple of weeks or be life threatening. For example, viral meningitis may improve without treatment, whereas bacterial meningitis can require intensive care.

Several types of bacteria can cause bacterial meningitis. The bacteria that cause bacterial meningitis are spread from person to person. Some bacteria are spread through the exchange of respiratory and throat secretions like saliva, or spit, during close contact (e.g., coughing or kissing) or lengthy contact, especially if the people live in the same household. The bacteria are not spread by casual contact or by simply breathing the air where a person with bacterial meningitis has been. Other meningitis-causing bacteria are not spread person to person, but can cause disease because the person has certain risk factors, such as a weak immune system or head trauma.

Healthy people can carry meningitis-causing bacteria in their nose or throat with no signs or symptoms of disease; this is called being a "carrier." Most carriers never become sick.

Infection happens when bacteria enter the bloodstream via respiratory and throat secretions and travel to the brain and spinal cord. Bacteria can also directly invade the meninges because of an ear or sinus infection or skull fracture. Bacterial meningitis is serious, comes on quickly—in a matter of hours, and requires immediate antibiotic treatment. Delaying treatment increases risk of permanent brain damage or death.

A number of factors increase the risk of contracting meningitis, including failure to complete a childhood vaccine schedule, living in a community setting like a college, working with animals, or having a weakened immune system (Mayo Clinic, 2016b). Children under age 5 and young adults are at higher risk.

A patient should have blood tests and a *lumbar puncture, or spinal tap,* for a diagnosis. A spinal tap is a test that analyzes a sample of a patient's cerebrospinal fluid. For this test, a needle is inserted into the patient's lower back to collect the fluid for analysis. X-rays and CT scans of the head, chest, or sinuses may reveal swelling.

Ways to prevent meningitis depend on the type of infection. Washing hands carefully is important to avoid exposure to viral infections. People who have been in contact with someone with bacterial meningitis are given antibiotics as a precaution.

Encephalitis

Encephalitis is a swelling of the brain. The usual cause is a viral infection, but bacteria can also cause encephalitis. Even if someone gets a virus that causes encephalitis, he or she will not automatically become infected. In fact, very few people who are infected with these viruses actually develop encephalitis. Some cases of encephalitis are mild, with symptoms that last only for a short time; a severe case of encephalitis, however, can be life threatening.

Signs and symptoms of encephalitis include sudden fever, headache, vomiting, and stiff neck and back. Other symptoms, such as seizures, require emergency treatment. Blood samples and a spinal tap are used to diagnose encephalitis. An MRI or CT scan and an EEG may be used to verify the diagnosis.

Most mild cases of encephalitis just run their course, and the patient gets better without treatment. Patients with severe encephalitis are usually hospitalized for treatment. The prognosis for encephalitis depends on whether the infection is mild, in which case patients fully recover. Severe infections can mean permanent disability or death.

Please note that although meningitis and encephalitis may seem similar, there are differences. Patients with meningitis may be uncomfortable, have low energy, or have severe headaches, but their cerebral function remains normal. With encephalitis, however, patients may have abnormalities in brain function, such as personality and behavior changes as well as changes in speech or movement.

West Nile Virus

West Nile virus (WNV) is spread to humans by infected mosquitoes. It is a seasonal epidemic in the United States, meaning that it flares up in the summer and continues into the fall. The best way to avoid WNV is to prevent mosquito bites by using insect repellent and wearing protective clothing.

There are no medications to treat or vaccines to prevent WNV infection. Symptoms develop between 3 and 14 days after being bitten by an infected mosquito. Most people who have WNV usually have no symptoms. Those with symptoms can have fever, head and body aches, skin rash, or swollen lymph glands. If WNV enters the brain, it can cause meningitis or encephalitis and serious symptoms, such as coma, convulsions, and paralysis. These symptoms occur rarely, however, usually in the elderly and those with weakened immune systems. In severe cases, patients need treatment that includes intravenous fluids, help with breathing, and nursing care.

Shingles

Both chicken pox and *shingles, or herpes zoster,* are caused by the varicella zoster virus, which is a herpes virus. About 30% of people who have had chicken pox get shingles (National Institute of Neurological Disorders and Stroke, 2016b). Yearly in the United States, there are about one million people affected by shingles. Persons most at risk are those who had chicken pox before age 1, people over 60 years old, and people with weakened immune systems. There is a vaccine that helps prevent shingles for those 60 and older.

After a person has chicken pox, the virus stays in the body near the spinal cord permanently, in an inactive state. It is not known why, but certain events, such as emotional stress, immune deficiency, or cancer, activate the virus, causing shingles. Once active, shingles becomes a second outbreak of chicken pox. The virus travels along nerve paths, destroying these paths as it goes, to the skin, where it causes a painful, blistering rash.

Before the rash develops, a patient may feel burning or itching where the rash forms. A few days later, spots appear on one side of the body, usually on one side of the trunk, stomach, arms, legs, or face. These spots turn into painful blisters that can last about a week. Eventually the blisters dry out, crust over, and fall off. Sometimes the blisters grow together, forming scabs that leave scars. Other signs and symptoms of shingles can be numbness, depression, fever, and headaches. Shingles lasts up to 30 days for most patients, and a second attack of shingles is rare.

Shingles is contagious and can spread from an affected person to babies, children, or adults who have not had chicken pox. Instead of developing shingles, however, these people have chicken pox.

A diagnosis is made by looking at the infected area; tests are rarely needed. Treatment for shingles includes antiviral medications. Sometimes shingles pain may last for months to years, even with treatment.

Degenerative Diseases

Some diseases of the nervous system cause degeneration or decline of neurons, nerves, and brain tissues. *Degenerative diseases* are nonreversible, meaning that body changes cannot be stopped or turned back. In addition, these diseases are progressive, meaning that they only get worse over time. The degenerative diseases discussed in this section are dementia, Alzheimer's disease, Parkinson's disease, amyotrophic lateral sclerosis (or Lou Gehrig's disease), and epilepsy.

Dementia

Dementia is not a single disease; instead, it is a general term used to describe symptoms caused by some brain diseases, such as Alzheimer's disease, brain tumors, or stroke, or by a head injury. Dementia can be caused by brain cell death that happens over time. Patients with dementia experience cognitive decline and may not think well enough to do daily tasks, such as getting dressed or eating. They may lose their ability to solve problems; their personalities may change; they may become stressed or experience hallucinations. Dementia is more common in the elderly, but it is not a normal part of aging; meaning that not all elderly people get dementia.

Memory loss is a common symptom of dementia. Memory loss by itself, however, does not mean dementia. Patients with dementia have problems with two or more brain functions, such as memory, perception, personality, and language.

Dementia usually gets worse over time and decreases the patient's life span. Most causes of dementia are not preventable, but quitting smoking as well as controlling high blood pressure and diabetes can reduce risk for some forms of dementia.

A neurologist can diagnose dementia by performing a physical examination and asking questions about the patient's health history. A mental health status examination is also performed to check mental function. Blood, spinal tap, EEG, CT or MRI scans, and urine are done to support a dementia diagnosis.

Treatment depends on the causes of dementia. Stopping or changing medications that cause confusion can lessen dementia's symptoms. There are medications that cannot cure dementia but do improve symptoms or slow down the progression of the disease. There is some evidence that exercises that stimulate thinking can lessen symptoms. As dementia progresses, some patients may need 24-hour care and help with daily activities such as eating and dressing.

Alzheimer's Disease

Alzheimer's disease (AD) slowly destroys memory and thinking. In most patients, AD symptoms first appear after the age of 65; however, it is possible to have symptoms as early as 40.

AD is the most common cause of dementia among the elderly; it affects over five million people in the United States and is the fifth leading killer. Every 70 seconds, someone in the United States develops AD (Alzheimer's Foundation of America, 2016). It occurs more frequently in women than in men, but that may be due to women living longer than men.

What causes AD is not fully known, but there may be a genetic link. However, in about 90% of cases, there is no clear genetic link. What is known is that AD develops over time. There can be brain damage a decade or more before AD symptoms appear.

AD causes abnormal protein clumps to develop, which leads to nerve fibers becoming tangled bundles and to neurons losing brain connections. Over time, neurons lose their ability to function and communicate with each other, and eventually they die.

As mentioned, Alzheimer's is a disease that progresses slowly; it does so in three stages. A patient in the early stage has no symptoms. In the middle stage, the patient has *mild cognitive impairment*, which means that problems with memory and other thinking problems are greater than normal for the patient's age. Before long, the damage spreads to different parts of the brain, and as more neurons die, the brain begins to shrink. By the final stage of AD, damage is widespread, and the brain shrinks significantly. This leads to an inability to complete simple tasks, and eventually to a need for total care.

A death related to AD can take as little as 3 to 4 years if the patient is older than 80, to as long as 10 or more years if the person is younger. Patients with AD are likely to develop other diseases, and most die from pneumonia.

Neurologists can diagnose AD with up to 90% accuracy. However, it can only be truly determined by an autopsy (medical examination of a dead body) to know the cause of death. A neurologist can diagnose "probable" AD by taking a health history and doing lab tests, a physical examination, brain scans, and psychological tests. The sooner a diagnosis of probable AD is made, the easier it is to manage symptoms.

There is no cure for AD. Until it can be cured or prevented, the number of AD patients will increase significantly if current population trends continue. The Alzheimer's Foundation of America (2016) estimates, based on national data trends, that by 2050, the number of Alzheimer's patients could more than triple to 16 million—almost equal to the population of Florida.

Parkinson's Disease

Parkinson's disease (PD) affects movement because brain neurons that control muscle movement are damaged. A neurotransmitter called *dopamine* sends signals to coordinate muscle movements. When dopamine-producing brain cells are damaged, they make less dopamine and cause PD motor symptoms. It is not understood why the dopamine-producing cells become damaged.

PD is characterized by progressive loss of muscle control, which leads to *tremors*, or shaking of the limbs and head; stiffness; slowness; and impaired balance. As symptoms worsen, the patient finds it increasingly difficult to walk, talk, and complete simple tasks.

PD usually begins around age 60, but early symptoms are not obvious and begin only gradually. In some patients, the disease progresses quickly. Although many patients become severely disabled, others experience only minor motor problems. No one can predict which symptoms will affect a patient, and the intensity of the symptoms also varies from patient to patient.

The signs and symptoms of PD arise in stages. In stage 1, symptoms affect only one side of the body. In stage 2, symptoms are on both sides. In stage 3, balance is impaired. In stage 4, assistance is needed to walk, and other symptoms become severe. Finally, with stage 5, the patient requires a wheelchair.

The 50,000 to 60,000 new cases diagnosed every year add to the already one million people who currently have PD, which means that PD is the most common movement disease in the United States; it is the 14th leading cause of death in the United States (National Parkinson's Foundation, 2016). Men are more likely to have PD than women, and it is more common in people of Western European descent than in those of Asian or African ancestry.

PD is probably caused by a combination of both genetic and environmental factors, such as living in a rural area, drinking well water, or being exposed to pesticides or wood pulp. At present, there is no cure for PD, but there is treatment for symptoms. Medication can slow the loss of dopamine and lessen symptoms of PD. Surgery is used when other treatments do not work.

Amyotrophic Lateral Sclerosis

Amyotrophic lateral sclerosis (ALS), or Lou Gehrig's disease, occurs because motor neurons die. When the motor neurons die, the brain's ability to start and control muscle movement is lost.

Muscle weakness is the first symptom of ALS. Then there is progression from weakness to paralysis of the limb and trunk muscles as well as muscles that control speech, swallowing, chewing, and breathing. When the breathing muscles become affected, the patient cannot breathe on his or her own and needs permanent ventilation support to survive. Because ALS attacks only motor neurons, the five senses are not affected. Although there is no cure or treatment that stops ALS and the disease is fatal, there are medications that modestly slow its progression. The life expectancy of an ALS patient is about 3 to 5 years from the time of diagnosis; however, about 10 percent do live for 10 years and more (National Institute of Neurological Disorders and Stroke, 2016a).

There is no one test to determine a diagnosis of ALS. Physical examination and diagnostic tests are used to rule out other diseases that mimic ALS. These tests include blood and urine tests, spinal tap, nerve biopsy, X-rays, and MRI scan. More than 12,000 people in the United States have a definite diagnosis of ALS (National Institute of Neurological Disorders and Stroke, 2016a). It is one of the most common neuromuscular diseases worldwide, and it can affect people of all races and ethnic backgrounds. ALS is more common in men than in women; however, the difference in incidence decreases as people get older. Most ALS patients are between the ages of 40 and 70, but some patients are in their 20s and 30s. ALS is more prevalent in patients of Northern European descent than in those of Asian or African ancestry.

Of the total number of US ALS cases, 90% are known as "sporadic," which means that the ALS affects anyone, anywhere. Only 10% are cases of inherited, or "familial," ALS (FALS). More research is needed to determine what genetic and/or environmental factors contribute to the development of ALS. It is known that military veterans, particularly those in the Gulf War, are approximately twice as likely to develop ALS (ALS Association, 2016).

Epilepsy

Seizures occur when neurons in the brain send out the wrong signals and cause movements and behaviors that can't be controlled, along with strange sensations and emotions. Seizures may be accompanied by *convulsions*, which are violent muscle spasms in the body; the patient also may lose consciousness. *Epilepsy* is a seizure disorder that is usually diagnosed only when a patient has had two or more seizures. Epilepsy has many causes, including illness, brain injury, alcoholism, and abnormal brain development. In some cases, the cause is unknown.

Nearly three million people in the United States have had a seizure or have been diagnosed with epilepsy. There are 200,000 new cases diagnosed each year; the highest numbers are for children under the age of 2 and adults over 65 (Epilepsy Foundation, 2016). Males are slightly more likely to have epilepsy than females. African Americans and persons with disabilities such as cerebral palsy are at greatest risk for epilepsy, as are patients who have had a stroke.

For about 80% of those with epilepsy and for whom treatment was started early, seizures can be controlled. Some patients, however, continue to have seizures even with treatment.

Most patients with epilepsy can live their lives without major problems if they receive treatment. For other patients, however, epilepsy is serious and affects many aspects of their lives, including their ability to carry out daily activities.

Brain scans and other tests can help diagnose epilepsy. There is no cure for epilepsy, but anticonvulsant medications control seizures for most patients. When medications don't work, then surgery or implanted devices such as nerve stimulators can help. Although epilepsy cannot be cured, it does eventually go away in some patients.

Many cases of epilepsy can be prevented by wearing seat belts and bicycle helmets and by other measures that prevent head injury. Treating cardiovascular disease, alcoholism, high blood pressure, infections, and other diseases that can affect the brain may also prevent epilepsy.

Stroke

The brain requires a constant supply of blood because blood carries oxygen and nutrients that the brain needs to function. A *stroke*, or cerebrovascular accident, occurs when a blood clot blocks a blood vessel that carries blood from the heart to the brain. It can also occur when a blood vessel breaks, stopping blood flow to the brain. In either case, the brain can't get the oxygen and nutrients that it needs, so brain cells die, causing brain damage.

The brain is divided into areas that control how the body moves and feels. When a stroke damages a certain area of the brain, that area no longer works as it did before the stroke. Whatever abilities that damaged area used to control, such as movement, vision, touch, and memory, can be permanently lost.

How a stroke patient is affected depends on the area damaged by the stroke and how much of the brain is injured. For example, patients who have a minor stroke may have only slight problems, such as lack of arm strength, whereas those who have a major stroke may be paralyzed on one side. Some patients recover completely from strokes, but most continue to have lifelong disability.

There are two kinds of stroke. The more common is *ischemic stroke*, which is caused by a blood clot that blocks a blood vessel in the brain. Unless nearby blood vessels deliver enough blood to the affected area, brain cells begin to die.

A stroke that is caused by a blood vessel that breaks and bleeds into the brain is a *hemorrhagic stroke*. Hemorrhagic strokes are a result of high blood pressure as well as brain aneurysms; both can weaken blood vessels. A *brain aneurysm* is a weak spot on the wall of a blood vessel that balloons out. As it gets bigger, the aneurysm bubbles and bursts, leaking blood into or outside the brain.

The following are common and sudden symptoms of stroke:

- Weakness of the face, arm, or leg on one side of the body

- Trouble seeing in one or both eyes

- Severe headache with no known cause

- Confusion; trouble speaking or understanding speech

- Trouble walking, or feeling dizzy

If you have these symptoms or see them in someone else, it's a medical emergency. See Figure 12.6 for a quick review of the warning signs of a stroke.

Treatment for stroke is more effective if given quickly: The patient needs to be at the hospital within 60 minutes of having a stroke. Unfortunately, only about 5% of those who suffer a stroke reach the hospital in time to receive the treatment they need (National Stroke Association, 2016).

Patients who suffer a major stroke are often partially paralyzed and have speech problems. With rehabilitation, these patients can try to regain the ability to walk, and to relearn self-care activities, such as eating and washing.

To diagnose a stroke, a neurologist reviews events, gets a health history, conducts a neurological exam, orders blood tests, and performs CT or MRI scans. The neurologist also does a brain angiography. For a *brain angiography*, a dye is injected into the blood vessels of the brain and an X-ray is taken. The angiography gives a picture of how blood flows through the vessels and indicates the size and location of blockages in the patient's brain.

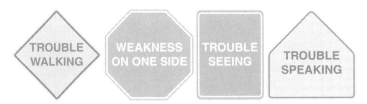

Figure 12.6 Warning Signs of a Stroke
If you believe that you—or that someone you know—is having a stroke, call 911 immediately.

Stroke kills more than 137,000 people a year in the United States. On average, someone dies of stroke every 4 minutes. It is the fourth leading cause of death, and causes more serious long-term disability than any other disease in the United States (National Stroke Association, 2016). Anyone at any time can have a stroke, but there are risk factors:

- *Age.* Chances of having a stroke double for each decade after age 55.
- *Race.* African Americans have a higher risk of death from a stroke than other racial groups.
- *Family health history.* Stroke risk is greater if a family member had a stroke.
- *Gender.* Stroke is more common in men than in women. However, more women than men die of stroke.
- *Prior stroke or other health problems.* Patient are at higher risk of stroke if they've already had one. Having had a heart attack or high blood pressure or diabetes is also a risk factor.

Up to 80% of strokes are preventable. A stroke can be prevented by managing diabetes, eating a balanced diet, controlling high blood pressure, exercising, not smoking, and not abusing alcohol.

Transient Ischemic Attack ("Mini-Stroke")

A *transient ischemic attack (TIA)* occurs when the blood supply to the brain is briefly stopped. Even though a TIA is often called a "mini-stroke," it is a warning to be taken seriously.

A TIA is caused by a moving clot in the brain that causes temporary blockage. TIA symptoms come on quickly and last for about a minute. Unlike a stroke, a TIA causes no permanent injury to the brain.

The signs and symptoms of a TIA are the same as for a stroke, and there is no difference in emergency medical care. Although a TIA stops before there is damage, there is no way to predict which clots will dissolve on their own. A TIA is a warning stroke and gives a patient time to act so as to prevent a permanent stroke.

Treatment for TIA depends on the location and cause of the clot. A patient who has had one or more TIAs is almost 10 times more likely to have a stroke than someone of the same age and sex who hasn't (National Stroke Association, 2016).

Sciatica

Sciatica is the pain, tingling, or numbness that goes along the longest nerve in the body, the sciatic nerve. This nerve controls many of the muscles in the lower legs and provides feeling to the thighs, legs, and feet. It runs from the back down to the buttock and down the back of each leg. The pain is caused by a pinched nerve root that connects to the sciatic nerve. It can be experienced as a mild ache to a sharp, burning sensation to a feeling of an electric shock.

Sciatica is a symptom, not a disease. The pain may be caused by a ruptured spinal disc, a narrowing of the spinal canal, or an injury. In many cases, no cause can be found. Depending on the cause, the pain from sciatica usually goes away on its own within a couple of months.

Risk factors for sciatica include health problems, lifestyle choices, age, and race. Sciatica most often occurs between the ages of 30 and 50 years. Other risk factors include a job that requires heavy lifting, sitting for long periods of time, and diabetes.

Although most patients recover from sciatica, often without any treatment, it can potentially lead to permanent nerve damage. Treatment, if needed, depends on the cause and can include physical therapy and exercises; medications such as steroids, opiates, or muscle relaxants; and in severe cases, surgery.

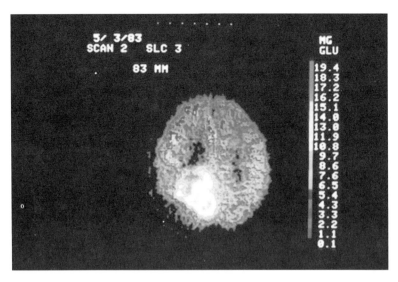

Figure 12.7   Brain Tumor

A PET scan (positron emission tomography) of a 62-year-old man with a brain tumor classified as a grade III astrocytoma. The PET scan displays an increased glucose metabolic rate shown by the irregular bright white area in the center of the scan.

Note. From the National Cancer Institute, Dr. Giovanni Dichiro, Neuroimaging Section, National Institute of Neurological Disorders and Stroke. This image is in the public domain and can be freely reused. Retrieved from https://commons.m.wikimedia.org/wiki/File:Pet_scan_of_brain_tumor.jpg

Tumors of the Central Nervous System

Brain and spinal cord tumors are found in tissue inside the skull or spinal column. A brain or spinal cord tumor is a mass of unnecessary cell growth. There are more than 120 types of brain and spinal cord tumors, and they do not discriminate—anyone can get them, regardless of age, gender, or race. More than 359,000 people in the United States are living with a brain tumor, and more than 195,000 are diagnosed with one each year (American Cancer Society, 2016). Spinal cord tumors are less common than brain tumors. Anyone can get spinal cord tumors, but they do affect young and middle-aged adults more often. Brain and spinal cord tumors destroy or damage cells by causing inflammation and by placing pressure on the brain, skull, spinal cord, and spinal column (see Figure 12.7).

No matter where they are located in the body, tumors are classified as benign (noncancerous) or malignant (cancerous). A benign tumor has slow-growing, normal-looking cells with clear edges, and it rarely spreads to other parts of the body. Often removed by surgery, benign tumors usually do not reappear. A malignant tumor is fast growing, invasive, and life threatening. These tumors are composed of cells that look different from normal cells. They quickly invade surrounding tissue and often have edges that are hard to define, which makes it difficult to surgically remove the entire tumor. They spread within the brain and spine by sending roots into nearby normal tissue.

There are two basic kinds of CNS tumors—primary and secondary. *Primary tumors* are growths that begin in the brain or spinal cord. They can be either malignant or benign and are identified by their type of cells and their location. Most primary tumors occur in adults. The cause of primary tumors is unknown.

Secondary tumors begin as cancer cells elsewhere in the body and then travel to the CNS. All secondary brain tumors are malignant, and are known as brain cancer. These brain tumors are the most common and occur mostly in adults. In general, the outcome is poor for most patients with secondary brain tumors because the cancer is not curable and eventually spreads to other areas of the body. Death often occurs within 2 years. Secondary spine tumors usually form within the bony covering of the spinal column, but may also invade the spinal canal from the chest or abdomen.

Some CNS tumors do not cause symptoms until they are large, then they quickly cause signs and symptoms. Other tumors have symptoms that develop slowly. The signs and symptoms depend on the tumor's size, location, and swelling, and how far it has spread. Common symptoms are headaches, seizures, and changes in the patient's mental function.

The tests that diagnosis a CNS tumor can include angiography, CT or MRI scans, EEG, biopsy of brain tissue, and spinal tap. Early treatment for CNS tumors often improves outcomes. The goals of treatment can be to cure or remove the tumor, relieve signs and symptoms, or provide comfort care.

Radiation of the whole brain is often used to treat tumors that have spread to the brain, especially if there is more than one tumor. Surgery is used for primary CNS tumors; some tumors are completely removed. Surgery may also be used for secondary CNS tumors when there is a single tumor and the cancer hasn't spread to other parts of the body. Those tumors that are deep inside the brain can be made smaller with surgery to help relieve symptoms.

Brain tumors occur more often in males than in females and are most common in middle-aged to elderly patients. They also occur more often in children under age 9 than in other children, and some tumors tend to run in families. Other risk factors for a primary CNS tumor include occupations where workers have repeated contact with certain chemicals, such as plastics. ·

Traumatic Brain Injury

Traumatic brain injury (TBI) is caused by a sudden trauma and results in damage to the brain. It can happen when the head suddenly and violently hits an object, but the object does not break through the skull, as in a punch. A penetrating injury occurs when an object pierces the skull and enters brain tissue, as in a bullet wound.

The signs and symptoms of TBI can be mild, moderate, or severe, depending on the amount of brain damage. Some symptoms appear immediately; others do not appear until days or weeks after the injury. A patient with mild TBI can lose consciousness for seconds or minutes and feel dazed weeks after the initial injury. Other symptoms of mild TBI include headache, blurred vision, fatigue, and trouble with concentration. A patient with severe TBI shows the same symptoms, but may also have a headache that gets worse, vomiting, and seizures. Anyone with severe TBI should receive medical attention immediately.

Fifty percent of all TBIs are from transportation crashes involving automobiles, motorcycles, bicycles, and pedestrians. These crashes are the major cause of TBI in people under age 75. For those 75 and older, falls cause the majority of TBIs. Approximately 20% of TBIs are due to violence, such as firearm assaults and child abuse, and about 3% are due to sports injuries. Half of all TBIs involve alcohol use. Over 90% of firearm TBIs result in death, whereas only 11% of TBIs from falls result in death.

There are different types of TBI. Concussion is the most minor and the most common type of TBI. A *concussion* is a head injury accompanied by a short loss of consciousness (see Figure 12.8). However, children and teens who continue to play sports while having concussion symptoms or

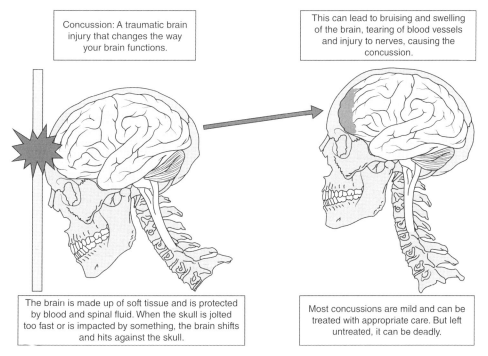

Figure 12.8 Concussion Anatomy

Note. Adapted from "Concussion Anatomy.png," by Max Andrews [CC BY-SA 3.0 (http://creativecommons.org/licenses/by-sa/3.0)], via Wikimedia Commons. Retrieved from https://commons.wikimedia.org/wiki/File%3AConcussion_Anatomy.png

who play too soon while the brain is still healing have a greater chance of getting another concussion. A repeat concussion that occurs while the brain is still healing from the first injury can be serious and affect a person for a lifetime. It can even be fatal.

Concussion signs and symptoms often show up soon after the injury. However, it may be difficult to know how serious the concussion is at first, and some symptoms may not show up for hours or days. The brain needs time to heal after a concussion and should be carefully monitored by a health care provider.

Other TBIs can be more severe than a concussion. A *skull fracture* is the cracking of the bone of the skull. In a depressed skull fracture, pieces of the broken skull press into the tissue of the brain; when something pierces the skull, the injury is called a penetrating skull fracture.

Skull fractures cause bruising of brain tissue, called a contusion. A *contusion* is swollen brain tissue mixed with blood from broken blood vessels. Another type of TBI is damage to a major blood vessel in the head that causes a *hematoma*, or an abnormal collection of blood outside a brain's blood vessel.

A TBI requires emergency medical care. Because little can be done to stop the initial brain damage caused by trauma, emergency health care providers try to stabilize the patient and focus on preventing further injury. Concerns include having proper oxygen supply and blood flow to the brain and the rest of the body, and controlling blood pressure. Many head-injured patients also having spinal cord injuries, so special care is taken in moving and transporting the patient.

A CT scan can show bone fractures as well as hematomas, contusions, and swelling of brain tissue. Sometimes when the brain is injured, fluids fill the brain space and cause swelling, called *intracranial pressure*. If a patient has a high amount of pressure, then a procedure is used that drains cerebrospinal fluid from the brain to bring down swelling.

Spinal Cord Injuries

A spinal cord injury is caused by a sudden, traumatic blow to the spine that fractures or dislocates vertebrae. The damage begins at the moment of the injury. Most injuries don't completely sever the spinal cord. Instead, there's damage where pieces of vertebrae tore into cord tissue or pressed on nerves. Some injuries allow almost complete recovery; others result in complete paralysis. Patients who survive a spinal cord injury usually have medical complications, such as chronic pain and bladder and bowel problems, along with an increased risk for respiratory and heart problems.

Spinal cord injuries are either complete or incomplete. An incomplete injury means that the ability of the spinal cord to send messages to or from the brain is not totally lost. People with incomplete injuries have some motor or sensory function below the injury. A complete injury is a total lack of sensory and motor function below the level of injury—that is, there is paralysis below the level of injury. *Paralysis* is the loss of muscle function in a part of the body. It occurs when something goes wrong with the way messages pass between the brain and muscles. Paralysis can be complete or partial, and it can be on one or both sides of the body. It can occur in just one area or be widespread. *Paraplegia* is paralysis of the lower half of the body, including both legs. *Quadriplegia* is paralysis of the arms and legs.

A spinal cord injury is a medical emergency. Immediate treatment reduces long-term effects. Later treatment usually includes medication, braces, and rehabilitation therapy. Surgery to relieve compression of the spinal tissue caused by surrounding broken bones is often necessary. Assistive devices like wheelchairs and specialized computer software may also help in improving a patient's functioning and independence.

Diseases of the Sensory System

The *sensory system* is part of the nervous system and is responsible for processing information from the senses. There are five senses in the sensory system:

1. *Sight or vision.* Light entering the eye forms an upside-down image on the retina at the back of the eye. The retina changes the light into nerve signals to the brain. The brain then turns the image right side up and tells us what we are seeing.

2. *Taste.* The tongue has small sensory cells called taste buds that react to chemicals in foods. Messages are sent from the taste buds to the brain to process taste.

3. *Touch.* Skin has sensory receptors that receive information related to touch, pressure, temperature, and pain. It sends this information to the brain for processing and reaction.

4. *Hearing.* Sound comes from sound waves entering the ears and causing the eardrums to vibrate. The vibrations are then sent to the ear bones and translated into nerve signals.

5. *Smell.* Special sensory cells, called olfactory sensory neurons, in the nostrils' mucous membranes react to chemicals we breathe in, and then send messages to the brain.

The sensory diseases discussed in this section are glaucoma, cataracts, age-related macular degeneration, diabetic retinopathy, tinnitus, Ménière's disease, and sensory processing disorder.

Eye Diseases

Some eye problems are minor, whereas others lead to permanent loss of vision. If a patient has some vision, then large-print books or special glasses can make life easier. If a patient has severe or total loss of vision, there are devices that help, such as braille books. Sometimes, vision loss can be prevented, which is why as people age, regular examinations and prompt treatment are critical to keeping eyes healthy.

The eye is a major organ of the sensory system, and although there are many eye diseases, three age-related diseases are the leading causes of low vision. Together, glaucoma, cataracts, and macular degeneration affect more than 10% of the US population (National Institute on Aging, 2016).

Glaucoma

Glaucoma is the leading cause of blindness in the United States (National Eye Institute, 2016a). It is caused by increased fluid pressure in the eye, which damages the optic nerve. There are no symptoms at first, but an eye exam can detect it. People at risk are African Americans over 40, all people over age 60, Mexican Americans, and people with a family history of glaucoma. All at-risk individuals should get an eye exam every 2 years. Treatment includes prescription eye drops and/or surgery.

Cataracts

By age 80, more that 50% of all people in the United States either have a cataract or have had cataract surgery (National Institute on Aging, 2016). A *cataract* starts slowly, but eventually causes the lens of the eye to be cloudy. Symptoms include blurry vision, lack of night vision, and double vision. New glasses, brighter lighting, or magnifying glasses can help at first. For some patients, surgery is used to remove the cloudy lens and replace it with an artificial lens. Wearing sunglasses and hats that block ultraviolet sunlight may help prevent cataracts.

Age-related Macular Degeneration

Age-related macular degeneration is a leading cause of vision loss in the United States for people over 60 years of age (National Eye Institute, 2016b). It is a disease that destroys central vision, which is necessary to see objects, read, and drive. This disease affects the part of the eye that sees small details. It is not painful, but does cause eye cells to die.

In some cases, macular degeneration starts slowly, so patients notice little change in their vision; for others, the symptoms come on fast and cause loss of vision in both eyes. Regular eye exams can detect macular degeneration before it causes vision loss. Treatment can slow the progress of this disease, but it can't restore lost vision.

Diabetic Retinopathy

Diabetic retinopathy is responsible for most blindness in US adults (American Academy of Ophthalmology, 2016). Caused by diabetes, diabetic retinopathy damages the tiny vessels inside the retina. The retina is the light-sensitive tissue at the back of the eye, and it needs to be healthy for a person to see clearly.

Patients might not notice at first, but symptoms develop into double vision, rings or flashing lights, eye pain, and trouble seeing. Those who have diabetes need to have an eye exam every year because finding and treating this disease early can save vision. Treatment includes surgery.

Ear Diseases

The ear is the organ for hearing and for balance. There are four major areas of concern related to ear problems: ear hygiene, noise injuries, age-related hearing loss, and ear emergencies. Complications with one or more of these areas can result in hearing problems and deafness; for example, about 30% of people by the age 65, and 50% by age 75, need hearing aids.

The ear has three main parts: outer, middle, and inner, and all of them are used in hearing. Sound waves come in through the outer ear, which is the visible external part. They reach the middle ear, where they make the eardrum vibrate, transmitting sound to the inner ear. The inner ear is responsible for not only the sense of hearing but also balance.

Ear infections are the most common illnesses in babies and young children. Most often, the infection affects the middle ear and is called *otitis media*. The canals inside the ears become clogged with fluid and mucus. This can affect hearing because sound cannot get through the fluid. The symptoms of an ear infection in children include earache, fever, crying, and irritability.

Ear infections often go away without treatment, but some infections in young babies may require antibiotics. Children who get frequent infections may need surgery to place small tubes inside their ears. The tubes relieve pressure in the ears so that the child can hear again.

Tinnitus

Tinnitus is a ringing, roaring, clicking, or hissing sound in the ears. Millions of people in the United States probably have tinnitus, but the exact number is difficult to determine because so many cases are left untreated (National Institutes of Health, 2011). Patients with severe tinnitus have trouble hearing, working, or even sleeping. Causes include hearing loss, exposure to loud noises, or medications for other diseases. Tinnitus may also be a symptom of other health problems, such as allergies; high or low blood pressure; tumors; and problems in the heart, jaw, and neck. Treatment for the condition depends on the cause and may include hearing aids, sound-masking devices, medications, and stress management to deal with the noise.

Ménière's Disease

Ménière's disease is the result of too much fluid in the inner ear. Its symptoms include dizziness, tinnitus, hearing loss, and ear pain that can last for several hours. These symptoms can appear suddenly, and as often as every day or as seldom as once a year. Ménière's disease usually affects just one ear.

Ménière's is a common cause of hearing loss, but what causes Ménière's is unknown. There is no cure, but patients can control symptoms by changing their diet or taking medication so that the body retains less fluid. Severe cases may need surgery.

Sensory Processing Disorder

Sensory processing disorder (SPD) causes difficulty with taking in and responding to sensory information. With SPD, the nervous system has trouble organizing messages that it receives from the senses into correct motor and behavioral responses. Someone with SPD finds it difficult to process and act on sensory information. This difficulty presents challenges in performing everyday tasks such as hearing, eating, smelling, and even walking.

SPD can affect only one sense or multiple senses. Some with SPD may over-respond to a sensation, whereas others may under-respond or not respond at all. For those whose sensory processing is impaired in muscles and joints, their posture and motor skills can be affected. The cause of SPD is unknown, but there is some evidence that both genetic and environmental factors are involved. Prenatal and birth complications may also play a role.

SPD is most often diagnosed in children, but those who reach adulthood without treatment can experience symptoms. Some research suggests that SPD is a distinct diagnosis, whereas others argue that it is a symptom of other developmental disorders, such as autism or attention deficit disorder.

There is no cure for SPD, but there are treatments available. Treatment for children is often a play-based intervention that takes place in sensory-rich environments. Treatment also includes occupational therapy and family-centered care.

Chapter Summary

- The nervous system is the major controlling, regulatory, and communication system in the body.
- The nervous system includes the central nervous system and the peripheral nervous system.
- The peripheral nervous system comprises the somatic and the autonomic nervous systems.
- The autonomic nervous system includes the sympathetic and parasympathetic nervous systems.
- The basic cell of the nervous system is the neuron.
- Many diseases of the nervous system are progressive and degenerative.
- The five main senses of the body are sight, smell, hearing, taste, and touch.

REVIEW QUESTIONS

1. Identify the organs of the central nervous system.
2. What are the differences among common, migraine, and cluster headaches?
3. What are the three major parts of the brain?
4. What is epilepsy, and how is it treated? What are risk factors for seizures?
5. How is Alzheimer's disease diagnosed?
6. What is sensory processing disorder, and how is it treated?
7. West Nile virus is usually a result of a bite from what insect?
8. What is the difference between paraplegia and quadriplegia?
9. What is the difference between a cataract and glaucoma?
10. What is more serious, a concussion or a contusion?

KEY TERMS

Age-related macular degeneration: Eye disease that destroys central vision

Alzheimer's disease (AD): Disease that causes brain cell death and results in a progressive decline in memory and thinking

Amyotrophic lateral sclerosis (ALS): Disease that affects and kills motor neurons, resulting in the brain's inability to start and control muscle movement

Autonomic nervous system: System of nerves that connect the central nervous system to organs and that are also involved in unconscious activities, such as breathing

Axon: Long fibers on a neuron, which carry impulses out of the neuron

Brain aneurysm: Weak spot in a blood vessel in the brain that balloons out and bursts

Brain angiography: Test in which dye is injected into the brain's blood vessels and then X-rayed

Brain stem: One of the three major parts of the brain; controls the flow of messages between the brain and the rest of the body, and is also responsible for basic vital life functions, such as breathing, heart rate, and blood pressure

Cataract: Clouding of the lens of the eye

Central nervous system (CNS): The brain and spinal cord

Cerebellum: One of the three major parts of the brain; coordinates and controls muscle activity, balance, and equilibrium

Cerebrospinal fluid: Fluid that protects the central nervous system

Cerebrum: Largest part of the brain; performs motor, sensory, and higher mental functions

Cluster headache: Intense pain on one side of the head

Concussion: Form of traumatic brain injury, which results in a short loss of consciousness

Contusion: Swollen brain tissue mixed with blood from broken blood vessels

Convulsion: Violent muscle spasms in the limbs or body

Degenerative diseases: In the context of the nervous system, diseases that cause nonreversible, progressive deterioration of neurons, nerves, and brain tissues

Dementia: Symptoms caused by brain diseases and sometimes by brain injury

Dendrites: Finger-like projections on neurons

Diabetic retinopathy: Eye disease caused by diabetes, which damages vessels inside the retina

Dopamine: Brain neurotransmitter that helps coordinate muscle movements

Encephalitis: Inflammation of the brain

Epilepsy: Seizure disorder, which is diagnosed only after a patient has had two or more seizures

Ganglia: Masses of nerve tissues outside the brain and spinal cord

Glaucoma: Damage to the optic nerve caused by pressure from excess fluid in the eye

Hematoma: An abnormal collection of blood outside a brain's blood vessel

Hemorrhagic stroke: Blood vessel breaking and bleeding into the brain

Intracranial pressure: Swelling caused by a brain injury that leads to fluids filling the brain space

Ischemic stroke: Blood clot blocking a blood vessel in the brain

Lumbar puncture, or spinal tap: Test that analyzes a sample of a patient's cerebrospinal fluid by inserting a needle into the patient's lower back to collect the fluid

Ménière's disease: Result of too much fluid in the inner ear

Meninges: Membranes that protect the central nervous system

Meningitis: Inflammation of the meninges, the membranes that surround the brain and spinal cord

Migraine headache: Repeating headache lasting 4–72 hours

Mild cognitive impairment: Memory and other thinking problems that are greater than normal for a patient's age

Motor output: The result of the nervous system sending signals to muscles, causing them to contract or relax, and also to glands, causing them to secrete hormones

Myelin sheath: Fatty protective membrane on the axon

Nerve impulse: Electrical signal

Nerves: Bundles of nerve fibers

Neural pathways: Neuron connections in the brain

Neuroglia: Cells that support, nourish, and protect neurons

Neurologist: Physician who specializes in neurology and is trained to diagnose and treat neurological diseases

Neurology: Medical specialty concerned with the nervous system

Neuron: Nerve cell

Neurotransmitters: Chemicals that help messages jump from one neuron to another

Node of ranvier: Gap in the myelin sheath of a neuron

Otitis media: Infection that affects the middle ear

Paralysis: Loss of muscle function in part of the body

Paraplegia: Paralysis of the lower half of the body

Parasympathetic nervous system: System of nerves that prepare the body for rest

Parkinson's disease (PD): Disease that causes destruction of neurons in the area of the brain that controls muscle movement

Peripheral nervous system (PNS): The nerves outside the central nervous system

Primary tumor: In the context of the nervous system, a growth that begins in the brain or spinal cord

Quadriplegia: Paralysis of the arms and legs

Sciatica: Pain along the path of the sciatic nerve

Secondary tumor: In the context of the nervous system, a tumor caused by cancerous cells elsewhere in the body that travel to the central nervous system

Seizure: Brief episode brought on when neurons in the brain send out the wrong signals and cause movements and behaviors that can't be controlled

Sensory input: Stimuli perceived by the senses (i.e., smell, sight, touch, taste, and hearing)

Sensory integration: The gathering and processing of sensory information by the nervous system

Sensory processing disorder (SPD): Disorder that causes difficulty with taking in and responding to sensory information

Sensory system: Body system responsible for the processing of information from the five senses

Shingles, or herpes zoster: Painful condition caused by a herpes virus

Skull fracture: Crack in the bone of the skull

Somatic nervous system: System of nerves that go to the skin and muscles

Stimuli (singular stimulus): Things that cause physiological changes in a cell, tissue, or organ

Stroke: Blood clot blocking a blood vessel that carries blood from the heart to the brain

Sympathetic nervous system: System of nerves that prepare the body for emergency situations

Tension headache: Most common type of headache in adults, caused by tight muscles in the shoulders, neck, scalp, and jaw

Tinnitus: Ringing, roaring, clicking, or hissing sound in the ears

Transient ischemic attack (TIA): Condition in which the blood supply to the brain is briefly stopped

Traumatic brain injury (TBI): Damage to the brain caused by a sudden trauma

Tremors: Shaking of the limbs and head

Vertebrae: Bones that protect the spinal cord

West Nile virus (WNV): Virus that is spread to humans by infected mosquitoes

CHAPTER ACTIVITIES

1. Draw the human body on flipchart paper and label the different parts of the nervous system. Be prepared to present your drawing in class.

2. You have been hired as a health educator by a community college. Many students on campus suffer from headaches. Your task is to identify 5 to 10 stress reduction techniques for college-age headache sufferers.

3. As a health promotion specialist at a local hospital, you will facilitate a support group for primary caregivers of loved ones with Alzheimer's disease. Write a two- to three-page paper on the physical, emotional, and social challenges of a caregiver whose loved one has Alzheimer's. As part of this assignment, identify health promotion strategies that address some of these challenges.

4. Conduct a 30-minute interview with a physical education teacher. The point of the interview is to discuss concussion awareness and prevention strategies. Write a two-page paper that summarizes your interview, and report your findings to the class.

5. You as a health promotion specialist will develop a one-page TIA prevention handout that addresses lifestyle factors such as diet, physical activity, weight management, alcohol consumption, and smoking cessation. Use visuals as well as words to illustrate your prevention messages. Be prepared to share your handout with others in class.

Bibliography and Works Cited

ALS Association. (2016). What is ALS? Retrieved from http://www.alsa.org/about-als/what-is-als.html

Alzheimer's Foundation of America. (2016). Alzheimer's disease. Retrieved from http://www.alzfdn.org/About Alzheimers/definition.html

American Academy of Dermatology. (2016). Shingles. Retrieved from https://www.aad.org/public/diseases /contagious-skin-diseases/shingles

American Academy of Neurology. (2016). Working with your doctor. Retrieved from http://patients.aan.com/go/workingwithyourdoctor

American Academy of Ophthalmology. (2016). What is diabetic retinopathy? Retrieved from https://www.aao.org/eye-health/diseases/what-is-diabetic-retinopathy

American Academy of Orthopedic Surgeons. (2013). *Spine basics.* Retrieved from http://orthoinfo.aaos.org/topic.cfm?topic=A00575

American Academy of Otolaryngology–Head and Neck Surgery. (2016a). Better ear health. Retrieved from http://www.entnet.org/?q=node/1250

American Academy of Otolaryngology–Head and Neck Surgery. (2016b). Ménière's disease. Retrieved from http://www.entnet.org/content/menieres-disease

American Cancer Society. (2016). Brain and spinal cord tumors in adults. Retrieved from http://www.cancer.org/cancer/braincnstumorsinadults/detailedguide/index

American Migraine Foundation. (2016). Living with migraines. Retrieved from https://americanmigrainefoundation.org/living-with-migraines/

Centers for Disease Control and Prevention. (2015). Brain injury basics. Retrieved from http://www.cdc.gov/headsup/basics/index.html

Centers for Disease Control and Prevention. (2016a). Bacterial meningitis. Retrieved from http://www.cdc.gov/meningitis/bacterial.html

Centers for Disease Control and Prevention. (201b). West Nile virus. Retrieved from http://www.cdc.gov/westnile/index.html

Christopher and Dana Reeve Foundation. (2016). Paralysis resource center. Retrieved from http://www.christopherreeve.org/site/c.mtKZKgMWKwG/b.4514599/k.901E/Newly_Paralyzed.htm

Epilepsy Foundation. (2016). About epilepsy: The basics. Retrieved from http://www.epilepsy.com/start-here/about-epilepsy-basics

Mayo Clinic. (2016a). Ear infection (middle ear). Retrieved from http://www.mayoclinic.org/diseases-conditions/ear-infections/basics/definition/CON-20014260?p=1

Mayo Clinic. (2016b). Meningitis. Retrieved from http://www.mayoclinic.org/diseases-conditions/meningitis/home/ovc-20169520

Mayo Clinic. (2016c). Sciatica. Retrieved from http://www.mayoclinic.org/diseases-conditions/sciatica/basics/definition/con-20026478

National Cancer Institute. (2016). SEER training modules: Nervous system. Retrieved from http://training.seer.cancer.gov/anatomy/nervous/

National Eye Institute. (2016a). Facts about glaucoma. Retrieved from https://nei.nih.gov/health/glaucoma/glaucoma_facts

National Eye Institute. (2016b). Age-related macular degeneration. Retrieved from https://www.nei.nih.gov/health/maculardegen

National Institute on Aging. (2016). What is a cataract? retrieved from http://nihseniorhealth.gov/cataract/whatisacataract/01.html

National Institute of Neurological Disorders and Stroke. (2016a). Amyotrophic lateral sclerosis (ALS) fact sheet. Retrieved from http://www.ninds.nih.gov/disorders/amyotrophiclateralsclerosis/detail_ALS.htm

National Institute of Neurological Disorders and Stroke. (2016b). NINDS shingles information page. Retrieved from http://www.ninds.nih.gov/disorders/shingles/shingles.htm

National Institutes of Health. (2011). NIH news in health: Ringing in your ears? Retrieved from https://newsinhealth.nih.gov/issue/Aug2011/Feature2

National Parkinson Foundation. (2016). What is Parkinson's? Retrieved from http://www.parkinson.org/understanding-parkinsons/what-is-parkinsons

National Stroke Association. (2016). Understand stroke. Retrieved from http://www.stroke.org/understand-stroke

Nemours Foundation. (2016). How the nervous system works. *KidsHealth.* Retrieved from http://kidshealth.org/en/parents/brain-nervous-system.html?ref=search#

Parikh, V., Tucci, V., & Galwankar, S. (2012). Infections of the nervous system. *International Journal of Critical Illness and Injury Science, 2*(2), 82–97. doi:10.4103/2229-5151.97273

Sensory Processing Disorder Foundation. (2016). About SPD. Retrieved from http://www.spdfoundation.net/about-sensory-processing-disorder/

US National Library of Medicine. (2016). Dementia. *MedlinePlus.* Retrieved from https://medlineplus.gov/dementia.html

Wolters Kluwer. (2016). Patient education: Encephalitis (The basics). *UpToDate.* Retrieved from https://www.uptodate-com.ezproxy.springfield.edu/contents/encephalitis-the-basics?source=search_result&search=encephalitis%20patents%20information&selectedTitle=1~150

CHAPTER 13

CARDIOVASCULAR SYSTEM AND RELATED DISEASES

CHAPTER OBJECTIVES

- Review the structure of the heart.
- Summarize the functions of the cardiovascular system.
- Discuss major types of cardiovascular diseases.
- Identify contributing causes of coronary artery disease.
- Explain the difference between myocardial infarction and cardiac shock.
- List healthy lifestyle changes that prevent cardiovascular diseases.
- Identify tests and procedures used to diagnose and treat cardiovascular diseases.

The cardiovascular system has three main functions: (a) the transport of nutrients, gases, hormones, and waste to and from the body's cells; (b) helping in the fight against diseases; and (c) the transport of blood throughout the body. Cardiovascular diseases, sometimes called heart diseases, involve the heart, blood vessels, and blood. The most common cause for these diseases is narrowing or blockage of the coronary arteries, the blood vessels that supply blood to the heart. Cardiovascular disease is the number one killer in the United States. It is also a major cause of disability. Although some risk factors for cardiovascular diseases cannot be controlled, people can make healthy lifestyle choices that reduce risk. These healthy lifestyle choices include managing blood pressure, lowering cholesterol levels, not smoking, and getting enough exercise.

Structure of the Cardiovascular System

The *cardiovascular system, or heart and circulatory system*, is the network that delivers blood throughout the body. *Blood* is the transport system that brings oxygen and nutrients to the body's cells and carries away waste materials. In addition, blood carries hormones that control the body's processing, and antibodies that fight invading microbes.

The heart is the pump that keeps the blood's transport system moving. Blood travels through a closed network of blood vessels. This network of blood vessels transports blood to the cells of organs and other body parts.

The cardiovascular system is made up of the heart and the circulatory system, which comprises the blood vessels, including the arteries, veins, and capillaries. There are actually two circulatory processes, with the heart acting as a double pump. The first is *pulmonary circulation*, which is circulation through a short loop from the heart to the lungs and back again. The second is *systemic circulation*, which sends blood from the heart to the other parts of the body and back again.

The Heart

The heart is the key organ of the cardiovascular system. A hollow, muscular pump, it beats from birth until death. Its main function is to send blood throughout the body. The *cardiac muscle*, or heart muscle, usually beats from 70 to 80 times per minute, but can go much faster when it needs to. It beats about 100,000 times a day, more than 30 million times per year, and about 3 billion times in an average lifetime of 75 years. As the cardiac muscle contracts, it pushes blood through the heart's cavities into the vessels and, finally, out to the rest of the body. It takes only about 20 seconds for the heart's cardiac muscle to pump blood to every cell in the body.

The nerves that connect to the heart tell it when to pump more or less blood depending on the body's needs. When we're sleeping, the heart pumps slowly to provide the small amount of oxygen needed by our bodies at rest. When we're exercising or frightened, the heart pumps faster in order to get more oxygen.

Considering how hard it works, the adult heart is a small organ, the size of a clenched fist, and it weighs about 11 ounces. Located in the middle of the chest, behind the breastbone and between the lungs, the heart is surrounded by a moist cavity called the *pericardial cavity*. The pericardial cavity is surrounded by the rib cage. The diaphragm is a muscle that lies below the heart. Surrounded by the pericardial cavity, rib cage, and diaphragm, the heart is well protected.

The heart does not look much like the hearts we see on Valentine's Day; it is more the shape of an upside-down pear (see Figure 13.1). It's a hollow shell with four cavities, or open spaces, that are surrounded by thick, muscular walls. The bottom of the heart is divided into two cavities called the *right and left ventricles*, which pump blood out of the heart. The ventricles meet at the bottom of the heart and form a point that leans to the left side of the chest. The left ventricle contracts harder, so you can feel the heart pumping on the left.

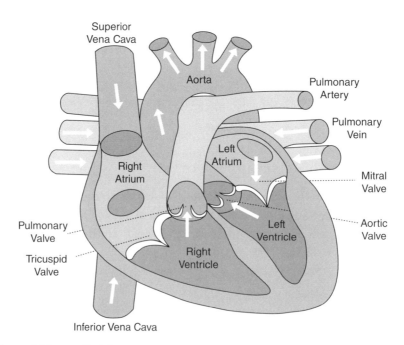

Figure 13.1 The Heart and Pulmonary Circulation

Note. Adapted from "Diagram of the Human Heart (Cropped).svg." Wikipedia Commons. Retrieved from http://commons.wikimedia.org/wiki/Image:Diagram_of_the_human_heart_%28cropped%29.svg

The upper part of the heart is also made up of two cavities, the right and left atria. The *right and left atria* take in the blood that enters the heart. Each side of the heart has one atrium and one ventricle. A wall, or *septum*, separates the left and right sides of the heart. A valve connects each atrium to the ventricle below it. The *mitral valve* connects the left atrium to the left ventricle. The *tricuspid valve* connects the right atrium to the right ventricle. There are also valves that separate the ventricles and the large blood vessels that carry blood leaving the heart. These valves are the *pulmonic valve*, which separates the right ventricle from the *pulmonary artery* that leads to the lungs, and the *aortic valve*, which separates the left ventricle from the *aorta, or main artery*, the body's largest blood vessel. There are also two large veins that carry deoxygenated blood into the heart: the *inferior vena cava*, which carries blood from the lower body; and the *superior vena cava*, which carries blood from the head, arms, and upper body. Figure 13.1 is a visual guide to the heart and pulmonary circulation.

Have you ever wondered about the sound that the heart makes—that "lub-dub" sound? The *cardiac cycle* makes that sound, and it has two parts. The first part begins when the ventricles contract, called *systole*, sending blood into the circulatory system. To prevent the flow of blood backwards into the atria during systole, the ventricular valves close, creating the first sound ("lub"). When the ventricles finish contracting, the aortic and pulmonic valves close to prevent blood from flowing back into the ventricles. This creates the second sound ("dub"). Then the ventricles relax, which is called *diastole*, and fill with blood from the atria. The diastole makes up the second part of the cardiac cycle.

A unique electrical system in the heart causes it to beat in its regular rhythm. The *sinoatrial node, or SA node*, a small area of tissue in the wall of the right atrium, sends out an electrical signal to start the contracting of the heart muscle. Each beat of the heart is set in motion by electrical signals. An electrical signal causes the atria to contract first; the signal then travels down to the *atrioventricular node, or AV node*. From here, the electrical signal travels through the right and left ventricles, causing them to contract and force blood out into the major arteries. In a normal, healthy heart, each beat begins with a signal from the SA node. This is why the SA node is sometimes called the heart's natural pacemaker. The *pulse, or heart rate*, is the number of signals the SA node produces per minute.

Blood Vessels

Blood vessels are hollow tubes that carry and circulate blood throughout the body. There are three different types of blood vessels. Blood vessels that carry blood away from the heart are *arteries*. They are the thickest blood vessels and have walls that contract to keep the blood moving away from the heart and through the body. Oxygen-rich blood is pumped from the heart into the aorta. This huge artery curves up and back from the left ventricle, then heads down in front of the spinal column into the abdomen. Two *coronary arteries* branch off at the beginning of the aorta and divide into a network of smaller arteries that provide oxygen and nourishment to the muscles of the heart.

The body's other main artery is the pulmonary artery, which carries oxygen-poor blood. From the right ventricle, the pulmonary artery divides into right and left branches on the way to the lungs, where blood picks up oxygen. As they get farther from the heart, the arteries branch out into *arterioles*, which are smaller, and then to capillaries. *Capillaries* are tiny, thin, and fragile; in fact, they are so thin that blood cells can only pass through them in single file.

Blood vessels that carry blood back to the lungs and heart are called *veins*. The walls of veins are so thin that you can see blood through the skin on some parts of your body. Look at your wrist and see the veins carrying blood back to your heart. The skin changes the light as the blood enters the body, making the red blood look blue from outside the skin.

Veins are not as strong as arteries, but they do have valves that prevent blood from flowing backward. Valves are like gates that allow blood to flow in only one direction. Vein valves keep blood flowing to the heart and allow blood to flow against gravity. For example, blood returning to the heart from a toe needs to flow against gravity up the leg.

A network of tiny capillaries connects the arteries and veins. Even though they are tiny, capillaries are important because they deliver nutrients and oxygen to cells. In addition, capillaries remove carbon dioxide and waste products from the cells.

If you could take all the blood vessels out of a child's body and lay them in one line, the line would be over 60,000 miles long (slightly more than the length of the state of Georgia). An adult's vessels would be about 100,000 miles long (slightly more than the length of the state of Oregon).

Blood

The human body would stop working without blood. The body's organs couldn't get the oxygen and nutrients they need to survive; we couldn't warm up or cool down or fight infections. Without enough blood, we'd weaken and die.

Blood is a living tissue made up of cells. The cells travel through the circulatory system, floating in a yellowish fluid called *plasma*, which is 90% water and contains nutrients, proteins, hormones, and waste products. Over half of blood is plasma. In Chapter 14 of this textbook, there is an in-depth discussion of the structure and function of blood as well as related diseases.

Function of the Cardiovascular System

The cardiovascular system works closely with other systems in the body, and in particular with the respiratory system (see Figure 13.2). These two systems work together in two ways. First, blood from the right side of the heart, dark red and low in oxygen, travels along pulmonary arteries to the lungs where it gets fresh oxygen and turns bright red. It flows along pulmonary veins back into the heart's left side.

Second, blood leaves the left side of the heart and travels through arteries that eventually divide into capillaries. The capillaries release nutrients, oxygen, hormones, and antibodies into the body's

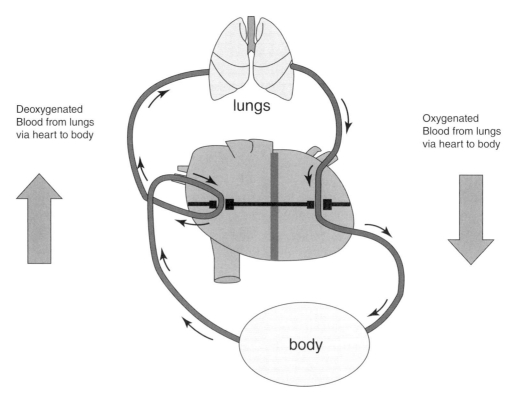

Figure 13.2   The Cardiovascular System and the Respiratory System

cells, and take in carbon dioxide and other waste products. The blood then travels in veins back to the right side of the heart, and the whole process begins again.

Diseases of the Cardiovascular System

Cardiovascular disease is a broad term that describes a range of diseases that affect the heart. These diseases include congenital heart defects, or heart defects that someone is born with; coronary artery disease; arrhythmias, or heart rhythm problems; heart infections; and diseases of the blood vessels. The medical study of the cardiovascular system and associated diseases is *cardiology*. A physician who has a medical specialty in cardiology is called a *cardiologist*.

Diseases of the cardiovascular system are sometimes called "heart diseases." Heart diseases are common—about 64 million Americans have some type of heart problem. More than 616,000 Americans die of a heart disease each year, accounting for 40% of all US deaths (American Heart Association, 2016b). Someone in the United States dies from heart disease every 34 seconds. Heart disease causes more deaths than all forms of cancer combined. In addition, heart disease affects all ages, not just older people.

Cardiovascular diseases are grouped into two categories: *congenital*, which means that the disease was present at birth, and *acquired*, which means that the disease developed some time after birth.

Congenital Heart Disease

Congenital heart disease (CHD), or congenital heart defects, are problems with the heart's structure and function that arise while the fetus is developing in the mother's womb. The cause of CHD is unknown—other diseases, medications, and genes may play a role.

CHD includes a wide range of diseases; however, all of these diseases are caused by how the heart muscle, chambers, or valves form. The most common type of birth defect, CHD causes more deaths in the first year of life than any other birth defect. At least 1 out of every 125 infants born each year has a heart defect, ranging from mild to severe (Dolbec & Mick, 2011). Some defects may be obvious at birth; others may not be detected until later in life. In the United States, more than one million adults are living with congenital heart defects (National Heart, Lung, and Blood Institute, 2011b).

There are factors that increase the risk of CHD, such as smoking while pregnant. Some of these risk factors can be prevented through good prenatal care. Protective factors include avoiding alcohol and drugs (including tobacco), eating a healthy diet, and having a rubella vaccine before pregnancy.

A life-threatening CHD is usually evident soon after birth, whereas less serious CHD is often not diagnosed until later in childhood or even adulthood. Symptoms of a life-threatening CHD include the following (National Heart, Lung, and Blood Institute, 2011b):

+ Bluish skin color

+ Swelling

+ Shortness of breath during feedings

+ Poor weight gain

+ Built-up fluid in the heart or lungs

Heart Murmur

Heart murmur is a common CHD. It is an unusual sound, like a blowing sound, that's heard when listening to the heart. Most heart murmurs are harmless and are not caused by heart problems. These murmurs are common in healthy children. Still others are acquired, which means that they are signs of a heart problem. Harmless heart murmurs do not require treatment. For acquired heart murmurs, treatment depends on the type of heart defect causing them. These defects cause problems with the heart's structure and function and are present at birth.

Tetralogy of Fallot

Tetralogy of Fallot is a complex and serious CHD that occurs in about 5 out of every 10,000 babies and affects boys and girls equally (National Heart, Lung, and Blood Institute, 2011c). With Tetralogy of Fallot, not enough blood can reach the lungs to get oxygen. This causes oxygen-poor blood to circulate in the body. The low level of oxygen leads to *cyanosis*, which is a bluish-purple color of the skin, lips, and fingernails. Tetralogy of Fallot is a disease caused by a combination of four heart defects:

1. A hole between the ventricles
2. A narrowing of the valve and artery that connect the heart with the lungs
3. A misplaced aorta that gets blood from both ventricles, not just one
4. A thickening of the wall of the right ventricle

These four heart defects of Tetralogy of Fallot can be repaired with at least one open-heart surgery soon after birth or in early infancy. The prognosis for this disease improves for most children who have had surgery. Many often survive to adulthood with regular medical follow-ups; however, without surgery, patients usually die by age 20.

Atherosclerosis, or Hardening of the Arteries

Although the term *cardiovascular diseases* refers to different types of heart or blood vessel problems, it usually means damage caused to the heart or blood vessels by *atherosclerosis, or hardening of the arteries*. Atherosclerosis is a common disease in the United States—so common that by the age of 12, an estimated 70% of children have developed the beginning stages of atherosclerosis (US National Library of Medicine, 2014b).

The cause of atherosclerosis is not completely understood. It may first appear when the inner layers of arteries become damaged and are thick, stiff, and narrow. This damage can be caused by aging as well as other factors, such as the following (US National Library of Medicine, 2014b):

• High blood pressure
• High cholesterol
• Diabetes
• Obesity
• Unhealthy diet, including high salt intake
• Lack of exercise
• Using tobacco products
• Family history of heart disease

When arteries become damaged, the body tries to repair them. This repair creates plaque in the walls of the arteries. *Plaque* is made of fat, cholesterol, calcium, and other substances that are naturally found in blood. Over time, plaque builds up in the arteries, making them hard, weak, and narrow (see Figure 13.3).

Plaque blocks and slows the flow of blood to organs and tissues, causing problems throughout the body. If the heart doesn't get enough blood, then tissues become starved of blood and oxygen, resulting in damage or tissue death.

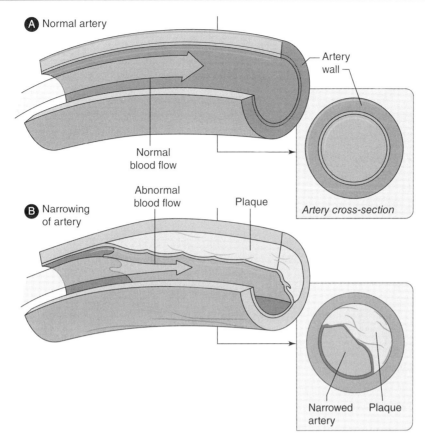

Figure 13.3 Atherosclerosis, or Hardening of the Arteries
Note. Adapted from the National Heart, Lung, and Blood Institute

In some cases, the plaque causes the wall of an artery to grow weak. This weakness causes a bulge in the artery, or an *aneurysm*. Aneurysms can break open, causing bleeding; they can be life threatening.

Some patients with atherosclerosis have no signs or symptoms until blood flow to part of the body becomes slow or blocked. If the arteries to the heart become too narrow, blood flow to the heart can slow down or stop. This can cause *angina*, or chest pain; shortness of breath; and other symptoms. Blocked arteries may also cause symptoms in the intestines, kidneys, legs, and brain.

Besides taking a health history and listening to the patient's heart and lungs with a stethoscope for blowing sounds, a health care provider might also order diagnostic tests for heart disease. See Table 13.1 for examples of diagnostic tests for cardiovascular diseases (US National Library of Medicine, 2014b).

Medication may also be prescribed to lower the patient's blood pressure or cholesterol levels and to prevent blood clots. If a patient has severe atherosclerosis, surgery to open or bypass blocked arteries may be necessary.

Although the etiology (cause) of atherosclerosis is not totally understood, there are certain traits, conditions, and behaviors that are risk factors for this disease. Atherosclerosis cannot be reversed once it has occurred, but there are health promotion and treatment strategies, such as lifestyle changes, that can control it. The lifestyle changes that reduce the risk or that can treat atherosclerosis are exercise, stopping smoking, avoiding fatty foods, limiting alcohol intake, managing stress, and having blood pressure checks every 1 to 2 years before age 50 and yearly after age 50 (US National Library of Medicine, 2014b). These lifestyle changes can prevent or slow the process from becoming worse. There are other risks factors, such as age and a family history of heart disease, that unfortunately cannot be controlled.

Table 13.1 Examples of Diagnostic Tests for Cardiovascular Diseases

Diagnostic Test	What It Does
Electrocardiogram (EKG or ECG)	Makes a graph of the heart's electrical activity. This test shows abnormal heartbeats, heart muscle damage, blood flow problems in the arteries, and heart enlargement.
Echocardiogram (EEG)	Uses ultrasound to create a picture of the heart and detect plaque in coronary arteries. The ultrasound also can be used to see how much blood is pumped out by the heart when it contracts.
Exercise or stress test (or treadmill test or exercise ECG)	Measures heart rate while the patient is exercising on a treadmill. This helps show how well the heart is working when it has to pump more blood.
Chest X-ray	Creates a picture of the heart, lungs, and other organs in the chest to see if there are any problems.
Nuclear scan	Shows the working of the heart muscle.
Cardiac catheterization (or coronary angiography or angiogram or arteriography)	Checks the inside of arteries for blockage by threading a tube through an artery in the groin, arm, or neck to reach the coronary artery; measures blood pressure and flow in the heart's chambers, collects blood samples from the heart, or injects dye into the coronary arteries.
Ventriculogram	Creates a picture of the left ventricle, which is the heart's main pumping chamber.
Intracoronary ultrasound	Uses a catheter that measures blood flow. It makes a picture that shows the condition of the artery wall.

Coronary Artery Disease (CAD)

The most common cardiovascular disease for adults in the United States is *coronary artery disease (CAD), or coronary heart disease*. It is the number one killer of both men and women in most racial and ethnic groups except for Asian Americans, and is a major cause of disability. Although often thought of as a "man's disease" because males have higher odds of developing CAD, the same number of women and men die each year from this disease (Sandmaier, 2007). Fifty percent of men and 67% of women who die suddenly of CAD have had no previous symptoms (American Academy of Family Physicians, 2014).

CAD is caused by plaque that has built up in the coronary arteries, which supply blood to the heart. When these arteries are blocked by plaque, the flow of blood to organs and other parts of the body is slowed, which causes problems.

The most common symptom of CAD is angina, chest pain that occurs because the heart doesn't get enough blood. Patients can also experience pain in the shoulders, arms, neck, jaw, or back. The pain feels like pressure or squeezing.

The first sign of CAD for some patients is not angina but a heart attack. A heart attack or myocardial infarction (MI) occurs when a coronary artery is blocked, either by plaque or by a blood clot that has formed around plaque that has broken off. If this blockage cuts off the blood flow completely, the part of the heart supplied by that artery begins to die (Figure 13.5). (MI is discussed further in the next section of this chapter.)

CAD can take years to develop. As coronary arteries become blocked, some patients may experience no symptoms (be asymptomatic), whereas others may experience angina, shortness of breath, heart attack, and even sudden death.

Checking the patient's blood pressure, cholesterol, and blood glucose levels helps a health care provider determine whether a patient has CAD. The provider will also check for a family's history of heart disease. If a patient is at high risk or already has symptoms, his or her health care provider performs several diagnostic tests, as described in Table 13.1.

Most people who have CAD take medication, such as beta-blockers, calcium channel blockers, and nitrates. These medications may have side effects for some patients, however. Beta-blockers can cause tiredness and sexual problems. Calcium channel blockers can cause constipation and leg swelling. Nitrates can cause headaches and redness in the face.

Angioplasty is a common surgical procedure for CAD. This procedure uses a tiny balloon to push open blocked arteries around the heart. The balloon is inserted in an artery in the arm or leg. To hold the artery open, a small metal rod called a *stent* is placed into the artery where the blockage was.

Angioplasty is generally safe, but there is the possibility of complications. The following are some of the risks of angioplasty and stent placement (National Heart, Lung, and Blood Institute, 2015):

- Allergic reactions to the drug used in the stent or the X-ray dye
- Bleeding or blood clotting
- Clogging of the inside of the stent
- Damage to a heart valve or blood vessel
- Heart attack
- Stroke
- Arrhythmia (irregular heartbeat)

Another surgical procedure for CAD is *bypass surgery.* Pieces of veins or arteries are taken from the legs and sewn into the arteries of the heart to bring blood past a blockage and increase the blood flow to the heart. Bypass surgery is usually done when angioplasty isn't possible.

Bypass surgery, like angioplasty and stent placement, carries risks. Most of these risks are low, however, and most patients do well. After angioplasty, patients can usually expect to return to their previous activity level within a few days. Recovery after bypass surgery does take longer. Regardless of the treatment options a patient may select—medications or surgery—CAD doesn't go away because there is no cure.

Patients can't do much about their family health history or age, but healthy lifestyle changes can help them avoid many of the risk factors for CAD. Figure 13.4 describes the healthy lifestyle choices a person can reasonably make to prevent not only CAD but other heart diseases as well.

The body needs time to respond to healthy lifestyle changes, and the benefits are often slow in coming. Even if a patient's lifestyle changes do not reduce risks and medication is needed, the patient still needs to keep to his or her healthy lifestyle changes for the medication to work.

Taking aspirin can help prevent CAD, but there are risks. Aspirin has been shown to lower the risk of a heart attack only for those who have already had one. It also can help keep arteries open in those who have had a heart bypass. However, the US Food and Drug Administration does not approve taking aspirin for preventing heart attacks in people who have never had one. Aspirin can have side effects, such as increasing chances of ulcers and kidney disease. It also can mix dangerously with other drugs, including some over-the-counter medicines. A patient should take aspirin only on his or her health care provider's specific recommendation (National Heart, Lung, and Blood Institute, 2015).

It's critical for CAD patients to realize that there's no quick cure. If a patient does *not* receive treatment, however, CAD will only worsen—leading to disability or death.

Myocardial Infarction, or Heart Attack

Myocardial infarction (MI), or heart attack, can be life threatening. MI occurs when plaque builds up and breaks in a coronary artery (see Figure 13.5). A blood clot then forms around the plaque and blocks the coronary artery. This blockage prevents oxygen-rich blood from getting to the heart muscle. When blood flow is blocked, the heart muscle becomes damaged. The damage causes not only scars but also

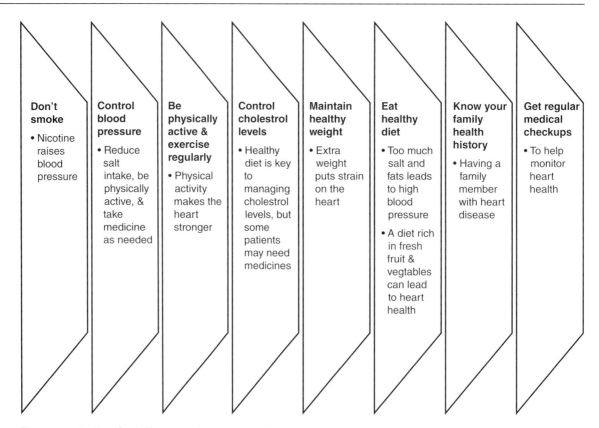

Don't smoke	Control blood pressure	Be physically active & exercise regularly	Control cholestrol levels	Maintain healthy weight	Eat healthy diet	Know your family health history	Get regular medical checkups
• Nicotine raises blood pressure	• Reduce salt intake, be physically active, & take medicine as needed	• Physical activity makes the heart stronger	• Healthy diet is key to managing cholestrol levels, but some patients may need medicines	• Extra weight puts strain on the heart	• Too much salt and fats leads to high blood pressure • A diet rich in fresh fruit & vegtables can lead to heart health	• Having a family member with heart disease	• To help monitor heart health

Figure 13.4 Healthy Lifestyle Choices to Help Prevent Heart Disease

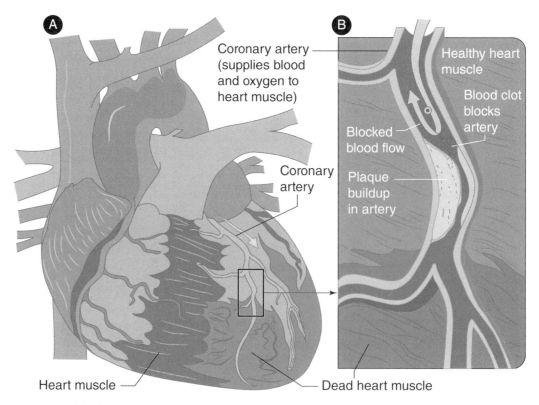

Figure 13.5 Myocardial Infarction (MI), or Heart Attack
Note. Adapted from the National Heart, Lung, and Blood Institute

death to the heart muscle. If blood flow remains blocked for 20 to 40 minutes in the coronary artery, then the heart muscle dies.

In the United States, about 3,000 people a day—one every 36 seconds—have a heart attack. Every year about 785,000 Americans have a first heart attack. Another 470,000 who have already had one or more heart attacks have another attack. Heart attacks are a common cause of death in the United States; they are responsible for one out of every six deaths (Centers for Disease Control and Prevention [CDC], 2016a). Although heart attacks can happen at any time, more heart attacks occur in the morning because higher levels of adrenaline are released from the adrenal glands during these hours.

When the heart actually stops during a heart attack, then it's referred to as a *sudden cardiac arrest (SCA)*. An SCA occurs when the heart suddenly stops pumping because of an electrical problem—not a blood flow problem as in a heart attack. An SCA can happen at the same time as a heart attack. It takes just 4 to 6 minutes after an SCA before a person experiences brain death, then complete death. In the United States, about a 1,000 people a day die from an SCA.

Some MIs are sudden and intense; however, most start slowly with mild pain. Some heart attacks are worse than others—it all depends on the area of the heart affected and on individual factors. In addition, symptoms of a heart attack vary among men and women. Women are more likely to die from heart attacks than men. No one knows for certain why. It may be that women don't seek treatment as soon as men. Or it might be because they don't recognize the symptoms, which can be different from the symptoms that men experience (WomenHeart, 2016). It may also be that women's smaller hearts and blood vessels are more easily damaged. Besides angina (chest pain), possible warning signs or symptoms of MI include the following (US National Library of Medicine, 2016):

- Pain in other areas of the upper body, such as the neck, shoulders, jaw, arms, or stomach
- Shortness of breath that lasts more than a few seconds
- *Syncope*, which is lightheadedness or temporary loss of consciousness due to a drop in blood pressure
- Nausea, sweating, fatigue, and feeling anxious
- *Heart palpitations*, or fast or out-of-rhythm heartbeats

An MI is usually treatable when diagnosed quickly. Without treatment, however, an MI can be fatal. About 40% of those people having an MI die before they get to the hospital. The chances of surviving depend on the treatment that is given within the first hour after an attack. Half of all people in the United States having an MI wait more than 2 hours before getting help. Some of these people feel that it would be embarrassing to have a false alarm. Others are afraid of having a heart attack and consequently deny the experience.

If someone is having a heart attack, immediate medical attention helps prevent disability or death. For those who experience both a myocardial infarction (MI) and sudden cardiac arrest (SCA), the survival rate outside of a hospital is less than 1–2% (CDC, 2016a). Given these tough odds of survival, anyone who is having a heart attack and/or an SCA needs to do the following (National Heart, Lung, and Blood Institute, 2011):

- **Call 911 immediately**, because emergency medical personnel can start treatment even before the patient gets to the hospital. Time is crucial because treatments that can stop an MI and SCA work best when given within the first hour.
- After calling for an ambulance and while waiting, the patient should chew and swallow one uncoated adult aspirin or four uncoated baby aspirins. The patient should not take the aspirin if he or she is allergic to aspirin.

Even if a patient is not sure that he or she is having an MI or SCA, the patient still needs to call 911. Delay is the primary reason for not getting adequate care.

Most of the risk factors for an MI are related to lifestyle choices, such as smoking, obesity, lack of exercise, stress, and alcohol abuse. Other risk factors are related to the patient's health history, the family's health history, and individual factors (National Heart, Lung, and Blood Institute, 2011; WomenHeart, 2016):

- Atherosclerosis (hardening of the arteries).

- Diabetes.

- High cholesterol levels.

- High blood pressure.

- Increasing age. About 83% of people who die from heart disease are 65 years of age or older.

- Race or ethnicity. African Americans, Mexican Americans, Native Americans, and Native Hawaiians are at greater risk for a heart attack than other races or ethnic groups.

- Gender. In the United States, more men have heart attacks, but heart disease is the leading cause of death for women.

The American Heart Association (2016) recommends that those at risk talk with family and loved ones about the warning signs or symptoms of a heart attack. These individuals also need to complete a heart attack survival plan and make a copy that can be easily found by family members and loved ones.

An MI damages heart tissue, which makes the heart less effective at pumping blood. After an MI, the patient's heart is permanently damaged. Treatment for MI therefore has three parts: (a) restoring the heart's balance between oxygen supply and demand, (b) pain relief, and (c) preventing future problems. To this aim, treatments for a heart attack include antiplatelet medication and/or aspirin, which helps prevent blood clots; anticoagulants, which prevent clotting in pathways; and nitrates, which help relieve symptoms. Surgery, such as angioplasty and bypass, is also an option following an MI.

It can take up to 8 weeks to recover after an MI, and as part of a patient's MI treatment plan, he or she will be enrolled in a *cardiac rehabilitation program*. A cardiac rehabilitation program provides information that helps patients understand their risk factors. The program also offers patients a guide to a healthy lifestyle that prevents future heart problems This guide helps patients learn how to reach and maintain a healthy weight through exercise and healthy eating. Patients also learn ways to control stress levels, blood pressure, and cholesterol levels. Cardiac rehabilitation programs typically last 3 to 6 months, and regular attendance is required because the more lifestyle changes a patient makes, the better his or her chances of preventing another heart attack.

Most people survive their first heart attack and lead normal lives. But having a heart attack does mean a commitment to lifestyle changes and taking medications that improve the patient's heart health. The extent to which a patient needs to make lifestyle changes and take medications depends on how badly his or her heart was damaged. Some of the lifestyle changes that can improve a patient's heart health are listed in Figure 13.4.

High Blood Pressure, or Hypertension

As already discussed, arteries are blood vessels that carry blood from the heart to the rest of the body. Normal arteries are smooth and flexible, and blood flows easily through them. As the blood moves through the arteries, it puts pressure on the artery walls; this is known as blood pressure. *Blood pressure* is the amount of pressure applied by the blood to the walls of the arteries. Blood pressure doesn't stay the same all the time; it changes over the course of the day. It lowers when a person is sleeping and rises when he or she is awake. Blood pressure also rises with excitement, stress, or activity, but for most of our waking hours, blood pressure stays the same when we're sitting or standing still.

As its name suggests, *high blood pressure (HBP), or hypertension*, is abnormally high pressure of the blood as it moves through the arteries. The heart has to work harder, and the arteries take a beating because of the higher pressure. HBP occurs for two reasons: First, blood volume is too high; second, blood vessels are too narrow due to a kidney hormone that causes blood vessels to narrow.

High blood pressure is common, and it is often called the "silent killer" because there are no symptoms until it causes damage. About one in three adults in the United States has HBP, or about 65 million US adults. It is more common in men than in women. About 65% of Americans ages 60 or older have HBP. Once HBP develops, the patient usually has it for the rest of his or her life (US Food and Drug Administration, 2015).

There are two types of HBP: primary and secondary. When the etiology (cause) is unknown, a patient has primary hypertension. Up to 95% of HBP cases are primary. When the etiology is known, a patient has secondary hypertension. Secondary hypertension is usually caused by other health problems or certain medications.

Regardless of the type of HBP, a patient can have it for years without knowing it. During this time, however, HBP can severely damage the body in several possible ways (US Food and Drug Administration, 2015):

- Weakening of the heart, leading to congestive heart failure—the inability of the heart to pump enough blood to meet the body's needs

- Aneurysms, or abnormal bulges in the wall of an artery

- Kidney failure when the blood vessels in the kidneys get too narrow

- Narrowing of the arteries in some places, limiting blood flow

- Bleeding in the blood vessels of the eyes, which can cause blindness

Given the damage that HBP can cause, it is important for people to know their blood pressure numbers, even when they are feeling healthy. Blood pressure is indicated by two numbers, separated by a slash when written (e.g., 120/80 mmHg). The first number is the *systolic blood pressure*, which is the peak blood pressure when the heart is squeezing blood out. The second number is the *diastolic blood pressure*. It's the pressure when the heart is filling up with blood—relaxing between beats. The abbreviation *mmHg* refers to millimeters of mercury, the unit used to measure blood pressure. Table 13.2 shows the range of blood pressure numbers applicable to most adults (ages 18 and older) who don't have a serious illness.

If both numbers stay above normal most of the time, a patient is at risk for health problems. The risk grows as blood pressure numbers rise. *Prehypertension* is an indication that the patient

Table 13.2 Categories for Blood Pressure Levels in Adults

Category	Systolic (top number)		Diastolic (bottom number)
Normal	Less than 120	and	Less than 80
Prehypertension	120–139	or	80–89
High blood pressure			
Stage 1	140–159	or	90–99
Stage 2	160 or higher	or	100 or higher

Note. From the National Heart, Lung, and Blood Institute

may end up with HBP unless he or she takes steps to prevent it. Some patients only have high systolic blood pressure, or *isolated systolic hypertension (ISH)*. ISH can cause as much harm as HBP.

HBP is diagnosed using a blood pressure test that is easy and painless. The health care provider uses a gauge, a stethoscope, and a blood pressure cuff. The cuff is wrapped around the patient's arm as the health care provider checks blood pressure. Patients can also check their blood pressure at home and keep track of the numbers for their health care provider.

If the blood pressure is 140/90 mmHg or higher over time, the health care provider will likely diagnose the patient with HBP. If the patient has diabetes or chronic kidney disease, however, a blood pressure of 130/80 mmHg or higher is considered HBP.

Patients with HBP need to treat and control it for life, which requires them to do three tasks: make lifestyle changes, take prescribed medications, and receive ongoing health care.

Treatment usually begins with healthy lifestyle changes that a patient can make to lower and control blood pressure (see Figure 13.4). Some patients can lower their blood pressure by following healthy lifestyle changes alone. For most patients, however, these changes are not enough, and they need to take medication, probably for the rest of their lives.

Patients with HBP often need more than one medication. These medications are called anti-hypertensive medicines. Some of the medications are diuretics, or "water pills," that help the kidneys flush extra water and salt from the body and decrease blood volume. Other drugs inhibit the effects of the kidney hormone that causes blood vessels to narrow, or help the heart beat slower and with less force.

The treatment goal is for a patient's blood pressure to stay at a normal level. If a patient receives HBP treatment and has repeat readings in the normal range, then his or her blood pressure is under control. However, the patient still needs to follow the treatment plan throughout his or her life. Sticking to the treatment plan is important because it helps prevent or delay health problems related to HBP and helps the patient live longer.

A family history of HPB is a risk factor, as well as certain traits, conditions, and lifestyle choices, including the following (American Academy of Family Physicians, 2015):

- Race or ethnicity—HBP is more common in African American adults than in White or Hispanic American adults
- Gender—birth control pills, pregnancy, or hormone therapy may cause HBP in some women
- Increasing age
- Certain medications
- Diet high in fat, salt, and cholesterol
- Lack of exercise
- Being overweight
- Tobacco use and alcohol abuse
- Lack of potassium in the diet
- Chronic stress
- Thyroid and chronic kidney diseases
- Other heart diseases

Patients who have one or more risk factors can take steps to prevent HBP. Healthy lifestyle changes (see Figure 13.4) can help maintain normal blood pressure; these individuals should also have their blood pressure checked frequently. Everyone 18 years of age and older should have his or her blood pressure checked at least once every 2 years.

Arrhythmia

Arrhythmia is an abnormal rhythm or pulse of the heart. There are different types:

Bradycardia: slow heart rate—less than 60 beats per minute

Tachycardia: fast heart rate—more than 100 beats per minute

Atrial fibrillation (AF): irregular heartbeat

AF is the most common type of arrhythmia; it occurs when rapid, disorganized electrical signals cause the heart's two upper chambers to fibrillate, which means to contract rapidly and irregularly.

As already discussed, the heart receives electrical signals that regulate its beat—that is, ensure that it contracts in an orderly way. Problems with the heart's electrical system—extra signals, signals that are blocked, or signals that travel in new and different pathways through the heart—cause abnormal heart rhythms, which in turn make it difficult for the heart to pump blood efficiently.

Almost everyone has experienced symptoms of arrhythmia, such as feeling the heart beating fast, a "fluttering" in the chest, or the heart "skipping a beat." Arrhythmias are extremely common and can happen at any age, especially as we grow older. Most cases are harmless, but some arrhythmias are extremely dangerous and require treatment. The following are common causes of arrhythmias (US National Library of Medicine, 2014a):

- Abnormal levels of potassium
- Heart attacks
- Heart diseases
- High blood pressure
- Diabetes
- Overactive thyroid gland
- Excessive use of alcohol or stimulants
- Tobacco use
- Stress
- Certain medications

In addition to these common causes, sometimes taking an anti-arrhythmic medication that is prescribed to treat one type of arrhythmia can cause another type of arrhythmia.

An arrhythmia can happen constantly, or it may come and go. A patient may or may not feel symptoms when the arrhythmia is present. Symptoms can be mild, or they may be severe or even life threatening. Symptoms of arrhythmia include the following (US National Library of Medicine, 2014a):

- Chest pain
- Fainting
- Dizziness
- Shortness of breath
- Sweating
- Tachycardia (fast heartbeat) or bradycardia (slow heartbeat)
- Syncope (lightheadedness)
- In extreme cases, collapse and sudden cardiac arrest

Health care providers diagnose an arrhythmia using the patient's personal and family health history, a physical exam, and an EKG.

Most arrhythmias are harmless and are left untreated. If a patient's arrhythmia does cause symptoms, then more aggressive treatment is needed. In addition to anti-arrhythmic medication, treatment may include electrical "shock" therapy: implanting a *heart pacemaker*, a device that helps the heart beat regularly.

The prognosis or outcome for arrhythmia depends on at least two factors. One factor is the kind of arrhythmia; some arrhythmias may be life threatening if they are not treated right away or do not respond well to treatment. Another factor is whether the patient has a heart disease, such as coronary artery disease (CAD). In fact, a major risk reduction strategy for arrhythmia is to make lifestyle changes that prevent CAD (see Figure 13.4).

Congestive Heart Failure (Heart Failure)

Although the term *congestive heart failure (CHF), or heart failure*, seems to imply that the heart stops beating, it in fact means that the heart isn't pumping blood as well as it should. With CHF, the weakened heart muscle can't supply the body's cells with enough blood. The heart keeps working, but the cells' need for blood and oxygen isn't being met. In other words, with CHF, the heart can't keep up with the body's cellular demands.

The heart tries to make up for the lack of blood supply by getting bigger or by pumping faster. The body also tries to help by taking blood away from less important organs to maintain flow to the more vital organs, the heart and brain. These temporary solutions mask the problem, but they don't fix it. CHF just continues and worsens. Eventually the heart and body can't keep up with the demand. This results in fatigue and difficulty breathing while doing daily activities like walking or climbing stairs.

Often chronic and progressive, CHF sometimes develops suddenly. It may affect only one side of the heart; this is referred to as right-sided CHF or left-sided CHF. It usually affects the left side first, then both sides of the heart are eventually involved. Symptoms of CHF include not only fatigue and difficulty breathing but also weight gain with *edema*, or swelling in the legs, ankles, or lower back.

Around 5.8 million people in the United States have CHF, and about half of those patients who develop heart failure die within 5 years of diagnosis (CDC, 2016b). Tests used to diagnose, find the cause of, and monitor CHF include echocardiogram, X-rays, MRIs, and blood tests.

The common causes of CHF are coronary artery disease (CAD), high blood pressure, and diabetes. Most cases of CHF can be prevented by the same healthy lifestyle changes (see Figure 13.4) that reduce the risks for heart disease.

In addition to making healthy lifestyle changes, a patient with CHF often needs medications. The medications treat the symptoms, prevent CHF from getting worse, and help the patient live longer. There are also surgeries and devices for patients with CHF, including angioplasty, a pacemaker that slows the heart rate, or a *defibrillator*, a device that sends electrical pulses to stop arrhythmia.

CHF is serious, and the only cure is a heart transplant. Almost 50,000 people die each year while awaiting a heart transplant (CDC, 2016b). The demand for heart transplants in the United States far exceeds the availability of donor organs.

For many patients with CHF, early diagnosis and treatment can improve quality of life and life expectancy. Unfortunately, however, for those patients who do develop severe CHF, medications, lifestyle changes, or other treatments are no longer helpful.

Heart Infections

Heart infections can cause heart diseases. There are three types of heart infections: *pericarditis*, an inflammation or swelling of the membrane surrounding the heart (pericardium); *myocarditis*, which affects the middle layer of the walls of the heart (myocardium); and *endocarditis*, which affects the heart's inner lining (endocardium). Varying slightly with each type of infection, the symptoms include fever; shortness of breath; fatigue; swelling in feet, legs, or abdomen; skin rashes; and changes in heart rhythm.

There are many causes of heart infections. The most common include bacteria that enter the bloodstream through everyday activities like eating or brushing teeth. An infection also can be caused by the tick-borne bacteria that are responsible for Lyme disease. Another common cause is viruses, including those responsible for influenza, mononucleosis, and measles. Viruses associated with sexually transmitted infections can travel to the heart muscle and cause an infection. Parasites that cause heart infections are found in uncooked foods and contaminated water, and can also be transmitted by insects. Some drugs can cause heart infections through an allergic or toxic reaction; these include antibiotics, such as penicillin, as well as illegal substances, such as cocaine. The needles used to administer medications or illegal drugs also transmit viruses or bacteria that cause heart infections.

Beyond taking the patient's health history and conducting a physical exam, a health care provider orders diagnostic tests that identify heart infections. These tests include blood tests, EEG, EKG, chest X-ray, CT scan, or MRI scan. Treatment for heart infections depends on the cause.

Diseases of the Veins

The veins in the body play an important role in circulation, carrying blood from different parts of the body back to the heart. But as people age, health problems can develop in the veins. In fact, one in three Americans over the age of 45 has some kind of vein disease (Agency for Healthcare Research and Quality, 2012). Early symptoms may seem minor. However, they can become more serious and even life threatening if not treated.

Varicose Veins

Varicose veins are veins that are swollen and bulge above the surface of the skin. They may be twisted, and are often blue or dark purple. Varicose veins are commonly found on the backs of the calves, on the inside of the leg, or on the feet, and are sometimes found on the groin. Generally, they are visible just under the surface of the skin. *Hemorrhoids* are swollen, inflamed veins around the anus or lower rectum and are a form of varicose vein. Spider veins are a smaller version of varicose veins.

Veins return blood back to the heart so that it can recirculate to the rest of the body. There are valves in veins that open to allow the blood to flow toward the heart. Sometimes the valves may stop working, allowing blood to flow back down into the veins. Blood then pools in the veins, causing *phlebitis*, or swelling and enlargement. The veins in the legs are especially at risk because they have to work against gravity to get the blood back to the heart. This is why most varicose veins are found in the legs.

Varicose veins can cause a painful feeling in the legs. There may be swelling of the feet, ankles, and one or both legs that gets worse throughout the day, but goes down overnight. This swelling is called *venous stasis*. The skin may feel warm and look red in the affected leg. In some severe cases, ulcers or blood clots may develop. A patient who has varicose veins can improve the symptoms by keeping a healthy weight, avoiding standing for long periods of time, raising his or her legs while sitting, and wearing loose clothing.

A health care provider may recommend that the patient with varicose veins wear compression stockings. The stockings help keep blood from pooling in the legs and reduce swelling when the patient is sitting or standing. If the patient's symptoms don't improve, there are more invasive treatment options, including surgery, laser therapy, and injection therapy.

Risk factors for varicose veins are family health history (varicose veins tend to run in families), gender (women are at greater risk), pregnancy, age (about 50% of people over the age of 50 have varicose veins), obesity, and occupation (standing for long periods of time without moving around) (Agency for Healthcare Research and Quality, 2012).

Deep Vein Thrombosis

Deep vein thrombosis (DVT) is a blood clot in a vein deep inside the body. These clots usually form in the leg veins. DVT is a fairly common condition, but also a dangerous one. If the blood clot breaks away and travels through the bloodstream, it can block a blood vessel in the lungs. This blockage, called a *pulmonary embolism*, can be fatal.

In addition to conducting a physical exam and taking a patient's health history, a health care provider can run diagnostic tests for DVT, including an ultrasound or *venography*, which involves injecting a dye into the vein and taking an X-ray so as to locate blood clots. If a patient is diagnosed with DVT, the main treatment goals include stopping the clot from getting bigger, preventing the clot from breaking off and traveling to the lungs, and preventing any future blood clots.

Elevation of the affected leg and compression can help reduce swelling and pain from DVT. Compression stockings can also reduce swelling in the leg after a blood clot has developed. Frequent exercising and stretching of the lower leg muscles if they have been inactive for long periods of time can help prevent DVT. For example, surgical patients need to get out of bed and move around as soon as possible after having surgery.

Several medications are used to treat or prevent DVT. The most common are anticoagulants, or blood thinners. *Anticoagulants* thin blood so that clots won't form.

DVT is a common problem in postoperative patients and those confined to bed. Risk for DVT increases if the patient has several factors at the same time. These risk factors include aging, inactivity, diseases that cause blood clotting, injury, surgery, pregnancy, obesity, varicose veins, and cancer. For some women, birth control pills or hormone therapy may also be risk factors.

Chapter Summary

- A complete heartbeat makes up a cardiac cycle, which has two parts. First, the ventricles contract (systole), sending blood into the circulatory system. When systole is finished, the aortic and pulmonic valves close to prevent blood from flowing back into the ventricles. Second, the ventricles relax (diastole) and fill with blood from the atria.

- Coronary artery disease is the most common cardiovascular disease for US adults. It is the number one killer of both men and women in most racial and ethnic groups and is a major cause of disability.

- When the heart actually stops during a heart attack, it is called sudden cardiac arrest (SCA). SCA occurs when the heart suddenly stops pumping due to an electrical problem (not a blood flow problem, as in a heart attack).

- High blood pressure, or hypertension, is abnormally high pressure of the blood as it moves through the arteries. The heart must work harder and the arteries take a beating because of the higher pressure.

- Atrial fibrillation (AF) is the most common type of arrhythmia; it occurs when rapid, disorganized electrical signals cause the heart's two upper chambers to fibrillate, which means to contract rapidly and irregularly.

- Congestive heart failure doesn't mean that the heart stops beating; instead, it means that the heart isn't pumping blood as well as it should.

- Although some risk factors for cardiovascular diseases, such as genetics, cannot be controlled, a person can reduce risk by making healthy lifestyle choices, such as managing blood pressure, lowering cholesterol, not smoking, eating a balanced diet, and exercising regularly.

- Varicose veins are swollen and bulge above the surface of the skin. They may be twisted, and are often blue or dark purple. Hemorrhoids are swollen, inflamed veins around the anus and are a form of varicose vein. Spider veins are a smaller version of varicose veins.

- Deep vein thrombosis (DVT) is a blood clot in a vein deep inside the body. These clots usually occur in the leg veins. DVT is a frequent problem for postoperative patients and those confined to bed.

REVIEW QUESTIONS

1.   What are the four chambers of the heart?

2.   What is the function of coronary arteries?

3.   Who should take aspirin for their heart health? Who should not take aspirin for their heart health?

4.   What does it mean to have a heart attack? A cardiac arrest?

5.   Identify treatment options for high blood pressure.

6.   What is atherosclerosis, and what are its causes?

7.   What tests are used to diagnose heart disease?

8.   Identify healthy lifestyle choices and discuss how they are protective factors against cardiovascular diseases.

9.   How do fat and cholesterol affect blood vessels?

10. Identify the differences among varicose veins, hemorrhoids, and spider veins.

KEY TERMS

Acquired: Refers to a disease or condition that develops some time after birth

Aneurysm: Weakness in the wall of an artery caused by plaque buildup

Angina: Chest pain

Angioplasty: Surgical procedure that uses a balloon to push open blocked arteries around the heart

Anticoagulants: Medication that thins blood so that clots won't form

Aorta, or main artery: The body's largest blood vessel, which carries oxygen-rich blood away from the heart

Aortic valve: Valve that separates the left ventricle from the aorta, or main artery

Arrhythmia: Abnormal rhythm or pulse of the heart

Arteries: Blood vessels that carry blood away from the heart

Arterioles: Vessels that are smaller than arteries

Atherosclerosis, or hardening of the arteries: Disease of the arteries that causes them to be thick, stiff, and narrow

Atrial fibrillation (AF): Condition brought on by rapid, disorganized electrical signals that cause the heart's two upper chambers to fibrillate, which means to contract rapidly and irregularly

Atrioventricular node, or AV node: Heart tissue that sends electrical signals that travel through the ventricles

Blood: The vitally important transport system that carries oxygen, nutrients, hormones, and antibodies to cells throughout the body and removes waste materials from the cells

Blood pressure: Amount of pressure applied by the blood to the walls of the arteries

Blood vessels: Hollow tubes that carry and circulate blood throughout the body

Bradycardia: Heart rate of less than 60 beats per minute

Bypass surgery: Procedure in which pieces of veins or arteries are taken from the legs and sewn into the arteries of the heart to bring blood past a blockage and increase the blood flow to the heart

Capillaries: The smallest branching blood vessels

Cardiac cycle: Complete heartbeat

Cardiac muscle: Heart muscle

Cardiac rehabilitation program: Program for patients with heart disease that provides prevention information and support

Cardiologist: A physician with a medical specialty in cardiology

Cardiology: The study of the circulatory system and of cardiovascular diseases

Cardiovascular disease: Broad term that describes a range of diseases that affect the heart

Cardiovascular system, or heart and circulatory system: Body system made up of the heart and blood vessels, including arteries, veins, and capillaries

Congenital: Refers to a disease or condition that is present at birth

Congenital heart disease (CHD): Health problems with the heart that develop before birth

Congestive heart failure (CHF), or heart failure: Inability of the heart to pump enough blood to meet the body's needs

Coronary arteries: Arteries that provide oxygen and nourishment to the muscles of the heart

Coronary artery disease (CAD), or coronary heart disease: Disease in which plaque builds up in the coronary arteries, which supply blood to the heart

Cyanosis: Bluish-purple color of the skin, lips, and fingernails

Deep vein thrombosis (DVT): Blood clot in a vein deep inside the body, usually in the leg veins

Defibrillator: Device that sends an electrical pulse to the heart to stop arrhythmia

Diastole: Relaxation of the heart's ventricles to allow in blood from the atria

Diastolic blood pressure: The blood pressure when the heart is filling up with blood—relaxing between beats

Edema: Swelling in the legs, ankles, or lower back

Endocarditis: Infection that causes inflammation in the heart's inner lining

Heart murmur: Unusual sound that's heard when listening to the heart

Heart pacemaker: Device that helps the heart beat regularly

Heart palpitations: Fast or irregular heartbeats

Hemorrhoids: Swollen, inflamed veins around the anus or lower rectum

High blood pressure (HBP), or hypertension: Abnormally high pressure of the blood as it moves through the arteries

Inferior vena cava: Large vein that carries deoxygenated blood from the lower body into the heart

Isolated systolic hypertension (ISH): Condition in which the patient has only high systolic blood pressure

Mitral valve: Valve that connects the left atrium to the left ventricle

mmHg: Abbreviation for millimeters of mercury, the unit used to measure blood pressure

Myocardial infarction (MI), or heart attack: Condition in which plaque totally blocks a coronary artery, or some plaque breaks off and causes a clot in a coronary artery

Myocarditis: Infection that causes inflammation in the middle layer of the walls of the heart

Pericardial cavity: Moist cavity that surrounds the heart

Pericarditis: Infection that causes inflammation of the membrane surrounding the heart

Phlebitis: Swelling and enlargement of the veins caused by the pooling of blood

Plaque: Substance made of fat, cholesterol, calcium, and other materials that builds up in arteries, making them hard, weak, and narrow

Plasma: Yellowish fluid that enables blood cells to travel through the circulatory system

Prehypertension: Elevated blood pressure indicating that the patient may end up with HBP unless he or she takes steps to prevent it

Pulmonary artery: Artery that leads to the lungs

Pulmonary circulation: The flow of blood through a short loop from the heart to the lungs and back again

Pulmonary embolism: Blood clot that breaks away, travels through the bloodstream, and blocks a blood vessel in the lungs

Pulmonic valve: Valve that separates the right ventricle from the pulmonary artery, which leads to the lungs

Pulse, or heart rate: The number of signals the SA node produces per minute

Right and left atria: Located in the upper part of the heart, the two cavities that hold the blood that enters the heart

Right and left ventricles: Located at the bottom of the heart, the two cavities that pump blood out of the heart

Septum: Wall that separates the left and right sides of the heart

Sinoatrial node, or SA node: Heart tissue that sends out electrical signals to start the contracting of the heart muscle

Stent: Small metal rod put into the artery where there is blockage

Sudden cardiac arrest (SCA): Stopping of the heart during a heart attack

Superior vena cava: Large vein that carries deoxygenated blood from the head, arms, and upper body into the heart

Syncope: Lightheadedness or loss of consciousness due to a drop in blood pressure

Systemic circulation: The flow of blood from the heart to other parts of the body and back again

Systole: Contraction of the heart's ventricles to send blood into the circulatory system

Systolic blood pressure: The peak blood pressure when the heart is squeezing blood out

Tachycardia: Heart rate of more than 100 beats per minute

Tetralogy of Fallot: Disease in which not enough blood is able to reach the lungs to get oxygen

Tricuspid valve: Valve that connects the right atrium to the right ventricle

Varicose veins: Veins that are swollen and bulge above the surface of the skin

Veins: Blood vessels that carry blood back to the lungs and heart

Venography: Diagnostic test that uses a dye that is injected into the vein to identify blood clots

Venous stasis: Swelling of the feet, ankles, and legs that gets worse throughout the day, but goes down overnight

CHAPTER ACTIVITIES

1. Conduct research and make a brochure on ways to prevent DVT, targeted to different settings. For example, you can chose to make a brochure for patients in hospitals or in long-term care facilities. Another option is to develop a brochure for airline travelers on long flights.

2. Many studies have shown a clear connection between healthy lifestyle choices and heart disease. Prepare a debate on whether health insurance companies should be allowed to charge higher premiums to people whose lifestyle choices put them at greater risk for heart disease.

3. Working in pairs, trace on paper how the blood flows through the heart.

4. Select a cardiovascular disease discussed in this chapter and identify healthy lifestyle choices that reduce risk. With a partner, design a one-page infographic using icons that send the message that healthy lifestyle choices reduce the risk for cardiovascular disease, and that show how. Use as few words as possible, but enough to explain your healthy lifestyle message.

5. You have been hired as a community health education specialist to work on the topic of heart health with seniors at a local senior center. Your task is to develop a heart health exercise program for seniors. The one-time program is 30 minutes in length and includes chair exercises, light stretching, and weight-bearing activities. Participants also learn about heart disease and its effects on health. How would you design this program? Write a two- to three-page paper that describes your 30-minute exercise program.

Bibliography and Works Cited

Agency for Healthcare Research and Quality. (2012). Your guide to preventing and treating blood clots. Retrieved from http://www.ahrq.gov/patients-consumers/prevention/disease/bloodclots.html

American Academy of Family Physicians. (2014). Coronary artery disease (CAD). *Family Doctor.org.* Retrieved from http://familydoctor.org/familydoctor/en/diseases-conditions/coronary-artery-disease.printerview.all.html

American Academy of Family Physicians. (2015). High blood pressure/overview. *Family Doctor.org.* Retrieved from http://familydoctor.org/familydoctor/en/diseases-conditions/high-blood-pressure.html

American Heart Association. (2016a). About heart attacks. Retrieved from http://www.heart.org/HEARTORG/Conditions/HeartAttack/AboutHeartAttacks/About-Heart-Attacks_UCM_002038_Article.jsp#.VqQcxporLtQ

American Heart Association. (2016b). What is cardiovascular disease? Retrieved from http://www.heart.org/HEARTORG/Caregiver/Resources/WhatisCardiovascularDisease/What-is-Cardiovascular-Disease_UCM_301852_Article.jsp#.VqQGzporLtQ

Centers for Disease Control and Prevention. (2016a). Heart disease. Retrieved from http://www.cdc.gov/heartdisease/index.htm

Centers for Disease Control and Prevention. (2016b). Heart failure fact sheet. Retrieved from https://www.cdc.gov/dhdsp/data_statistics/fact_sheets/fs_heart_failure.htm

Dolbec, K., & Mick, N. W., (2011). Congenital heart disease. *Emergency Medical Clinics of North America, 29,* 811–827. doi:10.1016/j.emc.2011.08.005

Franklin Institute. (2016). The heart: The engine of life. Retrieved from https://www.fi.edu/heart-engine-life

Mayo Clinic. (2016). Heart disease. Retrieved from http://www.mayoclinic.org/diseases-conditions/heart-disease/basics/definition/con-20034056

National Heart, Lung, and Blood Institute. (2011a). Don't take a chance with a heart attack: Know the facts and act fast. Retrieved from http://www.nhlbi.nih.gov/files/docs/public/heart/heartattackfsen.pdf

National Heart, Lung, and Blood Institute. (2011b). Heart & vascular disease. Retrieved from http://www.nhlbi.nih.gov/health/resources/heart#chol%20Heart%20and%20Vascular%20Diseases

National Heart, Lung, and Blood Institute. (2011c). What is Tetralogy of Fallot? Retrieved from http://www.nhlbi
.nih.gov/health/health-topics/topics/tof/

National Heart, Lung, and Blood Institute. (2015a). What is heart valve disease? Retrieved from http://www.nhlbi
.nih.gov/health/health-topics/topics/hvd

National Heart, Lung, and Blood Institute. (2015b). What is coronary heart disease? Retrieved from http://www
.nhlbi.nih.gov/health/health-topics/topics/cad

Sandmaier, M. (2007). *The healthy heart handbook for women*. National Heart, Lung, and Blood Institute.
Retrieved from https://www.nhlbi.nih.gov/files/docs/public/heart/hdbk_wmn.pdf

US Food and Drug Administration. (2015). High blood pressure (hypertension). Retrieved from http://www.fda
.gov/ForConsumers/ByAudience/ForWomen/ucm118529.htm

US National Library of Medicine. (2014a). Arrhythmia. *PubMed Health*. Retrieved from http://www.ncbi.nlm
.nih.gov/pubmedhealth/PMH0062940/

US National Library of Medicine. (2014b). Atherosclerosis. *PubMed Health*. Retrieved from http://www.ncbi
.nlm.nih.gov/pubmedhealth/PMH0062943/

US National Library of Medicine. (2016). Heart attack. *MedlinePlus*. Retrieved from https://www.nlm.nih.gov
/medlineplus/heartattack.html

Wolters Kluwer. (2016a). Patient education: Heart failure (The basics). *UpToDate*. Retrieved from https://www
.uptodate-com.ezproxy.springfield.edu/contents/heart-failure-the-basics?source=search_result&search=
heart%20failure&selectedTitle=3~150

Wolters Kluwer. (2016b). Patient education: Pericarditis in Adults (The basics). *UpToDate*. Retrieved from
https://www.uptodate.com/contents/pericarditis-in-adults-the-basics?source=search_result&search=
pericarditis&selectedTitle=1~150

Wolters Kluwer. (2016c). Patient education: Myocarditis (The basics). *UpToDate*. Retrieved from https://www
.uptodate.com/contents/myocarditis-the-basics?source=search_result&search=myocarditis&selectedTitle=
1~150

Wolters Kluwer. (2016d). Patient education: Endocarditis (The basics). *UpToDate*. Retrieved from https://www
.uptodate.com/contents/endocarditis-the-basics?source.=search_result&search=endocarditis&selected
Title=1~150

Wolters Kluwer. (2016e). Patient education: Varicose veins and other vein disease in the legs (The basics).
UpToDate. Retrieved from https://www.uptodate.com/contents/varicose-veins-and-other-vein-disease-in
-the-legs-the-basics?source=search_result&search=varicose%20veins%20adult&selectedTitle=2~150

WomenHeart. (2016). Am I having a heart attack? Retrieved from http://www.womenheart.org/?page=
Support_AmIHaving

BLOOD AND RELATED DISEASES

CHAPTER OBJECTIVES

- Review the functions of blood.

- Compare the functions of red blood cells, white blood cells, and platelets.

- List four main blood types and explain the Rh factor.

- Describe the complete blood count (CBC) test and explain why it is important to the diagnostic process.

- Summarize the role of the spleen in protecting the body against infection.

- Identify etiology, signs, symptoms, diagnostic tests, and treatment for selected blood disorders.

Blood carries gases, oxygen, and nutrients throughout the body. It also filters the body's waste, fights infections, heals wounds, and performs many other vital functions. In fact, blood performs so many vital functions that when something is wrong with blood, the entire body can be affected.

Whole blood has four main parts: plasma, red blood cells, white blood cells, and platelets. Blood diseases affect one or more of these parts and can be acute or chronic. Many blood diseases are inherited; others are caused by other diseases, side effects of medications, or a lack of certain nutrients.

What Is Blood?

Hematology is the study of blood in health and disease. It addresses problems with the red blood cells, white blood cells, platelets, blood vessels, bone marrow, lymph nodes, spleen, and proteins involved in bleeding and clotting. If a patient is diagnosed with a blood disease, his health care provider may refer him to a hematologist. A *hematologist* is a physician who has a specialty in blood diseases.

Without blood, the human body would weaken and die. Organs couldn't get the oxygen and the nutrients they need to survive, and we couldn't warm up or cool down. The average adult man has about 3 gallons, or 24 pints, of blood inside his body; the average adult woman has about 2.5 gallons, or 20 pints.

There is no substitute for blood. It can't be made or manufactured. According to the American Red Cross (2016), donors are the only source of blood for patients who need it, and more than 38,000 blood donations are needed every day. Another way to think about the demand is that in the United States, every 2 seconds a patient is in need of blood. Roughly, a donation equals about a pint, and one donation can help save the lives of up to three people.

Whole blood is living tissue made up of liquid and solids. It has four main parts: plasma, red blood cells, white blood cells, and platelets. The liquid, called *plasma*, is made of water, sugar, fat, salt, and protein. Plasma, which is 90% water, makes up 55% of blood volume. The main job of plasma is to carry blood cells throughout the body along with nutrients, waste products, antibodies, clotting factors, hormones, and proteins. The solid part of blood has three types of blood cells: red blood cells, white blood cells, and platelets (see Figure 14.1).

Red blood cells (RBCs) deliver oxygen from the lungs to tissues and organs. Known for their bright red color and a disc-like shape, RBCs are the most numerous cells in the blood. Every day, the body makes new RBCs to replace those that die or are lost from the body.

RBCs contain the iron-rich protein *hemoglobin*. Blood gets its bright red color when hemoglobin picks up oxygen in the lungs. As the blood travels through the body, hemoglobin helps RBCs pick up and carry oxygen from the lungs to all parts of the body. It also helps RBCs remove carbon dioxide from tissues and bring it to the lungs so that it can be exhaled. The test that measures the percentage of RBCs in a patient's blood is called the *hematocrit* and is a common diagnostic test.

RBCs start as immature cells in the bone marrow and grow into mature cells in about 7 days. Once mature, RBCs are released into the bloodstream. Unlike many other cells, RBCs have no nucleus so that they can easily change shape, helping them fit through various blood vessels in the body. However, although the lack of a nucleus makes RBCs more flexible, it also limits the cell's life span. RBCs survive on average only about 3 to 4 months.

White blood cells (WBCs) are the body's primary defense against infection and are part of the immune system. They can move out of the bloodstream and reach tissues being invaded by germs. Blood has fewer WBCs than RBCs; however, when WBCs are needed to fight infection, the body increases production.

There are several types of WBCs, and their life spans vary from a few days to months. The discussion in this chapter is limited to the *lymphocyte*, a major type of WBC. As discussed in Chapter 11, there are two major sets of these cells. T-cells help regulate the function of other immune cells and

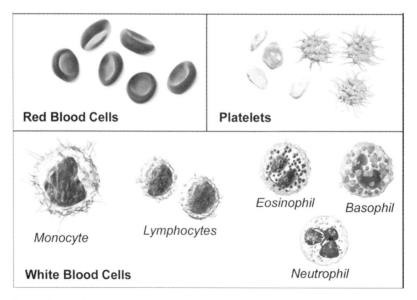

Figure 14.1 Three Types of Blood Cells

Note. From "Blausen Gallery 2014," by Blausen.com staff, Wikiversity Journal of Medicine, doi:10.15347/wjm/2014.010. ISSN 20018762. (Own work) [CC BY 3.0 (http://creativecommons.org/licenses/by/3.0)], via Wikimedia Commons. Retrieved from https://commons.wikimedia.org/wiki/File%3ABlausen _0425_Formed_Elements.png

directly attack various infected cells and tumors. B-cells make antibodies, which are proteins that target bacteria, viruses, and other foreign materials.

Unlike RBCs and WBCs, *platelets* are not cells, but instead are small bits of cells. Platelets' life span is about 6 days. Their function is to help blood form a clot if there is a cut in the skin. When a blood vessel breaks, platelets gather around the cut and stick to the lining of the injured blood vessel. Platelets with their sticky surface will then assist in forming clots to stop the bleeding. A *clot* covers the cut and prevents blood from leaking out. Although platelets alone can temporarily stop bleeding, *clotting factors*—certain minerals, proteins, and vitamins—are also needed to make a strong clot. Platelets and these clotting factors work together to form solid lumps to seal leaks and prevent bleeding inside and outside of the body. Clots also serve as the base for new tissue growth, thus promoting healing. The process of clotting, known as *coagulation*, is like putting together a puzzle with interlocking pieces. When the last piece is in place, then the clot is complete. If even one piece is missing, the final pieces can't come together to stop the bleeding.

A higher than normal number of platelets can cause unnecessary clotting, which leads to strokes and heart attacks; however, there are treatments that can help prevent these fatal events. Conversely, a lower than normal number of platelets can lead to extensive bleeding.

A *scab* is an external blood clot, and a *bruise* is an internal blood clot. Both scabs and bruises are signs of healing, but some blood clots can be dangerous. A blood clot that forms inside a blood vessel is dangerous because it stops the flow of blood and cuts off oxygen supply. In addition, when large blood vessels are cut, the body may not be able to repair itself through coagulation alone. In these cases, stitches or sutures are used to stop bleeding. *Stitches* are loops of thread used to join the edges of a skin cut.

RBCs, WBCs, and platelets develop in the bone marrow. *Bone marrow* is a spongy tissue located in the central cavity of bones. In newborns, all bones have active marrow. By young adulthood, however, only the spine, hip, and shoulder bones; ribs; breastbone; and skull contain the marrow that makes blood cells in adults.

The most undeveloped cells in the marrow are *stem cells*. Stem cells are unique in that they can develop into a number of different kinds of cells, including RBCs, WBCs, and platelets. In a healthy person, there are enough stem cells to keep making new blood cells all the time. Blood passes through the marrow and picks up the fully developed RBCs, WBCs, and platelets for circulation throughout the body.

The presence of stem cells in the blood is important because they can be collected by a special technique. If enough stem cells are harvested from a compatible donor, they can be transplanted into a patient.

Stem cell circulation, from marrow to blood and back, also occurs in the fetus. After birth, placental and umbilical cord blood can be collected, stored, and used for stem cell transplantation. (As mentioned, stem cells can also be collected from the blood and bone marrow of people of all ages.) The purpose of *stem cell transplantation* is to restore the marrow's function and to potentially treat many diseases. See Figure 14.2 for an overview of potential uses of stem cells in disease treatment.

Blood Transfusions

Each year, about 4.5 million Americans need a blood transfusion, the equivalent of one blood transfusion every 2 seconds in the United States. A blood transfusion is a simple procedure during which a patient receives whole blood or one of its parts through an *intravenous line (IV)*. An IV is a tiny tube that is inserted into a vein using a small needle.

Although whole blood can be transfused, it is rarely used. Instead, only parts of blood are transfused as needed. RBCs are most commonly transfused because these cells increase the blood's ability to carry oxygen and prevent fatigue and other health problems.

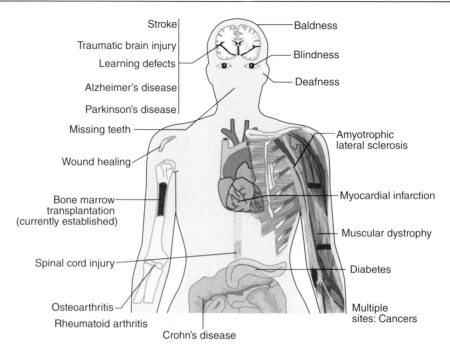

Stroke
Traumatic brain injury
Learning defects
Alzheimer's disease
Parkinson's disease
Missing teeth
Wound healing
Bone marrow transplantation (currently established)
Spinal cord injury
Osteoarthritis
Rheumatoid arthritis
Crohn's disease

Baldness
Blindness
Deafness
Amyotrophic lateral sclerosis
Myocardial infarction
Muscular dystrophy
Diabetes
Multiple sites: Cancers

Figure 14.2 Potential Uses of Stem Cells

Note. Adapted from "Medical Gallery of Mikael Häggström 2014," by Mikael Häggström, Wikiversity Journal of Medicine 1(2). doi:10.15347/wjm/2014.008. ISSN 20018762. (All used images are in public domain.) [Public domain], via Wikimedia Commons. Retrieved from https://commons.wikimedia.org/wiki/File%3AStem_cell_treatments.svg

As noted earlier, there is no synthetic substitute for blood, so the blood supply used for transfusion must be donated. One pint of donated blood can save up to three lives. There are three categories of blood donation (American Red Cross, 2016):

1. *Autologous.* When people know that they are going to need a transfusion, they sometimes donate their own blood beforehand.

2. *Directed.* A family member or friend with a compatible blood type donates blood to be used by a specific patient.

3. *Volunteer.* Most patients receive blood donated through blood drives, run by agencies like the American Red Cross. Even though 37% of the US population is eligible to donate blood, fewer than 10% each year give blood. In the United States, blood that comes from people who have been paid for it cannot be used for human transfusions.

Some people worry about getting diseases from infected blood, but the United States has one of the safest blood supplies in the world because of very strict blood screening. Also, the needles and other equipment used in blood donations are sterile and used only on one person and then thrown away.

If the situation is not a life-threatening emergency for the recipient, two tests are done to determine what donated blood the patient receives:

1. *Blood typing.* A lab technician draws a sample from a vein in the patient's arm using a sterile needle. The blood is then sent to the hospital's blood bank lab, where technicians test it for blood type.

2. *Cross-matching.* Once typing is complete, a compatible donor blood is chosen. As a final check, a blood bank technician mixes a small sample of the patient's blood with a small sample of the donor's blood to confirm that they are compatible.

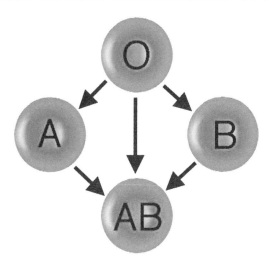

Figure 14.3 ABO Blood Donation

Note. From a person at the English language Wikipedia [CC-BY-SA-3.0 (http://creativecommons.org/licenses/by-sa/3.0/), GFDL (www.gnu.org/copyleft/fdl.html) or CC-BY-SA-3.0 (http://creativecommons.org/licenses/by-sa/3.0/)], from Wikimedia Commons.

Although all blood is made of the same basic elements, not all blood is alike. In fact, there are eight different common blood types, which are determined by the presence or absence of certain *antigens*, which are foreign substances in the body that trigger an immune response.

There are four main red blood cell types: A, B, AB, and O. Each can have or not have the antigen called Rh factor. (*Rh* is short for Rhesus.) The *Rh factor* can be either present (+) or absent (−). In general, Rh-negative blood is given to Rh-negative patients, and Rh-positive blood or Rh-negative blood is given to Rh-positive recipients. In an emergency, anyone can receive type O red blood cells. People with type O blood are known as "universal donors." Type AB individuals can receive red blood cells of any ABO type and are known as "universal recipients." In addition, AB plasma donors can give to all blood types. (See Figure 14.3.)

Like eye color, blood type is passed genetically from a person's parents. Whether a person's blood group is type A, B, AB, or O is based on the blood types of his or her mother and father. O+ is the most common blood type, yet not all ethnic groups have the same mix of these blood types. Hispanics, for example, have a high number of O's, whereas Asians have a high number of B's. The approximate percentage of blood types in the US population is listed in Table 14.1.

Table 14.1 Distribution of Blood Types in the US Population

Blood Type	% of Population
O+	38
O−	7
A+	34
A−	6
B+	9
B−	2
AB+	3
AB−	1

Note. From "Blood Types," by the American Red Cross, 2016. Retrieved from http://www.redcrossblood.org/learn-about-blood/blood-types

Ethnic or racial background plays an important role in blood transfusions. For example, sometimes if the donor and recipient are from the same racial background, the chance of a reaction can be reduced. That's why an African American blood donation may be the best hope for patients with sickle cell anemia, 98% of whom are of African American descent.

According to the American Red Cross (2016), there are three main reasons why a patient may need a blood transfusion:

1. *Loss of blood.* A patient may need a transfusion because of blood loss during surgery or from an injury or an illness.

2. *Inability to make enough blood.* As already mentioned, blood cells are made in the bone marrow; some diseases and treatments interfere with the marrow's ability to make blood. For example, cancer patients often need blood transfusions because chemotherapy decreases the bone marrow's production of blood cells.

3. *To prevent complications from an existing blood disease.* Patients with sickle cell anemia may benefit from regular transfusions to boost their blood's ability to carry oxygen. Patients with bleeding disorders, such as hemophilia, may need a transfusion to help prevent serious bleeding.

Most transfusions are performed in a hospital setting: at a patient's bedside, in the operating room, in the emergency room, or in the chemotherapy unit. About one in seven people entering a hospital needs blood (American Red Cross, 2016). If necessary, transfusions can also be performed in an outpatient care clinic or even at home.

A blood transfusion is relatively painless and takes about 1 to 4 hours, depending on how much blood is given. The recipient's blood pressure, body temperature, and pulse are taken throughout the procedure. He or she is also watched closely for any signs of an allergic reaction, including rash, fever, headache, or swelling.

Recipients who need many transfusions may require a *central line* (a tube inserted into a larger vein in the chest) or a *peripherally inserted central catheter or PICC line* (a longer tube inserted through a vein near the bend of the elbow). These lines allow easy access, and spare smaller veins the damage that comes from repeated punctures.

Serious reactions to transfusions are rare, but there are a few potential risks, including the following:

•   *Fever and/or allergic reaction.* The recipient's immune system can sometimes react to proteins in the donor's blood.

•   *Hemolytic reaction.* If a recipient's blood type and the donor's blood type do not match, the result can be a life-threatening condition called a *hemolytic reaction*, in which the recipient's immune system attacks the RBCs in the donated blood and destroys them.

Blood Tests

Blood tests are part of a routine checkup. According to the American Association for Clinical Chemistry (2016), they identify changes in a patient's health and help health care providers:

•   Diagnose diseases

•   Discover whether a patient has risk factors for certain diseases

•   Check whether medications are working for the patient

•   Determine how well the patient's blood is clotting

•   Evaluate how well the patient's body organs are working

A *blood test* is a laboratory analysis performed on a blood sample and is the most commonly performed medical test. *Venipuncture* is the collection of blood from a vein for laboratory analysis. Blood is drawn from a vein, usually from the inside of the elbow or the back of the hand. A needle is inserted into the vein, and the blood is collected in a syringe. If only a few drops of blood are needed, a *finger stick* is performed instead of drawing blood from a vein. In infants or young children, a sharp tool called a *lancet* may be used to puncture the skin and make it bleed. *Phlebotomy* is the term for drawing blood from a patient; a *phlebotomist* is the health care provider who takes the blood. In special circumstances or in emergencies, however, nurses, paramedics, and physicians can take blood from a patient.

One of the most common blood tests is the *complete blood count (CBC)*. The CBC is used to:

- Screen for diseases

- Help diagnose a disease

- Monitor the effectiveness of treatment

- Monitor treatment that is known to affect blood cells, such as chemotherapy

A CBC is a group of tests (including the red blood cell count and hematocrit) that provides information about the types and numbers of cells in a patient's blood. The CBC also measures the amount of hemoglobin, the oxygen-carrying protein in the blood. White blood cell count measures the number of WBCs. Platelet count measures the number of platelets.

A lab technician usually analyzes the blood test to see if the patient's results fall within the normal range. Blood test results are usually given as a range, rather than as a specific number, because what is normal for one person may not be normal for another. If a patient has CBC results that are within the normal range, he may not need another CBC until his health status changes. However, a CBC is regularly performed when a patient receives or has received treatment for a disease that affects blood cells, such as cancer.

In addition to the CBC, a health care provider may also perform a *blood smear*, which is a way of looking at blood cells under a microscope. In a normal blood smear, RBCs appear as regular, round cells with a pale center. Changes in the size or shape of these cells may suggest a blood disease.

Many health factors, including sex, age, race, and medical history, affect blood test results. Sometimes, diet, drugs, and how closely the patient follows pretest instructions can also affect test results.

Some blood tests give specific information about a disease, whereas others provide a more general overview of health problems. It is important to remember, however, that blood tests can have false-positive and false-negative results. For an interpretation of a blood test to be skilled and thorough, a health care provider must both understand the test results and have knowledge about the specific disease and the patient's experience.

Blood Disorders

Diseases of the blood or blood disorders can cause signs and symptoms anywhere in the body. The signs and symptoms are caused by low levels of red blood cells, abnormal blood vessels, or problems with blood clotting. With a disorder, blood is prevented from doing its job of carrying oxygen and nutrients to organs and allowing the body to warm up or cool down. Blood disorders discussed in this chapter are anemia, hemophilia, iron overload disease and hemochromatosis, blood cancers, and spleen disorders.

Anemia

Anemia is the most common blood disease, and there are more than 400 different types. Other, more popular names for anemia are "iron-poor blood," "low blood," or "tired blood." According to the

National Heart, Lung, and Blood Institute (2012), anemia affects more than 3.5 million Americans. It occurs in all age, racial, and ethnic groups. Although both genders are at risk, women who are menstruating or pregnant are at higher risk. Women of childbearing age are at higher risk because of blood loss from menstruation. Anemia can also develop during pregnancy because of low levels of iron and folic acid, and changes in the blood.

During the first year of life, some babies are at risk for anemia because of iron deficiency. At-risk infants include those who are born too early and those who are fed breast milk only or formula that isn't fortified with iron. Older adults are also at risk if they have certain health problems, such as autoimmune diseases, enlarged spleen, diabetes, heart failure, thyroid diseases, cancer, or infections.

Some types of anemia are mild and easily treated, and they can be prevented with a healthy diet. Other types are treated with dietary supplements. However, some types of anemia can be life threatening if not diagnosed and treated.

Some of the signs and symptoms of anemia can be easily overlooked or mistaken for other diseases (see Figure 14.4). In fact, many patients do not know that they have anemia until it is identified in a blood test.

According to the National Heart, Lung, and Blood Institute (2012), there are five main causes of anemia:

1. *Blood loss.* This is the most common cause of anemia. Heavy menstrual periods or bleeding in the digestive or urinary tract can cause blood loss. Surgery, trauma, or cancer also can cause blood loss.

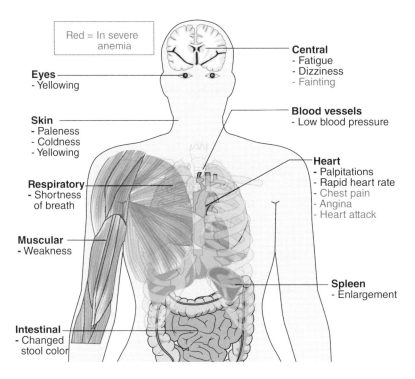

Figure 14.4 Symptoms of Anemia

Note. Adapted from "Medical Gallery of Mikael Häggström 2014," by Mikael Häggström, Wikiversity Journal of Medicine 1(2). doi:10.15347/wjm/2014.008. ISSN 20018762. [Public domain], via Wikimedia Commons. Retrieved from https://commons.wikimedia.org/wiki/File%3ASymptoms_of_anemia.png

2. *Lack of RBCs or damaged RBCs.* Both acquired and inherited factors can prevent the body from producing enough RBCs. *Acquired* refers to factors that a person is not born with but that develop. One example of an acquired factor is an enlarged spleen. *Inherited* refers to genetic factors that one or both of a person's parents passed on to him or her. An example of a disease caused by an inherited factor is sickle cell anemia.

3. *Diet.* A diet that lacks iron, folic acid, or vitamin B12 prevents the body from making enough RBCs.

4. *Hormones.* A kidney hormone stimulates bone marrow to make RBCs. A low level of this hormone can lead to anemia.

5. *Diseases and disease treatments.* Chronic diseases, such as heart failure, HIV/AIDS, and cancer, make it hard for the body to make enough RBCs. Certain cancer treatments damage the bone marrow or damage RBCs' ability to carry oxygen.

Iron Deficiency Anemia

Iron deficiency is a common cause of anemia. The term *anemia* usually refers to a condition in which a patient's blood has a lower than normal number of red blood cells. Anemia also can occur if red blood cells don't contain enough hemoglobin, an iron-rich protein that carries oxygen from the lungs to the rest of the body. The body needs iron to make hemoglobin. *Iron deficiency anemia* develops when the body starts using the iron it has stored because it is not getting enough iron. Over time, the stored iron gets used up. After the stored iron is gone, the body produces fewer RBCs. The RBCs it does produce have less hemoglobin than normal.

Iron deficiency anemia is usually caused by blood loss, but it can also be caused by poor absorption of iron. A patient might have poor absorption of iron for many reasons, including heavy menstrual periods, pregnancy, ulcers, colon cancer, gastric bypass surgery, and a diet low in iron. Other blood diseases and inherited diseases can also cause iron deficiency anemia.

The signs and symptoms of iron deficiency anemia are fatigue, shortness of breath, and chest pain. Other signs and symptoms include brittle nails, swelling of the tongue, cracks in the sides of the mouth, an enlarged spleen, and frequent infections. Severe iron deficiency anemia can cause heart problems, infections, and other complications.

Patients with iron deficiency anemia may have an unusual craving for nonfood items, such as ice, dirt, paint, or starch. This craving for and eating of these items is called *pica*. (Not all instances of pica are caused by anemia, however.) Sometimes, for example, children who have iron deficiency anemia eat lead paint chips and develop lead poisoning.

Other patients with iron deficiency anemia develop *restless legs syndrome (RLS)*. RLS causes a strong urge to move the legs, and strange and unpleasant feelings in the legs. Patients who have RLS often have a hard time sleeping due to constant leg movement.

Iron deficiency anemia can be successfully treated. The type of treatment depends on the cause and severity of the anemia and may include dietary changes, medicines, and surgery. Severe iron deficiency anemia requires treatment in a hospital, blood transfusions, iron injections, or intravenous iron therapy.

Pernicious Anemia

Pernicious anemia occurs when the body can't produce enough healthy RBCs because it doesn't have enough vitamin B12. It is caused when the gastrointestinal tract doesn't absorb enough vitamin B12 from food. *Vitamin B12, or folic acid,* is a nutrient found in some foods. The body needs this nutrient to make healthy RBCs and to keep the nervous system working properly.

Without enough vitamin B12, RBCs do not divide normally and are too large. They may also have trouble getting out of the bone marrow. Patients who have pernicious anemia lack the *intrinsic factor*, a protein made in the stomach. Technically, the term *pernicious anemia* refers to vitamin B12 deficiency due to a lack of intrinsic factor. However, other factors can also cause vitamin B12 deficiency, including infections, surgery, medicines, and diet.

Without enough RBCs to carry oxygen in the body, a patient with pernicious anemia can feel tired and weak. Severe pernicious anemia can damage the heart, brain, and other organs and cause nerve damage, memory loss, and digestive tract problems. Patients who have severe pernicious anemia are also at risk for weakened bones and stomach cancer.

The word *pernicious* means "deadly"; this form of anemia was often fatal in the past, before vitamin B12 treatments. Now, pernicious anemia usually is easy to treat with vitamin B12 pills or shots. With ongoing care and proper treatment, most patients with pernicious anemia recover and live normal lives. Without treatment, however, pernicious anemia leads to serious health problems.

Sickle Cell Anemia

Sickle cell anemia is caused by abnormal hemoglobin, which ultimately results in blocked blood flow. Normal hemoglobin gives RBCs a disc shape, but the RBCs with abnormal hemoglobin have a sickle or crescent shape; these cells are also stiff and sticky. The sickle cells block blood flow because they are unable to flow through small blood vessels (see Figure 14.5). This blockage of blood flow causes pain and organ damage, and raises the risk of infection.

Sickle cell anemia affects anywhere from 70,000 to 100,000 people in the United States, 98% of whom are of African descent (American Society of Hematology, 2016a). It is the most common form of an inherited blood disorder. Sickle cell anemia is inherited from both parents, and patients who have the disease are born with it. If a patient inherited the sickle cell gene from only one parent, he or she has *sickle cell trait*. Patients with sickle cell trait do not have the symptoms of sickle cell anemia. However, they can pass the sickle hemoglobin gene to their children.

Sickle cell anemia varies from person to person. Some patients who have this disease have chronic pain or fatigue. Almost all patients with sickle cell anemia have painful episodes or *crises*, which can last from hours to days and cause back pain as well as pain in the long bones and the chest. Some patients have one crisis every few years; others have many per year. The crises can be severe enough to require a hospital stay.

Many patients with severe sickle cell anemia receive blood transfusions every month. In the past, sickle cell patients often died between the ages of 20 and 40; however, because of improved treatment, today's patients can live into their 50s and beyond. Treatment is ongoing, and its goal is to manage and control symptoms. For most, there is no cure for sickle cell anemia. However, blood and marrow stem cell transplants may offer a cure for a small number of patients.

Bleeding Disorders

Normally, if you get hurt, your body forms a blood clot around the injured blood vessel to stop the bleeding. As noted earlier, when blood clots, it is called coagulation. For blood to clot, your body needs platelets, and proteins known as clotting factors. When blood clots stop the bleeding in injured blood vessels, it is known as *hemostasis*. Hemostasis has three major parts:

1. *Narrowing of blood vessels.* An injured blood vessel narrows so that blood flows out more slowly and clotting can start. At the same time, a pool or a lump of blood outside the blood vessel known as a *hematoma* forms and presses against the vessel, helping prevent further bleeding.

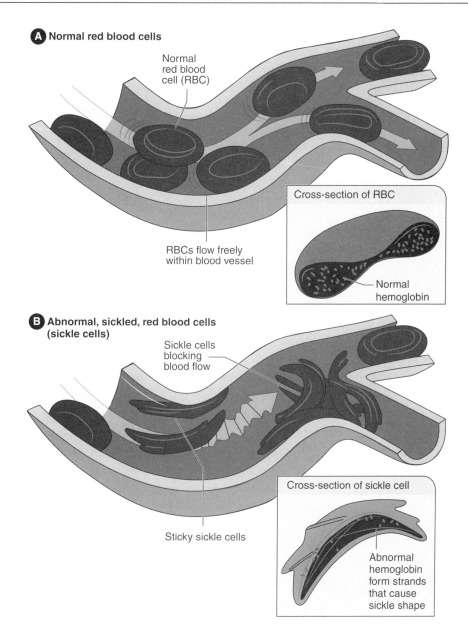

A Normal red blood cells

Normal
red blood
cell (RBC)

RBCs flow freely
within blood vessel

Cross-section of RBC

Normal
hemoglobin

B Abnormal, sickled, red blood cells
(sickle cells)

Sickle cells
blocking
blood flow

Sticky sickle cells

Cross-section of sickle cell

Abnormal
hemoglobin
form strands
that cause
sickle shape

Figure 14.5 Normal Red Blood Cells and Sickle Red Blood Cells
Note. From the National Heart, Lung, and Blood Institute

2. *Activity of platelets.* As soon as a blood vessel wall is damaged, platelets start to stick to the injured site. The "glue" that holds platelets to the blood vessel wall is a protein. As platelets grow and stick at the site, they form a mesh that plugs the injury.

3. *Activity of blood clotting factors.* The platelets change shape from round to spiny, and they release clotting factors to form a blood clot that blocks the hole in the injured blood vessel. Too much clotting, however, can block blood vessels that are not bleeding; consequently, the body limits clotting and dissolves clots that are no longer needed.

If something goes wrong during hemostasis, then excessive bleeding or excessive clotting can occur, both of which can be dangerous. When clotting is poor, even a slight injury to a blood vessel can cause major blood loss. When there is too much clotting, blood vessels can become clogged with clots. Clogged brain vessels can cause strokes; clogged heart vessels can cause heart attacks; and pieces of clots from veins in the legs, pelvis, or abdomen can travel through the bloodstream and cause a blocked pulmonary artery.

Symptoms of bleeding disorders include the following (Hemophilia Federation of America, 2016a):

- Easy bruising, or large bruises from a minor injury
- Bleeding gums
- Heavy bleeding for a long time from small cuts or dental work
- Unexplained nosebleeds that are hard to stop
- Heavy menstrual bleeding
- Anemia

Because many things can affect blood test results, such as stress or use of painkillers, a variety of blood tests are done to find out whether a patient has a bleeding disorder and what type. The health care provider also asks about the patient's symptoms and any family health history of bleeding disorders.

Hemophilia

There are many kinds of bleeding disorders, but one of the most common is hemophilia. *Hemophilia* is usually an inherited disorder that can range from mild to severe, depending on how much clotting factor is lacking in the blood. Patients with hemophilia have either a low level of clotting factors or none at all. The lower the level of clotting factors, the more serious the hemophilia. Without enough clotting factor, any cut or injury can mean excessive bleeding. In addition, patients with hemophilia may suffer from internal bleeding that can damage joints, organs, and tissues over time. Hemophilia occurs in about 1 out of every 5,000 male births in the United States, and affects all racial and ethnic groups (Hemophilia Federation of America, 2016b). About 20,000 males in the United States have this disorder (Centers for Disease Control and Prevention, 2016).

Hemophilia is caused by a problem in the genes that tell the body to make the clotting factors. These genes are located on the X chromosome. All males have one X and one Y chromosome (XY), and all females have two X chromosomes (XX). Males who inherit an affected X chromosome have hemophilia. A female who inherits one affected X chromosome becomes a carrier of hemophilia. A female who is a carrier can have symptoms of hemophilia, but often does not. In addition, she can pass the affected gene on to her children.

Major signs of hemophilia are bleeding that is unusually heavy and lasts a long time, or bleeding and bruising that occur without obvious cause. Other common signs and symptoms are joint swelling, severe pain, bleeding in the head and brain, and damage to body organs. If the bleeding is not stopped, it can be fatal.

To diagnose hemophilia, the health care provider performs blood tests. The tests determine whether the blood has low levels of any clotting factors, or whether the clotting factors are completely missing from the blood, or whether the blood is clotting properly; the blood tests also show the type of hemophilia. There are two types of hemophilia, A and B. The bleeding problems of hemophilia A and hemophilia B are the same. Only special blood tests can tell which type of the disorder the patient has. Knowing the type is important because aspects of the treatment plans for the two types are different.

The overall treatment for both types of hemophilia, however, is to replace the missing blood clotting factor so that the blood can clot properly. This is done by injecting commercially prepared clotting factor into the patient's arm. However, because hemophilia is a complex disease to treat, the best choice for treatment is a comprehensive hemophilia treatment center (HTC). An HTC provides care to address all issues related to the disorder.

Iron Overload Disease and Hemochromatosis

Iron overload disease is chronic and can be serious. It develops when the body absorbs too much iron over many years, and the iron builds up in organ tissues, such as the heart. Iron is an essential nutrient found in many foods. Healthy people usually absorb about 10% of the iron contained in the food they eat. However, the body has no natural way to rid itself of any excess iron, causing the excess to build up in the organs. Iron overload usually occurs when a genetic disorder causes the body to absorb too much iron. Too much iron can lead to hemochromatosis.

Patients with *hemochromatosis* absorb more iron than the body needs. Hemochromatosis affects everyone differently: Some patients have no symptoms; others experience joint pain, fatigue, weakness, weight loss, or stomach pain. Hemochromatosis also has no definitive symptoms—they are like those of many other diseases—so diagnosing this condition is difficult. If hemochromatosis is found early, treatment can slow its progress and prevent serious problems. However, if the disease is not treated early, it can cause arthritis, heart and liver problems, and gray-colored skin.

In the United States, more than one million people have the gene mutation that causes hemochromatosis. The gene mutation is most common among people whose ancestors came from Europe. The mutation is present at birth, but symptoms rarely appear before adulthood. Symptoms tend to occur in men between the ages of 30 and 50 and in women over age 50. The symptoms depend on which organs are being affected by the iron buildup. Not all people with this gene mutation develop iron overload, and not all people with iron overload develop hemochromatosis.

Patients with hemochromatosis can be treated by receiving frequent phlebotomies (removal of blood to decrease level of iron). How often patients have phlebotomies—and how many—depends on how much iron has built up in their body. Most patients have them once or twice a week for a year or more. After the iron is lowered to a safe level, the patient has phlebotomies only a few times a year. Without this treatment, hemochromatosis can cause death. The key to preventing hemochromatosis is early diagnosis and treatment.

Blood Cancers

Blood cancers affect the production and function of blood cells. These cancers usually start in the bone marrow where blood is made. With blood cancers, the normal development of blood cells is interrupted by the growth of an abnormal blood cell or a cancerous cell. Cancerous cells prevent blood from performing many of its functions, such as fighting off infections or preventing serious bleeding.

According to the National Cancer Institute (2016c), every 4 minutes someone is diagnosed with a blood cancer in the United States. About every 10 minutes, someone dies from a blood cancer. Another way to understand the impact in the United States is that nearly 155 people every day, or more than 6 people each hour, die from a blood cancer. The three main types of blood cancers that are discussed in this chapter—leukemia, lymphoma, and myeloma—caused the deaths of 56,630 Americans in 2015 (National Cancer Institute, 2016c).

Leukemia

Leukemia is a general term for several different blood cancers. The word *leukemia* means "white blood." Leukocytes, or white blood cells, fight infections and other foreign substances. Leukocytes are made in the bone marrow. Leukemia is caused by an uncontrolled increase in the number of leukocytes. The leukemia cells crowd out and replace normal blood and marrow cells. These cells also interfere with the production of healthy blood cells. The leukemia cells can spread to the bloodstream and lymph nodes. They can also travel to the brain and spinal cord and other parts of the body. Life-threatening symptoms can then develop as normal blood cells decline.

There are four major types of leukemia (see list). Their names are based on how quickly and where each develops in the bone marrow.

Four Major Types of Leukemia

Acute Myeloid Leukemia (AML)

Chronic Myeloid Leukemia (CML)

Acute Lymphocytic Leukemia (ALL)

Chronic Lymphocytic Leukemia (CLL)

Bone marrow has two main jobs. The first job is to make myeloid cells, and the leukemia is called *myeloid leukemia* if the cancerous cells develop in a marrow cell. The second job is to make lymphocytes, cells that are a part of the immune system. *Lymphocytic leukemia* occurs when the cancerous cells develop in a marrow cell that matures into lymphocytes. Regardless of whether the patient has myeloid or lymphocytic leukemia, once the marrow cell become leukemic, the leukemia cells grow and survive better than normal cells.

Leukemia can be either acute or chronic. Chronic leukemia is a slow-growing cancer that gradually gets worse over time. In acute leukemia, the cells are very abnormal and they increase very quickly, and the patient needs immediate treatment. Adults can get either type; children with leukemia most often have an acute type.

According to the National Cancer Institute (2016a), in 2015 there were close to 318,389 people living with leukemia in the United States; over 54,270 people were diagnosed with leukemia; and 24,450 were expected to die from this disease. Slightly more males than females are diagnosed with leukemia and die of leukemia. Although leukemia is among the most common childhood cancers, it most often occurs in older adults; the average age at diagnosis is 66 years. Leukemia is 10 times more common in adults than in children and adolescents. Death rates from leukemia are higher among the elderly. Leukemia is the seventh leading cause of cancer death in the United States (National Cancer Institute, 2016a).

People with leukemia have many treatment options, and treatment can often control the disease and its symptoms. Patients are affected and treated differently depending on the type of leukemia. Some types of leukemia can be cured, whereas other types are hard to cure.

Although the causes of leukemia are unknown, there are several risk factors, including smoking, previous cancer treatments, exposure to certain chemicals and radiation, certain genetic diseases, and family health history. However, most people with these risk factors don't get leukemia, and many people with leukemia have none of these risk factors.

Symptoms vary depending on the type and stage of leukemia, but they can include fever, pale skin, easy bleeding, tiny red spots on the skin, and joint pain. Figure 14.6 gives a detailed description of leukemia symptoms.

Lymphoma

Lymphoma is a blood cancer that affects the lymphatic system. The lymphatic system removes excess fluids from the body and produces immune cells. Lymphoma starts with a change to a lymphocyte, which is a type of white cell that fights infections. The change to the lymphocyte causes it to become a lymphoma cell. With this change, lymphoma cells pile up and form lymphoma cell masses. These masses gather in the lymph nodes or in other parts of the body. Over time, these cancerous lymphoma cells impair the immune system.

About half of the blood cancers that are diagnosed each year are lymphomas. Lymphoma is a general term for different types of blood cancer. *Hodgkin lymphoma* (HL) and *non-Hodgkin lymphoma* (NHL) are the two most common lymphomas. These lymphomas behave, spread, and respond to

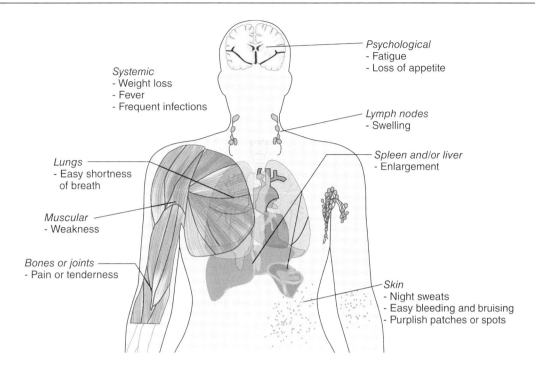

Figure 14.6 Symptoms of Leukemia

Note. Adapted from Mikael Häggström (All used images are in public domain.) [Public domain], via Wikimedia Commons. Retrieved from http://commons.wikimedia.org/wiki/File%3ASymptoms_of_leukemia.png

treatment differently. Health care providers usually distinguish between them only by looking at the cancer cells under a microscope. In some cases, sensitive lab tests may be needed to tell them apart.

About 12% of patients with lymphoma have HL. HL is one of the most curable forms of cancer. The cause for most cases of HL is not known, but what is known is that there is no way to prevent this lymphoma. HL is usually diagnosed when a person is in his or her 20s or 30s. It is less common in middle age and becomes more common again after age 60.

The major sign of HL is one or more enlarged (swollen) lymph nodes. The enlarged lymph node may be in the neck, upper chest, armpit, abdomen, or groin, and is usually painless. Other symptoms are cough and shortness of breath, fever, night sweats, fatigue, weight loss, and itchy skin.

Health care providers perform a test called a *lymph node biopsy* to find out if a patient has HL (National Cancer Institute, 2016b). A surgeon removes all or part of an enlarged lymph node (National Cancer Institute, 2016b). The lymph node is then examined by a pathologist. A *pathologist* is a physician who identifies diseases by studying cells and tissues under a microscope. Other tests for *staging*, or extent of spread, include blood tests, bone marrow tests, imaging tests such as a CT scan, and a lumbar puncture (spinal tap).

Hodgkin lymphoma can be cured in about 75% of all patients. The cure rate in younger patients is over 90%.

NHL is a cancer that starts in the cells of the immune system's. It begins when a type of white blood cell, called a T-cell or B-cell, becomes cancerous. The cell divides again and again, making more and more cancer cells. These cancer cells can spread to almost any part of the body. NHL can grow either quickly or slowly.

NHL is one of the most common cancers in the United States, making up 4% of all cancers (American Cancer Society, 2016). Although some types of NHL are among the more common childhood cancers, more than 95% of cases are adults (National Cancer Institute, 2016b). The NHLs seen in children are often very different from those seen in adults. Although NHL can occur at any age, about half of the patients are older than 65 because the risk of developing NHL increases with age.

Most of the time, it is not known why a person gets NHL. But there are risk factors, such as age, being male, being of European descent, certain chemicals, radiation treatment, autoimmune diseases, and obesity.

NHL can cause many symptoms, such as swollen lymph nodes, weight loss, fatigue, fever, coughing, trouble breathing, and chest and stomach pain.

At this time, there are no widely recommended screening tests for this cancer. Still, in some cases lymphoma can be found early. The best way to detect NHL early is by paying prompt attention to the signs and symptoms of this disease.

A lymph node biopsy is done to determine the NHL stage. Other tests for staging include blood tests, bone marrow tests, CT scan, and lumbar puncture. The following list describes how blood and bone marrow tests are done:

Blood tests: A small amount of blood is taken from the arm with a needle. The blood is collected in tubes and sent to a lab.

Bone marrow aspiration: A liquid sample of cells is taken from the marrow through a needle.

Bone marrow biopsy: A small amount of bone filled with marrow cells is removed through a needle.

The treatment and prognosis for patients with NHL depend on the exact type of the lymphoma and its stage. Treatment includes chemotherapy, radiation, stem cell transplantation, and surgery.

Whereas HL and NHL used to be considered fatal diseases, they are now curable. Many lymphoma patients are able to lead active lives as they receive treatment for their symptoms and are monitored by their health care providers.

Myeloma

Myeloma, or multiple myeloma (so named because myeloma occurs at different places in the bone marrow) is a blood cancer that starts in the bone marrow and targets plasma cells. Plasma cells are part of the immune system; they make antibodies that help the body fight infections and diseases. Sometimes, the body makes too many plasma cells in the bone marrow, and these cells are abnormal. The abnormal plasma cells, known as myeloma cells, prevent the marrow from making the right amount of antibodies, causing too many antibodies and leaving the body's immune system weak (see Figure 14.7).

Too many myeloma cells travel through the bloodstream and collect in other bones. Once in other bones, myeloma cells make substances that cause bone destruction, leading to bone pain and fractures. Myeloma cells also interfere with the function of red and white blood cells as well as cause kidney damage.

Although some patients with multiple myeloma have no symptoms, the following are the most common signs and symptoms of this disease: thirst, weakness, nausea, constipation, low blood count, kidney failure, infections, nerve damage, bone problems, frequent urination, and weight loss.

The American Cancer Society (2016) estimates that about 30,330 new US cases of multiple myeloma will be diagnosed in 2016. About 12,650 deaths are expected to occur (6,430 in men and 6,220 in women).

Myeloma is more common in African Americans, people over the age of 65, males, people with a family health history of myeloma, those who are obese, those who have been exposed to radiation, and those who work in petroleum-related industries.

Myeloma is usually found after an X-ray for a broken bone or after a routine blood or urine test. Personal and family health history, physical exam, blood tests, X-rays, and bone marrow tests are used to diagnose myeloma. If the biopsy shows that the patient has myeloma, then more tests, such as a CAT scan, are done to learn the stage of the disease.

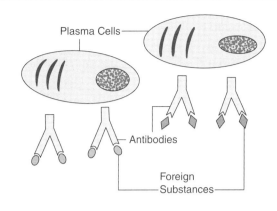

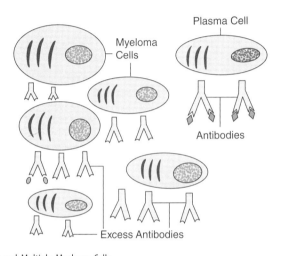

Figure 14.7 Normal Plasma Cells and Multiple Myeloma Cells

Note. Adapted from the National Cancer Institute, Visuals Online. Retrieved from http://visualsonline.cancer.gov/details.cfm?imageid=2718

Treatments slow myeloma cell growth and help ease symptoms. The treatment options depend on the patient's health and the type and stage of myeloma. Treatment for myeloma includes chemotherapy, radiation therapy, and stem cell transplantation.

Because the causes of myeloma are unknown, there is no exact way to prevent it. The only preventive measures are to be aware of the risks and symptoms, especially if there is a family health history of myeloma.

Sepsis

Sepsis, or septicemia, is a serious illness in which the body has a severe response to bacteria or other germs. The chemicals released into the blood to fight the infection trigger widespread inflammation, sometimes known as blood poisoning. This leads to blood clots and leaky blood vessels. They cause poor blood flow, which leaves the body's organs without nutrients and oxygen. In severe cases, one or more organs fail. In the worst cases, blood pressure drops, the heart weakens, and the patient may die.

Sepsis can happen to anyone, at any time, and from any type of infection, and can affect any part of the body. It can develop even after a minor infection. The risk of sepsis is higher in people with weakened immune systems, babies and very young children, the elderly, people with chronic illnesses, and people suffering from a severe burn or wound. Over one million cases of sepsis occur each year, and up to half of the people who get sepsis will die. That's more than the number of US deaths annually from prostate cancer, breast cancer, and AIDS combined.

Sepsis is difficult to diagnose and treat. It can develop suddenly and progress rapidly. Although a variety of strategies to detect and treat sepsis are used, sometimes it's too late to prevent grim outcomes. Part of the problem is that there is not a clear understanding of the underlying biological processes that make the immune system go haywire and trigger sepsis.

Physicians diagnose it using a blood test to see if the number of WBCs is abnormal. They also do lab tests that check for signs of infection.

Those with sepsis are usually treated in hospital intensive care units. Physicians try to treat the infection, sustain the vital organs, and prevent a drop in blood pressure. Many patients receive oxygen and intravenous fluids. Other types of treatment, such as respirators or kidney dialysis, may be necessary. Sometimes, surgery is needed to clear up an infection.

Ways to prevent sepsis include getting vaccinated against the flu, pneumonia, and any other infections that could lead to sepsis. People can prevent infections that can lead to sepsis by cleaning scrapes and wounds and by practicing good hygiene (e.g., washing hands, bathing regularly). If a person has an infection, he or she should look for such signs as fever, chills, rapid breathing and heart rate, rash, and confusion.

Spleen Disorders

The *spleen*, part of the lymphatic system, is a spongy, soft organ about as big as a human fist and shaped like a large lymph node. It is located near the upper left part of the stomach, just under the rib cage. The

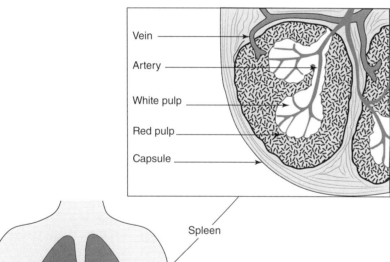

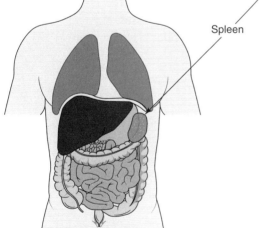

Figure 14.8 The Spleen

Note. Adapted from Wikicommons (public domain). Retrieved from http://training.seer.cancer.gov/module_anatomy/unit8_2_lymph_compo3_spleen.html

splenic artery brings blood to the spleen from the heart. Blood leaves the spleen through the *splenic vein*, which drains into a larger vein that carries the blood to the liver. The spleen has a covering, or capsule, that supports its blood vessels and lymphatic vessels (see Figure 14.8).

The spleen is made up of two kinds of tissue, *white pulp* and *red pulp*, and each has a specific function. The white pulp is part of the immune system, and its function is to make lymphocytes, which in turn produce antibodies.

The red pulp has four functions. First, it filters the blood, removing unwanted material. Second, other WBCs called phagocytes in the red pulp ingest germs, such as bacteria, fungi, and viruses. Third, red pulp monitors RBCs, destroying those that are damaged. Fourth, the red pulp is a reservoir for WBCs and platelets and helps keep bodily fluids in balance.

Many diseases can negatively affect the spleen. These include diseases of the blood and the lymph system, infections, certain cancers, and liver diseases. In healthy people, the spleen is usually small. However, certain diseases cause the spleen to swell or enlarge to several times its normal size. This condition is known as an enlarged spleen. An enlarged spleen is not a disease in itself but the result of another health problem. Causes of an enlarged spleen are infections, liver diseases, anemia, and certain cancers, such as leukemia and lymphoma. It can also be damaged by a bodily injury.

Symptoms of an enlarged spleen are usually not specific, but can include pain in the upper left stomach area or back. Patients should get medical help immediately if the pain is severe or gets worse when they take a deep breath.

A physical exam is an initial step to diagnosing an enlarged spleen. Usually a health care provider can feel an enlarged spleen, but X-rays and other imaging tests can determine how large the spleen is. Treating the disease that is causing the enlarged spleen usually takes care of the problem, but sometimes the spleen must be removed, in a surgical procedure called a *splenectomy*. When the spleen is removed, the body is less able to make antibodies. As a result, the body's ability to fight infections weakens, and patients are at high risk for infections. Despite these problems, however, the spleen is not necessary to survival. Other organs, such as the liver, make up for the loss by increasing their infection-fighting ability. These organs also screen for and remove RBCs that are damaged.

Chapter Summary

- Blood carries gases, oxygen, and nutrients throughout the body. It also filters the body's waste. Blood fights infections, heals wounds, and performs many other vital functions—so many vital functions that when something is wrong with the blood, a person's overall health is compromised.

- Hematology is the study of blood in health and disease; a hematologist is a physician who has a specialty in blood diseases.

- The average adult man has about 24 pints of blood inside his body; the average adult woman has about 20 pints. Roughly, a donation equals about a pint, and one donation can help save the lives of up to three people.

- The process of clotting, known as coagulation, is like a puzzle with interlocking parts. When the last part is in place, the clot forms—but if even only one piece is missing, the final pieces can't come together to stop the bleeding.

- Bone marrow stem cells are found circulating in the blood and in bone marrow in people of all ages, as well as in the umbilical cords of newborn babies. Stem cells are collected and used to treat many diseases, including leukemia and lymphoma.

- There are four main red blood cell types: A, B, AB, and O. In each type, the Rh factor, an antigen, can be either present (+) or absent (–).

- Anemia is the most common blood disease, and there are more than 400 different types.

- There are three main types of blood cancers: leukemia, lymphoma, and myeloma.

- Sometimes the spleen is removed by a splenectomy. When the spleen is removed, the body is less able to make antibodies. As a result, the body's ability to fight infections is weak. Other organs, such as the liver, can make up for this loss by increasing their infection-fighting ability.

REVIEW QUESTIONS

1.   What are the four main types of red blood cells? What is the Rh factor?

2.   Discuss the three types of blood donations.

3.   Explain why a patient may need a blood transfusion.

4.   List the five ways in which blood tests help health care providers determine a diagnosis.

5.   Explain anemia and identify causes for two types.

6.   What is iron overload disease, and how does it relate to hemochromatosis?

7.   What are three main types of blood cancers discussed in this chapter?

8.   What are the differences between blood tests and bone marrow tests?

9.   What groups are at risk for sepsis? Identify three ways to prevent sepsis.

10. What are the functions of the spleen? What are the negative consequences of a splenectomy?

KEY TERMS

Anemia: The most common blood disease, of which there are more than 400 different types

Antigens: Foreign substances in the body that trigger an immune response

Autologous (blood donation): A donation of a person's own blood when she knows in advance that she is going to need a blood transfusion

Blood cancers: Group of diseases that affect the production and function of blood cells

Blood smear: A way of looking at blood cells under a microscope

Blood test: Laboratory analysis performed on a blood sample

Blood typing: The confirmation of blood type by taking a blood sample from a patient and testing it

Bone marrow: Spongy tissue in the central cavity of bones that makes blood cells

Bruise: An internal blood clot

Central line: Tube inserted into a larger vein in the chest

Clot: Small "plug" made up of platelets and proteins known as clotting factors, which surrounds and covers an injured blood vessel

Clotting factors: Certain minerals, proteins, and vitamins that help make a strong clot

Coagulation: The process of clotting

Complete blood count (CBC): Group of diagnostic tests that gives information about the types and numbers of cells in a patient's blood sample

Crises: Painful episodes for patients with sickle cell anemia

Cross-matching: The selection of compatible donor blood

Directed (blood donation): A donation of blood to a specific patient by a family member or friend with a compatible blood type

Finger stick: Procedure performed when only a few drops of blood are needed

Hematocrit: Diagnostic test that measures the percentage of red blood cells in a patient's blood

Hematologist: Physician who specializes in blood diseases

Hematology: Study of blood in health and disease

Hematoma: A pool or a lump of blood outside a blood vessel that forms and presses against the vessel

Hemochromatosis: Chronic blood disease in which too much iron can cause serious health problems

Hemoglobin: Iron-rich, oxygen-carrying protein that is in red blood cells, and the name of the diagnostic test that measures the amount of hemoglobin in a patient's blood sample

Hemolytic reaction: Reaction that occurs when a patient's blood type and the donor's blood type do not match

Hemophilia: A bleeding disorder in which patients have either a low level of clotting factors or none at all

Hemostasis: The stopping of bleeding in injured blood vessels through clotting

Hodgkin lymphoma (HL): A type of lymphoma, a blood cancer that affects the lymphatic system

Intravenous line (IV): Tiny tube that is inserted into a vein using a small needle

Intrinsic factor: Protein made in the stomach that is often lacking in those with pernicious anemia

Iron deficiency anemia: A type of anemia that can be caused by blood loss but also by poor absorption of iron

Iron overload disease: Disease that develops when the body absorbs too much iron and it builds up in organ tissues

Lancet: Sharp tool used to puncture the skin and make it bleed

Leukemia: General term for different blood cancers

Lymph node biopsy: Diagnostic test used to find out if a patient has Hodgkin lymphoma

Lymphocyte: White blood cell

Lymphocytic leukemia: Type of blood cancer that develops in a bone marrow

Lymphoma: Blood cancer that affects the lymphatic system

Myeloid leukemia: Type of blood cancer that develops in the bone marrow

Myeloma, or multiple myeloma: Blood cancer that grows in the bone marrow and targets plasma cells

Non-Hodgkin lymphoma (NHL): Cancer cells in the immune system that can spread to almost any part of the body

Pathologist: A doctor who identifies diseases by studying cells and tissues under a microscope

Peripherally inserted central catheter (PICC): Tube inserted through a vein near the bend of the elbow

Pernicious anemia: Type of anemia that develops when the body does not make enough healthy red blood cells because it doesn't have enough vitamin B12

Phlebotomist: Health care provider who draws blood from patients

Phlebotomy: The procedure for taking blood from a patient

Pica: Unusual craving for and eating of nonfood items

Plasma: Liquid part of blood that carries blood cells, along with other substances, throughout the body

Platelets: Small bits of cells that help blood clot

Red blood cells (RBCs): The blood cells that deliver oxygen from the lungs to tissues and organs

Red pulp: Type of spleen tissue that filters blood, helps fight germs, monitors red blood cells, and keeps bodily fluids in balance

Restless legs syndrome: Condition that causes the patient to have a strong urge to move the legs and that often causes strange and unpleasant feelings in the legs

Rh factor: Type of antigen in the blood that can be either present (+) or absent (–)

Scab: An external blood clot

Sepsis, or septicemia: Serious illness in which the body has a severe response to bacteria and other germs

Sickle cell anemia: Genetic blood disease in which the hemoglobin shape is abnormal

Sickle cell trait: The inheritance of the sickle cell gene from only one parent

Spleen: Spongy, soft organ located near the stomach that helps in controlling the amount of blood in the body and in fighting infections

Splenectomy: Surgical removal of the spleen.

Splenic artery: Artery that brings blood to the spleen from the heart

Splenic vein: Vein through which blood leaves the spleen

Staging: The extent that a cancer has spread

Stem cells: Undifferentiated cells in the bone marrow that can develop into a number of different kinds of cells and can be used to treat many diseases

Stem cell transplantation: The collection of bone marrow stem cells from blood, bone marrow, and umbilical cord blood

Stitches: Loops of thread used to join the edges of a cut together to stop the bleeding

Venipuncture: Collection of blood from a vein for laboratory analysis

Vitamin B12, or folic acid: Nutrient found in some foods that helps the body make red blood cells and helps the nervous system work properly

Volunteer (blood donation): Blood donation by a volunteer at a blood drive

White blood cells (WBCs): The body's primary defense against infection

White pulp: Type of spleen tissue that makes lymphocytes

Whole blood: Living tissue comprising plasma, red blood cells, white blood cells, and platelets

CHAPTER ACTIVITIES

1. Research the controversy surrounding stem cell transplantation. Describe the procedure, its successes, and the obstacles to its use. Conduct an in-class debate on the pros and cons of stem cell transplantation and research.

2. Your instructor will give you a list of blood diseases not included in this chapter. Work in teams of two to four to research your assigned disease, including the symptoms of the disease, the changes that take place in the blood, available treatments, risk and protective factors, and current research on the disease. Your group can give a PowerPoint presentation on the selected disease and lead a class discussion.

3. Your instructor will be inviting a guest speaker from the American Red Cross to give a presentation on the importance of blood drives. Before the presentation, prepare three questions to ask the guest speaker.

4. You have been hired by the American Cancer Society as a community health education specialist. Your assignment is to develop health education materials for the three blood cancers discussed in this chapter. As part of the educational materials, develop a one-page infographic poster for each of the three cancers. Your target audience is low-health-literacy adults.

5. In groups of three to four, conduct research on the differences between sickle cell trait and sickle cell anemia. In addition, describe risk factors and diagnostic criteria for sickle cell trait. After this task is completed, create three case studies. One case study is of a patient with sickle cell anemia; the second is of a patient with sickle cell trait; and the third is of a patient with another form of anemia described in this chapter. Be prepared to present each case study and have classmates guess the blood disease.

Bibliography and Works Cited

American Association for Clinical Chemistry. (2016). Understanding your tests. Retrieved from https://labtestsonline.org/understanding/

American Blood Centers. (2012). About blood. Retrieved from http://www.americasblood.org/about-blood.aspx

America Cancer Society. (2016). Non-Hodgkin lymphoma. Retrieved from http://www.cancer.org/cancer/non hodgkinlymphoma/detailedguide/index

American Liver Foundation. (2015). Hemochromatosis. Retrieved from http://www.liverfoundation.org /abouttheliver/info/hemochromatosis/

American Red Cross. (2016). Blood types. Retrieved from http://www.redcrossblood.org/learn-about-blood /blood-types

American Society of Hematology. (2016a). Anemia. Retrieved from http://www.hematology.org/Patients /Anemia/

American Society of Hematology. (2016b). Blood basics. Retrieved from http://www.hematology.org/Patients /Basics/

Centers for Disease Control and Prevention. (2016). Blood disorders. Retrieved from http://www.cdc.gov /ncbddd/blooddisorders/index.html

Hemophilia Federation of America. (2016a). What is a bleeding disorder? Retrieved from http://www .hemophiliafed.org/bleeding-disorders/what-is-a-bleeding-disorder/

Hemophilia Federation of America. (2016b). What is hemophilia? Retrieved from http://www.hemophiliafed .org/bleeding-disorders/hemophilia/

Leukemia and Lymphoma Society. (2013). Blood and marrow stem cell transplantation. Retrieved from http://www.lls.org/sites/default/files/file_assets/PS40_BloodMarrow_booklet_6_16reprint.pdf

Mayo Clinic. (2016a). Enlarged spleen (splenomegaly). Retrieved from http://www.mayoclinic.org/diseases -conditions/enlarged-spleen/basics/definition/CON-20029324

Mayo Clinic. (2016b). Leukemia. Retrieved from http://www.mayoclinic.org/diseases-conditions/leukemia /basics/definition/con-20024914

Merck. (2016). Merck manual: Consumer version: Blood disorders. Retrieved from http://www.merckmanuals .com/home/blood-disorders

National Cancer Institute. (2016a). Leukemia—patient version. Retrieved from http://www.cancer.gov/types /leukemia

National Cancer Institute. (2016b). Lymphoma—patient version. Retrieved from http://www.cancer.gov/types /lymphoma

National Cancer Institute. (2016c). Plasma cell neoplasms (including multiple myeloma)—patient version. Retrieved from http://www.cancer.gov/types/myeloma

National Heart, Lung, and Blood Institute (2011). What is hemochromatosis? Retrieved from http://www.nhlbi .nih.gov/health/health-topics/topics/hemo

National Heart, Lung, and Blood Institute. (2012). What is anemia? Retrieved from https://www.nhlbi.nih.gov /health/health-topics/topics/anemia.

National Institute of General Medical Sciences. (2016). Sepsis fact sheet. Retrieved from https://www.nigms.nih .gov/Education/Pages/factsheet_sepsis.aspx

National Institute of Neurological Disorders and Stroke. (2015). NINDS restless legs syndrome information page. Retrieved from http://www.ninds.nih.gov/disorders/restless_legs/restless_legs.htm

Office on Women's Health (2012). Bleeding disorders fact sheet. Retrieved from https://www.womenshealth.gov /publications/our-publications/fact-sheet/bleeding-disorders.html

Rubarth, L. B. (2011). Blood types and ABO incompatibility. *Neonatal Network, 30*(1), 50–53.

US National Library of Medicine. (2016). Spleen removal. *Medline Plus.* Retrieved from https://www.nlm.nih .gov/medlineplus/ency/article/002944.htm

CHAPTER 15

RESPIRATORY SYSTEM AND RELATED DISEASES

CHAPTER OBJECTIVES

- Describe the functions of the respiratory system.

- List respiratory system organs and describe their role in respiration.

- Identify and discuss respiratory infections.

- Explain differences between common cold and flu symptoms.

- Compare and contrast acute bronchitis with chronic bronchitis.

- Define COPD and identify causes, risk factors, and treatment options.

- Describe what happens to the respiratory system during an asthma attack.

- Review the role of tobacco products and secondhand smoke in lung cancer.

- Summarize different treatment options for respiratory failure.

The primary function of the respiratory system is to supply the blood with oxygen. Once supplied, blood then delivers oxygen to all parts of the body. The respiratory system supplies oxygen to the blood through breathing. When we breathe, we inhale oxygen and exhale carbon dioxide.

The respiratory system has three main parts: airways, lungs, and muscles. Related diseases can affect one or all three of these main parts. The diseases can be caused by genetics or by environmental factors, such as tobacco smoke, air pollution, and pollens.

Structure and Function of the Respiratory System

The *respiratory system* is a group of organs that supply oxygen to the blood. The blood then delivers oxygen to all of the body's cells because they need oxygen to function. Oxygen enters the respiratory system when we inhale (breathe in). We exhale (breathe out) carbon dioxide, a waste product that can be harmful to tissues and organs if it collects in the body. The three main parts of the respiratory system are airways, lungs, and muscles.

Airways

Airways are pipes that carry oxygen-rich air to the lungs. They also carry carbon dioxide out of the lungs. The airways include the nose; mouth; larynx; trachea; and bronchi with their branches, the bronchioles.

Air first enters the nose and the mouth. Because cold and dry air irritates the lungs, one function of the nose and the mouth is to wet and warm the air. Nose hairs

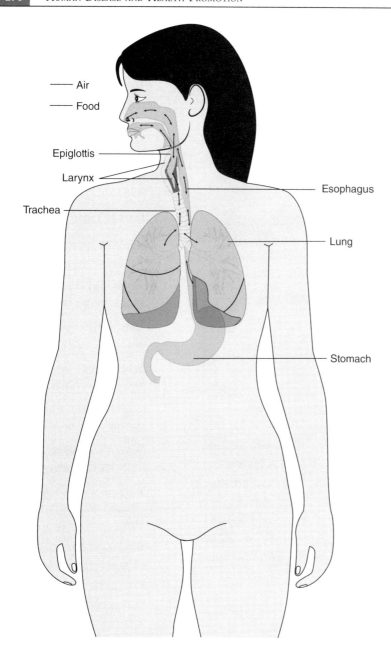

Air

Food

Epiglottis

Larynx

Trachea

Esophagus

Lung

Stomach

Figure 15.1 The Airways

Note. Adapted from the National Cancer Institute

and mouth saliva also trap germs and particles. The air then travels through the larynx, or voice box, and down the trachea, or windpipe. As its name suggests, the voice box is responsible for making sounds. A flap of tissue called the *epiglottis* covers the windpipe when we swallow. This prevents food and liquid from entering the airways (see Figure 15.1). The trachea splits into two tubes, the right and left bronchi, which enter and carry oxygen farther into the lungs. The two bronchi have tiny tube-like branches called bronchioles, which carry oxygen even deeper into the lungs.

Tiny hairs called *cilia* are coated with sticky mucus and protect the airways. Cilia filter out germs and particles that enter the airways when breathing in air, as well as help warm it. They sweep germs and particles up to the nose or mouth. From there, the germs and particles are coughed, swallowed, or sneezed out of the body.

Lungs

Lungs are the main organs of the respiratory system and allow the exchange of oxygen and carbon dioxide in the blood. The lungs are a pair of spongy, air-packed organs that fill the inside of the *thorax*, or chest cavity. The left lung is a little smaller than the right lung to allow room for the heart.

The lungs have five lobes. The right lung is divided into three lobes: superior, middle, and inferior. The left lobe has two lobes: superior and inferior (see Figure 15.2).

Each lung has two layers of membrane called the *pleura*. One layer of the pleura envelops the lungs, and the other lines the inner chest wall. In between the two layers of membrane is a fluid that allows the lungs to smoothly expand and contract with each breath.

Both lungs are attached to a network of tubes that bring oxygen from the air into the blood. Within each lung, the bronchi branches into thousands of bronchioles. The bronchioles end in tiny spongy air sacs called *alveoli*. The alveoli are where the crucial exchange of carbon dioxide for oxygen takes place in the lungs. The exchange works in the following way: Capillaries cover the outside walls of the alveoli. These capillaries have blood that is high in carbon dioxide. The carbon dioxide moves from the capillaries into the alveoli, where it mixes with air and is exhaled. At the same time, oxygen is inhaled and is passed into the capillaries. The red blood cell protein *hemoglobin* helps move oxygen from the alveoli to the capillaries.

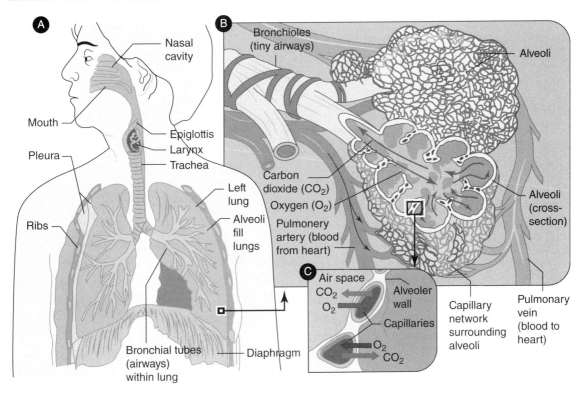

Figure 15.2 The Respiratory System

Figure A shows the location of the respiratory structures in the body. Figure B is an enlarged view of the airways, alveoli (air sacs), and
capillaries (tiny blood vessels). Figure C is a close-up view of gas exchange between the capillaries and alveoli. CO_2 is carbon dioxide, and O_2
is oxygen.

Note. Adapted from the National Cancer Institute

The average adult's lungs have about 600 million alveoli, and a dense network of capillaries surrounds each alveoli. The capillaries connect to arteries and veins that move blood through the body. There are so many capillaries in the lungs that if you placed them end to end, they would cover almost 1,000 miles.

As the largest organ in the body, lungs need a significant surface area for gas exchange. It is deceiving how large the lungs are because they have so many folds. However, if the folds were stretched out, the total surface area of the lungs is about the size of a tennis court. Lungs are unique in their size and shape; only the brain is more complex in design and function.

As its name implies, respiration is the central function of the respiratory system. *Respiration*, which takes place in the lungs, is the exchange of oxygen in the air for carbon dioxide from the blood. There are two distinct parts to respiration:

- *Inhalation:* breathing in, or flow of air into lungs, which brings fresh oxygen
- *Exhalation:* breathing out, or flow of air out of lungs, which removes carbon dioxide

The air we breathe in is made up of several gases, including *oxygen*, which is the most important to our survival. Cells need oxygen for energy and growth; without it, the cells die. Lungs first breathe in air, then extract the oxygen and pass it on to the bloodstream, where it is rushed off to tissues and organs. We breathe in and out about 22,000 times a day, processing about 300 cubic feet or over 8,000 liters of air (National Geographic Society, 2016).

Carbon dioxide is the waste gas that is created during the body's energy-producing process. It is gotten rid of when we breathe out. Without the vital exchange of oxygen and carbon dioxide, cells would die, and the body would suffocate.

Muscles

Breathing is complicated, even though we do it in our sleep. The act of breathing is done by the *diaphragm*, the dome-shaped muscle between the chest cavity and the stomach area. The diaphragm, along with the *intercostal muscles*, or rib muscles, are the main muscles used for inhalation.

The *respiratory rate*, or breathing rate, is the number of inhalations and exhalations per minute. Normal respiratory rates for an adult at rest range from 8 to 16 breaths per minute. The breathing rate is faster in children and faster in women than in men.

The rate at which we breathe is controlled by the brain, which is quick to sense any changes in the body and in the environment. The brain is the body's biggest user of oxygen and the first organ to suffer if there is a shortage. It has a respiratory control center that checks breathing by sending signals down the spine and to the muscles involved in breathing. The signals make sure that the breathing muscles contract and relax, allowing for breathing to continue automatically.

Various factors can affect someone's respiratory rate. A person can change his or her respiratory rate, such as by breathing faster or holding the breath. Emotions can also change breathing rate; for example, when a person is scared, he or she inhales more and exhales less. Respiratory rate also depends on physical activity and air quality. For example, a person breathes more with physical activity and less with air pollution.

Diseases of the Respiratory System

A *respiratory disease*, or lung disease, is any problem in the airways or lungs that results in a person's having difficulty breathing. There are three main types of respiratory diseases, all of which can occur together:

- *Airway diseases.* These usually cause a narrowing of the airways.
- *Lung tissue diseases.* These affect lung tissue structure and cause scarring or inflammation of the tissue. The scarring or inflammation makes it hard for the lungs to fully expand to take in oxygen and release carbon dioxide.
- *Lung circulation diseases.* These diseases cause an inability of the lungs to take in oxygen and release carbon dioxide. They affect blood vessels in the lungs and can also affect heart function.

Many respiratory diseases are caused by multiple factors. Some of these factors are intrinsic, meaning they belong naturally to the person. Examples of *intrinsic factors* include gender and genetic background. Other factors are extrinsic, meaning that they come from the outside and are not a natural part of the person. Examples of *extrinsic factors* include exposure to air pollutants and tobacco smoke.

Pulmonology is the branch of medicine that deals with the structure, function, and diseases of the lungs. *Pulmonologists* are physicians who study a subspecialty of internal medicine to treat respiratory diseases.

Respiratory Tract Infections

Infections can affect any part of the respiratory system and are divided into upper respiratory tract infections and lower respiratory tract infections (see Figure 15.3).

Upper Respiratory Tract Infections

Although there is dispute over the exact boundary between the upper and lower respiratory tracts, the upper respiratory tract is usually thought to be the airway above the vocal cords, and includes the nose, sinuses, pharynx, and larynx.

Sore Throat or Pharyngitis   A *sore throat* is pain or scratchiness in the throat that often worsens with swallowing. It is the primary symptom of *pharyngitis*—inflammation of the pharynx, or throat. The terms *sore throat* and *pharyngitis* are often used to describe the same illness, but sore throat is only one symptom of pharyngitis. There can also be difficulty swallowing and eating, swollen glands in the neck, swollen tonsils with pus, and a hoarse voice; the symptoms depend on the cause. Although anyone can get pharyngitis, there are risk factors, including the following (US National Library of Medicine, 2015b):

• Age, with children and teens being most at risk

• Allergies or chronic sinus infections

• Exposure to toxic chemicals, air pollution, and tobacco products

• Living or working in close quarters

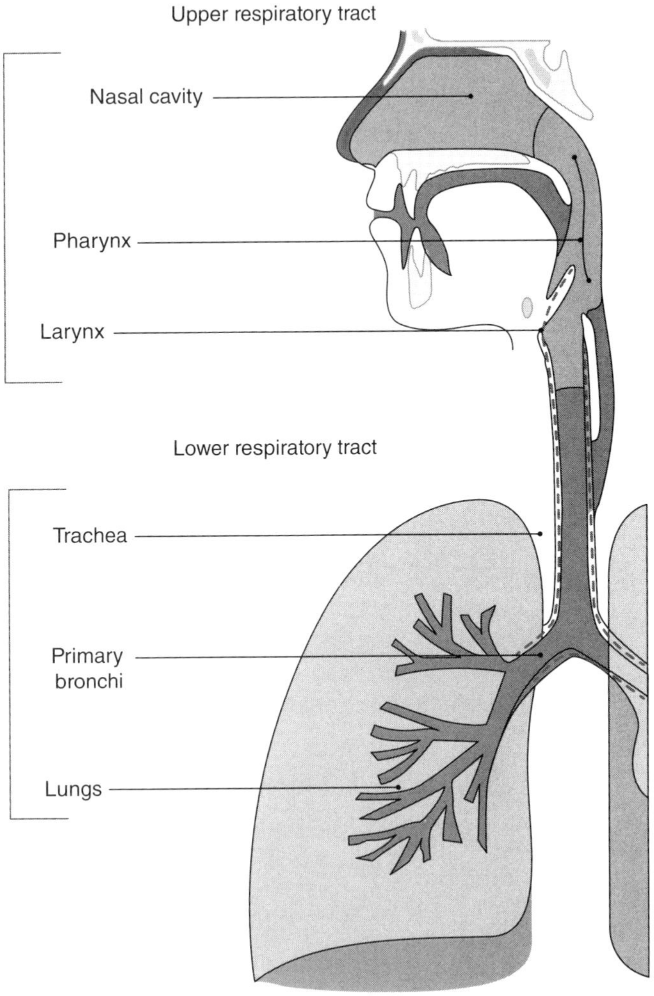

Pharyngitis caused by viral infection is the most common, and it can last 5 to 7 days. Viral pharyngitis does not require medical treatment. For treating pharyngitis from bacterial infections, antibiotics are often prescribed. Penicillin is the antibiotic treatment frequently prescribed for a *strep throat*, the most common bacterial infection associated with a sore throat.

Figure 15.3 Upper and Lower Respiratory Tract Infections

Note. Adapted from Lord Akryl [Public domain], via Wikimedia Commons. Retrieved from http://cancer.gov

Laryngitis   *Laryngitis* is an inflammation of the larynx caused by overuse or infection. Inside the larynx are the *vocal cords*, which are two folds of mucous membrane covering muscle and cartilage. Normally, the vocal cords open and close smoothly, forming sounds through their movement and vibration. But with laryngitis, the vocal cords become inflamed and cause the voice to sound hoarse. Laryngitis may be acute or chronic. The signs and symptoms include voice loss, sore throat, and cough. Most cases of laryngitis are not serious, but chronic voice loss can signal a more serious health problem.

Risk factors for laryngitis include respiratory infections, exposure to toxic chemicals, air pollution, and tobacco products. Overusing the voice by singing or shouting can also cause laryngitis.

Children with laryngitis may need medical attention if they have noisy breathing sounds, difficulty swallowing, and a high fever. These symptoms may indicate *croup*, an inflammation of the larynx and the airway just beneath it. These symptoms can also indicate *epiglottitis*, which is inflammation of windpipe tissue and can be life threatening.

Tonsillitis   *Tonsils* and *adenoids* are glands of the immune system; they trap germs coming in through the mouth and nose. The tonsils are on both sides of the back of the mouth, and the adenoids are higher up, behind the nose.

Sometimes tonsils and adenoids become infected. *Tonsillitis* causes a severe sore throat and fever. Swallowing is painful, and glands in the neck become swollen and sore. The adenoids are usually infected at the same time as the tonsils, and they become enlarged and sore. Infected adenoids make breathing difficult and can cause earaches. The first treatment for infected tonsils and adenoids is antibiotics. Tonsillitis is dangerous when there are at least five episodes in one year or if it does not respond to antibiotics. If there are frequent tonsillitis episodes, then surgery is needed. Surgery to remove the tonsils is called a *tonsillectomy*, and usually the adenoids are removed at the same time. It is the second most common surgery performed on children (American Academy of Otolaryngology, 2016). If left untreated, tonsillitis can damage other body organs, including the heart.

Common Cold   The *common cold* is an acute upper respiratory infection caused by a virus. It is called the common cold because there are over one billion colds in the United States each year, with adults having about three a year.

Colds can occur any time of the year, but they are most frequent in winter or rainy seasons. Symptoms are runny nose and sneezing. People are most contagious for the first 2 to 3 days of a cold and are not contagious after the first week. Cold symptoms appear about 2 or 3 days after contact with the virus, but they sometimes take up to a week. According to the Centers for Disease Control and Prevention ([CDC], 2016b), most cold viruses are not transmitted easily through the air, but you can catch a cold when:

- A person with the virus sneezes, coughs, or blows his or her nose near you
- You touch your nose, eyes, or mouth after touching something that has the virus on it
- You have hand-to-hand contact with an infected person

The best treatment for a cold is to rest and drink fluids. Most cold symptoms usually go away within a week, but can last for 2 weeks. Over-the-counter cold medications ease symptoms, but do not make the cold go away faster. Antibiotics should not be used to treat a cold virus because they do not kill viruses and can make the situation worse. There are ways to help lower the chances of getting a cold, such as washing hands often with water or using hand sanitizer.

Influenza   *Influenza, or flu*, is an infection caused by influenza viruses. The flu can cause mild to severe symptoms or even lead to death. Those at greatest risk for serious health problems if they get the flu are the elderly, children, pregnant women, and patients with certain diseases or conditions, such as asthma.

The influenza virus infects the nose, throat, and lungs, and symptoms include the following (CDC, 2016c):

- Fever
- Cough
- Body aches
- Vomiting
- Sore throat
- Runny nose

Table 15.1 Cold Symptoms Versus Flu Symptoms

Signs	Cold	Flu
High fever		X
Cough and sore throat	X	X
Body ache, headache, and tiredness		X
Sneezing	X	
Stuffy nose	X	X
Breathing problems		X

Note. Adapted from "Influenza (Flu)," by the Centers for Disease Control and Prevention, 2016. Retrieved from https://www.cdc.gov/flu/index.htm

- Tiredness
- Diarrhea

The flu is spread by droplets, and when people with the flu cough, sneeze, or talk, they spread those droplets onto the mouths or noses of people who are nearby. Less often, a person might get the flu by touching an object, such as a doorknob, that has the flu virus on it and then touching their own mouth, eyes, or nose.

Most otherwise healthy adults can infect others beginning 1 day before having symptoms and up to 7 days after becoming sick. Some people, especially young children and people with weakened immune systems, can infect others for an even longer time.

As many as one in five Americans gets the flu each year, and although the virus can be mild in some years, it can be severe or even deadly in others. How severe the flu will be from one season to the next is hard to determine, because of such factors as what flu viruses are spreading, how much flu vaccine is available, and how effective it is. The CDC (2016c) recommends three steps to fighting the flu:

- Get a flu vaccine
- Stop the spread when sick by avoiding close contact, washing hands often, and covering mouth and nose when sneezing or coughing
- Take antiviral drugs if prescribed because they can make symptoms milder

The flu and the common cold have similar symptoms, and it can be difficult to know the difference between them. In general, the flu is worse than the common cold. Unlike the flu, colds generally do not put a person at risk for serious health problems, such as pneumonia, bacterial infections, or hospitalizations (see Table 15.1).

When someone has the flu, he or she usually has a fever. A *fever* is a body temperature higher than 97° to 99° Fahrenheit. A fever is not an illness but a part of the body's defense against infection. Most bacteria and viruses that cause infections do well at the body's normal temperature. A slight fever makes it harder for them to survive and also activates the body's immune system.

Treatment for a fever depends on the cause. A health care provider may recommend drinking enough liquids to prevent dehydration and using over-the-counter medications.

Sinusitis   *Sinusitis* is inflammation of the sinuses. *Sinuses* are hollow cavities within the bones surrounding the nose (see Figure 15.4). There are four groups of sinus cavities: maxillary, ethmoid, frontal, and sphenoid. Sinuses make mucus that drains into the nose.

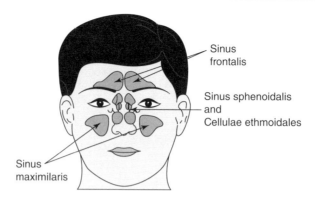

Sinus
frontalis

Sinus sphenoidalis
and
Cellulae ethmoidales

Sinus
maximilaris

Figure 15.4 The Sinus

Symptoms of sinusitis include fever, weakness, cough, and congestion. There can be mucus drainage in the back of the throat called *postnasal drip*. About 37 million Americans are affected by sinusitis every year. It is usually more uncomfortable than dangerous, but in rare cases, infection can spread from the sinuses to the bones or the brain.

Sinusitis can be acute or chronic. Acute sinusitis often starts as a cold, which then turns into a bacterial infection. The point at which the common cold ends and a sinus infection begins is not always clear. Allergies, pollutants, nasal problems, and certain diseases cause sinusitis.

Acute sinusitis often goes away in a few weeks, either on its own or after treatment with medications, vaporizers, and nasal sprays. Chronic sinusitis, by contrast, is usually not caused by infection. It does not respond to treatment, so surgery is often necessary. Regardless of whether the sinusitis is acute or chronic, the primary treatment goal is to decrease inflammation and improve sinus drainage.

To prevent sinusitis, sinuses need to be kept clear by blowing the nose, using decongestants, and drinking fluids. Patients with allergies should avoid *allergens*, or substances that cause an allergic reaction, to prevent sinusitis.

Lower Respiratory Tract Infections

The lower respiratory tract is made up of the trachea (windpipe), the bronchi and bronchioles, and the alveoli, which make up the lungs. These structures pull in air from the upper respiratory system, absorb the oxygen, and release carbon dioxide in exchange. Other structures in the lower respiratory tract, the thoracic cage (rib cage) and the diaphragm, protect and support these functions. Lower respiratory tract infections are less common than upper respiratory infections. However, lower respiratory tract infections are usually more serious and are a leading cause of death among infectious diseases.

Pneumonia   *Pneumonia*, or bronchopneumonia, is an infection in one or both of the lungs. Bacteria, viruses, fungi, and toxic chemicals cause pneumonia. The infection inflames the lungs' air sacs and alveoli, causing them to fill up with fluid or pus. The symptoms of pneumonia—fever, chills, cough, trouble breathing, and chest pain—can range from mild to severe.

There are many different types of pneumonia, but most fall into three general categories related to how a person got pneumonia. *Community-acquired pneumonia (CAP)* occurs outside of hospitals and other health care settings. CAP is the most common type of pneumonia; about four million people get this type of pneumonia each year. *Hospital-acquired pneumonia (HAP)*, or nosocomial pneumonia, is pneumonia contracted while patients are in the hospital. HAP tends to be more serious than CAP because the patient is already sick. *Healthcare-associated pneumonia* refers to pneumonia that patients contract in health care settings other than hospitals, such as a nursing home.

People most at risk for pneumonia are older than 65 or younger than 2 years of age. Those who already have health problems, such as heart failure, diabetes, or HIV/AIDS infection, are also at risk. If a patient has pneumonia, he or she needs to limit contact with family, loved ones, and friends.

Pneumonia is the most common cause of infectious death in the United States, with more than 10 million cases every year and about 500,000 hospitalizations (National Heart, Lung, and Blood Institute, 2016a). Many factors affect how serious pneumonia is, such as the type of germ causing the infection, and the patient's age and overall health. Most people are treated at home if their symptoms are mild. Patients with severe symptoms, such as pneumonia in both lungs, need treatment in a hospital. Severe pneumonia may require 3 weeks or more before a patient is fully recovered.

To diagnose pneumonia in a patient, a health care provider takes a health history, conducts a physical examination, and orders a chest X-ray and a sputum test. A *sputum test* is a sample of a patient's sputum, or spit, that is tested for infection. Treatment for pneumonia depends on the cause. If it is bacterial, then antibiotics are used; if it is viral, then antiviral medications are used.

There are vaccines to prevent pneumococcal pneumonia, a common type of bacterial pneumonia. Other preventive measures include washing hands frequently and not smoking.

Tuberculosis   *Tuberculosis (TB)* is an infection caused by bacteria that attack the lungs and damage other parts of the body. TB causes more deaths in the world than any other infectious disease. About two billion people are infected with TB worldwide, about 15 million of whom are in the United States (CDC, 2016d). TB is transmitted through the air when an infected patient coughs, sneezes, or talks. It is not usually transmitted through the TB patient's personal items (e.g., clothing).

There are two types of TB. *Latent tuberculosis* refers to TB in a healthy person whose immune system usually fights and controls the infection. If an infected person is unhealthy with a weak immune system, then the bacteria cause *active tuberculosis* and spread to other parts of the body. When TB becomes active, it kills 60% of those who are not treated. In the United States, about 20,000 TB infections become active every year (CDC, 2016d). The treatment for active TB requires taking several medications for long periods of time. When active TB patients follow their treatment plan, 90% of them survive.

To diagnose active TB, a health care provider relies on symptoms and the patient's history of exposure to TB. Diagnostic tests for TB include a *mantoux test*, which is a type of skin test; sputum samples; blood tests; and X-rays.

Some TB patients may have few or no symptoms. Others experience a cough that lasts 3 weeks or longer, coughing up blood or mucus, weight loss, weakness, and fever.

Many health care providers often hospitalize TB patients to observe them during treatment. Patients who have been treated for at least 2 weeks are usually no longer contagious. But for those patients who do not take their medications as prescribed or who do not follow their treatment plan, the bacteria become resistant to treatment and put others at risk for infection.

TB is preventable. Adequate ventilation and improving crowded conditions can decrease the spread of TB, as can having infected patients cover their mouth and nose when coughing or sneezing. Identifying infected people early and treating them with medications is another way to prevent its spread. A vaccine is available for some infants and is recommended for those who live in parts of the world that have high TB infection rates, such as Asia.

Chronic Obstructive Pulmonary Disease

Chronic obstructive pulmonary disease (COPD) is a group of diseases—for example, emphysema and chronic bronchitis—that make breathing difficult. When you breathe in, each air sac fills with air like a small balloon, and when you breathe out, the sacs collapse. In COPD, air sacs lose their

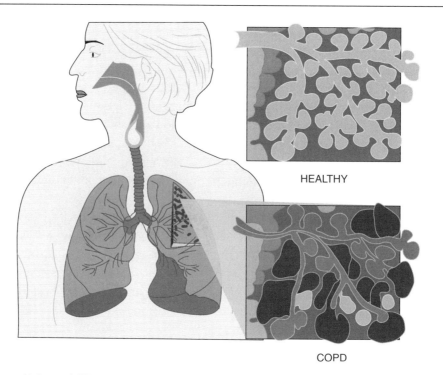

HEALTHY

COPD

Figure 15.5 Lungs, Air Sacs, and COPD

Note. Adapted from "COPD Versus Healthy Lung.jpg," by Jtravers at en.wikipedia [Public domain], from Wikimedia Commons. Retrieved from http://commons.wikimedia.org/wiki/File%3ACopd_versus_healthy_lung.jpg

shape and become floppy (see Figure 15.5). While other major causes of death have been decreasing, COPD mortality (death) rates have risen. COPD is the third leading cause of death in the United States (CDC, 2016a). Twelve million Americans are diagnosed with COPD, and millions more are unaware they have it.

Tobacco use is the main cause of COPD in the United States. Secondhand smoke, work-related pollution (e.g., fumes), and genetic factors can also cause COPD. What is surprising is that as many as one out of six Americans with COPD has never smoked. The groups more likely to report COPD are those ages 65 to 74 years, non-Hispanic Whites, women, those with lower incomes, current or former smokers, and those with a history of asthma.

COPD may cause no symptoms in the beginning. As the disease gets worse, however, symptoms become severe. The severity of COPD symptoms depends on how much lung damage there is. If a patient keeps smoking, the damage worsens faster than if he or she stops smoking. Common symptoms of COPD include frequent coughing with a lot of mucus, known as a *smoker's cough*; difficulty breathing; fatigue; and wheezing.

Diagnosis of COPD involves not only taking a patient's health history and doing a physical examination but also measuring lung function. Lung function tests measure how much and how fast a patient can breathe and how well the lungs deliver oxygen to the blood. A *spirometry* is a lung function test that measures how much and how fast a patient can breathe in and out, and detects COPD before symptoms develop. Other diagnostic tests for COPD include a chest X-ray, chest CT scan, and blood tests that measure the oxygen level in the blood.

Although there is no cure, early detection and treatment of COPD slow the disease and improve quality of life. What is critical to treatment is avoiding tobacco smoke and other air pollutants. Coughing and wheezing can be treated with a *bronchodilator*, medication that relaxes the muscles around the airways, which makes breathing easier. Most bronchodilators are taken with a device called an *inhaler*. In addition, patients with low blood oxygen levels are given supplemental oxygen or can have surgery. Other COPD treatments are pulmonary rehabilitation, which is a type of physical therapy in which the patient is taught to breathe more easily, and surgery.

The best way to avoid getting COPD is to try to avoid irritants to the lungs: tobacco use, secondhand smoke, air pollution, and respiratory infections.

Emphysema

Emphysema is a type of COPD that causes damage to the lungs' air sacs by filling them with air high in carbon dioxide. Because the air sacs are damaged, the lungs lose their ability to empty easily. Not enough air is exhaled to allow oxygen to enter, so the air sacs stretch and burst.

Emphysema is a crippling and weakening disease that causes chronic lung obstruction and destruction. It is also a *progressive disease*, meaning that it gets worse over time. As it progresses, the lungs cannot absorb oxygen or release carbon dioxide, causing breathing to be difficult. Difficulty breathing is called *dyspnea*, and those with dyspnea either have *tachypnea* (fast breathing) or *apnea* (inability to breathe).

Nearly two million Americans have emphysema, and it causes about 10,000 deaths per year. It is the most common cause of death from respiratory diseases. Most with this disease are men age 65 and older.

The cause of emphysema is not fully understood, but smoking is responsible for most cases. Exposure to air pollution can also cause emphysema. Rarely, emphysema is caused by an inherited lack of a protein. When this is the cause, the disease is called Alpha-1 antitrypsin deficiency emphysema.

Because emphysema progresses so slowly, there are few symptoms in the early stages of the disease. Symptoms rarely appear until a person has smoked a pack of cigarettes a day for more than 20 years or until 30% to 50% of lung tissue is lost. Over time, most patients with emphysema develop short, deep breathing that clears out carbon dioxide building up in the lungs.

At first, people with emphysema have shortness of breath only during exercise, but eventually they are short of breath during daily activities (e.g., walking). As time goes on, there is shortness of breath for much of the day, even while sleeping. At its worst, emphysema causes "air hunger," which is the constant feeling of being unable to catch one's breath. The person has a suffocating, painful feeling and distress from the inability to breathe. Other symptoms of emphysema include wheezing, smoker's cough, swelling of the chest, weight loss, and weakness.

To diagnose emphysema, the health care provider asks the patient about his or her smoking history and exposure to air pollution, as well as about family health history. The physical examination includes looking for dyspnea and how the chest moves during breathing, and listening for wheezing and smoker's cough. In most patients, emphysema is diagnosed by CT scans, X-rays, or lung function tests.

No treatment can cure emphysema, but it can reduce symptoms, complications, and disability. The single most important factor for healthy lungs is to stop smoking. Although stopping smoking is most effective in the early stages of emphysema, it also can slow the loss of lung function in later stages.

There are different medications that help relieve symptoms of emphysema, including broncho-dilators, antibiotics, and oxygen therapy. Other treatments available for patients with advanced emphysema include pulmonary rehabilitation; *lung volume reduction surgery*, in which parts of diseased lung are removed; and lung transplant. A lung transplant is usually only for patients whose life expectancy is less than 2 to 3 years.

Patients with mild emphysema who quit smoking and adopt healthy habits can enjoy a normal lifestyle for a long time. Even patients with advanced emphysema have a good chance of surviving for 5 years or more if they quit smoking. In patients with emphysema who continue to smoke, however, the disease may reduce their life span by 10 years or more.

Bronchitis

Bronchitis is an inflammation of the bronchi. The inflammation narrows the bronchi, making breathing difficult and causing a person to cough. The cough is caused by irritation to the bronchi or by mucous that needs to be cleared.

The two main types of bronchitis are acute, which lasts less than 6 weeks, and chronic, which occurs frequently for more than 2 years. *Acute bronchitis, or chest cold,* is common in the United States: Millions of cases are diagnosed every year, most often in the fall and winter.

Most acute bronchitis cases are caused by viral infections, the same viruses that cause colds and the flu. A patient develops acute bronchitis after a cold or the flu. At first, it affects the nose, sinuses, and throat, then it spreads to the bronchi.

The main symptom of acute bronchitis is constant coughing with sputum. Bronchitis also causes *wheezing*, which is a whistling sound when breathing; chest pain; fatigue; a low fever; and dyspnea. Some patients can feel fine and have no fever, yet they have a cough that lasts for several weeks after the cold or the flu goes away. With acute bronchitis, symptoms can last for up to 10 days, but even after the infection has cleared, the patient may have a dry, nagging cough that can last up to 8 weeks.

Most patients with acute bronchitis do not need antibiotics. Vapors, sprays, and cough medications give temporary relief from coughing. Although a single episode of acute bronchitis usually is not a concern, it can lead to pneumonia in some people.

Chronic bronchitis is more serious than acute because it is a constant inflammation of the bronchi and requires regular medical treatment. This constant inflammation causes *hypoxia*, or insufficient oxygen in the tissues. Chronic bronchitis is caused by repeated attacks of acute bronchitis that last for at least 3 months. A sign of chronic bronchitis is a long-term, heavy cough with sputum that has pus. Chronic bronchitis is a type of COPD.

Smoking and air pollution are common causes of chronic bronchitis. Treatment helps with symptoms, but chronic bronchitis never goes away completely. Early diagnosis and treatment, combined with quitting smoking and avoiding air pollution, do improve quality of life.

Treatment for bronchitis relieves symptoms and eases breathing. Medications for bronchitis, such as bronchodilators and steroids, open the bronchi and help clear away mucus. For some patients with chronic bronchitis, oxygen therapy and pulmonary rehabilitation can relieve symptoms.

The elderly, infants, and young children are at greater risk for bronchitis, as well as those who smoke or who live with a smoker. Air pollution, infections, having a lung disease, and allergies can worsen the symptoms of chronic bronchitis, especially for smokers. Women are more than twice as likely as men to be diagnosed with chronic bronchitis.

Asthma

Asthma is a chronic swelling and narrowing of the bronchial tubes, which makes breathing difficult (see Figure 15.6). The swelling and narrowing are caused by three factors:

- *Inflammation.* The bronchial tubes become red, irritated, and swollen.
- *Bronchospasms.* The muscles around the bronchial tubes tighten and narrow.
- *Hyperactivity or hypersensitivity.* The bronchial tubes are sensitive to triggers.

Asthma rates have increased steadily in the United States over the past 15 years. There are more than 20 million people diagnosed with asthma; 9 million are children under 18. It is the most common chronic childhood disease in the United States. Women are more likely than men to have asthma and are more likely to die from it. There are about 5,000 asthma deaths annually (Asthma and Allergy Foundation of America, 2016).

Before an asthma episode

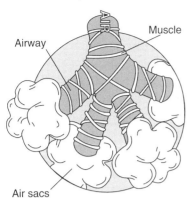

After an asthma episode

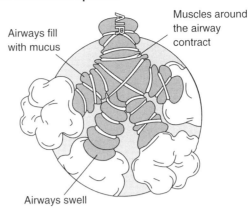

Figure 15.6 Asthma Attack

During an asthma episode, inflamed airways react to environmental triggers, such as smoke, dust, or pollen. The airways narrow and make extra mucus, making it difficult to breathe.

Note. From FDA/Renée Gordon; vectors by Mysid. [Public domain], via Wikimedia Commons

Asthma affects individuals differently; however, it is most severe in children. This is because children have smaller and narrower bronchial tubes than adults. Children also breathe at higher rates than adults and are more sensitive to irritants and poor air quality.

A family history of asthma increases the chances that a person will have asthma. If a person has a parent with asthma, he or she is three to six times more likely to have asthma than someone who does not have an asthmatic parent (Asthma and Allergy Foundation of America, 2016). Although family health history does play a part, it is still unknown why some people get asthma and others do not. In addition to having asthma, some patients can experience a form of bronchitis called asthmatic bronchitis. Why some asthmatic patients experience bronchitis while others do not is also unknown.

Asthma is divided into two types: allergic asthma and nonallergic asthma. Allergies and asthma are closely related, and allergens (allergy-causing substances) in the environment are a major cause of asthma.

Regardless of the type, people with asthma have it all the time. Asthma attacks occur only when something bothers the bronchial tubes. During an *asthma attack*, the sides of the bronchial tubes swell and shrink. Muscles around the bronchial tubes tighten, and less air gets in and out of the lungs. Mucous clogs up the bronchial tubes even more (see Figure 15.6). During severe episodes, airways become extremely narrow, causing little airflow, and can lead to death. There are four major symptoms of an asthma attack:

• Shortness of breath after exercise, when resting, or at nighttime

• Coughing after exercise or exposure to cold air

• Wheezing or whistling sounds

• Chest tightness

Asthmatics have an attack when they are exposed to *asthma triggers*, but not all asthmatics react to the same triggers. How bad the attack is depends on how many triggers cause the symptoms and how sensitive the patient's lungs are to them. There are many different types of asthma triggers; the following are the most common:

Asthma Triggers

- Allergies
- Physical exercise
- Dust mites
- Tobacco smoke
- Air pollution
- Cockroaches
- Pets
- Certain foods
- Hormone changes
- Respiratory infections
- Stress and strong emotions
- Temperature changes
- Pollens and molds

For a diagnosis of asthma, the health care provider records the patient's health history, does a physical examination, and performs the following tests:

- *Spirometry*—measures the amount of air the patient can breathe in and out as well as how fast he or she can blow air out

- *Chest X-ray or electrocardiogram*—shows whether another disease or a foreign object is causing symptoms

Asthma is a chronic disease, so medications can treat asthma but not cure it. The medications work by opening up the bronchial tubes. Some medications are in pill form; others are breathed in with an inhaler or a *nebulizer*, which is a machine that makes a mist of the medication. Asthma medications fall into two groups: long-term control and quick relief. Medications for long-term control are taken daily over a long period of time. They help prevent symptoms from starting and are used to reduce inflammation, relax bronchial tube muscles, and improve lung function. Quick-relief medications are used once symptoms start, and they give relief in minutes. They do this by quickly relaxing tightened muscles around the bronchial tubes. Quick-relief medications are only to prevent an asthma attack when symptoms worsen or to stop attacks once they have started.

It is not fully understood how to prevent, treat, and cure asthma. In most cases, what causes the asthma is unknown, but it can be managed by knowing the warning signs of an attack, staying away from triggers, and following a treatment plan.

Lung Cancer

Lung cancer develops when cancer cells in the lung tissues grow out of control. These cancer cells grow into tumors that then disturb the way the lungs work. There are two main types of lung cancer: primary and secondary. Primary lung cancer starts in the lung and then spreads to other organs, such as the brain. Secondary lung cancer starts somewhere else in the body, such as the colon, and spreads to the lungs. This spreading of cancer cells to other organs is known as *metastasis*.

Lung cancer is the leading cause of cancer death for men and women in the United States, killing more than 161,000 Americans every year (National Cancer Institute, 2012). More Americans die each year of lung cancer than from breast, prostate, and colorectal cancers combined. The risk is slightly higher for a man to have lung cancer in his lifetime than it is for a woman. It occurs mainly in people who are 65 years old and older.

Tobacco use is the greatest risk factor for lung cancer. The longer a person uses tobacco and the more he or she uses, the greater the risk. If a person quits before cancer develops, the damaged lung tissue gradually improves. An estimated 45 million adults in the United States are current smokers, and until their tobacco use is sharply decreased, lung cancer will continue to be the number one cause of cancer death in the United States. Ironically, lung cancer is also the most preventable form of cancer, because more than 87% of the cases are caused by tobacco use (National Cancer Institute, 2012). Stopping tobacco use could nearly wipe out lung cancer.

Persons exposed to tobacco smoke or secondhand smoke are also at risk for developing lung cancer. Hundreds of thousands of nonsmokers who were exposed to secondhand smoke have developed lung cancer. Each year, about 3,000 nonsmoking adults die of lung cancer as a result of breathing secondhand smoke (National Cancer Institute, 2012). Secondhand smoke causes 30 times as many lung cancer deaths as caused by all other air pollutants combined. According to the American Heart Association (2015), studies show that a person breathing secondhand smoke is exposed to the same tar, nicotine, cyanide, formaldehyde, arsenic, ammonia, methane, carbon monoxide, and other harmful substances as the person smoking a cigarette. The US Environmental Protection Agency ranks secondhand smoke as one of the most dangerous cancer-causing substances.

Exposure to secondhand smoke is a particularly serious health risk for children. It is so serious that if you or a member of your household smokes around children, the children inhale the equivalent of 102 packs of cigarettes by age 5. Effects of secondhand smoke on children include increased risk for ear and respiratory infections as well as increased risk for *sudden infant death syndrome (SIDS)*. SIDS is the sudden death of an infant under 1 year of age that remains unexplained after a thorough investigation. SIDS deaths occur unexpectedly and quickly to apparently healthy infants, usually when he or she is sleeping.

In addition to tobacco use, other risks for lung cancer include family health history as well as exposure to *carcinogens*, or cancer-causing agents like radon, asbestos, and air pollution. If people are exposed to these carcinogens and smoke, their risk is greatly increased.

There are no warning signs for early lung cancer, and by the time most patients have symptoms, the cancer is serious. Symptoms of lung cancer include the following (National Cancer Institute, 2012):

- Cough that doesn't go away
- Difficulty breathing, and wheezing
- Chest pain
- Pneumonia that doesn't go away
- Coughing up blood
- Weight loss
- Hoarseness
- Fatigue

To diagnose lung cancer, a health care provider gets information on the patient's health history, smoking habits, and exposure to environmental hazards. The patient also is given a physical examination and diagnostic tests. The following are examples of diagnostic tests for lung cancer (National Cancer Institute, 2012):

- *Chest X-ray*—imaging test that shows abnormal growths in lungs.
- *CT scan*—imaging test that shows signs of cancer that don't show up on X-rays.
- *Sputum sample*—sample of sputum studied to detect cancer cells.

- *Bronchoscopy*—procedure in which a tube called a *bronchoscope* is passed through the nose or mouth and down into the lungs. This scope sees into the lungs and removes tissue.

- *Fine-needle aspiration*—procedure in which a needle is passed through the chest wall into the lung to remove tissue or fluid.

- *Thoracotomy*—surgical removal of lung tissue.

There are two options for treating lung cancer. One option tries to cure the cancer; the other stops the cancer from spreading and reduces symptoms. Patients may be given just one option or a combination of both. What treatment the patient receives depends on three factors:

- The type of lung cancer

- Where the cancer is and whether it has spread to other parts of the body

- The patient's age and overall health

Surgery is used to remove lung tissue with cancerous tumors. Sometimes a large part of a lung or all of it is removed. If the cancer has not spread, surgery can cure the patient. Radiation therapy uses high-energy rays to shrink or kill cancer cells. Often radiation therapy helps a patient feel less pain and discomfort. Chemotherapy uses anticancer medications that attack cancer cells and normal cells. Targeted therapy uses medications to block the growth and spread of cancer cells.

Typically, the earlier a cancer is diagnosed, the more successful the treatment. At the time of diagnosis, if the cancer has not spread to any other body parts, it is called *localized cancer.* Only 16% of lung cancers, however, are diagnosed at an early, localized stage. Patients with localized lung cancer have a 5-year survival rate of 49% (National Cancer Institute, 2012). This means that these patients have cancer just in the lungs and that they have a 49% chance of surviving 5 years after diagnosis.

Patients whose cancer has spread within the chest have a 5-year survival rate of 16% (National Cancer Institute, 2012). And those patients whose lung cancer has spread to other organs have a 5-year survival rate of 2%. As mentioned, the 5-year survival rate refers to the number of patients still alive 5 years after diagnosis, whether they are disease-free, in remission, or under treatment. Unfortunately, this does not mean that 5-year survivors have been permanently cured of lung cancer.

The best way to prevent lung cancer is to stop smoking or not start at all. All types of smoking—cigarettes, cigars, and pipes—increase the risk for lung cancer. The following are other ways to reduce risk for lung cancer (National Cancer Institute, 2012):

- Avoid secondhand smoke

- Test for radon in the home or workplace

- Protect yourself from dust and chemical fumes

- Avoid asbestos

- Eat a healthy diet, and exercise

Screening can find cancers early, when they may be easier to treat. However, there is controversy about lung cancer screening. For example, there is a public health debate about whether screening smokers with X-rays or mucus samples saves lives. There is research that does support CT scans for older people who smoke heavily, because scans do save lives (National Cancer Institute, 2012). However, there is no agreement as to who should or should not get a CT scan screening.

Cystic Fibrosis

Cystic fibrosis (CF) is an inherited disease that is frequently fatal. It is also chronic and progressive, affecting multiple systems, especially the lungs, digestive tract, and pancreas. In patients with CF, there is a defect in the glands that make mucus and sweat. Mucus is a slippery substance that lubricates and protects the respiratory, digestive, and reproductive systems. It prevents tissues from drying out. In patients with CF, their mucus is abnormally thick and sticky. This mucus clogs airways, causing breathing problems, bacterial infections, and lung damage. Sweat is moisture that cools the body. CF patients lose large amounts of salt when they sweat, upsetting the mineral balance in their blood.

About 30,000 children and young adults in the United States have CF, and every year, about 2,500 babies are born with CF (American Lung Association, 2016). The disease occurs mostly in Whites whose ancestors came from northern Europe, although it does affect to a lesser degree all races and ethnic groups. It is the most common deadly inherited disease affecting Whites in the United States. In addition, there are about 12 million Americans without symptoms who have an abnormal "CF gene." These people are usually unaware that they are carriers. That's because a person with CF must inherit two defective CF genes—one from each parent—to have symptoms.

A baby born with two defective CF genes usually has symptoms during its first year, but most (80%) are not diagnosed until their third birthday. A small number are not diagnosed until age 18 or older because older patients tend to have a milder form of the disease.

The disease progresses shortly after birth, and an infant with CF has a lung infection as a first symptom. The lung infection causes chronic coughing, wheezing, and inflammation. Eventually, a repeating cycle of infection and inflammation develops. Over time, mucus buildup and infections cause permanent lung damage, including scar tissue and cysts. Other CF symptoms include salty-tasting skin, and some infants with CF also have a blockage in the intestine.

As CF patients grow older, they have digestive problems because the thick, sticky mucus blocks the function of the pancreas. The pancreas makes enzymes that help digest food, so when mucus blocks the ducts of the pancreas, these enzymes can't reach the intestines to aid digestion. With the thick buildup of mucus in the intestines and in the lungs, patients experience diarrhea, malnutrition, poor growth, weight loss, frequent respiratory infections, breathing difficulty, and eventually permanent lung damage. Progressive lung disease is the cause of death in most CF patients.

There is a DNA blood test to help detect CF. The test detects the gene known to cause CF. Another test for CF is a sweat test that looks for a high salt level in the patient's sweat. Other diagnostic tests include blood tests, chest X-rays, lung function tests, and sputum cultures.

There is no cure for CF, so the goal of treatment is to clear mucus, control lung infections, and prevent obstruction in the digestive system. Because CF affects different people in different ways, treatment is tailored to the needs of each patient and may include the following (American Lung Association, 2016):

- Daily airway clearance techniques
- Antibiotics for infections
- Pain relievers
- Decongestants
- Inhaled medications
- Vitamin supplements
- Medications that thin mucus
- Lung transplant

Although treating symptoms does not cure the disease, it does improve quality of life for most patients. Treatment has over the years increased the average life span of CF patients to around age 36.

One CF treatment that holds promise is gene therapy. Because CF is a genetic disease, the only way to prevent or cure it would be to use gene therapy at an early age. Ideally, gene therapy repairs or replaces the defective gene before symptoms cause permanent damage.

Prenatal genetic tests enable parents to find out whether a baby is likely to have CF. However, these tests are expensive and carry risks for the mother, and are not used for all pregnant women. In families with CF, brothers, sisters, and first cousins of the CF patient should be tested to see if they carry a defective gene, especially if they have chronic lung or digestive problems.

Lung Failure

Lung failure, or respiratory failure, occurs when not enough oxygen passes from the lungs into the blood. It also occurs if the lungs can't remove carbon dioxide from the blood. Both of these problems, a dangerously low oxygen level and a dangerously high carbon dioxide level in the blood, can occur at the same time.

Almost any disease that affects breathing can lead to lung failure. For example, patients who have diseases or injuries that affect the muscles, nerves, bones, or tissues that support breathing are at risk. Other examples of diseases that cause lung failure are COPD, asthma, CF, and pneumonia because they block airways, damage lung tissue, and weaken muscles that control breathing.

Symptoms of lung failure include dyspnea, tachypnea, and air hunger (feeling as though you can't breathe in enough air). In severe cases, there is *cyanosis*, which is a bluish color to the skin, lips, and fingernails. Eventually, the brain and heart malfunction, resulting in severe drowsiness and abnormal heartbeats, both of which can lead to death.

A health care provider detects lung failure based on symptoms and a physical examination. A blood test confirms the diagnosis when it shows a dangerously low level of oxygen or a dangerously high level of carbon dioxide. Chest X-rays and other diagnostic tests are done to determine the cause of lung failure.

A goal to treating lung failure is to get oxygen to the lungs and other organs and to remove carbon dioxide from the body. Another goal is to treat the underlying cause. By treating the underlying cause, the symptoms of lung failure can become less severe.

Lung failure can be acute or chronic. Acute lung failure occurs quickly and requires emergency treatment. It is usually treated in an intensive care unit. Chronic lung failure occurs more slowly and lasts longer. It can be treated at home or at a long-term care center.

The outlook for lung failure depends on three factors: the underlying cause, how quickly treatment begins, and the patient's overall health. Oxygen is given at first, usually more than is needed, but then the amount is adjusted over time. Patients with severe lung diseases need long-term breathing support, such as portable oxygen therapy. In the case of chronic lung failure, portable oxygen therapy takes the form of extra oxygen given through two small plastic tubes (cannula) that are placed in both nostrils or through a mask that fits over the nose and mouth.

If the patient still has trouble breathing, then oxygen is given through a *tracheostomy*. This is a surgically opened hole that goes through the front of the neck and into the windpipe. A breathing tube is placed in the hole to help the patient breathe.

If the oxygen level in the patient's blood doesn't increase, or if she still has trouble breathing, then a *ventilator* is used. A ventilator is a machine that supports breathing. It blows air with increased oxygen content into the lungs. The patient uses the ventilator until she can breathe on her own.

Chapter Summary

- The respiratory system is a group of organs that supply oxygen to the blood and remove carbon dioxide.
- There are three main parts to the respiratory system: airways, lungs, and muscles.
- A respiratory disease is any problem in the lungs that results in difficulty breathing.

- Pulmonology is the branch of medicine that deals with the structure, function, and diseases of the respiratory system. Pulmonologists are physicians who treat the respiratory system.

- Chronic obstructive pulmonary disease is a group of diseases in which air sacs lose their shape and become floppy.

- Lung cancer, although preventable, is the leading cause of cancer death for men and women in the United States. Tobacco use is the greatest risk factor for lung cancer.

REVIEW QUESTIONS

1. Through what organs does air travel? How does oxygen move from the lungs to the blood?

2. How are cold symptoms different from flu symptoms?

3. If you are an asthmatic, what can you do to prevent an asthma attack?

4. Identify and explain two COPDs.

5. What is the role of tobacco products and secondhand smoke in respiratory diseases?

6. Explain the importance of identifying patients with active TB, and list treatment options.

7. What happens when a TB patient does not comply with his or her treatment plan?

8. What are the risk and protective factors for lung cancer?

9. List and explain three types of pneumonia.

10. What are the health risks for children who are exposed to secondhand smoke?

KEY TERMS

Acute bronchitis, or chest cold: Inflammation of the bronchi that lasts less than 6 weeks

Adenoids: Part of the immune system, glands that are behind the nose

Airways: Pipes in the body that carry oxygen to the lungs and carry out carbon dioxide.

Allergen: Substance that causes an allergic reaction

Alveoli: Tiny spongy air sacs at the end of the bronchioles

Apnea: Inability to breathe

Asthma: Chronic swelling and narrowing of the bronchial tubes, which can cause serious difficulty breathing

Asthma attack: Reaction in which the sides of the bronchial tubes swell and shrink, making breathing difficult

Asthma trigger: Anything that causes asthma attacks

Bronchitis: Inflammation of the bronchi

Bronchodilator: Medication that relaxes the muscles around the airways

Bronchoscope: Tube used in a bronchoscopy to see into the lungs and remove tissue

Bronchoscopy: Procedure in which a tube is passed through the nose or mouth and down into the lungs

Bronchospasms: Tightening of the muscles around the bronchial tubes

Carbon dioxide: Waste gas

Carcinogen: Cancer-causing agent

Chronic bronchitis: Constant inflammation of the bronchi

Chronic obstructive pulmonary disease (COPD): Group of diseases in which air sacs lose their shape and become floppy

Cilia: Tiny hairs that are coated with sticky mucus to protect the airways

Common cold: Acute upper respiratory infection caused by a virus

Croup: Inflammation of the larynx and the airway just beneath it

Cyanosis: Bluish color to the skin, lips, and fingernails

Cystic fibrosis (CF): Genetic disease that causes a defect in the glands that make mucus and sweat

Diaphragm: Dome-shaped muscle that assists in the job of breathing

Dyspnea: Difficulty breathing

Emphysema: Disease that causes damage to air sacs by filling them with air high in carbon dioxide

Epiglottis: Flap of tissue that covers the windpipe when a person swallows

Epiglottitis: Inflammation of the epiglottis, the tissue that covers the windpipe

Exhalation: Part of respiration that results in the flow of air out of lungs

Extrinsic factors: Factors that are not a natural part of a person

Fever: Body temperature that is higher than normal

Fine-needle aspiration: Procedure in which a needle is passed through the chest wall into the lung

Hemoglobin: Iron-rich, oxygen-carrying protein in red blood cells

Hyperactivity or hypersensitivity: In the context of the respiratory system, bronchial tubes' high sensitivity to asthma triggers

Hypoxia: Insufficient oxygen in the tissues

Inflammation: Redness, irritation, and swelling

Influenza, or flu: Infection caused by influenza viruses

Inhalation: Part of respiration that results in the flow of air into lungs

Inhaler: Device used to take bronchodilators

Intercostal muscles: Located in the rib cage, the main muscles used for inhalation

Intrinsic factors: Factors that belong naturally to a person

Laryngitis: Inflammation of the larynx, or voice box

Lung cancer: Disease that develops when cancer cells in the lung tissues grow out of control

Lung failure: Failure of the lungs to pass sufficient oxygen into the blood or to remove carbon dioxide from the blood, or both

Lungs: Parts of the respiratory system that exchange oxygen and carbon dioxide in the blood

Lung volume reduction surgery: Surgical removal of diseased lung tissue

Mantoux test: Diagnostic skin test for tuberculosis

Metastasis: Spread of cancer cells from one organ to another

Nebulizer: Machine that makes a mist of a medication

Oxygen: The gas in air that is most important to our survival, because cells need it for energy and growth

Pharyngitis: Inflammation of the pharynx, or throat

Pleura: Layers of tissue that cover each lung

Pneumonia: Infection in one or both of the lungs

Postnasal drip: Mucus drainage in the back of the throat

Progressive disease: A disease that gets worse over time

Pulmonologist: Physician who studies a subspecialty of internal medicine to treat respiratory diseases

Pulmonology: Branch of medicine that deals with the structure, function, and diseases of the respiratory system

Respiration: The exchange in the lungs of oxygen for carbon dioxide

Respiratory disease: Any problem in the lungs that results in having difficulty breathing

Respiratory rate: The number of inhalations and exhalations per minute

Respiratory system: Group of organs that work together to supply oxygen to the blood and remove carbon dioxide

Sinuses: Hollow air spaces within the bones surrounding the nose

Sinusitis: Inflammation of the sinuses

Smoker's cough: Frequent cough with a lot of mucus

Sore throat: Pain or scratchiness in the throat that often worsens with swallowing

Spirometry: Lung function test that measures how much and how fast a patient can breathe in and out, and detects chronic obstructive pulmonary disease

Sputum test: Diagnostic test that takes a sample of a patient's sputum, or spit

Strep throat: The most common bacterial infection associated with a sore throat

Sudden infant death syndrome (SIDS): Sudden death of an infant under 1 year of age that remains unexplained after a thorough investigation

Tachypnea: Fast breathing

Thoracotomy: Surgical procedure in which the chest is cut open and tissue is removed from the lungs

Thorax: Chest cavity, occupied by the lungs and heart

Tonsillectomy: Surgical removal of the tonsils and usually the adenoids

Tonsillitis: Inflammation of the tonsils, usually caused by infection

Tonsils: Part of the immune system, glands that are on both sides of the back of the mouth

Tracheostomy: Surgically opened hole that goes through the front of the neck and into the windpipe

Tuberculosis (TB): Bacterial infection that attacks the lungs and damages other parts of the body

Ventilator: Machine that supports breathing

Vocal cords: Two folds of mucous membrane inside the larynx

Wheezing: Whistling sound when breathing

CHAPTER ACTIVITIES

1.   Identify 5 to 10 examples of popular over-the-counter (including alternative) medicines for cold and flu. Compare the ingredients of these medications. Finally, write a two- to three-page paper identifying the pros and cons of taking versus not taking these medications.

2.   Your instructor will divide the class into pairs. Student A counts the number of breaths that student B takes in one minute while in a seated position. Record this number as the resting respiratory rate. Now have student B do a physical exercise for 1 minute. Count the number of breaths student B takes for 1 minute after exercising. Compare the two numbers and discuss why the number of breaths increased dramatically after student B exercised. Now, have student B do this exercise with a mask or scarf that makes breathing more difficult. Compare the experiences of being able to exercise with healthy lungs versus unhealthy lungs.

3.   You and your classmates will each be conducting an interview with someone who uses a tobacco product. Beforehand, brainstorm with your class to come up with questions; the whole class will agree on the final list. As part of the interview, ask the person if he or she has had difficulty quitting. Report your findings to the class.

4.   Research international public health campaigns to stop the use of tobacco products. Identify countries that have the strongest antismoking campaigns and give examples of their strategies.

5.   You are hired by a school department to conduct an antismoking workshop for elementary grade students. Identify three to five activities for this age group that can be in the workshop.

Bibliography and Works Cited

American Academy of Otolaryngology–Head and Neck Surgery. (2016). Tonsils and adenoids. Retrieved from http://www.entnet.org/content/tonsils-and-adenoids

American Academy of Pediatrics. (2016). The dangers of secondhand smoke. *HealthyChildren.org*. Retrieved from https://www.healthychildren.org/English/health-issues/conditions/tobacco/Pages/Dangers-of-Secondhand-Smoke.aspx

American Heart Association. (2015). Smoking: Do you really know the risks? Retrieved from http://www.heart.org/HEARTORG/HealthyLiving/QuitSmoking/QuittingSmoking/Smoking-Do-you-really-know-the-risks_UCM_322718_Article.jsp#

American Lung Association. (2016). Cystic fibrosis. Retrieved from http://www.lung.org/lung-health-and-diseases/lung-disease-lookup/cystic-fibrosis/

Asthma and Allergy Foundation of America. (2016). Asthma. Retrieved from http://www.aafa.org/page/asthma.aspx

Centers for Disease Control and Prevention. (2015). Bronchitis (chest cold). Retrieved from http://www.cdc.gov/getsmart/community/for-patients/common-illnesses/bronchitis.html

Centers for Disease Control and Prevention. (2016a). Chronic obstructive pulmonary disease (COPD). Retrieved from https://www.cdc.gov/copd/index.html

Centers for Disease Control and Prevention. (2016b). Common cold and runny nose. Retrieved from https://www.cdc.gov/getsmart/community/for-patients/common-illnesses/colds.html

Centers for Disease Control and Prevention. (2016c). Influenza (flu). Retrieved from https://www.cdc.gov/flu/index.html

Centers for Disease Control and Prevention. (2016d). Tuberculosis (TB) disease: Symptoms & risk factors. Retrieved from https://www.cdc.gov/Features/TBsymptoms/

Mayo Clinic. (2015). Laryngitis. Retrieved from http://www.mayoclinic.org/diseases-conditions/laryngitis/basics/definition/con-20021565?METHOD=print

National Cancer Institute. (2012). What you need to know about lung cancer. Retrieved from http://www.cancer.gov/publications/patient-education/wyntk-lung-cancer

National Emphysema Foundation. (2016). COPD and emphysema afflict millions. Retrieved from http://www.emphysemafoundation.org/index.php/the-lung/copd-emphysema

National Geographic Society. (2016). Lungs. Retrieved from http://science.nationalgeographic.com/science/health-and-human-body/human-body/lungs-article/

National Heart, Lung, and Blood Institute. (2012). The respiratory system. Retrieved from http://www.nhlbi.nih.gov/health/health-topics/topics/hlw/system

National Heart, Lung, and Blood Institute. (2016a). Explore pneumonia. Retrieved from http://www.nhlbi.nih.gov/health/health-topics/topics/pnu/types.html

National Heart, Lung, and Blood Institute. (2016b). What causes respiratory failure? Retrieved from http://www.nhlbi.nih.gov/health/health-topics/topics/rf/causes

National Institute of Environmental Health Sciences. (2016). Lung diseases. Retrieved from http://www.niehs.nih.gov/health/topics/conditions/lung-disease/index.cfm

National Jewish Health. (2016). Sinusitis: Overview. Retrieved from https://www.nationaljewish.org/healthinfo/conditions/sinusitis/

US National Human Genome Research Institute. (2013). Learning about cystic fibrosis. Retrieved from http://www.genome.gov/10001213

US National Library of Medicine. (2015a). Rapid shallow breathing. *Medline Plus.* Retrieved from https://medlineplus.gov/ency/article/007198.htm

US National Library of Medicine. (2015b). Pharyngitis – sore throat. *Medline Plus.* Retrieved from https://medlineplus.gov/ency/article/000655.htm

CHAPTER 16

THE DIGESTIVE SYSTEM AND RELATED DISEASES

CHAPTER OBJECTIVES

• Describe the structure and function of the digestive system.

• Discuss common diagnostic tests for diseases of the digestive system.

• Explain common signs and symptoms of digestive system diseases.

• Review common diseases of the liver, gallbladder, and pancreas.

• Give examples of differences among hepatitis A, B, and C.

• Identify cancers of the digestive system.

• Summarize the relationship between oral health and overall health.

The digestive system is a series of hollow pipes and more than a half dozen organs that break down food and liquids into smaller nutrients that are absorbed into the body. This system also moves unused waste out of the body. To make nutrients and to move waste are complex processes that also involve the circulatory system. The nutrients from the digestive system are carried by blood throughout the body to nourish cells and provide energy. Digestive system diseases occur when there is a faulty function during digestion.

Function of the Digestive System

With 30 feet of hollow pipes and more than a half dozen organs, the adult digestive system, or gastrointestinal system, manages over a thousand pounds of food each year. In adults, the digestive system processes about three gallons of digested food, liquids, and digestive juices every day. *Digestion* is the process by which food and liquids are broken down into nutrients so that the body can use them to build, nourish, and replace cells and to supply energy to muscles. Digestion also moves waste by separating out unneeded materials and flushing them out of the body.

Gastroenterology is the branch of medicine that studies the function, structure, and diseases of the digestive system. *Gastroenterologists* are physicians with extra training to practice this internal medicine subspecialty.

Structure of the Digestive System

The digestive system is in the abdominal cavity. The *abdominal cavity* is the largest hollow space in the body, between the diaphragm and pelvis, and contains the abdominal organs. The digestive system includes the following:

- Digestive tract
- Gallbladder
- Pancreas
- Liver
- Parts of the nervous and circulatory systems

The *digestive tract,* or gastrointestinal (GI) tract, breaks down food and liquids into essential nutrients and is responsible for absorption. It's a group of hollow organs joined into a long, twisting tube from the mouth to the anus. These organs are the mouth, esophagus, stomach, small intestine, large intestine (or colon), rectum, and anus (see Figure 16.1).

Each organ of the digestive tract has a lining called the *mucosa.* The mucosa has tiny glands that make the juices needed to digest food. The digestive tract also has a layer of muscle that breaks down food and moves it along.

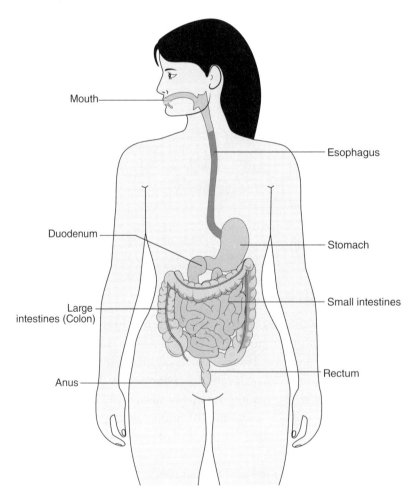

Figure 16.1   Digestive Tract

Note. Adapted from "Tractus Intestinalis Esophagus.svg," by Olek Remesz (wiki-pl: Orem, commons: Orem) (Own work) [CC-BY-SA-2.5-2.0-1.0 (http://creativecommons.org/licenses/by-sa/2.5-2.0-1.0)], via Wikimedia Commons. Retrieved from http://commons.wikimedia.org/wiki/File%3ATractus_intestinalis_esophagus.svg

Digestion begins in the mouth. In the mouth, food and liquids are either cooled or warmed to match body temperature. Food needs to be a mashed-up liquid for the digestive system to break it down into nutrients (e.g., proteins, carbohydrates, and fats). Teeth chew and grind food, while the tongue works it into a ball for swallowing.

Over a quart of saliva is secreted each day by three pairs of salivary glands in the mouth. *Saliva* contains the enzymes that start digestion. The enzymes are secreted not only in the mouth but also at other points along the digestive tract. Digestive enzymes break down food into smaller parts so that the body can absorb it.

The organs of the digestive tract have muscles that move their walls so that food and liquid are forced through the system. Muscle movement forces food and liquid to travel from one organ to the next. The first muscle movement occurs when food or liquid enters the mouth through the lips and is swallowed. Although we start to swallow by choice, once it begins, swallowing becomes automatic and is led by the nerves.

Swallowing pushes chewed food as a small lump into the esophagus. The *esophagus*, a hollow tube 10 inches long, connects the throat above to the stomach below. Where the esophagus and stomach meet, there is a ring-like muscle called a *sphincter,* which closes the passage between the two organs. As food nears the closed sphincter, the sphincter opens, and food passes to the stomach.

The *stomach* is a J-shaped pouch that has three tasks. First, it stores swallowed food and liquid. Second, it produces *gastric juices.* When food enters the stomach, it mixes with gastric juices so that bacteria are killed and proteins are broken down. A thick mucus layer coats the stomach lining and helps keep the acidic gastric juices from dissolving its tissue. Food stays in the stomach for about an hour, during which time it is made into a thick, creamy paste called *chyme.*

The stomach's third task is to empty the chyme slowly into the small intestine. Several factors affect how the stomach empties, including the kind of food. For chyme to leave the stomach, another sphincter at the end of the stomach opens into the *duodenum,* the first part of the small intestine. Most of the digestion of food and liquids takes place in the duodenum, where chyme mixes with more enzymes from the pancreas and with bile, which is produced by the liver. A green-brown juice, *bile* has acids for melting fats into a watery substance. Bile is stored between meals in the *gallbladder,* a pear-shaped sac. At mealtime, it is squeezed out of the gallbladder through tubes. After the chyme leaves the duodenum, it continues through the *small intestine,* a 20-foot tube-shaped organ, where food, liquids, and minerals are absorbed.

The lining of the small intestine has several folds that are covered with millions of tiny finger-like bumps called villi. The *villi* push food molecules, water, and minerals to the linings of the small intestine, where there are specialized cells. These cells help absorbed nutrients cross the small intestine's lining into the bloodstream. Once absorption occurs, nutrients are carried off by the bloodstream to other parts of the body for storage or further chemical change.

Whatever is not digested by the small intestine becomes waste, and it goes into the large intestine. About 5 feet long, the *large intestine, or colon,* surrounds the small intestine like an upside-down U. It stores waste, which is eaten by billions of harmless bacteria and mixed with dead cells. The colon is also where water is absorbed back into the body and feces are formed. *Feces* are mostly water, dietary fiber, undigested food, and other waste. After it is formed, feces are moved into the 5-inch-long *rectum,* where they are stored briefly and removed from the body through the anus by a bowel movement. The *anus* is a ring of muscles and the outer opening of the rectum. The frequency of bowel movements for normal, healthy people usually varies from three per day to three per week.

Other organs of the digestive system are the pancreas, gallbladder, and liver; they make juices that help in digestion. The *pancreas* is located behind the stomach and makes enzymes. These enzymes are pumped into the duodenum through tubes. Another tube also connects the gallbladder, which stores bile, to the duodenum.

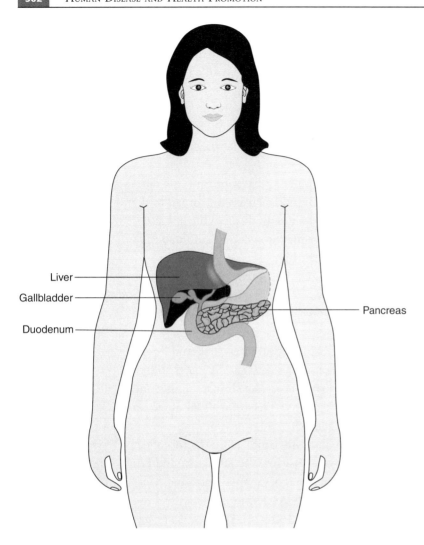

Liver

Gallbladder

Duodenum

Pancreas

Figure 16.2 Liver, Gallbladder, Duodenum, and Pancreas

Note. Adapted from the National Institute of Diabetes and Digestive and Kidney Diseases

The body's main chemical factory is the *liver*, which performs hundreds of different functions (see Figure 16.2). One of the most important functions of the liver is the making of *bile*. Bile mixes with the fat in food. Acids from the bile dissolve fat into the watery contents of the intestine, much as detergents dissolve grease from a frying pan, so that the intestinal and pancreatic enzymes can digest the fat molecules.

Two types of nerves help control the action of the digestive system. *Extrinsic,* or outside, nerves are outside the walls of the digestive organs. They connect the digestive organs to the brain and spinal cord. These nerves release two chemicals: acetylcholine and adrenaline. *Acetylcholine* makes the organ muscles squeeze to push food and liquids through the digestive tract. It also causes the stomach and pancreas to make more digestive juices. *Adrenaline* has the opposite effect. It relaxes the muscles of the stomach and intestine and decreases the flow of blood to these organs, slowing or stopping digestion.

Intrinsic, or inside, nerves are in the walls of the esophagus, stomach, small intestine, and colon. These nerves act when these organs are stretched by food. They release different chemicals that speed up or slow down the movement of food and the production of juices.

Common Symptoms and Diagnostic Tests of the Digestive System

There are many diseases of the digestive system, ranging from mild to serious. The medical term for this area of the body is the *abdomen,* and health care providers describe pain in the area as abdominal pain. The following are common symptoms related to the digestive system:

Symptoms Related to Diseases of the Digestive System

Abdominal pain—pain between the chest and pelvic area; can be dull or sharp cramps

Bloody stool—dark red or black feces

Bloated stomach—feeling full around the abdomen; swelling and cramping

Diarrhea—abnormally frequent and liquid feces

Gas/flatulence—air in the intestine that passes through the anus

Incontinence—inability to control the release of urine or feces

Nausea—feeling sick to the stomach; feeling the need to vomit

Vomiting—forcing what's in the stomach up through the esophagus and out the mouth

Constipation—infrequent bowel movement or difficulty with bowel movement due to dry, hard feces

Heartburn/acid indigestion—burning pain in throat or chest

Common diagnostic tests for diseases of the digestive system discussed in this chapter are listed here. Please refer to these lists in the discussions of symptoms and diagnostic tests:

Common Diagnostic Tests for Diseases of the Digestive System

Endoscopy—procedure using an endoscope to look inside body passageways; if anything looks abnormal, the endoscope has tools at its end that can gather a tissue sample for lab analysis

Colonoscopy—examination of the inside of the colon with an endoscope

Sigmoidoscopy—examination of the inside of the rectum and lower part of the colon with an endoscope

Upper GI endoscopy—examination of the lining of the esophagus and stomach with an endoscope

Barium swallow test—test in which patients drink a liquid containing barium, which coats the lining of the esophagus, stomach, and small intestine; any abnormality in the lining of these organs is revealed and X-rayed

Endoscopic ultrasound (EUS)—ultrasound with a probe put down the throat into the digestive tract; used to see how a cancer has spread or to guide the taking of a tissue sample

Laparoscopy—procedure in which an endoscope is inserted into the abdomen through an incision (cut) to take pictures of organs

Diseases of the Digestive System

Diseases of the digestive system are common, but sometimes people are embarrassed about having one, which makes it difficult to deal with and to talk to others about. This difficulty often leads to suffering in silence. What's more, digestive system diseases are placing a growing health care burden on Americans, causing high numbers of clinic visits and hospitalizations. Treatment, however, can often be as simple as making lifestyle changes or taking over-the-counter medications.

Gastroesophageal Reflux Disease

The sphincter at the end of the esophagus opens to let food pass into the stomach. It then quickly shuts to prevent the return of food and stomach juices back into the esophagus. However, sometimes the sphincter does not close completely and allows stomach juices to leak back into the esophagus. The stomach's juices are acidic and can inflame, destroy, and scar the lining of the esophagus. Once in the esophagus, the juices can flow from the mouth into the lungs. When there are stomach juices in the esophagus, mouth, or lungs, the condition is called *gastroesophageal reflux disease (GERD),* or acid reflux. GERD has many causes, such as caffeine, nicotine, alcohol, and chocolates. Overeating, pregnancy, and certain medications can also cause GERD.

Heartburn or acid indigestion is the most common symptom of GERD. Other symptoms include dry cough, sore throat, hoarseness, and chest and back pain. When stomach juices regularly back up into the esophagus, the condition is referred to as chronic GERD, which causes the eating away of the esophagus lining, resulting in bleeding and scar tissue.

Life-threatening diseases (e.g., cancer) have symptoms similar to those of GERD, so patients with GERD symptoms should seek prompt medical attention. Diagnosis is based on the patient's health history, signs and symptoms, and diagnostic tests, such as a barium swallow test.

Anyone, including infants and children, can have GERD, but it tends to increase with age. In mild cases, patients can manage their symptoms with lifestyle changes, such as avoiding alcohol and tobacco, not eating spicy or fatty foods, eating smaller meals, losing weight if needed, and sleeping with the head raised about 6 inches.

If symptoms persist despite lifestyle changes, then over-the-counter medications can help. In more severe cases, surgery is recommended. If left untreated, GERD leads to more serious health problems, including inflammation of the esophagus, stomach ulcers, and increased risk of esophageal cancer.

Peptic Ulcers

Peptic ulcers (PUs) are open sores that may bleed. If a PU develops in the stomach lining, it is called a *gastric ulcer*; a PU in the duodenum lining is called a *duodenal ulcer*. PUs can also develop in the lining of the esophagus. Eighty percent of PUs are duodenal and occur mostly in men ages 20 to 50.

People can have both gastric and duodenal ulcers at the same time and have more than one ulcer in a lifetime. PUs occur when the acidic digestive juices eat away at the inner lining of the esophagus, stomach, or small intestine.

The most common cause of PUs is infection with the *H. pylori* bacteria. It is not clear how *H. pylori* spreads, but it may be spread by unclean food or water or by close person-to-person contact, such as kissing. The second most common cause of a PU is the long-term and frequent use of pain relievers, including aspirin or ibuprofen. The pain reliever acetaminophen does not cause PU. Other medications that can cause ulcers are those used to treat osteoporosis. It's a myth that spicy foods or a stressful job can cause a PU, but both can make symptoms worse.

A burning stomach pain is the most common symptom of PU. The pain starts between meals or during the night, stops if the patient eats or takes antacids, and lasts from minutes to hours. It can come and go for several days or weeks. Other symptoms of PU include weight loss, bloating, burping, and vomiting. Less often, ulcers cause severe symptoms, such as constant sharp abdominal pain, vomiting of blood, and bloody stools.

The diagnostic tests for PU include those for *H. pylori* infection. *H. pylori* can be detected in a blood test, stool test, or breath test. An endoscopy or biopsy can also identify *H. pylori*.

PU can be cured with treatment that involves antibiotics to kill the *H. pylori* bacteria and other medications that reduce acid level, relieve pain, and encourage healing. Neither antacids nor milk can heal PU, although they can help with symptoms. Surgery is rare and used only if the ulcers do not heal, cause holes, or block food from moving out of the stomach. Surgery removes the ulcers and reduces the amount of acid in the stomach. PUs can be treated successfully, but if not treated, they can lead to internal bleeding, infection, and scar tissue.

Lifestyle changes that relieve symptoms of and prevent PUs include making healthy food choices, managing stress, avoiding tobacco products, and limiting alcohol intake. An important prevention step can be to switch pain relievers. People should always use caution with pain relievers, however, particularly if they are used regularly.

Abdominal Hernia

A *hernia* occurs when an organ or tissue sticks out through an opening into another area where it should not be. This causes a bulge under the skin. There are different types of hernias in various places throughout the body, each requiring a specific treatment. Some people are born with hernias; others develop them later in life. People born with weak abdominal muscles are more likely to get a hernia. Hernias get bigger if a person has weak muscles or increases pressure in the abdomen by straining. The straining can be caused by aging, bowel movements, lifting heavy objects, coughing, obesity, previous surgery, or pregnancy.

Abdominal hernias are the most common type of hernia. They cause some of the intestine to stick out through an opening in the abdominal wall. This can occur in different areas, and the hernia is given a different name depending on the location. The *hiatal hernia* is an example of a common abdominal hernia that occurs mostly in people who are age 50 or older and obese. Hiatal hernias involve the stomach, which slips upward through an opening in the diaphragm and passes into the chest. Digestive juices leak through the diaphragm and reach the esophagus. Unlike other types of hernias, there is no bulge on the outside of the body. When these hernias are small, there usually are few or no symptoms. If they are large, some patients have heartburn, chronic burping, and chest pain.

Health care providers diagnose hernias by conducting a physical examination and health history. There are tests to determine the cause of hernias, including chest X-ray, barium swallow, and endoscopy.

The outlook for a hiatal hernia is good, and most patients do not require treatment. If there are symptoms, then lifestyle changes are needed, such as losing weight if obese and avoiding alcohol or tobacco products. Taking antacids to reduce heartburn also helps some patients. Hiatal hernias are treated successfully with medication and lifestyle changes 85% of the time. If these don't help, then surgery may be needed.

It is difficult to prevent abdominal hernias, but keeping a healthy weight and eating a diet high in fiber reduce risks. Avoiding alcohol and tobacco products as well as activities that cause abdominal strain can also prevent abdominal hernias.

Gastroenteritis and Food Poisoning

Gastroenteritis, or stomach flu, is an inflammation of the lining of the stomach and intestines. Causes range from bacteria, viruses, and parasites to food reactions and unclean water.

Gastroenteritis is not the same as the flu. Real flu affects the respiratory system, and the cause is influenza viruses. Gastroenteritis attacks the stomach and intestines, causing diarrhea, abdominal pain, vomiting, muscle pain, headaches, and fever. If the gastroenteritis is caused by bacteria, then antibiotics can treat the bacterial infection; antibiotics won't work against virus infections. The bacteria that cause gastroenteritis include *E. coli* from food poisoning, and salmonella, which is from improper handling of food.

Viral gastroenteritis, caused by a virus, is the second most common illness in the United States. There are many viruses that cause gastroenteritis, but it is often a *norovirus* infection, a frequent cause of foodborne illness worldwide. Mostly adults are affected by noroviruses. They get these viruses by eating or drinking contaminated food or water or by being in close contact with an infected person. For children, it's usually the *rotavirus* that causes viral gastroenteritis. They get infected when they put their fingers or other objects contaminated with the virus into their mouths. Each gastrointestinal virus has a season when it's most active. In the United States, for example, norovirus and rotavirus infections are more widespread between October and April.

The difference between gastroenteritis and *food poisoning* is that gastroenteritis is an infection in the lining of the stomach and intestines, whereas food poisoning is a bacterial gastroenteritis that is specifically caused by eating food that was not properly cleaned. Food poisoning also refers to chemical food poisoning, such as that caused by eating a poisonous mushroom. In general, gastroenteritis describes what the patient has, and food poisoning describes how the patient got it. Food-borne illnesses, which include food poisoning, sicken about one in six Americans every year, leading to 128,000 hospitalizations and about 3,000 deaths (Centers for Disease Control and Prevention [CDC], 2016a). People who are at risk for gastroenteritis include young children, those who live in close quarters, and anyone with a weakened immune system.

Depending on the cause, gastroenteritis symptoms appear within hours to 3 days after infection and can range from mild to severe. Symptoms usually last a day or two, but can last up to 10 days. The main complication of gastroenteritis is *dehydration,* which is a severe loss of water and salts needed for normal body functions. If dehydration occurs, hospitalization might be needed to replace lost fluids intravenously.

A diagnosis of gastroenteritis is based on symptoms, physical examination, and sometimes a review of similar cases in the community. A stool test can detect rotavirus or norovirus, but not the other viruses that cause gastroenteritis.

There is no treatment for gastroenteritis, so prevention is key. In addition to avoiding contaminated food and water, thorough and frequent hand washing is the best defense. Other ways to prevent gastroenteritis include the following (Mayo Clinic, 2016b):

- Vaccinating children against the rotavirus

- Avoiding close contact with anyone who has gastroenteritis

- Avoiding sharing personal items

- Using only well-sealed bottled drinking water and avoiding raw or undercooked foods (when one is traveling in other countries with high rates of gastroenteritis)

Appendicitis

The *appendix* is a finger-like pouch attached to the large intestine and located in the lower right area of the abdomen (see Figure 16.3). It is not known what the appendix does, but removing it does not seem to affect a person's health.

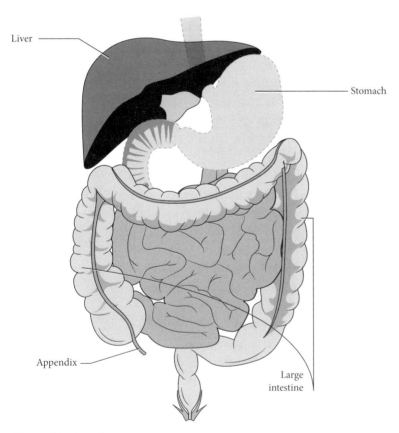

Figure 16.3 Appendix

Note. Adapted from Pearson Scott Foresman [Public Domain], via Wikimedia Commons

When a person has *appendicitis*, germs in the appendix multiply rapidly, causing it to become inflamed and filled with pus. An inflamed appendix bursts if not removed. Bursting spreads infection throughout the abdomen and causes a dangerous condition called *peritonitis.* Appendicitis causes more emergency abdominal surgeries than any other health problem.

The cause of appendicitis is not always clear, but it can develop because of infection or injury to the abdomen. It can also be caused by food waste, parasites, growths, or feces that block the opening of the appendix.

Most patients with appendicitis have sudden abdominal pain that gets worse over time, lasting up to 18 hours. It begins near the belly button and then moves to the lower right. Other symptoms include loss of appetite, vomiting, constipation or diarrhea, fever, and abdominal swelling.

Appendicitis is a medical emergency and requires quick diagnosis and treatment so that the appendix does not burst. A health care provider diagnoses appendicitis by taking a patient's health history and conducting a physical examination. Laboratory and imaging tests are used to confirm appendicitis if a person does not have

abdominal pain. If a patient has severe abdominal pain, then a surgical procedure called an *appendectomy* may be needed. Nonsurgical treatment may be used if surgery is not available or if the diagnosis is unclear. Nonsurgical treatment includes antibiotics to treat infection and a diet low in fiber until the infection goes away.

Those between the ages of 10 and 30 are most at risk for appendicitis. With adequate care, patients can recover from appendicitis and not need to make lifestyle changes. Full recovery from surgery takes about 4 to 6 weeks.

Diverticulosis and Diverticulitis

As people age, small pouches called *diverticula* form along the wall of the colon and stick outward, causing *diverticulosis*. In the United States, the majority of Americans over age 60 have diverticulosis.

Most people with diverticulosis have few or no symptoms, and often learn that they have it only through tests ordered for something else, such as a screening colonoscopy. If there are symptoms, they are mild cramps, constipation, or diarrhea. Diverticulosis is diagnosed with a colonoscopy. Treatment includes a high-fiber diet and anticramping drugs to relieve symptoms.

When diverticulosis is associated with inflamed or infected pouches, then it is called *diverticulitis*. The most common symptom of diverticulitis is abdominal pain, and there is sometimes fever, vomiting, cramping, and constipation. When serious, diverticulitis leads to bleeding and blockages. To make a diagnosis, a health care provider performs a physical examination and imaging tests. Treatment includes antibiotics, pain relievers, and a liquid diet. A serious case may require surgery.

Crohn's Disease

Crohn's disease is one of a group of diseases called *inflammatory bowel disease (IBD)*. IBD is a general term for different diseases that cause inflammation in the digestive tract. *Crohn's disease* is one of the most common IBDs. Crohn's affects any area from the mouth to the anus, but it mostly affects where the small and large intestine meet. Crohn's inflames all the layers of the intestinal wall. In turn, this inflammation leads to ulcers and bleeding (see Figure 16.4). It also prevents the intestine from absorbing nutrients from food.

There are 700,000 people in the United States who suffer from Crohn's disease, and about 8,000 new cases are diagnosed every year (Crohn's and Colitis Foundation of America, 2016a). It commonly starts between the ages of 13 and 30, with most people getting the disease in their 20s. Crohn's affects males or females equally. African Americans are less at risk for the disease; people of Jewish descent are at more risk.

The causes of Crohn's disease are not well understood. Diet and stress aggravate Crohn's, but they do not cause it. Crohn's may be due to a virus or parasite that triggers an abnormal immune system reaction, causing the digestive tract to overreact. That is why Crohn's is described as a disease of both the digestive and immune systems.

Crohn's is more common in those who have family members with the disease, so heredity may play a role. However, most people with Crohn's have no family history of the disease. Environmental factors like living in an urban area or in northern climates may play a role in developing Crohn's.

Signs and symptoms range from mild to severe and can develop gradually or come on suddenly, without warning. There are long periods of having no signs and symptoms. But even a mild case of Crohn's is difficult to ignore. The most common symptoms are abdominal pain and bloody diarrhea. Other symptoms include frequent bowel movements (up to 20 a day), weight loss, fever, fatigue, dehydration, and ulcers. Other areas that can become inflamed include the eyes, skin, and joints.

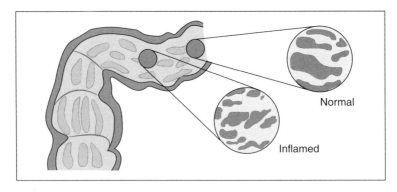

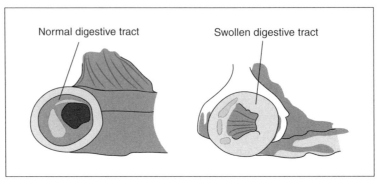

Figure 16.4 Crohn's Disease
Top: In Crohn's disease, parts of the digestive tract become inflamed and scarred.
Bottom: When scar tissue builds up, the passage can become narrow.
Note. Adapted from the National Institute of Diabetes and Digestive and Kidney Diseases

Crohn's can cause complications, such as intestinal blockages and anemia. Children with the disease can have growth problems.

Crohn's disease is not the same in everyone. Some patients have severe pain and frequent diarrhea. Others have only occasional diarrhea and little pain. Those who smoke have worse symptoms and are more likely to need surgery than nonsmokers with Crohn's. Eating well, getting enough rest, and learning to manage stress can lessen symptoms.

Because it is similar to other digestive tract problems, Crohn's often goes undiagnosed. The health care provider diagnoses Crohn's with a physical examination, health history, lab tests, imaging tests, and a colonoscopy. Because Crohn's has a range of signs and symptoms, there is no single test used for diagnosis.

There is no cure for Crohn's and no one treatment plan for all patients. Treatment goals are to decrease the inflammation, relieve symptoms, and correct nutritional problems. Medications, nutritional supplements, and sometimes surgery to repair or remove affected portions of the digestive tract can be part of a treatment plan. About 70% of people with Crohn's eventually require surgery. Up to 60% of patients who have surgery will have symptoms again within 10 years (Crohn's and Colitis Foundation of America, 2016a).

Ulcerative Colitis

Ulcerative colitis (UC) is another type of IBD and is a result of an abnormal immune system response. It is an inflammation of the lining of the colon and rectum. The disease starts in the rectum and spreads to the colon, or it starts in the colon. UC causes ulcers to form in the lining of the colon.

With UC, there is usually a series of symptoms that often get worse and then a period of no symptoms. Its main symptom is frequent episodes of bloody diarrhea, which can last for weeks.

Although UC usually is not fatal, it is a serious disease that causes life-threatening health problems, such as colon cancer.

No one is sure what triggers UC, but the digestive tract becomes inflamed when the immune system overresponds to a virus or bacteria. Researchers no longer believe that stress is the main cause, although stress can often worsen symptoms.

UC tends to develop in those ages 15 to 30. About 1.4 million Americans have been diagnosed with UC, and it affects about the same number of women and men. The following are risk factors for UC (Crohn's and Colitis Foundation of America, 2016b):

- *Age.* UC usually begins before the age of 30.
- *Race or ethnicity.* Those of Jewish descent have the highest risk.
- *Family health history.* Although most patients with UC have no family history of this disease, risk is higher if a close family member has it.

Major symptoms for UC include abdominal pain, bloody stools, and diarrhea. Additional symptoms are ulcers, weight loss, and fever. About half of UC patients have only mild symptoms, whereas others have more severe, frequent attacks that require hospitalization.

UC is diagnosed with a physical examination and health history along with a colonoscopy. A biopsy determines the presence of ulcers and other symptoms. Stool tests detect a virus or bacteria, and blood tests detect anemia, a complication of UC.

The treatment goals for UC are to control and to prevent attacks as well as to help the colon heal. Treatments include anti-inflammatory medication, bland diet, and surgery. Surgery is used as a last resort, but it will cure UC and lessen the risk of colon cancer. It requires the entire removal of the colon, including the rectum. After surgery, an opening in the abdominal wall is made that connects the small intestine to the anus for bowel function.

There are possible complications with UC if left untreated, including severe bleeding and an increased risk of colon cancer. Due to the high risk of colon cancer associated with UC, a risk that increases each decade after UC is diagnosed, colon cancer screening with a colonoscopy is recommended. Because the cause of UC is unknown, means of preventing it are also unknown.

The differences between Crohn's disease and ulcerative colitis can be difficult to understand. The two diseases share many symptoms, but are treated differently medically and surgically. The diagnosis of one rather than the other remains difficult. At times, a final diagnosis is possible only after treatment makes the type of disease obvious. The following list outlines the general differences between Crohn's disease and ulcerative colitis:

Differences Between Crohn's Disease and Ulcerative Colitis

Crohn's Disease	Ulcerative Colitis
Happens anywhere between the mouth and the anus	Limited to the colon
Healthy parts of the intestine in between inflamed areas	Continuous inflammation of the colon
Affects all the linings of the colon	Affects only the innermost lining of the colon

Irritable Bowel Syndrome

Irritable bowel syndrome (IBS) is a disturbance in the functioning of the digestive tract. It causes problems with bowel movements. IBS is not a disease but a syndrome (a group of symptoms). IBS occurs when muscles in the colon contract faster or slower than normal. This causes chronic abdominal pain, gassiness or bloating, and diarrhea. Other symptoms of IBS include constipation, mucus in the stool, and the feeling of incompletely passing stools.

IBS is different from inflammatory bowel disease (IBD). It has some symptoms in common with IBD, but the two conditions involve very different treatments. For example, IBS does not cause the destructive inflammation found in IBD, so in many ways it is a less serious health problem. Patients with IBS are not at higher risk for colon cancer, and they seldom require hospitalization or surgery.

One in six adults in the United States—twice as many women as men—has IBS. It affects people of all ages, most often at times of emotional stress. IBS is so common in the United States that it is one of the top ten most frequently diagnosed health problems (International Foundation for Functional Gastrointestinal Disorders, 2015).

The cause of IBS is not fully understood. Sometimes it arises after an infection in the intestines, but there may be other triggers. IBS was once thought to be caused by stress, but now it is believed that IBS is caused by the interaction between the brain and the digestive tract.

The colon reacts to the information it receives from the nerves by contracting its muscles and secreting fluids. Patients with IBS have irregular patterns of colon muscle contraction. The term "irritable" is used because the nerves that control the muscles are unusually sensitive and active. Ordinary stimulation—eating, stress, hormonal changes, or medications—can trigger a response in patients with IBS that causes spasms. Sometimes spasms slow the bowel movement and cause constipation. At other times, spasms can cause diarrhea. Spasms can also cause other symptoms, such as cramps and bloating. The discomfort from spasms is often relieved with a bowel movement.

Symptoms commonly occur after the patient eats a large meal, or they may be stress related. There can be times when symptoms flare up as well as periods when they disappear. Patients with IBS are more likely to have other functional disorders, such as chronic fatigue syndrome, or psychological symptoms of anxiety and depression.

A diagnosis of IBS requires a health history and physical examination. Diagnostic tools such as blood and stool tests, endoscopy, X-rays, and psychological tests are helpful to rule out other diseases.

IBS treatment targets the symptoms, but choosing a treatment can be difficult because people have different symptoms. The first line of treatment for IBS is education for mild cases, with symptoms managed by dietary changes and stress management techniques. Although stress does not cause IBS, it can worsen symptoms, so stress management can be helpful. Medications can relieve symptoms in more severe cases. IBS may be a lifelong condition for some patients, but it does not cause permanent damage to the intestines, and it does not lead to more serious diseases (e.g., cancer).

Hemorrhoids

One of the most common anal problems is hemorrhoids. *Hemorrhoids* are swollen and inflamed veins around the anus or in the lower rectum. There are two types of hemorrhoids: external and internal. External hemorrhoids are located under the skin around the anus; blood clots form and cause bleeding, swelling, or a hard lump around the anus. When the blood clot dissolves, extra skin is left behind. This skin can become irritated or itch.

Internal hemorrhoids develop in the lower rectum and stick out through the anus. The most common symptom of internal hemorrhoids is bright red blood on the stool, on toilet paper, or in the toilet bowl after a bowel movement.

Hemorrhoids are not dangerous, but they often cause pain, discomfort, and anal itching. Some people with hemorrhoids never have symptoms; for others, symptoms go away within a few days. Most hemorrhoids shrink back inside the rectum on their own, but severe hemorrhoids stick out permanently and require treatment.

About 75% of adults in the United States have hemorrhoids at some point in their lives. Hemorrhoids are common among adults ages 45 to 65 and among pregnant women (American Society of Colon and Rectal Surgeons, 2016). Risk factors for hemorrhoids include chronic constipation or diarrhea, straining during bowel movements, sitting on the toilet too long, and lack of fiber in the diet. Another factor is the weakening of tissue in the rectum and anus that can occur with age. Pregnancy can also cause hemorrhoids by increasing pressure in the abdomen, which enlarges the veins in the lower rectum and anus.

The health care provider performs a physical examination to look for hemorrhoids in a patient. Additional tests include colonoscopy, sigmoidoscopy, or a barium swallow test.

Eating a high-fiber diet and taking a fiber supplement can relieve symptoms. Other helpful changes include drinking more water, exercising, and not straining during bowel movements. Ointments can relieve pain and itching, but these should be used for only a short time because they can damage skin. Large hemorrhoids that do not respond to treatment can be surgically removed.

Hepatitis

Hepatitis is the inflammation of the liver and is usually caused by a virus. Heavy alcohol use, toxins, some medications, and certain diseases can also be the cause. Hepatitis can be acute (lasting less than 6 months) or chronic (lasting 6 months and longer). *Viral hepatitis*, caused by a virus, is the leading cause of liver cancer and the main reason for liver transplantation. According to the CDC (2016b), over four million Americans are living with chronic hepatitis; unfortunately, most do not know they are infected. There are several types of viral hepatitis, but this chapter's discussion is limited to the more widespread types: hepatitis A, hepatitis B, and hepatitis C (see Table 16.1).

Hepatitis A is caused by the hepatitis A virus (HAV). It is the least serious type of hepatitis and spreads when infected feces matter enters the mouth. HAV is common and usually spreads by direct personal contact and by having contact with objects handled by the infected person. People can have the HAV infection for 2 to 3 weeks before they feel sick, meaning that they can infect others without knowing.

Most healthy people who have HAV recover within a month or two. There is no cure and no treatment for HAV other than bed rest, no alcohol, and medication to help relieve symptoms. HAV never becomes chronic, and once a person has had it, he or she becomes immune to future infection.

More serious is *hepatitis B,* which is caused by the hepatitis B virus (HBV). It is serious because HBV causes lifelong chronic infection and severe liver problems. HBV is about a hundred times more contagious than HIV/AIDS. The virus is spread when blood and bodily fluids (e.g., sweat, tears, saliva, semen, and vaginal secretions) from an infected person enter the body of someone who is not protected. HBV is not spread by food or water as HAV is, but through sexual contact, kissing, shared toothbrushes, tattooing, body piercing, acupuncture, and sharing needles or needle sticks, or from an infected mother to her baby during birth. People can be infected with the HBV up to 6 months before having symptoms, meaning that they can infect others during that time without knowing. Anyone can get HBV, and in the United States every year, there are about 200,000 new cases and about 5,000 HBV-related deaths (CDC, 2016c).

Most people infected with HBV recover in a few months, and after infection, they become immune to the virus. About 10%, however, become carriers of the virus and can infect others for the rest of their lives even though they may have no symptoms. There are about one million carriers of HBV in the United States (CDC, 2016c).

Hepatitis C is caused by the hepatitis C virus (HCV) and is the most widespread blood-borne infection in the United States (CDC, 2016d). At first, a person develops an acute infection, with

Table 16.1   Comparison of Hepatitis A, B, and C

Hepatitis	A (HAV)	B (HBV)	C (HCV)
How is it spread?	Ingestion of fecal matter from • Close contact with an infected person • Sexual contact with an infected person • Contaminated foods or drinks	Contact with infected blood and body fluids from • Mother to baby • Sexual contact • Sharing needles or needle sticks	Contact with blood and body fluids of an infected person from • Sharing needles or needle sticks Less common: • Sexual contact • Mother to baby
Symptoms of acute infection	Symptoms of all types of viral hepatitis are similar and can include one or more of the following: • Fever • Fatigue • Loss of appetite • Nausea • Vomiting • Abdominal pain • Jaundice		
Persons at risk	• Travelers to regions with HAV • Sex partners of infected persons • Household members of infected persons	• Infants born to infected mothers • Sex partners of infected persons • Injection drug users • Household contacts of infected persons • Health care workers exposed to blood on the job • Travelers to regions with HBV	• Injection drug users • HIV-infected persons • Infants born to infected mothers
Chronic infection	No chronic disease	10% chronic Can cause: • Liver damage • Cirrhosis • Liver cancer	85% chronic Can cause: • Liver damage • Cirrhosis • Liver cancer
Vaccine	Yes	Yes	No
Outcome	Most with acute disease recover with no lasting liver damage; rarely fatal.	Most with acute disease recover with no lasting liver damage; acute is rarely fatal. Chronically infected patients can develop chronic liver disease.	Acute is uncommon. Up to 70% of chronically infected patients develop chronic liver disease.

Note. Adapted from Centers for Disease Control and Prevention, 2016b, 2016c, 2016d

symptoms that can range from mild to severe. For reasons not known, up to 25% of people get rid of the virus without treatment. The rest who become infected with HCV develop a lifelong chronic infection that leads to severe liver problems. HCV usually spreads when blood from an infected person enters the body of someone not infected. Most people become infected by sharing needles to inject drugs. Having sexually transmitted diseases or HIV, or engaging in sex with multiple partners can also increase the risk.

HCV infection occurs in about 25% of people who are HIV-positive. What is even more alarming is that out of those who are HIV-positive and are injection drug users, the infection rate rises from 25% up to 90% (CDC, 2016d). An estimated 3.2 million people in the United States have chronic HCV, and most are unaware of their infection. Each year, about 17,000 Americans become infected and about 12,000 die from HCV-related liver diseases. There is no cure for HCV, although medication relieves symptoms.

Viral hepatitis symptoms are similar no matter whether the hepatitis is an A, B, or C type. These symptoms include jaundice, or yellowing of the skin and whites of the eyes; fever; lack of appetite; feeling tired; dark urine; abdominal pain; diarrhea; and nausea.

Blood tests are used to diagnose viral hepatitis. Liver function tests determine if the liver is damaged; sometimes, a liver biopsy is done to check for organ damage. Ultrasounds can check for any progress toward cancer, especially in cases of chronic HBV and HCV infection.

The best way to prevent HAV and HBV infection is to get vaccinated; however, there is no vaccine to prevent HCV infection. Besides vaccines, ways to prevent viral hepatitis include the following (CDC, 2016b, 2016c, 2016d):

- Washing hands after using the bathroom and before fixing food or eating
- Using latex condoms
- Avoiding tap water when traveling
- Not getting tattoos, body piercings, or acupuncture from an unlicensed setting
- Not sharing needles to inject drugs
- Not sharing personal items

Cirrhosis

Cirrhosis is the scarring of healthy tissue in the liver; when the whole liver is scarred, it then shrinks and gets hard. Scar tissue cannot do what healthy liver tissue does, which is to make protein, help fight infections, clean the blood, help digest food, and store energy.

Cirrhosis is caused by chronic liver diseases that damage liver tissue (see Figure 16.5). It takes years for liver damage to lead to cirrhosis, but once the liver is damaged, cirrhosis is permanent.

Cirrhosis occurs twice as frequently in males as in females; chronic alcoholism is the leading cause of cirrhosis in the United States (American Liver Foundation, 2016). The amount of alcohol that causes cirrhosis is different for each person. Chronic hepatitis C is the second leading cause of cirrhosis in the

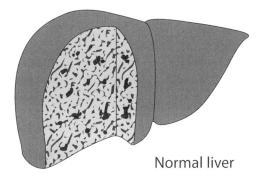

Normal liver

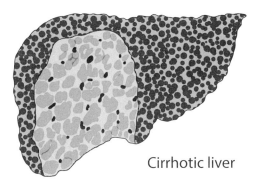

Cirrhotic liver

Figure 16.5 Cirrhosis

Stages of liver damage leading to cirrhosis

Note. Adapted from the National Institute of Diabetes and Digestive and Kidney Diseases

United States. Hepatitis C causes the liver to swell, which over time leads to cirrhosis. About one in four people with chronic hepatitis C develops cirrhosis. Other causes include chronic hepatitis B, obesity, malnutrition, toxins, and congestive heart failure.

There are usually no symptoms of cirrhosis in its early stage. Yet over time, cirrhosis causes many symptoms, including abdominal pain, itching, swelling, nausea, and weight loss. Some of the complications from cirrhosis include jaundice, gallstones, bruising, and bleeding easily. There can also be fluid buildup along with painful swelling of the legs and abdomen, as well as mental confusion. If left untreated, cirrhosis eventually leads to death.

Cirrhosis is diagnosed by a review of the symptoms, blood tests, health history, and physical examination. A liver biopsy checks how much of the liver has been damaged.

Treatment for cirrhosis depends on the cause and the degree of liver damage. The goals of treatment are to prevent further liver damage and reduce complications. Depending on the disease that is causing cirrhosis, medications or lifestyle changes are part of treatment. When cirrhosis cannot be treated, then a liver transplant is needed.

It is possible to prevent further liver damage with proper management of cirrhosis. Ways to manage cirrhosis include having a healthy lifestyle, limiting salt intake, stopping drinking alcohol, practicing safe sex, and not sharing needles or personal items with others.

Gallstones

Gallstones are small, pebble-like substances that develop in the gallbladder where bile is stored. They look like stones and can be as small as a grain of sand or as large as a golf ball. The gallbladder can develop just one large stone, hundreds of tiny stones, or a combination of the two.

There are two types of gallstones, but about 80% of the stones are cholesterol. Cholesterol stones are yellow-green and are made mostly of hard cholesterol (see Figure 16.6).

If gallstones travel from the gallbladder, they block the passageway and, therefore, the normal flow of bile to the small intestine. Bile then builds up in the passageway and causes inflammation. If this happens, it causes severe, steady pain in the upper right abdomen and upper back. The pain starts suddenly and lasts anywhere from minutes to several hours. Other symptoms include fever, jaundice, vomiting, and sweating. These symptoms combined are referred to as a *gallbladder attack*, and an attack can occur more than once over weeks, months, or even years. Some people have attacks that are

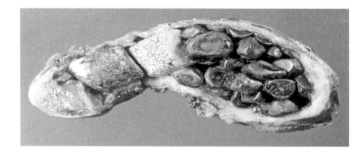

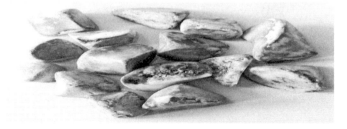

Figure 16.6 Cholesterol Gallstones

Note. From the National Institute of Diabetes and Digestive and Kidney Diseases so severe that they last more than several hours. When this happens, the condition is referred to as *acute cholecystitis* and can lead to infection. Acute cholecystitis requires hospitalization for observation and treatment that often includes surgery.

Many people with gallstones have no symptoms, however. Often the gallstones are found when a test is performed for some other problem. These "silent gallstones" are not likely to cause symptoms, and there is no treatment.

Gallstones affect well over 25 million people in the United States. Nearly one million new cases of gallstones are diagnosed every year. According to the National Institutes of Health (2015), gallstones are found most often in:

- Women over 20 years of age, pregnant women, and men over 60 years of age
- Overweight or obese people
- People who have rapid weight loss
- Patients who use birth control pills, cholesterol-lowering drugs, and certain other medications
- Native Americans
- Hispanics of Mexican origin

To diagnose gallstones, the health care provider conducts a physical examination, health history, and routine blood tests. Other diagnostic tests include abdominal ultrasound.

Once a patient has one gallstone attack, there is about a 70% chance of having another one. Many health care providers suggest surgery to remove the gallbladder to prevent future attacks. The surgery is safe, patients generally do well, and it is effective. Without surgery, the gallbladder might burst open, causing more problems.

Pancreatitis

The pancreas secretes digestive enzymes into the small intestine to help digest fats, proteins, and carbohydrates. Normally, digestive enzymes do not become active until they reach the small intestine, where they begin digestion. If these enzymes are active inside the pancreas, however, they start eating the pancreas itself, causing inflammation.

There are two types of pancreatitis. *Acute pancreatitis* is sudden inflammation of the pancreas that lasts for a short time. Some patients have more than one attack, but they can recover fully after each one. Most cases of acute pancreatitis in the United States are due to gallstones or heavy alcohol use. An estimated 50,000 to 80,000 cases of acute pancreatitis occur in the United States each year. The disease occurs more often in women than in men and usually after age 40 (National Pancreas Foundation, 2014).

Acute pancreatitis begins with severe, constant pain in the upper abdomen that lasts for a few days. Other symptoms include swollen abdomen, nausea, vomiting, and fever. Diagnosis is based on a physical examination as well as blood and urine tests. Treatment may include a hospital stay for intravenous (IV) fluids, antibiotics, and pain medication. If there is no damage to other organs, then acute pancreatitis usually improves on its own. However, some patients have acute pancreatitis that is severe. These patients develop heart, lung, or kidney failure. In the most severe cases, bleeding occurs in the pancreas, leading to shock and sometimes death.

Chronic pancreatitis does not improve and leads to a slow destruction of the pancreas. It is usually caused by heavy alcohol use. Symptoms include nausea, vomiting, weight loss, and oily stools. Treatment may include a hospital stay for IV fluids, pain medications, and nutritional support. After that, the patient may need to take enzyme medication and follow a special diet. It is also important not to smoke or drink alcohol. The prognosis is better if pancreatitis is caused by gallstones than if it is related to alcoholism.

Malabsorption Syndrome

Malabsorption syndrome occurs when the small intestine has difficulty absorbing vitamins and nutrients from food. Many diseases, including HIV/AIDS, cause malabsorption syndrome, as do certain medications, surgeries, and lactose intolerance. A person with *lactose intolerance* cannot digest foods with lactose, the sugar found in milk and in foods made with milk.

The symptoms of malabsorption syndrome include fatigue, weight loss, bloating, diarrhea, and abdominal pain. Because fat is not absorbed in the intestines, feces look fatty and pale and have a foul smell.

Diagnosis and treatment depend on the specific disease causing the malabsorption syndrome. Diagnostic tests include physical examination as well as blood, stool, and urine tests. For treatment, the patient's diet is controlled, and he or she takes vitamin and nutritional supplements. Possible complications from chronic malabsorption are anemia, gallstones, and malnutrition. Malnutrition develops when the body does not get the vitamins, minerals, and other nutrients it needs to stay healthy.

Cancers of the Digestive System

Cancers of the digestive system account for about 20% of all cancers. If you add up all the cancers of the digestive system, the number of new cases totals more than 250,000 annually. These cancers also cause 1.5 million deaths per year (National Cancer Institute, 2016a). Given the number of different cancers of the digestive system, this section is divided into two parts. The first part gives an overview of colorectal cancer; the second part is limited to key points about the less widespread cancers of the esophagus, liver, and pancreas.

Colorectal cancer starts in the colon or the rectum. These cancers are also referred to separately as *colon cancer* or *rectal cancer*, depending on where they start. Colorectal cancer is the fourth most common cancer in the United States. In 2015, about 143,000 Americans were diagnosed with this cancer, and it affected men and women equally (National Cancer Institute, 2016a). Colorectal cancer is more common in people over 50, and the risk increases with age. Deaths from colorectal cancer have fallen in the past decade due to earlier screening along with better treatments, but the cause is still unknown.

A person is more at risk for colorectal cancer if there are *polyps,* which are growths inside the colon and rectum. Most polyps are not cancerous, but some do become cancer. A family history of colorectal cancer puts a person at higher risk, as does inflammatory bowel disease. Symptoms include bloody or narrow stools, a change in bowel habits, weight loss, and abdominal pain. Everyone who is 50 or older should be screened for colorectal cancer. The most thorough examination of the colon is a colonoscopy.

Standard treatments include surgery, chemotherapy, radiation therapy, or a combination. Treatment depends partly on the stage of the cancer. At the earliest stage, colorectal cancer is treated with surgery, often during a colonoscopy. Surgery can usually cure the cancer when it is found early. For later stages, more complicated surgery is needed, as well as chemotherapy and radiation.

Cancer of the esophagus, or esophageal cancer, is found in the lower part of the esophagus, near the stomach. When it spreads, it travels from the esophagus to other parts of the body, such as the liver or lungs. Cancer of the esophagus may be related to having GERD, using tobacco products, heavy alcohol use, or obesity. In addition, certain groups—men, the elderly, and African Americans—are at greater risk for esophageal cancer.

Primary *liver cancer* starts in the liver. Metastatic liver cancer starts somewhere else and spreads to the liver. Risk factors for liver cancer include having hepatitis B or C, heavy alcohol use, cirrhosis, obesity, and diabetes. Symptoms include a lump or pain on the right side of the abdomen and jaundice. However, symptoms may not appear until the cancer is advanced, making it harder to treat.

The cause of *cancer of the pancreas, or pancreatic cancer,* is unknown. It is more common in people with diabetes or chronic pancreatitis, smokers, and those with a family history of the disease. Pancreatic cancer is slightly more common in women than in men. The risk increases with age. Because pancreatic cancer is often advanced when first diagnosed, few cancer tumors can be removed by surgery. In more than 80% of patients, the tumors have spread and cannot be completely removed at the time of diagnosis. Ninety-five percent of the people diagnosed with this cancer will not be alive 5 years later (National Cancer Institute, 2016d).

Final Note: Benefits of Good Oral Health

The relationship between good oral health and a healthy body might not be obvious. However, proper flossing and brushing and professional teeth cleaning help those with chronic diseases and help ward off infection. A healthy mouth and healthy body go hand in hand. Good oral health does improve overall health and reduces the risks for serious diseases. The following are examples of why having good oral health is important to overall health:

- Tooth decay and gum disease are associated not only with an unsightly mouth but also with chronic bad breath. It is much easier to eat properly, get restful sleep, and concentrate without aching teeth.

- Chronic inflammation from gum disease has been associated with cardiovascular problems, such as heart disease and stroke.

- Poor oral health is linked to infections in other parts of the body.

- People with uncontrolled diabetes often have severe gum disease. Having diabetes can make it difficult to fight off infection and puts a person at risk for gum disease. With infection, a diabetic will find it more difficult to control blood glucose levels.

- Women may experience increased gum disease during pregnancy. Some research evidence suggests a relationship between gum disease and preterm, low-birth-weight infants.

Chapter Summary

- The digestive system is a series of hollow pipes and organs that break down food and liquids into nutrients that are absorbed into the body. This system also moves unused waste out of the body.

- Digestion is the process in which food and liquids are broken down into essential nutrients so that the body can use them to build, nourish, and replace cells as well as supply energy to muscles. Digestion also moves waste by separating out unneeded materials and flushing them out of the body.

- Crohn's disease and ulcerative colitis are part of a disease group called inflammatory bowel disease (IBD). IBD is a general term given to different diseases that cause inflammation in the digestive tract.

- Irritable bowel syndrome is different from inflammatory bowel disease. It has some symptoms in common with IBD, but the two conditions involve very different treatments.

- Viral hepatitis is the leading cause of liver cancer and the most common reason for liver transplantation. Over four million Americans are living with chronic hepatitis, and most do not know they are infected.

- Cancers of the digestive system account for about 20% of all cancers. If you add up all the cancers of the digestive system, the number of new cases totals more than 250,000 annually. These cancers cause 1.5 million deaths per year.

- Good oral hygiene, including proper flossing and brushing and professional teeth cleaning, helps those with chronic diseases and helps wards off infection.

REVIEW QUESTIONS

1. Explain the differences between the digestive system's extrinsic and intrinsic nerves.

2. List and describe common symptoms of digestive system diseases.

3. List and describe common diagnostic tests for digestive system diseases.

4. Compare and contrast hepatitis A, B, and C.

5. What are the causes of a hernia?

6. What is the purpose of a screening colonoscopy?

7. What are hemorrhoids, and what causes them?

8. What is the function of the gallbladder?

9. How does oral health affect the overall health of the body?

10. What is the difference between gastric and peptic ulcers?

KEY TERMS

Abdomen: Medical term for stomach

Abdominal cavity: The largest hollow space in the body, which contains the abdominal organs

Abdominal hernia: Condition in which some of the intestines stick out through an opening in the abdominal wall

Acetylcholine: Chemical that helps organs push food and liquids through the digestive tract

Acute cholecystitis: Severe gallbladder attack causing the gallbladder to be even more inflamed

Acute pancreatitis: Sudden inflammation of the pancreas that lasts for a short time

Adrenaline: Chemical that relaxes stomach and intestine muscles to slow or stop digestion

Anus: Ring of muscles that leads to the outer opening of the rectum

Appendectomy: Surgical removal of the appendix

Appendicitis: Condition in which the appendix becomes inflamed and fills with pus

Appendix: Finger-like pouch attached to the large intestine

Bile: Fluid made in the liver that has acids for melting fats

Cancer of the esophagus, or esophageal cancer: Cancer cells that are found in the esophagus

Cancer of the pancreas, or pancreatic cancer: Cancer cells that start in the pancreas

Chronic pancreatitis: Inflammation of the pancreas that does not improve

Chyme: Partially digested food that stays in the stomach for about an hour and is turned into thick and creamy paste

Cirrhosis: Scarring of the liver

Colon cancer: Cancer that starts in the colon

Colorectal cancer: Cancer that starts in the colon or the rectum

Crohn's disease: Inflammatory bowel disease that inflames all the layers of the intestinal wall

Dehydration: Severe loss of water and salts needed for normal body functions

Digestion: The process by which food and liquids are broken down into essential nutrients

Digestive system: A series of hollow pipes and more than a half dozen organs that (a) break down food and liquids into nutrients that are absorbed into the body and (b) move unused waste out of the body

Digestive tract: Group of hollow organs that break down food and liquids into nutrients and are responsible for absorption

Diverticula: Small pouches that form along the wall of the colon

Diverticulitis: Inflammation of the diverticula, usually when diverticulosis is present

Diverticulosis: Condition in which the diverticula stick outward

Duodenal ulcer: Peptic ulcer in the duodenum

Duodenum: Sphincter at the end of the stomach, and the first part of the small intestine

Esophagus: Long, hollow tube that connects the throat above with the stomach below

Extrinsic nerves: Nerves outside the digestive organs that help control the digestive system

Feces: Water, undigested food, and other waste

Food poisoning: Bacterial gastroenteritis caused by eating certain foods or chemicals

Gallbladder: Organ that stores bile

Gallbladder attack: Condition that arises when gallstones get stuck in a passageway to the small intestine, causing pain, fever, jaundice, vomiting, and sweating

Gallstones: Small, pebble-like substances that develop in the gallbladder

Gastric juices: Fluids produced by the stomach to help kill bacteria and break down proteins

Gastric ulcer: Peptic ulcer in the stomach

Gastroenteritis: Inflammation of the lining of the stomach and intestines

Gastroenterologist: Physician with extra training to practice the internal medicine subspecialty of gastroenterology

Gastroenterology: Branch of medicine that studies the function, structure, and diseases of the digestive system

Gastroesophageal reflux disease (GERD): Disease caused by the flow of stomach juices into the esophagus, mouth, or lungs

Hemorrhoids: Swollen and inflamed veins around the anus or in the lower rectum

Hernia: Condition in which an organ or tissue sticks out through an opening into another area where it shouldn't be and causes a bulge under the skin

Hepatitis A: Inflammation of the liver caused by hepatitis A virus (HAV)

Hepatitis B: Inflammation of the liver caused by the hepatitis B virus (HBV)

Hepatitis C: Inflammation of the liver caused by the hepatitis C virus (HCV)

Hiatal hernia: Condition in which part of the stomach slips upward through an opening in the diaphragm and passes into the chest

Inflammatory bowel disease (IBD): General term given to a group of diseases that cause inflammation in the digestive tract

Intrinsic nerves: Nerves in the walls of the esophagus, stomach, small intestine, and colon that help control the digestive system

Irritable bowel syndrome: Problems in the function of the digestive tract that cause problems with bowel movements

Lactose intolerance: The inability to digest foods with lactose, the sugar found in milk and in foods made with milk

Large intestine, or colon: Organ that stores waste, absorbs water back into the body, and forms feces

Liver: The organ that is the body's main chemical factory and performs hundreds of different functions, including making bile and breaking down unwanted chemicals (e.g., alcohol)

Liver cancer: Cancer cells that start in the liver

Malabsorption syndrome: Condition in which the small intestine has difficulty absorbing nutrients

Mucosa: Lining of the digestive tract organs

Norovirus: Viral infection that adults often get from eating or drinking contaminated food or water or from close contact with an infected person

Pancreas: An organ that makes enzymes, located behind the stomach

Peptic ulcer (PU): Open sore that may bleed

Peritonitis: Condition in which an inflamed appendix bursts and spreads infection throughout the abdomen

Polyps: Growths inside the colon and rectum that may become cancerous

Rectal cancer: Cancer that starts in the rectum

Rectum: A long tube where feces is stored and removed from the body through the anus

Rotavirus: Viral infection that children often get from putting objects contaminated with the virus into their mouths

Saliva: Liquid secreted in the digestive system and that has the enzymes that start digestion

Small intestine: Tube-shaped organ where food, liquids, and minerals are absorbed

Sphincter: Ring-like muscle where the esophagus and stomach meet

Stomach: An organ that helps with digestion by storing swallowed food and liquids, releasing gastric juices, and emptying chyme into the small intestines

Ulcerative colitis (UC): Inflammation that causes ulcers in the lining of the colon

Villi: Tiny bumps on the linings of the small intestine that push food molecules, water, and minerals to the linings of the small intestine

Viral hepatitis: Inflammation of the liver caused by a virus

CHAPTER ACTIVITIES

1. Form small groups and role-play the process of digestion. One student is the food, and the other students in the group are different organs in the digestive tract, such as the mouth, esophagus, stomach, small intestine, large intestine or colon, rectum, and anus. Each organ needs to state its function as the food moves along the tract.

2. Form pairs and brainstorm ways to prevent the transmission of viral hepatitis A, B, and C.

3. Use pictures in your textbook or other sources to make your own drawing of the digestive system. Label the important parts of the digestive system and color each part a different color.

4. Create, write, and present a case study of a patient with a digestive system disease. The case study needs to identify a treatment plan that includes primary, secondary, and tertiary prevention strategies. Given the circumstances described, class members will attempt to determine the best prevention strategies. Often, there is no one right strategy, so student presentations should promote class discussion.

5. You have been hired to create and conduct a stress reduction workshop for residents at a local assisted living residence. Many of the residents have stress-related digestive problems. As part of your workshop, develop a mindfulness or guided meditation activity that is designed to reduce stress. Share this activity with others in your class.

Bibliography and Works Cited

American Gastroenterological Association. (2016a). GERD. Retrieved from http://www.gastro.org/patient-care /conditions-diseases/gerd

American Gastroenterological Association. (2016b). Diverticulosis and diverticulitis. Retrieved from http:// patients.gi.org/topics/diverticulosis-and-diverticulitis/

American Liver Foundation (2016). Cirrhosis information. Retrieved from http://www.liverfoundation.org/

American Society of Colon and Rectal Surgeons. (2016). Hemorrhoids. Retrieved from https://www.fascrs.org /patients/disease-condition/hemorrhoids

Centers for Disease Control and Prevention. (2016a). Foodborne germs and illnesses. Retrieved from http://www .cdc.gov/foodsafety/foodborne-germs.html

Centers for Disease Control and Prevention. (2016b). Viral hepatitis—hepatitis A information. Retrieved from http://www.cdc.gov/hepatitis/HAV/index.htm

Centers for Disease Control and Prevention. (2016c). Viral hepatitis—hepatitis B information. Retrieved from http://www.cdc.gov/hepatitis/HBV/index.htm

Centers for Disease Control and Prevention. (2016d). Viral hepatitis—hepatitis C information. Retrieved from http://www.cdc.gov/hepatitis/hcv/cfaq.htm

Crohn's and Colitis Foundation of America. (2016a). What is Crohn's disease? Retrieved from http://www.ccfa .org/what-are-crohns-and-colitis/what-is-crohns-disease/

Crohn's and Colitis Foundation of America. (2016b). What is ulcerative colitis? Retrieved from http://www.ccfa .org/what-are-crohns-and-colitis/what-is-ulcerative-colitis/

International Foundation for Functional Gastrointestinal Disorders. (2015). Intro to IBS. Retrieved from http:// www.aboutibs.org/site/what-is-ibs/intro-to-ibs/

Mayo Clinic. (2016a). Peptic ulcer. Retrieved from http://www.mayoclinic.org/diseases-conditions/peptic-ulcer /basics/definition/con-20028643

Mayo Clinic. (2016b). Viral gastroenteritis (stomach flu). Retrieved from http://www.mayoclinic.org/diseases -conditions/viral-gastroenteritis/basics/definition/CON-20019350

National Cancer Institute. (2016a). Colorectal cancer—patient version. Retrieved from http://www.cancer.gov /types/colorectal

National Cancer Institute. (2016b). Esophageal cancer—patient version. Retrieved from http://www.cancer.gov /types/esophageal

National Cancer Institute. (2016c). Liver and bile duct cancer—patient version. Retrieved from http://www .cancer.gov/types/liver

National Cancer Institute. (2016d). Pancreatic cancer—patient version. Retrieved from http://www.cancer.gov /types/pancreatic

National Geographic Society. (2016). Digestive system. Retrieved from http://science.nationalgeographic.com /science/health-and-human-body/human-body/digestive-system-article.html

National Institute of Diabetes and Digestive and Kidney Diseases. (2013). Your digestive system and how it works. Retrieved from https://www.niddk.nih.gov/health-information/health-topics/Anatomy/your-digestive-system/Pages/anatomy.aspx

National Institute of Diabetes and Digestive and Kidney Diseases. (2015). Appendicitis. Retrieved from http://www.niddk.nih.gov/health-information/health-topics/digestive-diseases/appendicitis/Pages/overview.aspx

National Institutes of Health. (2015). Galled by the gallbladder? Your tiny, hard-working digestive organ. *News in Health.* Retrieved from https://newsinhealth.nih.gov/issue/feb2015/Feature2

National Pancreas Foundation. (2014). About acute pancreatitis. Retrieved from https://www.pancreasfoundation.org/patient-information/acute-pancreatitis/

US National Library of Medicine. (2014a). Digestive diseases. *MedlinePlus.* Retrieved from https://www.nlm.nih.gov/medlineplus/ency/article/007447.htm

US National Library of Medicine. (2014b). Malabsorption. *MedlinePlus.* Retrieved from https://www.nlm.nih.gov/medlineplus/ency/article/000299.htm

WebMD. (2016). The mouth-body connection: 6 ways oral hygiene helps keep you well. Retrieved from http://www.webmd.com/oral-health/gum-disease-health

Wolters Kluwer. (2016a). Patient education: Acid reflux (gastroesophageal reflux disease) in adults (The basics). *UpToDate.* Retrieved from http://www.uptodate.com/contents/acid-reflux-gastroesophageal-reflux-disease-in-adults-beyond-the-basics

Wolters Kluwer. (2016b). Patient education: Hiatal hernia (The basics). *UpToDate.* Retrieved from https://www.uptodate.com.ezproxy.springfield.edu/contents/15877?search=&source=graphics_search&imageKey=PI/78791#graphicRef78791

CHAPTER 17

URINARY SYSTEM, MALE REPRODUCTIVE SYSTEM, AND RELATED DISEASES

CHAPTER OBJECTIVES

- Identify the major structures and functions of the urinary system.

- Summarize how urine is made.

- Explain common symptoms of urinary problems.

- Describe common diseases of the urinary system.

- Review the major structures of the male reproductive system.

- Describe common diseases of the male reproductive system.

The urinary system maintains body fluids within normal limits by regulating the amount of water that is excreted in the urine. It rids the body of waste products that build up as a result of cellular metabolism. Other ways that the urinary system helps the body include regulating electrolytes in the body fluids and maintaining normal pH of the blood. In addition, the urinary system controls red blood cell production and helps maintain normal blood pressure.

Function of the Urinary System

The *urinary system, or renal system*, is made up of the organs, tubes, muscles, and nerves that work together to create, store, and excrete urine. The word *renal* means "related to the kidneys." The kidneys are the organs that do the most work. Urine is the fluid waste made by the kidneys.

This system's main function is to maintain homeostasis—an internal balance of chemicals and water in the body. It keeps homeostasis by getting rid of wastes and excess fluids, keeping vitamin and mineral levels in check, and controlling acid levels in blood.

Homeostasis requires the urinary system to work with the lungs, skin, liver, and intestines. Although these organs also excrete body wastes, the major task of excretion still belongs to the urinary system. If it fails, the other organs cannot take over. *Excretion*, or urination, is the process by which waste and other non-useful materials are eliminated from the body. Adults urinate (pee) about a quart and a half of urine each day, depending on the amount of fluid taken in and fluid lost through sweating and breathing. Certain types of medications and liquids (e.g., alcohol) also affect how much a person urinates.

Urology is the branch of medicine that studies diseases of the male and female urinary system and the male reproductive organs. *Urologists* treat diseases of the urinary tract in both males and females. They also treat male reproductive organs. Urologists are physicians who are trained in the internal medicine subspecialty of urology.

The kidney is part of the urinary system, but it has its own medical specialty: nephrology. *Nephrology* is the study of the function, diseases, and treatment of the kidneys. A *nephrologist* is a physician who treats diseases of the kidney and is trained in the internal medicine subspecialty of nephrology.

Structure of the Urinary System

The urinary system's structure includes kidneys, ureters, bladder, sphincter muscles, and urethra (see Figure 17.1). The structure is the same in males and females, although certain parts are slightly different between the sexes.

As already mentioned, the *kidneys* do the important work of the urinary system. There are two kidneys; each is reddish-brown, fist-sized, and bean-shaped. There is one kidney on each side of the body, just below the rib cage and in the middle of the back.

The kidneys clean the blood by getting rid of waste and extra fluids, maintain the balance of salt and minerals in the blood, make red blood cells, help keep blood pressure normal, and promote strong bones. The blood and fluids enter the kidney through the *renal artery*.

All the blood in the body passes through the kidneys about 20 times every hour. The kidneys remove urea and other waste from the blood. *Urea* is produced during digestion, when foods with protein, such as meat, are broken down in the body. It is then carried in the bloodstream to the kidneys. In each kidney, there are about a million small, ball-shaped filtering units called nephrons. *Nephrons* separate the good from the bad.

Once filtered, most of the water, sugar, vitamins, and salts are taken back into circulation by blood. Together with the clean blood, they leave the kidneys through the *renal veins*.

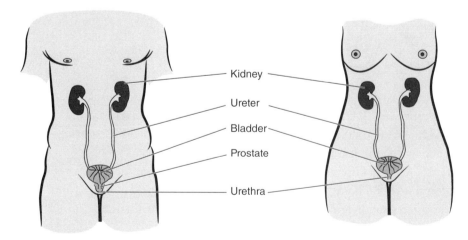

Figure 17.1 Urinary System

Note. Adapted from the National Institute of Diabetes and Digestive and Kidney Diseases (NIDDK) and the National Cancer Institute. This figure does not have a copyright statement. The NIDDK encourages people to share this content freely. Retrieved from https://www.niddk.nih.gov/health-information/health-topics/diagnostic-tests/imaging-urinary-tract/Pages/imaging-urinary-tract.aspx

Unhealthy substances—urea, uric acid, excess salt, and other waste—as well as water form into *urine,* or pee, as they pass through the nephrons. It is the nephrons in the kidneys that make urine. Urine travels from the kidneys down into two thin tubes, or *ureters,* to the bladder. The ureters are about 8 to 10 inches long; one ureter extends from each kidney. Muscles in the ureter walls constantly tighten and relax to force urine away from the kidneys down to the bladder. Small amounts of urine are emptied into the bladder from the ureters about every 10 to 15 seconds.

The *bladder* is a hollow muscular organ shaped like a balloon; it sits in the pelvis and stores urine. A normal, healthy bladder can hold up to two cups of urine comfortably for 2 to 5 hours. As the bladder fills with urine and gets closer to its limit, nerves from the bladder send a message to the brain that the bladder is full, and the urge to empty the bladder grows. When a person urinates, the brain signals the bladder muscles to tighten while at the same time signals the sphincter muscles to relax. To prevent urine leaks, *sphincter muscles* close tightly around the opening of the bladder into the *urethra,* the tube that allows urine to pass outside the body.

The only difference between the female and male urinary system is the length of the urethra. In females, the urethra is about 1 to 2 inches long and sits between the clitoris and the vagina. In males, it runs the length of the penis, is about 8 inches long, and opens at the end of the penis. Like the female urethra, the male urethra gets rid of urine; it also releases semen during ejaculation.

Common Signs, Symptoms, and Diagnostic Tests of the Urinary System

Common health problems of the urinary system include urinary tract infections, bladder cancer, kidney stones, and chronic kidney disease. Aging causes most urinary system diseases. As part of the aging process, our kidneys change, losing the ability to concentrate urine or remove wastes from the blood. Aging causes the muscles in the ureters, bladder, and urethra to lose strength. The bladder also shrinks with age, causing older people to urinate more often. In some older people, the ability to control urination is completely lost. Illness or injury causes damage to the kidneys. This damage can prevent the kidneys from filtering blood completely or can block the passage of urine.

Urinary system diseases involve one or both kidneys, one or both ureters, the bladder, and the urethra. In men, the prostate or one or both testicles can also be involved. There are many common signs and symptoms of urinary system diseases, including the following (US National Library of Medicine, 2016a):

- Darkening of the skin
- Frequent headaches
- Itchiness
- *Nocturia* (frequent urination at night)
- *Pleura* (frequent urinating)
- *Hematuria* (blood in the urine)
- Nausea, vomiting, and loss of appetite
- Swelling of hands and feet
- Muscle cramps or back pain
- Tiredness
- High blood pressure
- *Dysuria* (burning feeling when urinating)

- *Urgency* (constantly feeling the need to urinate)
- Dribbling or other changes with urination

Urinary diseases are often difficult to diagnose and treat. Some of these diseases rarely cause symptoms until they are advanced. Other times, symptoms are so general that they can be similar to those of other diseases.

Routine urinalysis is a lab test that involves having the patient urinate into a special container. This urine is referred to as a *urine sample,* and it is then analyzed at a lab. Depending on the test, the urine sample is often done using the *clean-catch method,* which prevents the sample from becoming contaminated by germs, or by putting a tube, or *catheter,* through the urethra into the bladder.

Other urine tests include *urine cultures,* in which bacteria from a urine sample are grown in a lab. Urine cultures help diagnose urinary tract infections (UTIs). A *urodynamic test* looks at two functions: how urine is stored in the bladder, and how urine flows from the bladder through the urethra. This test is used for patients with muscle or nerve problems in the lower part of the urinary system. It is done by putting a tube through the urethra into the bladder. The bladder is then filled with water, X-ray dye, or a gas. Another tube is put into the rectum or vagina to measure the pressure put on the bladder when straining or coughing. X-ray pictures are taken when the bladder fills and empties.

A health care provider can diagnose urethra and bladder diseases by looking through a flexible tube called a *cystoscope,* which is a type of endoscope. Most cystoscopes have a light and a small camera at their end to see inside the bladder and urethra. They also have a small clipping device on its tip, to get a tissue sample of the bladder.

Other tests include *ultrasonography,* which gives information about any changes in the kidneys. A kidney biopsy is used to diagnose kidney diseases and causes of acute kidney failure. A biopsy is also done on a transplanted kidney to look for signs of rejection.

Diseases of the Urinary System

Diseases of the urinary system include any diseases that affect the kidneys, ureters, bladder, or urethra. Some urinary diseases develop quickly; others develop more slowly. Urinary diseases can be caused by other diseases as well as by infection, inflammation, injury, and cancer.

Urinary Tract Infections

Urinary tract infections (UTIs) occur anywhere along the urinary tract. Bacteria enters the urethra and then into the bladder. The bacteria cause infections that can spread from the bladder to the kidneys. The infections have different names, depending on what part of the urinary tract is infected (US National Library of Medicine, 2016):

- *Urethritis*—infection in the urethra
- *Cystitis*—infection in the bladder
- *Pyelonephritis*—infection in one or both kidneys

There are certain risk factors for UTIs. The biggest risk factor is being female—about half of all women have a UTI sometime in their life. Moreover, half of those who have had it once get it again within a year. Women get UTIs more often because their urethra is shorter and closer to the anus than it is in men. They are likely to get a UTI infection after sexual activity and when using a diaphragm or spermicide for birth control. Menopause also increases the risk of a UTI. Other factors that increase risk include the following:

- Certain diseases (e.g., diabetes)
- Problems emptying bladder completely

- Pregnancy

- Aging

- Kidney stones

- Surgery involving the urinary system

Cystitis is an inflammation of the bladder, and it is usually caused when bacteria gets into the bladder. Once in the bladder, bacteria stick to the bladder and multiply, leading to an inflammation of the tissue lining. The symptoms of cystitis include hematuria, dysuria, pleura, urgency, fever, cramps, and back pain. These symptoms, although unpleasant, are treatable.

When bacteria travel up the ureters and into the kidneys, the result is *pyelonephritis*. Signs and symptoms of pyelonephritis include fever, chills, pain, night sweats, fatigue, nausea, and reddened skin. Older adults may also experience mental confusion. In some cases of pyelonephritis, there can be so many bacteria and white blood cells that it causes pus-filled urine.

Urethritis is usually caused by sexually transmitted infections (STIs). Much less often, it is caused by an injury or exposure to chemicals (e.g., spermicide). The main symptoms of urethritis are dysuria and pleura as well as redness around the opening of the urethra. Men with urethritis often have a yellow discharge from the urethra.

To diagnose a UTI, a urine sample is collected for a urinalysis as well as for a urine culture. Blood tests and an ultrasound can be used to look at the kidneys and bladder to detect a UTI.

In the case of a mild infection, antibiotics can prevent it spreading to the kidneys. Antibiotics can stop symptoms for a short time. Symptoms of a bladder infection usually disappear within 24 to 48 hours after treatment begins. If it is a kidney infection, it may take a week or longer for symptoms to go away.

Some patients have UTIs that keep coming back even with treatment. Such infections are called chronic UTIs. In the case of a chronic UTI, stronger antibiotics are needed. If a structural problem is causing the infection, surgery is recommended.

A complication of a UTI is a life-threatening blood infection called *sepsis*. Sepsis occurs among those at greatest risk: young children, very old adults, and those with a compromised immune system. Other complications from UTIs include kidney damage and chronic kidney infection.

Unfortunately, there is no way to prevent UTIs, but lifestyle changes (e.g., drinking fluids) can help. Cleanliness of the genitals reduces the risk of bacteria getting in the urethra. The genitals need to be cleaned and wiped from front to back to reduce the chance of bacteria reaching the urethra. It is also important to keep the genitals clean during sexual activity by urinating before and after.

Bladder Cancer

Each year in the United States, about 77,000 people are found to have *bladder cancer*, and most are over 70 years old. It is the fifth most common type of cancer (American Cancer Society, 2016). Bladder cancer cells spread by breaking away from the original cancerous tumor and traveling through the blood vessels to the liver, lungs, and bones. In addition, bladder cancer cells spread through lymph vessels to nearby lymph nodes.

It is not understood why some people get bladder cancer while others do not, but there are certain risk factors. These include smoking, specific toxins in the workplace, past personal history of bladder cancer, family history of bladder cancer, some cancer treatments, and being a White male (American Cancer Society, 2016). However, many people with bladder cancer have none of these risk factors, and many others who have these risk factors do not develop it.

Bladder cancer symptoms cause hematuria, urgency, incontinence, and dysuria. These symptoms are similar to other health problems and make bladder cancer difficult to diagnose.

In addition to a physical examination and a health history, the tests that help diagnose bladder cancer include urinalysis, cystoscopy, and biopsy. For a small number of patients, the entire area with cancer is removed during a biopsy. In these cases, bladder cancer is diagnosed and treated at the same time.

If the cancer spreads from its original place to another part of the body, the new tumor has the same kind of abnormal cells and the same name as the original tumor. For example, if bladder cancer spreads to the liver, the cancer cells in the liver are actually bladder cancer cells. It is treated as bladder cancer, not as liver cancer.

Treatments for bladder cancer are biological therapy, chemotherapy, radiation therapy, and surgery. The treatment choice depends not only on the age and general health of the patient but also on the location of the tumor.

Biological therapy as treatment for bladder cancer patients uses bacteria to help the immune system kill cancer cells. Chemotherapy treats bladder cancer before or after surgery. Radiation therapy is high-energy rays that kill cancer cells and is sometimes given instead of surgery or chemotherapy.

Surgery for bladder cancer involves removing some or all of the bladder. Once the bladder is removed, then a new way is needed for urine to exit or to be stored. After the bladder is removed, the surgeon uses a piece of the intestines to make a new path for urine to exit or to be stored. However, even if the surgery is successful, bladder cancer often returns.

Kidney Problems

Each day, both kidneys filter about 200 quarts of blood and remove 2 quarts of waste through excretion (National Cancer Institute, 2016). Body waste is sent through the blood to be filtered by the kidneys for nutrients. As mentioned earlier, the nephrons filter materials that the body can still use, such as sodium and potassium, and return them back into the bloodstream.

Most kidney diseases attack the nephrons. If the nephrons become damaged, they lose their ability to filter and remove the body's waste and fluids. Causes of nephron damage include injuries, medications, or a family history of kidney disease. Certain chronic diseases, such as diabetes or high blood pressure, can also cause nephron damage.

Although normal kidney function decreases as we age, a decrease for any other reason is a cause for concern. Toxins and extra fluids can build up in the blood and lower hormone production, resulting in serious health problems. About 1 in 10 adults nationwide, or about 20 million people, have at least some signs of kidney damage (National Institute of Diabetes and Digestive and Kidney Diseases, 2014).

Kidney disease usually does not cause signs and symptoms until the problem becomes serious. If there are symptoms, they may include nausea; swelling of feet, hands, or face; back pain; bloody urine; high blood pressure; and urgency in peeing.

The only way to be sure if there is a kidney problem is to be tested, and those diseases that are caught early can be treated. Left untreated, however, kidney diseases can lead to permanent damage or even kidney failure. When this happens, treatment options may be limited to removal of a kidney.

Kidney Stones

Kidney stones are like small rocks that form in the kidney. These stones are produced when waste in the urine clumps together. Crystals form when there is too much waste. The crystals attract other elements to join and form a stone that grows larger. After it is formed, a stone stays in the kidney, or it passes through the urinary tract. For most people, taking in enough liquid washes them out, or other chemicals in the urine stop a stone from forming.

There are four main types of kidney stones, and each has a different cause and treatment. About 80% are calcium stones, which are usually caused by too much calcium or vitamin D, some medicines, genetics, or other kidney problems.

Some kidney stones are as small as a grain of sand, and others are as large as a pebble; some are smooth, and others are sharp. A few are as large as a golf ball.

Small stones pass through the urinary system and out of the body without causing too much pain. Larger stones, however, block the flow of urine, causing extreme pain. Kidney stones do not usually cause any symptoms until they start to pass. These symptoms include

- Stomach and back pain

- Vomiting

- Hematuria (blood in urine)

- Fever and chills

Kidney stones are diagnosed with a health history and physical examination, as well as urine, blood, and imaging tests. Once out of the body, stones are analyzed to determine why a patient has them and how to reduce risk of future stones.

Treatment for kidney stones depends on the location and size of the stones. Patients are usually asked to drink plenty of water and are given pain medication to help smaller stones pass more easily. Another treatment is sound waves that blast the stones into smaller pieces that are then more easily passed. Sometimes, an endoscope is put into the ureter to get rid of the stones that are stuck. In severe cases, surgery is required.

Each year, more than 500,000 people go to emergency rooms for kidney stones (Urology Care Foundation, 2015). The number of adults and children in the United States with kidney stones has increased over the past 30 years so that it is now estimated that 1 in 10 people will have kidney stones at some time in his or her life (Urology Care Foundation, 2015).

The peak age for stones is between 20 and 50 years of age. Although anyone can have kidney stones, Whites are more likely to have them than African Americans, and men are much more likely than women. Having a history of kidney stones increases the risk to 50% for developing another one within 5 to 7 years. Those who eat a lot of animal protein or do not drink enough liquids, especially water, are also at high risk for kidney stones.

To prevent stones from forming, people should drink plenty of fluids; eat less salt, sugar, meat, and eggs; and keep a normal body weight. It is not advised to reduce calcium intake without medical supervision. Studies have shown that limiting calcium in the diet may not stop kidney stones from forming and may harm bones (Urology Care Foundation, 2015).

Kidney Disease

Kidney disease, or renal disease, occurs when waste builds up in the blood because of damaged nephrons. Too much protein in the urine is one of the earliest signs of nephron damage and is easy to detect through a urine test. However, too much protein is often unnoticed because not many people get regular urine testing. Consequently, kidney disease is underdiagnosed in the United States (National Kidney Foundation, 2010).

There are different types of kidney disease. When damage to nephrons occurs quickly, it is known as *acute kidney failure* (AKF) or acute renal failure (ARF). There are many causes for AKF, including kidney injury, blocked urine flow, infections, pregnancy complications, or damage from toxins. Athletes who do not drink enough fluids while competing can get AKF because of sudden breakdown of muscle tissue.

It is more common, however, for nephrons to slowly get worse over time, causing *chronic kidney disease* (CKD). CKD arises when there is kidney damage that lasts for more than 3 months. It is grouped into five stages based on how well the kidneys are able to filter blood. In stage one, for example, the kidneys still can filter out most wastes; in stage five, severe damage causes the kidneys to fail.

Often called a "silent killer," CKD does not usually cause symptoms to show until the damage is done. Early CKD often has no symptoms, although some patients may have nocturia, dry skin, back pain, and trouble sleeping. If CKD gets worse, wastes build up in the blood and cause high blood pressure, anemia, malnutrition, weak bones, depression, and numbness.

Twenty-six million adults in the United States have CKD, and millions more are at risk (National Kidney Foundation, 2010). Those with high blood pressure, diabetes, cardiovascular disease, and a family history of kidney failure are most at risk for CKD. Additional risk factors include obesity, smoking, autoimmune diseases, infections, toxins, and kidney damage.

CKD occurs more often in women than men. It can strike people of any race, but African Americans are especially at risk—they are four times more likely to have CKD than Whites (National Kidney Foundation, 2010). CKD can also strike anyone at any age, but the elderly are most at risk.

Besides taking a health history and doing a physical examination, health care providers diagnose CKD by using blood and urine tests, CAT scan, MRI, and kidney biopsy. The glomerular filtration rate (GFR) is the best test to measure the level of kidney function and determine the stage of kidney disease. If the GFR number is low, then the kidneys are not working as well as they should.

The goal of CKD treatment is to prevent or slow down damage to the kidneys. If another disease such as high blood pressure is causing CKD, then managing that disease is important. Patients often take two or more medicines to lower blood pressure, control blood glucose, and lower blood cholesterol; this helps not only treat CKD but also manage the causes. Patients also may need to take a *diuretic,* a medication to get rid of excess water.

Some patients live with CKD for years without needing intensive treatment; others quickly progress to kidney failure. When kidney function has fallen below a certain point, the condition is referred to as *kidney failure,* or renal failure.

Kidney failure causes serious harmful effects throughout the body, and there are only two treatment choices: dialysis or kidney transplant. Most patients with kidney failure receive dialysis. Health care providers do not always agree about when patients with kidney failure need dialysis.

There are two options with dialysis. In *hemodialysis* (HD), a patient sits in a chair while blood is carried into a machine that filters the waste and then returns the clean blood back into the patient's body. HD cleans the blood by using a special filter called a *dialyzer.* During HD, blood moves through the inside of thousands of dialyzer fibers. Needed blood cells and proteins that are too big to pass through the fibers go back to the body. Wastes and extra water go through the fibers and are removed from the body. HD is most often done at a medical center three times a week for at least 3 to 4 hours each treatment.

Peritoneal dialysis (PD) does not use a machine as hemodialysis does; instead, the body is the filter. In PD, solutions are pumped into the stomach through a catheter that is put in the stomach wall. The catheter helps draw out the waste from the blood. It stays in the body all the time and hangs out a few inches. The catheter drains into a bag that is cleaned by the patient and is covered up when not in use. Unlike hemodialysis (HD), PD eliminates the need to sit in a clinic for several hours. The choice between HD or PD depends on the patient's wishes and overall health, as well as on available resources. Survival rates for both treatments are about the same.

A *kidney transplant* requires major surgery to put a donor kidney into the body of a person who has severe kidney failure. It is often a better treatment than dialysis for severe kidney failure because it lets the patient live as close to a normal life as possible.

A transplant is just a treatment, not a cure, and there are major drawbacks to a kidney transplant. Waiting for a donated kidney can take years. The reason for waiting is that not just any kidney works. The new kidney has to match the blood and tissue type of the recipient. Otherwise, the patient's body rejects the kidney, causing it to stop working. Matching blood and tissue type is carefully done through blood tests. Even so, rejection can occur at any time—even years after a transplant.

The three possible sources for a *kidney donation* are (a) a living blood relative (parent, sibling); (b) a living loved one (spouse, friend); or (c) a deceased donor.

If a living blood relative or loved one wants to donate a kidney, he or she is tested to see if his or her kidney is a good match. Patients who do not have a family member or loved one to donate a kidney are put on a waiting list. This waiting list allows patients to receive a kidney from a donor who has just died. How long patients wait for a donated kidney depends on finding a good match. Some people wait several years for a good match; others are matched within a few months.

Kidney transplantation requires surgery that puts a healthy kidney from another person into a patient's body. This one new kidney takes over the work of two failed kidneys. A surgeon places the new kidney inside the stomach and connects the artery and vein of the new kidney to the patient's artery and vein. The ureter from the new kidney is connected to the bladder. The new kidney starts making urine as soon as blood starts flowing through it, but sometimes it needs a few weeks before it starts working. Unless they cause health problems, the patient's own kidneys are left in place.

Risk of kidney disease can be reduced by controlling blood pressure and blood sugar, maintaining proper weight, not smoking, drinking plenty of water, exercising regularly, and avoiding excessive use of over-the-counter medications that harm the kidneys (e.g., ibuprofen).

Kidney Cancer

A *kidney tumor* is an abnormal growth in the kidney. These tumors are either benign or malignant. The most common kidney tumor is a blister-like *cyst*. Cysts do not progress to cancer and usually do not need treatment. If the kidney tumor is solid, then it is cancerous more than 80% of the time.

Every year in the United States, about 62,700 new cases of kidney cancer will be diagnosed, and about 14,240 people will die from it (Urology Care Foundation, 2016c). Kidney cancer is more common in males and is usually diagnosed between the ages of 50 and 70. It is among the 10 most common cancers in both men and women (Urology Care Foundation, 2016c).

The most common type of kidney cancer is *renal cell carcinoma (RCC)*. Although RCC usually grows as a single tumor within one kidney, there can be two or more tumors in one kidney or even tumors in both kidneys at the same time. Children are more likely to develop a kidney cancer called *Wilms' tumor*, probably caused by the poor development of kidney cells.

For reasons that are unclear, the number of people having kidney cancer has been rising since the 1990s (Urology Care Foundation, 2016c). The risks for kidney cancer include smoking, high blood pressure, obesity, workplace exposure to toxins, family history of kidney cancer, chronic kidney disease, dialysis, and a diet that is high in fried meat.

Kidney tumors often do not cause symptoms and are detected only during a medical visit for another health problem or during a routine screening. Pain on the side that does not go away, a lump felt near the stomach, weight loss for no reason, and hematuria are early symptoms of kidney cancer.

Unfortunately, no blood or urine tests detect kidney tumors. Besides a physical examination and health history, an ultrasound or CT scan is used in the diagnosis. If it is cancer, the patient is tested to see if the cancer has spread beyond the kidney. These tests include CT scan or MRI, chest X-ray, and blood tests. A bone scan is also used if the patient has bone problems or abnormal blood test results.

Chemotherapy, hormone therapy, and radiation therapy are not effective treatments for kidney cancer, so a nephrectomy, or tumor removal, is recommended. In performing a nephrectomy, the surgeon removes either some of the diseased tissue of the kidney or the entire kidney. The decision to remove some or all of a kidney depends on several factors, including whether there is more than one tumor. The removal of one kidney generally has no health consequences as long as the remaining kidney works well.

In many cases, the cause of kidney cancer is not known; in other cases, even when the cause is known, the cancer may not be prevented. However, there are ways to reduce risks for kidney cancer.

Smoking causes a large number of cases, so stopping smoking may lower risk. If obesity and high blood pressure are causes, then maintaining a healthy weight, eating a diet high in fruits and vegetables, exercising, and managing high blood pressure may reduce risk. Finally, avoiding workplace exposure to toxins, such as asbestos, also may reduce risk.

Function and Structure of the Male Reproductive System

This section of the chapter describes the male reproductive system's function and structure as well as related diseases. Most of the male reproductive system—the penis, scrotum, and testicles—is outside of the man's pelvis (see Figure 17.2). The functions of the male reproductive system are to (a) produce, care for, and transport sperm and semen; (b) deposit sperm in the female reproductive system; and (c) produce and secrete male sex hormones. The following are the major male reproductive organs:

- Anus—opening at the end of the digestive tract where feces leave the body.
- Bladder—organ that holds urine.
- Penis—outer male reproductive organ.
- Rectum—lower end of the large intestine that leads to the anus.
- Urethra—tube where urine passes from the bladder out of the body. The male urethra also ejaculates semen.
- Scrotum—bag of skin that holds the testicles.
- Testicles—pair of male glands that make semen.

The *penis* is the male organ for sexual intercourse. It has three parts: the root, which attaches to the wall of the pelvis; the shaft or body; and the glans, which is the cone-shaped head of the penis. The glans

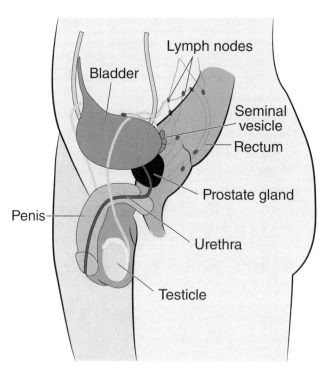

Figure 17.2 Male Reproductive System

Note. Adapted from the National Cancer Institute, Visuals Online. This image is in the public domain and can be freely reused. Retrieved from https://visualsonline.cancer.gov/details.cfm?imageid=9422

is covered with a loose layer of skin called foreskin. This skin is sometimes removed in a circumcision. The opening of the urethra is at the tip of the penis.

Circumcision is a medical procedure that is usually done during a baby boy's first few days of life. Although circumcision is not medically necessary, parents who choose to have their children circumcised often do so based on religious and cultural beliefs or concerns about hygiene.

The inside of the penis has spongy tissue that has thousands of large spaces. The nervous system fills these spaces with blood when the man is sexually aroused. When the penis fills with blood, it becomes rigid and erect, which helps in penetration during sexual intercourse. The skin of the penis is loose and elastic to adapt to changes in penis size during an erection. *Erection* is the temporary lengthening, thickening, and hardening of the penis.

Semen carries sperm and is ejaculated or discharged through the end of the penis when the man reaches *orgasm, or sexual climax*. When the penis is erect, the flow of urine is blocked from the urethra, allowing only semen to be ejaculated at orgasm.

The scrotum is the loose sac of skin that hangs behind the penis. It holds the testicles or testes, as well as many nerves and blood vessels. In a sexually mature male, the two testicles make and store millions of tiny sperm cells.

The scrotum acts as a climate control system for the testicles. The testicles are oval organs about the size of large olives that lie in the scrotum. For normal sperm development, the testicles must be at a temperature slightly cooler than body temperature. Special muscles in the scrotum allow it to contract and relax, moving the testicles closer to the body for warmth or farther away from the body to cool. The brain and the nervous system give the scrotum the cue to change the temperature.

Most men have two testicles. The testicles are responsible for producing *testosterone*, the primary male sex hormone. This hormone not only helps in making sperm but also causes males to have deeper voices, bigger muscles, and body and facial hair.

The *epididymis* is a long, coiled tube that rests on the back side of each testicle and moves and stores sperm cells. When sperm are stored in the epididymis, they have time to mature. Once mature, sperm can swim on their own.

The internal organs of the male reproductive system are called the *accessory organs*. The accessory organs include the *vas deferens*, a long tube that travels from the epididymis into the pelvic cavity, to just behind the bladder. The vas deferens transports mature sperm to the urethra for ejaculation. The *ejaculatory ducts* are formed by the joining of the vas deferens with the seminal vesicles. The *seminal vesicles* are sacs or glands that attach to the vas deferens near the base of the bladder. These vesicles make semen, which gives sperm their energy and helps them move.

The *prostate gland* is walnut sized and is located below the bladder in front of the rectum. This gland makes additional fluid to help in ejaculation and nourish sperm.

Cowper's glands are pea sized and are on the sides of the urethra just below the prostate gland. These glands make a fluid that acts like grease in the urethra, helping the flow of fluids.

Diseases of the Male Reproductive System

Because most of the male reproductive organs are on the outside of the body, signs and symptoms are usually obvious at an early stage. Penis and testicular diseases are the two major types of diseases that affect the male reproductive external organs and can affect a man's sexual functioning and fertility.

Epididymal Cysts

An *epididymal cyst* is a sperm-filled cyst in the epididymis. Small epididymal cysts, sometimes known as spermatic cysts, are common, particularly for men in their 40s and 50s. Although the main cause of these cysts is unknown, risk factors are trauma or inflammation.

The cysts develop slowly and are usually painless. A single cyst may feel like an extra lump above the testicle or an enlargement on one side of the scrotum. In many cases, there are multiple painless cysts that can feel like a tiny bunch of grapes on top of and behind the testicles. Symptoms include pain, swelling, or redness of the scrotum.

These cysts are often discovered by a man's self-examination of the testicles or by a health care provider during a physical examination. An ultrasound may be used to confirm the diagnosis.

Epididymal cysts usually stay small and do not need treatment. Rarely do the cysts become large and cause pain, in which case they are removed.

Testicular Cancer

Testicular cancer can be in one or both testicles. Most testicular cancers begin in the cells that make sperm. The exact cause of this cancer is not known, but there are risk factors—for example, abnormal testicle development, a history of testicular cancer, and a history of undescended testicles (the condition in which one or both testicles fail to move into the scrotum before birth). Other possible risk factors include exposure to certain toxins, HIV infection, and a family history of testicular cancer.

Testicular cancer is the most common form of cancer in American men between the ages of 15 and 36 years (American Society of Clinical Oncology, 2016a). This does not mean that men at other ages cannot get this disease, but it is less common. White men are five times more likely than Black and Asian American men to develop this cancer.

There are often no symptoms, and if there are, symptoms are pain in the testicles, back, or groin; swelling of a testicle; fluid in the scrotum; and growth of breast tissue. If the cancer has spread, there can be symptoms in other parts of the body, such as the lungs, abdomen, back, or brain.

A physical examination can detect a lump or mass in one of the testicles. Other diagnostic tests include CT scan, blood tests, chest X-ray, and ultrasound. Testicular cancer has three main treatment options: surgery, radiation, and chemotherapy. Surgical treatment removes the testicle and may remove nearby lymph nodes. Radiation therapy uses high-energy rays after surgery to prevent the cancer from returning. Chemotherapy uses drugs to kill cancer cells. If not treated, testicular cancer spreads to other parts of the body, including the abdomen, lungs, and spine.

Testicular cancer is one of the most treatable and curable cancers, even when the cancer has spread. The survival rate for men in the early stage of some types of testicular cancer is almost 100% (American Society of Clinical Oncology, 2016a). The survival rate for more advanced forms is slightly lower, depending on the size of the tumor and when treatment was started.

There is no way to prevent testicular cancer. Some health care providers recommend regular testicle self-examination to identify the disease at its earliest stage; however, not all health care providers agree on the effectiveness of testicle self-examination. The US Preventive Services Task Force (USPSTF, 2011) recommends against routine screening for testicular cancer because there is no known effective screening technique. This recommendation does not apply if there is a personal health history of an undescended testicle (American Society of Clinical Oncology, 2016a).

Varicoceles

The *spermatic cord*, a cord that suspends the testes within the scrotum, carries blood to and from the testicles. A *varicocele* is a swelling of a vein along this cord. The swelling is similar to varicose veins in the legs.

Varicoceles are more common in men ages 15 to 25 years. The condition usually develops slowly and is most often seen on the left side of the scrotum. There are no significant risk factors for developing varicoceles; however, being overweight may increase risk.

Varicoceles can cause testicular shrinkage, low sperm count, and poor sperm quality. Low sperm count and poor sperm quality lead to *infertility*, a term used when a man has not been able to get a woman pregnant after at least 1 year of trying. Varicoceles occur in approximately 15% of normal males and are usually not important clinically, unless they are associated with infertility.

Some men with varicoceles have no symptoms. Others have symptoms that include enlarged, twisted veins in the scrotum that cause swelling or painless lumps in the testicles. A varicocele feels like a "bag of worms" surrounding the testicle, and may be accompanied by a constant pulling, dragging, or dull pain in the scrotum.

To diagnose varicoceles, the health care provider examines the groin area and feels for a growth along the spermatic cord. The testicle on the side of the varicocele may also be smaller than the one on the other side. For treatment, a jock strap or snug underwear may help get rid of the pain. If pain continues, then surgery may be needed.

Undescended Testicle

As noted earlier, an *undescended testicle* is one that fails to move down into the scrotum before birth. Most of the time, children's testicles descend by the time they are 9 months old. Testicles that do not naturally descend into the scrotum are considered abnormal. Undescended testicles are common in infants who are born early.

There are usually no symptoms associated with an undescended testicle, except that the testicle is not found in the scrotum. A physical examination and imaging tests confirm that one or both of the testicles are not in the scrotum. Most cases improve without treatment, and once a testicle is found in the scrotum, it is considered descended. If testicles do not descend by the time the child is a year old, then medical treatment is needed. Surgery at this age reduces the chances of permanent damage to the testicles. In some cases, no testicle is found, even during surgery. This is referred to as a *vanished testicle, or absent testicle* and may be caused by a problem that arose while the fetus was still developing in the mother.

An undescended testicle is also more likely to develop cancer, even if it is brought down into the scrotum. The other testicle is also more likely to develop cancer, even if it descended properly. If the undescended testicle is found later in life, the health care provider may recommend removal due to the high risk of cancer.

Infertility

As noted, male infertility refers to a man's inability to impregnate a woman after at least 1 year of trying (US National Library of Medicine, 2016). To conceive a child, a man's sperm must combine with a woman's egg following sexual intercourse.

Many diseases, including hormone problems as well as lifestyle and environmental factors, cause infertility. Issues that lead to male infertility include health problems that affect how the testicles work. Other problems are hormone imbalances and blockages in the male reproductive organs. In about 50% of cases, the cause of male infertility is unknown. One third of infertility cases are caused by male reproductive issues, one third by female reproductive issues, and one third by both male and female reproductive issues or by unknown factors.

About 10% to 15% of men who are infertile have a complete lack of sperm (US National Library of Medicine, 2016). The most common cause of this condition is varicocele. When the cause for male infertility is known, treatments include medications, surgery, or *assisted reproductive technologies (ART)*. ART is a general term used for artificial or partially artificial methods used to achieve pregnancy.

Prostate Problems

The prostate is a small gland in men that sits low in the pelvis, below the bladder and just in front of the rectum. It wraps around the urethra (refer to Figure 17.2). The prostate helps make semen, the fluid that carries sperm from the testicles through the penis.

A young man's prostate is about the size of a walnut, and it slowly grows larger with age. As it grows, it may squeeze the urethra and cause problems with urination. Sometimes men in their 30s and 40s have prostate problems; for others, symptoms do not develop until they are in their 50s. An infection or a tumor can also make the prostate larger.

A health care provider may find a prostate problem during a routine checkup or by performing a *digital rectal exam (DRE)*. In a DRE, the health care provider inserts a gloved and lubricated finger into the rectum to feel the prostate and to check for anything abnormal.

Another test that helps diagnose prostate problems is the *PSA blood test. Prostate-specific antigen (PSA)* is a substance made by the prostate. It is found in increased amounts in the blood of men who have prostate cancer, enlarged prostate, an infection, or swelling of the prostate. The PSA blood test measures the amount of PSA, but it cannot determine whether the problem is cancer or another disease.

Men with a high PSA level are more likely to have prostate cancer than men with low levels, but there are no normal and abnormal ranges of PSA in the blood. One in four men with a high PSA level actually has prostate cancer.

The three most common prostate problems are prostatitis, enlarged prostate, and prostate cancer. One of these problems does not lead to another; for example, having an enlarged prostate is not a risk factor for prostate cancer. It is also possible to have more than one of these problems at the same time.

Prostatitis

Prostatitis is a swelling of the prostate gland and is usually caused by a bacterial infection. It affects at least 50% of all men at some time during their lives (US National Library of Medicine, 2016). Prostatitis is not a risk factor for any other prostate diseases. There are several types of prostatitis; this discussion is limited to the most common.

Acute bacterial prostatitis usually starts suddenly from a common bacterial infection in the urine that leaks into the prostate. It can cause fever, chills, pain when urinating, and blood in the urine. Most cases of acute bacterial prostatitis are treated with antibiotics and pain medication.

Chronic bacterial prostatitis is a bacterial infection that keeps coming back. The symptoms are similar to those of a urinary tract infection (UTI). The cause can be a defect in the prostate that lets bacteria collect in the urinary tract. Antibiotic treatment is best for chronic bacterial prostatitis. Long-term, low-dose antibiotics may help relieve symptoms in cases that do not get better.

Chronic pelvic pain syndrome (CPPS) is the most common but least understood type of prostatitis. Found in men of any age from late teens to the elderly, CPPS has symptoms that come and go without warning. CPPS causes pain in the lower back, in the pelvic area, or at the tip of the penis. Men with this type of prostatitis often have painful ejaculation. They may feel the need to urinate frequently, but pass only small amounts of urine. Infection-fighting cells are often present, but no bacteria can be found. Treating CPPS usually requires a combination of pain medicines, surgery, and lifestyle changes, depending on the type and severity of symptoms.

Benign Prostatic Hyperplasia

Benign prostatic hyperplasia (BPH), or enlarged prostate, causes the prostate to press on the urethra, leading to urination and bladder problems (see Figure 17.3). *Benign* means there is not cancer, and *hyperplasia* means abnormal cell growth.

The cause of BPH is unknown, but it happens to almost all men as they get older. Factors linked to aging and the testicles may play a role in the growth of the gland. BPH is not linked to cancer and does not increase the risk of getting prostate cancer; however, signs and symptoms for BPH and prostate cancer are similar.

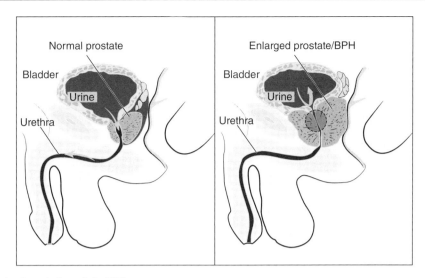

Figure 17.3 Benign Prostatic Hyperplasia (BPH)

Note. Adapted from the National Cancer Institute. This image is in the public domain and can be freely reused. Retrieved from https://commons.wikimedia.org/wiki/File:Benign_prostatic_hyperplasia.jpg

More than half of men in their 60s and most men in their 70s and 80s have signs and symptoms of BPH. In fact, according to the Urology Care Foundation (2016b), BPH is so common that all men most likely will have an enlarged prostate if they live long enough. Signs and symptoms of the condition include:

- Dribbling of urine
- *Incontinence* (cannot control urine flow)
- Bloody urine
- Difficulty and pain with urination
- Needing to urinate often
- Slowed start of the urinary stream

To diagnose BPH, the health care provider takes a health history and conducts a physical examination and a digital rectal exam (DRE). Urinalysis, urine culture, and PSA test also are used to diagnose BPH.

The choice of BPH treatment is based on symptoms and depends on whether there are other health problems. Many men with BPH have mild symptoms; others are in pain, particularly those over 60. BPH cannot be cured, but treatment relieves symptoms. The three treatment options are watchful waiting, medication, and surgery. Watchful waiting is recommended when symptoms are mild; the health care provider has regular follow-up with the patient but does not give treatment until problems get worse.

One type of medication for BPH relaxes muscles near the prostate, and the other type shrinks the prostate gland. Some evidence shows that taking both drugs together may work best to keep BPH from getting worse.

Many herbs have been tried for treating BPH, such as saw palmetto, which may ease BPH symptoms and is recommended as an alternative medication. Although some studies have shown that it helps with symptoms, further research is still needed.

The number of prostate surgeries has gone down over the years, but it is still a common treatment. Surgery is used when symptoms are severe or when drug therapy does not work. Prostate surgery is recommended if the patient has incontinence, regular blood in the urine, persistent UTIs, kidney failure, or bladder stones. Most men who have prostate surgery have improvement in urine flow rates and symptoms. However, even after surgical treatment, BPH may return over time. Other treatments include radio waves, microwaves, or lasers, which are used to treat urinary problems caused by BPH. These methods use different kinds of heat to reduce extra prostate tissue.

Prostate Cancer

Prostate cancer are cancer cells in the tissues of the prostate. It is the most common cancer in American men after skin cancer. Prostate cancer grows slowly when compared to most other cancers. Cell changes may begin 10, 20, or even 30 years before a tumor gets big enough to cause symptoms. By the time symptoms appear, the cancer may already be advanced.

By age 50, some precancerous or cancer cells may exist, but very few men have symptoms of prostate cancer. More than half of all American men have some cancer in their prostate glands by the age of 80 (American Society of Clinical Oncology, 2016b). Most of these cancers never cause symptoms or present a serious threat to health. Only about 3% of American men will die of prostate cancer. The following are risk factors:

- Age: men age 50 and older
- Family health history: men whose fathers or brothers had prostate cancer
- Race: most common among African American men
- Diet: eating high-fat food with few fruits and vegetables

At the start, prostate cancer does not cause symptoms. As the cancer grows, there may be trouble peeing or the need to urinate often, especially at night. There may be pain or burning while urinating; blood in the urine or semen; pain in the back, hips, or pelvis; and painful ejaculation.

Prostate cancer can spread to the lymph nodes of the pelvis or spread throughout the body. It tends to spread to the bones, meaning that bone pain, especially in the back, can be a symptom of advanced prostate cancer.

The symptoms are similar to the symptoms of BPH. To diagnose prostate cancer, the health care provider takes a personal and family health history and does a physical examination along with a DRE and a PSA test. An ultrasound exam may also be needed. If these tests show evidence of cancer in the prostate, the health care provider confirms this with a biopsy.

Treatment for prostate cancer depends on whether cancer is in just the prostate or whether it has spread to other parts of the body. It also depends on the patient's age and overall health. For prostate cancer that has not spread to other parts of the body, treatment includes watchful waiting, surgery, radiation therapy, and hormone therapy.

The main goal of a cancer screening test is to reduce the number of deaths from the disease. There are two screening tests used for prostate cancer: PSA blood test and digital rectal exam (DRE). The US Preventive Services Task Force (USPSTF, 2015) found that among adult men, only a very small number, if any, would benefit from a PSA screening. Therefore, the USPSTF recommends against PSA screening for prostate cancer.

Erectile Dysfunction

Hormones, blood vessels, nerves, and muscles work together to cause an erection. The brain starts an erection by sending nerve signals to the penis when it senses sexual stimulation. Touch may cause an erection, as well as other triggers, such as what the man sees or hears, or sexual thoughts. *Erectile dysfunction (ED)* refers to trouble getting or keeping an erection. Although ED becomes more common as males age, it is not a natural part of aging.

ED can be a sign of health problems, particularly those that affect the heart and blood vessels. Unhealthy lifestyle can also contribute to ED; that is, anything that is bad for the heart, such as smoking, is also bad for sexual health. It was once thought that ED was caused by mental or emotional problems, but it is known that most ED has a physical cause; however, depression and anxiety can still cause ED.

There are several treatments for ED. For many men, the answer is as simple as taking prescription medications, getting counseling, more exercise, losing weight, or not smoking. When these treatments fail, then medicines injected directly into the penis can help.

Another way to have an erection is to use a special vacuum tube. The penis is inserted into the tube, which is connected to a pump. As air is pumped out of the tube, blood flows into the penis and makes it larger.

If all other options fail, some men need *penile implant* surgery to treat ED. A surgeon implants a device that inflates to create an erection. This operation cannot be reversed, meaning that once a man has a penile implant, he must use the device to have an erection.

Chapter Summary

- The urinary system filters waste and extra fluid from blood.
- Problems in the urinary system include kidney failure, urinary tract infections, kidney stones, prostate enlargement, and bladder control problems.
- Urology is the branch of medicine that studies the diseases of the male and female urinary system and the male reproductive organs. Nephrology is the study of kidney function.
- Diseases of the urinary system include any diseases that affect the kidneys, ureters, bladder, or urethra.
- The main functions of the male reproductive system are to (a) produce, care for, and transport sperm and semen; (b) deposit sperm in the female reproductive tract; and (c) produce and secrete male sex hormones.
- Male infertility refers to a man's inability to get a woman pregnant after at least 1 year of trying.

REVIEW QUESTIONS

1. Describe the structure and function of the ureter, bladder, and urethra.
2. What are the differences among dysuria, nocturia, pleura, urgency, and hematuria?
3. How is urine made?
4. What is the difference between hemodialysis (HD) and peritoneal dialysis (PD)?
5. What causes kidney stones, and what are treatment options?
6. What is the difference between acute renal failure and chronic renal failure?
7. What will happen if both kidneys fail to function?
8. What should you do to take care of your urinary system? Can you identify at least one prevention strategy for kidney disease?
9. What causes the prostate to enlarge?
10. What are some causes of male infertility?

KEY TERMS

Accessory organs: Internal organs of the male reproductive system

Acute bacterial prostatitis: Common bacterial infection in the prostate gland

Acute kidney failure (AKF), or acute renal failure (ARF): Condition that arises when damage to nephrons occurs quickly

Assisted reproductive technologies: Artificial or partially artificial methods used to achieve pregnancy

Benign prostatic hyperplasia (BPH): Enlargement of the prostate gland, which causes it to press on the urethra

Biological therapy: Treatment that helps the immune system kill bladder cancer cells

Bladder: Hollow organ shaped like a balloon that stores urine until a person is ready to urinate

Bladder cancer: Cancer cells that form in the tissues of the bladder

Catheter: Small tube put through the urethra into the bladder

Chronic bacterial prostatitis: Chronic bacterial infection in the prostate gland

Chronic kidney disease (CKD): Condition that arises when nephrons slowly get worse and kidney damage lasts for more than 3 months

Chronic pelvic pain syndrome (CPPS): Type of prostatitis infection that is present, but without detectable bacteria

Circumcision: Removal of the foreskin

Clean-catch method: Method of collecting of a urine sample in a way that ensures it is germ-free

Cowper's glands: Glands that produce a fluid that acts like grease in the urethra, helping the flow of fluids

Cystitis: Urinary tract infection in the tissue lining of the bladder

Cystoscope: Type of endoscope that is used to diagnose some urethra and bladder diseases

Dialyzer: Special filter used in hemodialysis that cleans the blood

Digital rectal exam (DRE): Procedure done as part of prostate exam

Diuretic: Medication to get rid of excess water in the body

Dysuria: Burning feeling when urinating

Ejaculatory ducts: Ducts formed by the joining of the vas deferens and the seminal vesicles

Epididymal cysts: Sperm-filled cysts, or swelling in the epididymis

Epididymis: Tube on the backside of each testicle that moves and stores sperm cells

Erectile dysfunction (ED): Trouble getting or keeping an erection

Erection: The temporary lengthening, thickening, and hardening of the penis

Excretion/urination: The process by which waste and other nonuseful materials are eliminated from the body

Hematuria: Blood in the urine

Hemodialysis (HD): Procedure in which a patient's blood is carried into a machine that filters the waste and then returns the clean blood back into the patient's body

Incontinence: Inability to control the flow of urine

Kidney disease: Disease that occurs when waste builds up in the blood because of damaged nephrons

Kidney donation: Donation of a kidney from a living blood relative, a living loved one, or a deceased donor

Kidney failure: Condition in which kidney function has fallen below a certain level

Kidneys: Organs that clean the blood, maintain the balance of salt and minerals in the blood, make red blood cells, help keep blood pressure normal, and promote strong bones

Kidney stones: Small rocks made of waste in the urine and that form in the kidney

Kidney transplant: Surgical procedure that puts a donor kidney into a person with severe kidney failure

Kidney tumor: Abnormal growth in the kidney

Male infertility: The inability of a man to get a woman pregnant after 1 year of trying

Nephrologist: Physician who treats diseases of the kidney and is trained in the internal medicine subspecialty of nephrology

Nephrology: Medical specialty that specializes in the study of the function, diseases, and treatment of the kidneys

Nephrons: Small filtering ball-shaped units in each kidney

Nocturia: Frequent urinating at night

Orgasm, or sexual climax: For men, the point at which semen is discharged through the end of the penis

Penile implant: A surgically inserted device that inflates to create an erection

Penis: The male organ for sexual intercourse

Peritoneal dialysis (PD): Procedure in which solutions are pumped into the stomach through a tube that help draw out the waste from the blood and remove it from the body

Pleura: Frequent urinating

Prostate cancer: Cancer cells in the tissues of the prostate

Prostate gland: Gland that makes additional fluid to help in ejaculation

Prostate-specific antigen (PSA): Substance made by the prostate

Prostatitis: Inflammation of the prostate gland

PSA blood test: Measures the amount of prostate-specific antigen (PSA)

Pyelonephritis: Urinary tract infection of one or both kidneys

Renal artery: Artery through which blood and fluids enter the kidney

Renal cell carcinoma (RCC): The most common type of kidney cancer

Renal veins: Veins that transport substances useful to the body along with clean blood out of the kidneys

Routine urinalysis: Lab test that involves having the patient urinate into a special container

Semen: A liquid that carries sperm and is discharged from the penis

Seminal vesicles: Sacs with glands that make semen

Sepsis: Life-threatening blood infection

Spermatic cord: A cord that suspends the testes within the scrotum and carries blood to and from the testicles

Sphincter muscles: Muscles that prevent urine to leak from the bladder

Testicular cancer: Cancer cells that start in the tissues of testicles

Testosterone: Hormone responsible for male traits and for assisting in the production of sperm

Ultrasonography: Diagnostic test that gives information about the kidneys

Undescended testicle: Testicle that fails to move into the scrotum before birth

Urea: Waste material produced when food proteins are broken down

Ureters: Two thin tubes that allow urine to travel from the kidneys down to the bladder

Urethra: Tube that allows urine to pass outside the body

Urethritis: Urinary tract infection of the urethra

Urgency: Constant feeling of the need to urinate

Urinary system, or renal system: The organs, tubes, muscles, and nerves that work together to create, store, and excrete urine

Urinary tract infection (UTI): Bacterial infection that can occur anywhere along the urinary tract

Urine: Fluid waste made by the kidneys, containing urea, uric acid, excess salt, and other waste, as well as water

Urine culture: Test in which bacteria from a urine sample are grown in a lab

Urine sample: Sample of urine for a urinalysis

Urodynamic test: Test that looks at how urine is stored and how it flows from the bladder through the urethra

Urologist: Physician who has a specialty in the treatment of urinary tract diseases in males and females as well as of diseases in the male reproductive system

Urology: Branch of medicine that focuses on the diseases of the male and female urinary system and the male reproductive organs

Vanished testicle, or absent testicle: A testicle that cannot be found, even during surgery

Varicocele: A swollen vein of the spermatic cord

Vas deferens: Long tube that transports mature sperm to the urethra for ejaculation

Wilms' tumor: Kidney cancer that develops in children

CHAPTER ACTIVITIES

1. In pairs, label the parts of the male and female urinary system and the male reproductive system. Along with your labels, describe the function(s) of each part.

2. Trace the route of sperm from the epididymis to the outside of the body using the correct terms for the male reproductive system organs and glands.

3. Brainstorm the factors (e.g., environmental, hormonal, physical) and risk reduction measures that affect fertility in males.

4. Your instructor will invite a guest speaker from a dialysis unit to give a presentation on filtration, reabsorption, and secretion related to the functioning kidney and a kidney in hemodialysis. Following this presentation, keep an accurate record of your intake and output of fluids for a 24-hour period—that is, how often you drink fluids and how often you urinate. You should also observe whether you urinate more during the day or at night. Bring your results to class for analysis and discussion. As part of discussion, identify how kidneys change across the lifespan and how different diseases affect urination.

5. A senior center has hired you as a health educator. A need of your target audience is UTI prevention in males and females. In pairs, brainstorm a design for a UTI prevention awareness campaign for this population. What are the five key messages or key points of the campaign?

Bibliography and Works Cited

American Cancer Society. (2016). Bladder cancer. Retrieved from http://www.cancer.org/cancer/bladdercancer/

American Society of Clinical Oncology. (2016a). Testicular cancer. Retrieved from http://www.cancer.net/cancer-types/testicular-cancer

American Society of Clinical Oncology. (2016b). Prostate cancer. Retrieved from http://www.cancer.net/cancer-types/prostate-cancer

Figler, B. D. (2016). *Evaluation of kidney and urinary tract disorders*. Kenilworth, NJ: Merck.

Johns Hopkins Medicine. (2016). Overview of urogenital disorders. *Health Library*. Retrieved from http://www.hopkinsmedicine.org/healthlibrary/conditions/kidney_and_urinary_system_disorders/overview_of_urogenital_disorders_85,P01466/

Mayo Clinic. (2016). Urinary tract infection (UTI). Retrieved from http://www.mayoclinic.org/diseases-conditions/urinary-tract-infection/basics/risk-factors/con-20037892

National Cancer Institute. (2016a). Seer training modules: Introduction to the urinary system. Retrieved from http://training.seer.cancer.gov/anatomy/urinary/

National Cancer Institute. (2016b). Understanding prostate changes: A health guide for men. Retrieved from http://www.cancer.gov/types/prostate/understanding-prostate-changes

National Institute of Diabetes and Digestive and Kidney Diseases. (2014a). The kidneys and how they work. Retrieved from http://www.niddk.nih.gov/health-information/health-topics/Anatomy/kidneys-how-they-work/Pages/anatomy.aspx

National Institute of Diabetes and Digestive and Kidney Diseases. (2014b). Treatment methods for kidney failure: Kidney transplantation. Retrieved from https://www.niddk.nih.gov/health-information/health-topics/kidney-disease/treatment-methods-for-kidney-failure-transplantation/pages/facts.aspx

National Kidney Foundation. (2010). About chronic kidney disease: A guide for patients and their families. Retrieved from https://www.kidney.org/sites/default/files/docs/11-50-0160_jai_patbro_aboutckdv2lr.pdf

National Kidney Foundation. (2016a). Dialysis. Retrieved from https://www.kidney.org/atoz/content/dialysisinfo

National Kidney Foundation. (2016b). Glomerular filtration rate (GFR). Retrieved from https://www.kidney.org/atoz/content/gfr

Nemours Foundation. (2016). Male reproductive system. Retrieved from http://kidshealth.org/en/parents/male-reproductive.html

Radiological Society of North America. (2016). Varicocele embolization. Retrieved from http://www.radiologyinfo.org/en/info.cfm?pg=Varicocele

Urology Care Foundation. (2015). What are kidney stones? Retrieved from http://www.urologyhealth.org/urologic-conditions/kidney-stones

Urology Care Foundation. (2016a). What are spermatoceles (spermatic cysts)? Retrieved from http://www.urologyhealth.org/urologic-conditions/spermatoceles

Urology Care Foundation. (2016b). What is benign prostatic hyperplasia (BPH)? Retrieved from http://www.urologyhealth.org/urologic-conditions/benign-prostatic-hyperplasia-(bph)

Urology Care Foundation. (2016c). What is kidney cancer? Retrieved from http://www.urologyhealth.org/urologic-conditions/kidney-cancer

US National Library of Medicine. (2016a). Kidney diseases. *MedlinePlus*. Retrieved from https://www.nlm.nih.gov/medlineplus/kidneydiseases.html

US National Library of Medicine. (2016b). Male reproductive system. *MedlinePlus*. Retrieved from https://www.nlm.nih.gov/medlineplus/malereproductivesystem.html#topics

US Preventive Services Task Force. (2011). Testicular cancer: Screening. Retrieved from https://www.uspreventiveservicestaskforce.org/Page/Document/UpdateSummaryFinal/testicular-cancer-screening

US Preventive Services Task Force. (2015). Prostate cancer: Screening. Retrieved from http://www.uspreventiveservicestaskforce.org/Page/Document/UpdateSummaryFinal/prostate-cancer-screening

Wolters Kluwer. (2016a). Patient education: Urinary tract infections in adults (The basics). *UpToDate.* Retrieved from https://www-uptodate-com.ezproxy.springfield.edu/contents/urinary-tract-infections-in-adults-the -basics?source=search_result&search=urinary%20tract%20infection&selectedTitle=1~150

Wolters Kluwer. (2016b). Patient education: Urinary tract infections in adolescents and adults (Beyond the basics). *UpToDate.* Retrieved from https://www-uptodate-com.ezproxy.springfield.edu/contents/urinary -tract-infections-in-adolescents-and-adults-beyond-the-basics?source=related_link

CHAPTER 18

FEMALE REPRODUCTIVE SYSTEM AND RELATED DISEASES

CHAPTER OBJECTIVES

- Explain the structure and function of female reproductive system organs.

- List physical changes associated with female puberty, the childbearing years, and menopause.

- Summarize causes, diagnosis, and treatment of common diseases related to the female reproductive system.

- Give examples of pregnancy complications.

- Distinguish among sexually transmitted infections.

Many health issues affect the female reproductive system, but we do not necessarily know what causes them. However, there are ways to treat many of these issues with medications, surgery, or lifestyle changes. The specific health issue, its signs and symptoms, and the patient's age and desire to have children are all factors that guide treatment choices.

Gynecology is the branch of medicine that deals with the functions and diseases specific to the female reproductive system. A gynecologist focuses only on the care of the reproductive system, whereas an obstetrician focuses on women during and shortly after pregnancy. An obstetrician is also concerned with the health of the fetus. Training is often combined to form a single medical specialty: obstetrics and gynecology (OB-GYN), and almost all gynecologists are obstetricians. Gynecologic oncologists are board-certified OB-GYNs who have additional training in gynecologic cancer.

Structure of the Female Reproductive System

The organs of the female reproductive system allow females to make ova, or eggs. (The singular form is ovum.) The fertilization of ova by sperm is known as reproduction. In

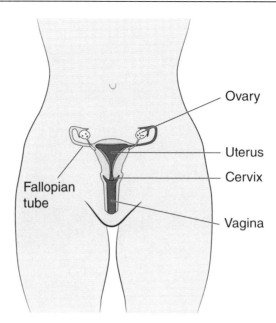

Figure 18.1 Female Reproductive System
Note. Adapted from Womenshealth.gov

addition to reproduction, these organs provide a safe place for the *fetus* to grow, develop, and be born. After birth, the breasts produce milk to feed the baby.

The organs of the female reproductive system are found both inside and outside the body. Those found inside the body are the ovaries, fallopian tubes, and uterus (see Figure 18.1).

The *ovaries* are oval-shaped glands on either side of the uterus; their function is to produce hundreds of undeveloped ova. Every female is born with a lifetime supply of ova, stored in the ovaries and, after puberty, released every month into the bloodstream. They pass out of the body during *menstruation*.

Ovaries also produce the female sex hormones estrogen and progesterone. *Estrogen* is responsible for the development of breasts and other sex characteristics and starts the beginning of puberty. *Progesterone* builds up the lining of the uterus for the fertilized ova. Both estrogen and progesterone are important in preparing a woman's body for pregnancy.

Each ovary is connected to the uterus by a *fallopian tube*. Ova travel from the ovaries to the uterus via the fallopian tubes. At the other end of each fallopian tube is a fringed area that looks like a funnel. When mature ova pop out of an ovary, they enter the fallopian tube, where they meet tiny hairs in the tube's lining, called cilia. *Cilia* push the ova down the narrow tunnel toward the uterus. *Conception* is the moment when fertilization begins in the fallopian tubes. The fertilized ovum then travels to the uterus, where it attaches into the lining of the uterine wall.

The *uterus, or womb*, is where a fetus, or unborn baby, develops, from the embryo stage (the end of the eighth week after conception, when the major structures have formed) until its birth. The uterus has a thick lining and strong, muscular walls. These walls expand and contract to handle a growing fetus and then help push the baby out during labor.

The uterus has two parts. The body expands to hold a developing baby; the *cervix* is a ring of muscle at the end of the uterus. The cervix allows sperm to enter the uterus, and menstrual blood and babies to go through into the vagina. Until birth, the baby is held in place by the cervix. During birth, the cervix expands, and the baby is pushed through it.

Reproductive organs found outside the body are the vagina (see Figure 18.2) and the breasts (see Figure 18.3). The *vagina* connects the cervix to the outside of the woman's body. It is the hollow tube that receives the man's penis during sexual intercourse. During menstruation, blood flows out of that tube. Because it has muscular walls, the vagina can expand or contract. The vagina's walls are lined with mucous membranes, which keep it protected and moist.

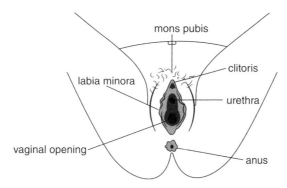

Figure 18.2   Vagina
Note. Adapted from Womenshealth.gov

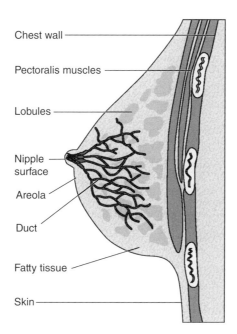

Figure 18.3   Breast
Note. Adapted from "Illu Breast Anatomy.jpg," by Maksim, Wikicommons. This work is in the public domain. Retrieved from https://commons
.wikimedia.org/wiki/File:Illu_breast_anatomy.jpg

The vagina's opening has folds of external skin covered in pubic hair. The external skin is called the labia, which also covers the clitoris. The *labia* surrounds the outside of the vagina. The *clitoris* is the sensory organ located just above the vagina. Together these organs are known as the *vulva*. The urethra is used for urination and also opens into the vulva, but it is separate from the vagina.

The female has two breasts in the upper part of the body (see Figure 18.3). The breasts' primary function is to feed a baby by secreting milk following childbirth. To do this, each breast has anywhere from 15 to 20 *lobules* of glandular tissue, arranged like the petals of a daisy. These lobules are further divided into smaller lobules called *mammary glands* that produce milk. Mammary glands have small tubes or ducts that open out at the nipple for breastfeeding newborn babies. The *nipple* is located near the tip of each breast and is surrounded by a circular area of darker skin called the *areola*.

Function of the Female Reproductive System

As its name implies, the main function of the female reproductive system is to reproduce the species. It does this by producing ova and, during each menstrual cycle, moving an ovum to the place where it can be fertilized by a sperm. Once an ovum is fertilized, the reproductive system offers an environment for it to develop and grow into a baby. If fertilization does not take place, then menstruation occurs. In addition, this system makes female sex hormones that cause the development and release of ova.

Other functions include providing sexual pleasure for the woman and her partner(s), influencing sexual behavior, giving off scents to attract partners, and helping the body store nourishment for offspring. The female reproductive system also coordinates with the urinary system, allowing a woman to urinate.

When a baby girl is born, her ovaries contain thousands of ova, which remain inactive until puberty begins. The reproductive system changes over time as a girl develops into an adult. These changes, known as *puberty*, begin between the ages of 10 and 14 years. During puberty, the pituitary gland, located in the brain, starts making hormones that stimulate the ovaries to make female sex hormones. The secretion of these sex hormones causes a girl to develop into a sexually mature woman. Some of the shifts that occur to a female body at puberty include not only the start of menstrual periods but also growth of pubic and underarm hair, widening of hips, breast development, and emotional changes.

Toward the end of puberty, females release ova as part of a menstrual cycle, or monthly period. With every cycle, a woman's body prepares for a potential pregnancy. About once a month, an ovary sends an ovum into one of the fallopian tubes. Unless the ovum is fertilized by a sperm while in the fallopian tube, it dries up and leaves the body about 2 weeks later through the uterus—this is menstruation. Commonly known as "having a period," blood and tissues from the inner lining of the uterus combine to form the menstrual flow, which lasts from 3 to 7 days. A female's first period is called a *menarche*. It can take up to 2 years from menarche for a female's body to develop a regular menstrual cycle. During that time, her body is adjusting to the hormones puberty brings. On average, the menstrual cycle for an adult woman is 28 days, but the range can be slightly shorter or longer. The cycle stops while a woman is pregnant.

Many women experience *premenstrual syndrome (PMS)*, or discomfort in the days before their periods. At least 85% of menstruating women have at least one PMS symptom monthly (US National Library of Medicine, 2016b). PMS includes physical and emotional symptoms, such as acne, bloating, fatigue, backaches, sore breasts, headaches, food cravings, irritability, and depression. It is usually at its worst during the 7 days before a female's period starts, and disappears once it begins. Some women also experience abdominal cramps caused by chemicals in the body that make the muscles in the uterus contract.

Women can have other health issues with their periods that include pain, heavy bleeding, and skipped periods. *Amenorrhea* is the lack of a menstrual period by age 15 or in women who have not had it for 90 days. Not having periods can mean that the ovaries have stopped making normal amounts of estrogen. Causes of amenorrhea are pregnancy, breastfeeding, extreme weight loss, exercising, eating disorders, or stress. Diseases can also cause amenorrhea.

Dysmenorrhea are painful periods with severe cramps or back pain. Although some pain during a period is normal, extreme pain is not. Menstrual cramps in younger women are usually caused by too much of a certain hormone; in older women, the pain is sometimes caused by issues in the pelvic organs. Treatment for dysmenorrhea depends on its severity and cause.

Abnormal uterine bleeding is bleeding that is different from normal periods. It includes bleeding between periods, after sex, or after menopause. Abnormal bleeding can have many causes; some are serious, others minor. Treatment for abnormal bleeding depends on its severity and cause.

Fertilization

When the male ejaculates, sperm travel in semen from the penis into the vagina. One ejaculation contains between 75 million and 900 million sperm. They "swim" up from the vagina through the cervix and uterus to meet the ovum in the fallopian tube and cause *fertilization*. It takes only one sperm to fertilize the ovum. About a week after the sperm fertilizes the ovum, the fertilized ovum attaches to the uterus, which is called *implantation.*

Once there is implantation, the embryonic stage begins, and the fertilized ovum divides into an *embryo.* After approximately 8 weeks, the embryo is about the size of an adult's thumb, but almost all of its parts—brain, nerves, heart, blood, stomach, intestines, and skin—have formed.

During the fetal stage, development of the embryo continues as cells multiply, move, and change. The embryo now becomes a fetus, which floats in *amniotic fluid* inside the *amniotic sac.* The amniotic fluid and sac protect the fetus against bumps and jolts to the mother's body.

The fetus needs many things from its mother as it develops, including protection, oxygen, food, water, and waste removal. It receives oxygen and nourishment from the mother's blood via the *placenta,* a temporary sac-shaped organ that sticks to the lining of the uterus and holds and attaches the fetus. The fetus is connected to the placenta by the *umbilical cord.*

Pregnancy lasts about 9 months. When the baby is ready for birth, the walls of the uterus contract, causing labor pains. Mucus and amniotic fluid comes out through the vagina when the mother's "water breaks." The contractions cause the cervix to widen enough for the baby to come through. The baby is pushed out along the *birth canal,* a narrow, bone-walled passageway from the womb through the cervix, the vagina, and the vulva. The baby is pushed forcibly through the birth canal, sometimes needing the assistance of metal forceps or suction devices. The baby's head usually comes first, then the umbilical cord comes out. As mentioned, the umbilical cord connects the fetus in the womb to its mother. The cord runs from an opening in the fetus's stomach to the placenta in the womb. The umbilical cord is cut after the baby is delivered. After the umbilical cord is cut, a stump of tissue remains attached to the baby's belly button (navel). The stump gradually dries and shrivels until it falls off, usually 1 to 2 weeks after birth.

The last stage of the birth process, the *afterbirth,* involves the delivery of the placenta, including the umbilical cord. Contractions of the uterus push the placenta out, along with all its membranes and fluids.

Infertility

Infertility is the inability of a woman to get pregnant after at least 1 year of trying, or 6 months if a woman is 35 or older (Centers for Disease Control and Prevention [CDC], 2016c). Female infertility can result from physical problems as well as lifestyle and environmental factors. If a woman has repeated miscarriages, it is also called infertility. A *miscarriage, or spontaneous abortion,* is an unplanned loss of a pregnancy.

Ten percent of women ages 15 to 44 in the United States have difficulty getting pregnant or staying pregnant (CDC, 2016c). Many cases of female infertility are related to issues with menstruation, including irregular or absent periods. Another issue is *premature ovarian failure,* meaning that the ovaries stop functioning before natural menopause. Besides these health issues, there are other causes of infertility, including age, substance abuse, stress, diet, exercise, weight, and sexually transmitted infections (STIs). Providers recommend specific treatments for infertility based on test results and how long partners have been trying to get pregnant. The age and overall health of partners is also taken into consideration.

One third of infertility cases are caused by female reproductive issues, one third by male reproductive issues, and one third by both male and female reproductive issues or by unknown factors. When it is possible to find the cause, infertility can be treated with a combination of medication, surgery, or assisted reproductive technology, including artificial insemination.

Assisted reproductive technology (ART) is a general term used for artificial or partially artificial methods used to achieve pregnancy. *Artificial insemination* is one type of ART, in which the woman is injected with specially prepared sperm. Another ART is to remove ova from a woman's body, then mixing them with sperm to make embryos. The embryos are then put back into the woman's body.

Menopause

Menopause is defined as the point when a woman has not had a period for 12 months in a row (American Sexual Health Association, 2016). It is a normal part of life, just like puberty, and signals the end of a woman's ability to reproduce. Every woman will experience menopause, but not all women do so in the exact same way. Most women experience menopause around age 50 to 58, though it can happen earlier. Smoking causes early menopause, as does never having had a baby, exposure to toxins, heart disease, epilepsy, or having received treatment for depression. Having had pelvic surgery, such as a hysterectomy, can also cause early menopause. *Hysterectomy,* the surgical removal of the uterus and often the cervix, ovaries, and fallopian tubes, makes periods stop. Once a woman has a hysterectomy, she cannot become pregnant.

During menopause, the woman's body no longer produces the hormones necessary for the reproductive cycle to work. When the body no longer makes female hormones, a woman is *menopausal.* After a full year without a period, a woman has been "through menopause." *Postmenopause* follows menopause and lasts for a lifetime.

The time before menopause is *perimenopause.* There is no real agreement about how long this period lasts or when exactly it begins. Regardless, for 5 to 10 years before monthly periods stop, the body responds to hormonal changes that eventually lead to menopause. Signs of perimenopause include occasionally missed periods, periods that are longer or shorter, and changes in the volume of menstrual blood. Eventually periods become less frequent, then stop altogether.

Common signs and symptoms of perimenopause are changes in menstrual periods; hot flashes, or sudden feeling of heat in the body; vaginal dryness; night sweats; trouble sleeping; headaches; moodiness; and a decrease in sex drive. Women can also experience vaginal pain during sexual intercourse. A woman can find out if she is going through menopause through a hormone test.

For treatment during perimenopause, some providers suggest birth control pills to help with menstrual period issues. If the patient is bothered by symptoms like hot flashes, night sweats, or vaginal dryness, health care providers might suggest taking, low-dose antidepressants and vaginal estrogen. They may also suggest *hormone replacement therapy (HRT).* Taking female hormones helps with menopause symptoms and prevents the bone loss that occurs with menopause. HRT has risks, however. That is why the US Food and Drug Administration suggests that women who want to try HRT use the lowest dose possible for the shortest time it's needed. The menopausal symptoms also can return when the patient stops taking HRT.

Common Diagnostic Tests and Procedures of the Female Reproductive System

Some diseases of the female reproductive system can be detected early, if not prevented. Preventive health care includes having regular gynecological exams and screening tests.

If a woman is over 21, chances are she has had an annual *gynecological examination*. These exams help women stay healthy. The first annual exam should be done by age 18, or earlier if she is sexually active. A woman should have these exams any time if she has severe pelvic pain or abnormal bleeding, or when the vagina swells or is itchy.

The gynecological exam includes listening to the heart and lungs, and visual examination and palpation (feeling) of both breasts and the abdomen for any issues. The health care provider also does a two-handed *pelvic exam* (see Figure 18.4). For the younger female patient, however, there is no pelvic exam.

The pelvic exam checks the size, mobility, shape, position, surface, texture, and amount of tenderness of internal and external reproductive organs. To do a pelvic exam, the provider inserts gloved fingers into the vagina to feel the ovaries and uterus. A gentle exam of the internal reproductive

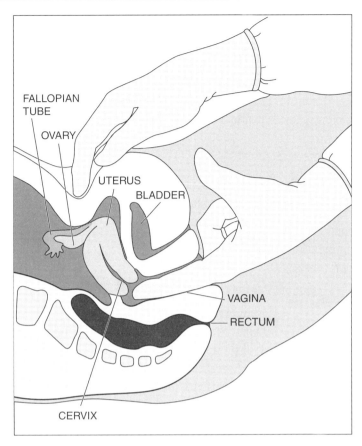

Figure 18.4 Pelvic Exam

Note. Adapted from the National Cancer Institute, n.d., AV-0000-4114, unknown author, public domain, via Wikimedia Commons. Retrieved from https://commons.wikimedia.org/wiki/File:Pelvic_exam_nci-vol-1786-300.jpg

organs is done while the provider presses on the patient's abdomen with his or her other hand. Some providers also examine the rectum with the finger while the other remains in the vagina. The pelvic exam alerts the provider to cysts, growths, and other health issues.

During the gynecological examination, the provider also does a Pap test. A *Pap test* detects abnormal cells in the cervix. To perform a Pap test, the provider uses a brush that scrapes cells from the cervix for examination under a microscope. Abnormal cells can indicate cancer or precancer in the cervix. Not all abnormal cells are found to be cancerous, however. There is no consensus among national health organizations—the American Cancer Society (2016), the American Congress of Obstetricians and Gynecologists (2016), or the US Service Prevention Task Force (2012)—as to whether women should have an annual Pap test screening. These organizations do agree, however, that a Pap test screening is not necessary for women who have had a hysterectomy or who are 65 years or older and have had an adequate screening history.

Other testing and screening during a gynecological exam depends on the age of the patient and any risk factors. A *bone mineral density (BMD) test* checks for osteoporosis (thinning and weakening of the bones) using X-rays. A BMD is recommended for those age 65 and older. A BMD is also recommended if the patient is between the ages 60 and 64, weighs less than 154 pounds, and does not take estrogen.

Breast cancer screenings find issues before any symptoms appear, when there is a better chance of successful treatment. Tests used for breast cancer screening are mammograms and clinical breast exams. Mammograms use an X-ray exam of the breasts to look for abnormal changes. A *screening mammogram* is for women with no breast cancer symptoms, and it involves two X-rays of each breast. Screening mammograms can show lumps or tumors that cannot be felt. Generally, only women ages 50 to 74 years should get a screening mammogram every 2 years, unless there are risk factors, such as a family history of breast cancer. A *diagnostic mammogram* is used to check for breast cancer after a lump or other signs of breast cancer have been found.

Some women perform a breast self-exam. A breast self-exam should not take the place of routine clinical breast exams and mammograms, however. Studies have not demonstrated that breast self-exam alone reduces the number of deaths from breast cancer.

Pregnancy Tests

A pregnancy test detects a hormone in the urine or blood that is only present when a woman is pregnant. Most of these tests can determine whether a woman is pregnant about one week after a missed period. Over-the-counter home pregnancy urine tests are easy to use, inexpensive, and accurate. Blood tests can tell sooner than urine tests, but the woman needs to have a provider perform this test.

Birth Control Methods

Women can choose different types of birth control methods, including implants, pills, and surgery. Yet despite these choices, almost 50% of all pregnancies in the United States are not planned (Planned Parenthood, 2016). One out of every two American women between the ages of 15 to 44 has at least one unplanned pregnancy in her lifetime (CDC, 2015). Culture, religion, personal behavior, education, and economic factors all play a role in this high number.

Both natural and artificial birth control methods try to prevent pregnancy. Natural birth control methods have no side effects, but are less effective than artificial methods. The following lists describe natural and artificial birth control method.

Examples of Natural Types of Birth Control

1. *Abstinence*—not having sexual intercourse.

2. *Natural family planning/rhythm method*—not having sex, or using barrier methods, on days most likely to get pregnant. The woman needs to know her menstrual cycle, check her vaginal discharge, and record her body temperature each day in order to predict the date of ovulation.

3. *Withdrawal*—keeps sperm from entering the vagina. The male removes his penis from the vagina before ejaculation.

Examples of Artificial Types of Birth Control

1. Barrier methods use *spermicide*, a chemical jelly, foam, cream, or suppository. It is put into the vagina before sexual intercourse to kill sperm.

    a. *Contraceptive sponge*—soft foam disc that covers cervix to block sperm

    b. *Diaphragm, cervical cap*—silicone cup that blocks sperm from entering the cervix

    c. *Female condom*—thin sheath worn by the woman inside her vagina

    d. *Male condom*—thin sheath placed over an erect penis

2. Hormonal methods use hormones to stop ovaries from releasing ova.

    a. *Oral contraceptives*—medication that causes changes in the uterus and cervix

    b. *Skin patch*—adhesive pad placed on the skin that releases hormones into the bloodstream and thickens vaginal discharge

    c. *Hormone injection*—a shot that contains hormones that stop the body from releasing ova and thicken the mucus of the cervix

d. *Vaginal ring*—thin, flexible ring releases hormones that thickens vaginal discharge

e. *Emergency contraception pill*—medication that prevents pregnancy up to 5 days after unprotected sex

3. Implantable devices use hormones to stop the ovaries from releasing ova.

a. *Implantable rod*—flexible rod put in the upper arm

b. *Intrauterine devices (IUD)*—small T-shaped device that goes into the uterus (One type of IUD is made of copper that is toxic to sperm, and another type releases a hormone.)

4. The following are permanent or surgical birth control methods.

a. *Sterilization implant*—nonsurgical method of sterilizing women

b. *Surgical sterilization*—surgical procedure that closes the fallopian tubes by cutting, tying, or sealing them

Each method has its pros and cons, and even the most effective birth control can fail (see Table 18.1). But chances of getting pregnant are lowest if the method chosen is always used correctly and every time during sexual intercourse.

Table 18.1 Female Birth Control Methods

Method	Failure Rate (number of pregnancies expected per 100 females)	Side Effects
Abstinence	0	None
Sterilization surgery	Less than 1	Pain, bleeding, complications from surgery
Sterilization implant	Less than 1	Pain, ectopic pregnancy
Implantable rod	Less than 1 Might not work for overweight women	Acne, weight gain, ovarian cysts, depression, hair loss, sore breasts, changes in period, lower sex drive
Emergency contraception/ morning-after pill	1 Must be used within 72 hours of having unprotected sex	Vomiting, headaches, irregular bleeding, breast tenderness
Skin patch	5 May not work as well in overweight women	Spotting or bleeding between periods Greater exposure to estrogen than with other methods
Vaginal ring	5	Spotting or bleeding between periods, swelling and irritation of the vagina, vaginal discharge
Male condom	11–16	Allergic reactions
Diaphragm or cervical cap with spermicide	15	Allergic reactions, urinary tract infections
Sponge with spermicide	16–32	Allergic reactions and irritation, difficulty with removing it
Withdrawal	19	None
Female condom	20	Irritation of vagina, allergic reactions
Natural family planning	25	None
Spermicide alone	30 Works best if used with barrier method, such as a condom	Irritation of vagina Allergic reactions Urinary tract infections
No method	85	None

Abortion

Abortion is the procedure, either chemical or surgical, for ending a pregnancy early. An abortion is usually done in the first trimester of the pregnancy. There are two options for getting an abortion. One is an in-clinic procedure performed by a health care provider in a hospital, physician's office, or health center. When performed by a health care provider during the first trimester, abortions are generally safe and rarely have serious complications. Another option is to take the "abortion pill," which is the popular name two different medications used to end a pregnancy (Planned Parenthood, 2016). In general, the pill is used up to 70 days or 10 weeks after the first day of a woman's last period. Women who need an abortion and are more than 10 weeks' pregnant can have a surgical in-clinic abortion.

Abortion generally does not reduce a woman's ability to get pregnant in the future. Abortions are very common; 3 out of 10 women in the United States have an abortion by the time they are 45 years old (Planned Parenthood, 2016).

A *medical abortion* uses a chemical that blocks the hormone needed for pregnancy. It causes the lining of the uterus to become thin, and is only done in the first nine weeks of pregnancy. For most women, medical abortion feels like a bad menstrual period with strong cramps, diarrhea, and upset stomach. A medical abortion is about 97% effective.

Surgical abortion removes the lining of the uterus and is performed by a health care provider. For most women, this type of abortion feels like strong menstrual cramps. There are two types of surgical abortions; both use suction to empty the uterus. *Manual vacuum aspiration* is done in the first 12 weeks of pregnancy. *Dilation and evacuation (D&E)* is done after the first month of pregnancy and before the end of the 13th week. A surgical abortion is nearly 100% effective.

Health Problems with Pregnancy

Health problems during pregnancy can affect the mother's health, that of the fetus, or both. A high-risk pregnancy is one in which there is greater health risk to the mother or her fetus than a normal pregnancy. An example is an ectopic pregnancy. An *ectopic pregnancy* occurs when the fetus grows outside the uterus, usually in one of the two fallopian tubes. These pregnancies are a medical emergency and can be fatal for the woman if the fallopian tube ruptures. The following are some other examples of health problems during pregnancy:

- *Pregnancy with multiples.* Women who have babies after age 30 or are taking fertility drugs have an increased chance of giving birth to more than one baby. Pregnancy with multiples can cause premature births and low birth weights as well as carry higher risk of disabilities.

- *Preeclampsia.* This condition causes high blood pressure, and protein buildup in the urine of pregnant women. Preeclampsia can result in kidney failure, seizures, and death, as well as early delivery. It can be life threatening for the mother and unborn baby.

- *Gestational diabetes.* A woman who did not have diabetes can develop it during pregnancy.

- *High blood pressure.* This condition can make it hard for blood to reach the placenta.

- *Preterm labor.* Labor that begins before 37 weeks of pregnancy puts both the mother and baby at increased risk for health problems.

- *Miscarriage.* Signs of miscarriage include vaginal bleeding, cramping, or fluid and tissue passing from the vagina. The loss of pregnancy after the 20th week is a *stillbirth.*

Prenatal care is medical care that a woman receives during pregnancy and that helps identify issues before they become serious. During these visits, the woman is examined, and the growth of the baby is checked. Even before considering becoming pregnant, a woman should see a health care provider for *preconception care.* Lifestyle changes for women who want to become pregnant include stopping smoking and alcohol use, reaching a healthy weight, and gaining control of chronic diseases.

Pregnancy and Delivery

A normal pregnancy is approximately 40 weeks, and it is divided into three trimesters. In the *first trimester* (weeks 1–12), the sperm fertilizes the ovum, causing cells to form the fetus and the placenta.

In the *second trimester* (weeks 13–28), a woman can find out the sex of her infant. Muscle tissue, bone, and skin have formed; movement begins; and the fetus sleeps and wakes regularly. The survival rate for babies born at 28 weeks is about 92%, although those born at this time can have serious health problems.

By the *third trimester* (weeks 29–40), bones are soft and yet almost fully formed, and the eyes open and close. Infants born before 37 weeks are *preterm* and are at increased risk for health problems. At 37 weeks, the fetus is full term and can usually survive without support if delivered. However, unless there is a medical issue, it is best to wait until at least 39 weeks to deliver. This gives the lungs, brain, and liver more time to develop.

Labor is a three-stage process that results in the birth of the baby and the expulsion of the placenta. The first stage begins with the woman's contractions and continues until she is dilated fully, which means the cervix has stretched open to prepare for birth. The second stage is the active stage, in which the woman begins to push downward. There is complete dilation of the cervix. This stage ends with the actual birth. The third stage begins with the birth and ends with the completed delivery of the placenta.

Just as pregnancy is different for every woman, the signs of labor and the length of time for each stage are different from woman to woman. Some women when giving birth do fine with just natural pain-relief methods. Natural methods include deep breathing, warm baths, and massages. Many women blend natural methods with medications to ease pain. Sometimes a woman may have an *induced labor,* in which medications are used to bring on labor if the health of the mother or the fetus is at risk.

There are two methods of delivery: cesarean and vaginal. A *cesarean delivery* (or C-section) is surgery in which a fetus is delivered through an incision in the mother's abdomen and uterus. This surgery is necessary if a woman is carrying more than one fetus or if the labor is not going well. Other reasons for a C-section include the baby's health being in danger, or a chance of a breech birth. A *breech birth* means that the baby is upside down and that the feet are delivered first.

Women who have a C-section are given pain medication—an epidural block, a spinal block, or general anesthesia. An *epidural block* is an injection in the spine that numbs the lower part of the body. A *spinal block* also numbs the lower part of the body by an injection directly into the spinal fluid.

C-section delivery is safe, but it can increase the risk of having difficulties with future pregnancies. For this reason, a vaginal birth is generally the preferred method of delivery.

Breastfeeding

Breastfeeding is the feeding of human breast milk to a baby. It is done either directly from the breast or by *expressing,* which is pumping out breast milk and bottle-feeding it to the baby. It is recommended by the Office of Women's Health (2014) that breast milk be given to babies for at least the first 6 months of life and then a combination of solid foods and breast milk until the baby is at least 1 year old. *Weaning* is the switching from breast milk or formula to other foods and fluids.

Breastfeeding is the recommended method for feeding babies because the milk has the right balance of nutrients to help a baby grow. Some nutrients in breast milk help protect babies against common childhood illnesses and infections. Breastfeeding also improves the survival rate of babies during their first year of life, including lower risk of sudden infant death syndrome (SIDS).

There are some cases, however, when it is best for a mother not to breastfeed. If a mother has HIV, for example, the infection can be passed to the baby through breast milk. Certain medications, illegal drugs, and alcohol can also be passed through the breast milk to the baby.

Diseases of the Female Reproductive System

For purposes of discussion in this chapter, common female reproductive system diseases are split into three groups: diseases that cause abnormal uterine bleeding, diseases that cause inflammation, and cancers.

Diseases That Cause Abnormal Uterine Bleeding

Endometriosis is a disease in which uterine tissue grows somewhere else—for example, in the ovaries. This out-of-place tissue causes pain, infertility, and heavy periods. Although many women have cramping during their menstrual period, women with endometriosis have severe menstrual pain that increases over time. It affects about 1 out of 10 women (Office of Women's Health, 2015a). Some women have no symptoms at all, and for them, having trouble getting pregnant may be their first sign. Endometriosis is one of the top three causes of infertility.

The cause of endometriosis is unknown, and it cannot be prevented, but there are risk factors for developing the condition, including the following:

- A family history of endometriosis
- Menarche at a young age
- Frequent periods or periods that last 7 or more days
- Never having had children

Endometriosis is usually diagnosed in women in their 30s and 40s and is determined by signs and symptoms, pelvic exam, ultrasound, and laparoscopy. Treatment is usually pain medications with hormone therapy or surgery. Treatment depends on severity and on whether the patient hopes to become pregnant. If the patient wants a pregnancy, then surgery increases the chance of success. Regardless of the treatment, endometriosis is chronic, but signs and symptoms can improve after menopause.

Hormonal imbalance causes *polycystic ovary syndrome* (PCOS). It is the most common hormonal problem among women of reproductive age and a leading cause of infertility (Endocrine Society, 2016). PCOS occurs when a woman's ovaries or adrenal glands make more male hormones than normal. The term *polycystic* means "many cysts," and with PCOS there are clusters of small cysts in the ovaries. These cysts are fluid-filled bubbles that contain immature ova. Symptoms of PCOS include the following:

- Irregular or absent menstrual periods
- Infertility
- Excess body or facial hair
- Acne or patches of brown or black skin
- Pelvic pain
- Baldness

Women who are obese are more likely to have PCOS. Those with PCOS are at higher risk of diabetes, metabolic syndrome, heart disease, and high blood pressure.

The cause of PCOS is unknown, although it does run in families. There is no cure, but medications control symptoms. Birth control pills help women have normal periods and reduce male hormone levels; other medications reduce hair growth, control blood pressure, and lower cholesterol. Lifestyle changes including exercise and healthy eating can also control PCOS signs and symptoms.

Cervical polyps are finger-like growths in the uterus. They are bright red or purple and feel spongy. The cause of cervical polyps is not fully understood, but they can develop with chronic inflammation in the cervix or high levels of sex hormones.

Cervical polyps are common, particularly in perimenopausal women who have been pregnant. Most women have only one polyp, but some women have two or three.

Polyps may not cause symptoms, but the symptoms are heavy periods, abnormal bleeding from the vagina, and a yellowish mucus. Usually diagnosed during a pelvic exam, polyps are confirmed by a cervical biopsy.

A health care provider can remove polyps during a simple outpatient procedure. Most polyps are not cancerous and are easy to remove. They do not usually grow back. A way to prevent polyps is to treat cervical infections early.

Uterine fibroids are tumors that grow in the uterus and are made up of muscle and tissue. Fibroids grow as a single tumor or in clusters. A single fibroid may be 1 inch or less or can grow to more than 8 inches across.

Fibroids are the most common noncancerous tumors in women of childbearing age, affecting up to 25% of all women (Office of Women's Health, 2015b). The cause of fibroids is unknown, but African American women and overweight women are at greatest risk. By the age of 50, up to 80% of Black women and up to 70% of White women have fibroids (Office of Women's Health, 2015b). Women who have given birth are at lower risk.

For some women, fibroids cause heavy and painful periods, bleeding between periods, frequent urination, pain during sex, lower back pain, infertility, and early labor. Other women have no symptoms and do not need treatment. A health care provider can find fibroids during a pelvic exam or by using imaging tests. Treatment includes medications to control pain and bleeding, as well as hormone therapy. In more severe cases, surgery is an option. Fibroids are the major reason for having a hysterectomy, and if both ovaries are removed, the woman enters menopause. Often, fibroids stop growing or shrink after menopause.

Diseases That Cause Inflammation

Vaginitis is inflammation of the vagina, and most women deal with some type of vaginitis during their lifetime (Office of Women's Health, 2015c). Often called vaginal symptoms, vaginitis is not a sign of a serious disease, and the majority of symptoms are not due to sexually transmitted infections. Vaginitis is diagnosed when the provider examines the patient's vagina and surrounding areas for inflammation. A sample of any discharge is taken for testing. Causes of vaginitis include the following:

- *Bacterial vaginosis*—infection and inflammation of the vagina caused by bacteria. It is the most common vaginal infection in women of childbearing age. Symptoms include fishy-smelling discharge, especially after intercourse, as well as itching, burning, and swelling in the vagina.

- *Trichomoniasis* (trich)—infection with trichomonas, a protozoan organism. Trich is a common sexually transmitted infection. Symptoms are yellow discharge and pain during intercourse.

- *Vaginal candidiasis* or *yeast infection*—fungus infection with itching, burning, swelling, and a thick white discharge.

Treatment for vaginitis includes antibiotic or antifungal medications taken orally, put on the vagina as creams or gels, or inserted as a *vaginal suppository*. A suppository is medication inserted into the vagina, where it melts. The following approaches reduce the risk of vaginitis:

- Be abstinent.
- Do not douche.
- Limit the number of sex partners.
- Correctly use prescribed medications.

Cancers

There are different types of *uterine cancer*, with endometrial cancer being the most common. *Endometrial cancer* is cancer of the *endometrium*, the innermost lining of the uterus that grows each month during childbearing years. It does this to support an embryo if a woman becomes pregnant. If pregnancy does not occur, then the endometrium is shed during the menstrual period.

Risk factors for uterine cancer are use of estrogen without progesterone, diabetes, hypertension, and later age of menopause (after age 52). But one of the greatest, most common risk factors for uterine cancer is obesity (Foundation for Women's Cancer, 2016). Women who are obese have higher circulating levels of estrogen, which increases risk.

The major warning sign for uterine cancer is abnormal vaginal bleeding. Recognizing this symptom helps in early diagnosis and treatment. In older women, any bleeding after menopause may be a symptom of uterine cancer. About 75% of women diagnosed with uterine cancer have already gone through menopause. Younger women are also at risk, and should note heavy vaginal bleeding as a symptom. Other symptoms of uterine cancer include:

- Bleeding between periods
- Persistent pelvic pain
- Watery vaginal discharge
- Pain during sexual intercourse

When a woman experiences these symptoms, a physical and pelvic examination is done by her provider. If the examination is abnormal, she should have an endometrial biopsy, ultrasound, or a D&C (dilation and curettage) procedure.

Although uterine cancer is treated with radiation therapy, chemotherapy, or hormonal therapy, the common treatment is surgery. Several types of surgery can be done, including a hysterectomy. The treatment can also include more than one option depending on the age and health of the patient and on the type, stage, and location of the cancer.

Cervical cancer is abnormal cervix cells that grow out of control. Over time, it can spread into nearby tissues. The cancer cells spread by breaking away from the cervical tumor and traveling to the lymph nodes, lungs, liver, or bones. In the United States, there is a conservative estimate of almost 13,000 new cases of cervical cancer every year, and more than 4,000 deaths (National Cervical Cancer Coalition, 2016).

Early cervical cancer usually does not cause symptoms, but when it is in later stages, there can be abnormal vaginal bleeding, pelvic pain, and pain during intercourse. If a patient has symptoms of cervical cancer, the provider may use two additional diagnostic tests: a cervical exam with a colposcope that can examine tissue closely, and a biopsy to remove cervix tissue for lab analysis. If cervical cancer is caught early, it can be cured.

The *human papillomavirus (HPV)* infection is the cause of almost 90% of cervical cancers. Sixty percent of sexually active women have been infected with HPV sometime in their life (CDC, 2016b).

Most infections clear up on their own, but an HPV infection that does not go away can cause cervical cancer. Other risk factors for cervical cancer are cigarette smoking, having sex at an early age, multiple sexual partners, and sexual partners who have multiple partners.

A woman's risk of cervical cancer is reduced by having regular cervical cancer screening tests and getting an HPV vaccine before becoming sexually active. The HPV vaccine is recommended for girls ages 11 or 12 and can be given to females ages 9 to 26 (CDC, 2016b).

Cancer of the ovary is not common, but it causes more deaths than other female reproductive cancers. One out of every 72 women can expect to develop *ovarian cancer* at some time in her life (CDC, 2014). This cancer mainly develops in older women: 50% of women diagnosed with it are 63 years or older (Ovarian Cancer National Alliance, 2016).

The three main types of ovarian cancer all begin in the ovaries and can rapidly spread to other organs. The sooner ovarian cancer is found and treated, the better the recovery. When the cancer is found at an early stage, about 94% of patients live longer than 5 years after diagnosis (Ovarian Cancer National Alliance, 2016). Ovarian cancer is hard to detect early, however, and there is no cure. Women with this cancer may have no or mild symptoms until it is in an advanced stage. If there are symptoms, these may include:

• Pelvic and back pain

• Weight gain or loss

• Vaginal bleeding

• Abnormal periods

Diagnostic tests for ovarian cancer are physical and pelvic examinations, lab tests, ultrasound, or a biopsy. Treatment is usually surgery followed by chemotherapy, hormone therapy, or radiation. If there is surgery, it is often a *laparotomy*, which means the ovaries, uterus, fallopian tubes, supporting ligaments, and possibly pelvic and lymph nodes are removed.

The risk factors for ovarian cancer are age over 55, never having been pregnant, a family history of cancer, and a past history of other cancers. For prevention, if a woman does have a family history or past history of cancer, it is recommended that her ovaries be removed after ending childbearing or by age 35.

Breast Health

Part of breast health is to know the way breasts normally feel and to look for changes. A woman's breasts change at different times of her life. Some of these changes are part of the natural process of aging; other changes can be a sign of a problem, including breast cancer. There are steps that a woman can take to have healthy breasts, including screening mammograms and clinical breast exams.

If a woman finds a lump and the lumpiness is felt throughout the breast and feels like the other breast, then it is probably normal breast tissue. By contrast, lumps that feel harder or different from the rest of the breast or the other breast are a concern. When this type of lump is found, it may be a sign of breast cancer or benign breast diseases.

Changes in breasts are not necessarily signs of cancer. Minor and serious breast health problems can have the same symptoms. However, some benign breast changes do increase the risk of breast cancer. That is why it is important for a woman who has a breast lump, pain, discharge, or skin rash to see her health care provider right away.

Benign breast diseases describe a range of noncancerous breast problems. Some of these problems cause pain, and treatment can help; others need no treatment. According to the Susan G. Komen for the Cure (2013), the following are examples of benign breast diseases:

• *Cysts* are lumps filled with fluid. They are not removed unless painful; they do not increase the risk for breast cancer.

- *Fibroadenomas* are lumps that feel like marbles and move around easily when pushed. They do not increase the risk for breast cancer and are usually painless.

- *Intraductal papillomas* are wart-like growths near the nipple. They are removed with surgery and do not increase breast cancer risk unless there is abnormal cell growth.

Breast Cancer

Breast cancer is cancer cell growth in the breast tissues. These cancer cells grow and divide, invade nearby breast tissue, form a tumor, and then can spread to other parts of the body. A cancerous tumor is hard to move under the skin and feels solid, with irregular edges.

There are different types of breast cancer; their names are based on which cells turn cancerous. Some types are noninvasive, and the cancer cells do not spread into nearby breast tissue. Other types spread and grow in the fatty tissues of the breast. Still others start within the breast but then spread to vital organs. Whatever the type, breast cancer alone does not kill, because breasts are not vital organs. The cancer kills only when it spreads to vital organs.

Breast cancer is the second most common type of cancer in women, affecting one in eight women during their lives. For reasons unknown, the number of cases has doubled in the United States since the 1940s. Although the number of cases is increasing and breast cancer is the second leading cause of cancer deaths in women, second only to lung cancer, there is hope. The hope lies in the fact that the number of deaths is decreasing due to new technologies and earlier detection.

Although no one knows why some women get breast cancer, there are a number of risk factors. Some of these risks—aging, having dense breasts, or having periods before age 12—cannot be changed. There are, however, risk factors for breast cancer that can be changed: excessive use of alcohol, obesity, long-term use of hormone replacement therapy, taking birth control pills, or having your first child after age 35 (National Breast Cancer Foundation, 2015).

Having a risk factor does not mean a woman will get breast cancer. Most women have some risk factors, and most women do not get breast cancer. In fact, most women who develop breast cancer have no special risk factors.

There are warning signs for breast cancer. Some people do not have any signs or symptoms and find out that they have breast cancer only after a routine screening mammogram. As shown in the following list, some of the warning signs for breast cancer are the same as for benign breast diseases:

- Lump
- Skin dimpling
- Change in skin color or texture
- Change in the appearance of the nipple—for example, pulling in
- Clear or bloody fluid that leaks out of the nipple

Breast cancer is diagnosed through a physical examination and taking a health history. Providers may also perform a breast ultrasound, mammogram, MRI, and breast biopsy to determine a diagnosis.

There are two goals in breast cancer treatment. The first is to get rid of the cancer; the second is to prevent it from returning. Treatment depends on the type and size of the cancer, how far it has spread, and the woman's age and health.

Those with breast cancer often have more than one treatment option. Treatment can include surgery, radiation therapy, chemotherapy, and hormone therapy. A *lumpectomy* is surgery that removes cancer tumors. Removal of part or all of the breast is a *mastectomy*. Radiation therapy destroys cancer cells in the breast tissue and is used after removal of the tumor or breast. Chemotherapy is used early to slow or stop the cancer from spreading. Hormone therapy is used mostly in women over age 50 against tumors that respond to estrogen.

Two ways to possibly reduce the risk for breast cancer are to exercise regularly and avoid excessive alcohol consumption. More extreme ways to prevent breast cancer for women with a very high risk is to remove the breasts, reducing risk up to 90%. Injections that stop hormone production by the ovaries or stop the effects of estrogen can be used in high-risk women, reducing risk up to 50% (National Breast Cancer Foundation, 2015).

Sexually Transmitted Infections

A person gets *sexually transmitted infections (STIs)* by having sexual contact with an infected person. The causes of STIs are bacteria, parasites, and viruses. There is no way to know that a person is infected, because many STIs have no symptoms; however, STIs can still be passed from person to person even without symptoms. They spread during vaginal, anal, or oral sex or during genital touching. Many STIs have only mild symptoms or none at all. When symptoms do develop, they often are mistaken for something else, such as a UTI.

In the United States there are about 19 million new STI diagnoses each year (CDC, 2016e). These infections affect men and women of all backgrounds and economic levels. Almost half of new infections are among young people ages 15 to 24. Women are particularly affected by STIs. They experience more frequent and more serious health problems from STIs than men.

Not all STIs are spread the same way, and each STI causes different health problems. Overall, untreated STIs can cause cancer, pelvic inflammatory disease, infertility, pregnancy problems, widespread infection to other body parts, organ damage, and even death.

There is no one screening test for all STIs. STI screening tests involve a physical examination as well as blood, urine, fluid, or tissue samples. Which STI test and how often to be tested depends mainly on the woman's sexual history and her partner's.

There are more than 30 types of STIs, and most are treatable. Treatment depends on the STI type. For some STIs, just taking medications can cure it; for STIs that cannot be cured, treatment relieves symptoms. For all STIs, abstinence is the primary way to lower risk. Other than abstinence, ways to reduce the risk include the following:

- *Mutual monogamy*—agreement between two uninfected partners to have sex only with each other
- Reduce the number of sex partners
- Get vaccines to prevent Hepatitis B and HPV
- Use condoms correctly and with every sexual contact

Chapter 3 of this book reviews STIs in detail, including chlamydia, gonorrhea, syphilis, and HIV/ AIDS. Table 18.2 is limited to an overview of the most common STIs that affect women.

Table 18.2 Sexual Transmitted Infections (STIs)

STI	Description
Bacterial vaginosis	Caused when too much of certain bacteria change the normal balance of bacteria in the vagina. Most women have no symptoms. Those with symptoms have vaginal itching, pain when urinating, and vaginal discharge.
Chlamydia and gonorrhea	Caused by bacteria that infect the cervix or the urethra. Often no symptoms, or there is vaginal, discharge, itching, pain, or sore throat. Can be cured with antibiotics. Women under the age of 25 who have had sex should be tested for chlamydia at least once per year.
Syphilis	Caused by bacteria. Can infect many parts of the body. A painless sore in the genital area can be an early sign. If found early, it is treated easily. If not treated, signs may disappear, but can return years later in advanced stages.

(continued)

Table 18.2 *Continued*

STI	Description
Genital herpes	Caused by a virus. Some women have no symptoms. Symptoms go away and then return. Symptoms include small bumps, blisters, vaginal discharge, muscle pain, fever, pain when urinating, itching, burning, or swollen glands in genital area. Treatment helps with symptoms, but there is no cure.
Human immunodeficiency virus/acquired immunodeficiency syndrome (HIV/AIDS)	When HIV infection is advanced, it is called AIDS. HIV enters the bloodstream through bodily fluids and invades and kills cells of the immune system, which will lead to AIDS. There is no cure. Because it can take several years after infection with HIV to develop AIDS, many infected people do not know their status.
Human papillomavirus (HPV)	Viral infection that causes genital warts and leads to cervical cancer. Most infections have no symptoms.
Trichomoniasis (Trich)	Caused by bacteria. Symptoms are discharge and vaginal pain. Cured with antibiotics.
Pubic lice (crabs)	Parasitic insect; an infected person finds lice in the genitals. Causes itching in the genital area.

Chapter Summary

- There are several functions of the female reproductive system. The main function is to reproduce the species by producing the ova that are necessary for reproduction.
- The uterus offers an environment for a baby to develop and grow before birth.
- Types of birth control methods can be divided into two major categories: natural and artificial.
- Artificial insemination is an infertility treatment in which the woman is injected with specially prepared sperm. Assisted reproductive technology (ART) is a group of different methods used to help infertile couples.
- Breasts change over the lifetime of a woman, including developing benign lumps, discharge, and tissue masses. Although many women fear cancer, changes in the breast are not necessarily cancer.
- Having a risk factor does not mean a woman will get breast cancer. Most women have some risk factors, and most women do not get breast cancer. Further, most women who develop breast cancer have no special risk factors.
- The causes of STIs are bacteria, parasites, and viruses. Women experience more frequent and more serious health problems from STIs than men.

REVIEW QUESTIONS

1. What are signs and symptoms of premenstrual syndrome?
2. List some of the factors that increase the risk of breast cancer.
3. Explain why breastfeeding is important to both mother and child.
4. What are the two different types of mammograms?
5. Explain the differences among endometriosis, polycystic ovary syndrome, and uterine fibroids.
6. Identify risk factors for sexually transmitted infections. What are some ways to prevent them?
7. Name and describe two benign breast diseases.
8. Summarize three cancers of the female reproductive system.
9. Discuss health problems associated with pregnancy.
10. Name and describe the stages of menopause.

KEY TERMS

Abnormal uterine bleeding: Bleeding from the vagina that is different from normal menstrual periods

Abstinence: Not having sex

Afterbirth: Last part of the birthing process, in which the placenta along with its membranes and fluids are expelled from the body following the delivery of the baby

Amenorrhea: Lack of a menstrual period in young women or in older women who may have gynecological problems

Amniotic fluid: Fluid in which the fetus floats

Amniotic sac: Sac that holds the amniotic fluid and fetus

Areola: Circular area of pigmented skin at the end of each breast

Artificial insemination: Infertility treatment in which the woman is injected with specially prepared sperm

Assisted reproductive technology (ART): Artificial or partially artificial methods used to achieve pregnancy

Bacterial vaginosis: Inflammation of the vagina caused by bacteria

Benign breast diseases: Group of conditions marked by changes in the breast that are not cancerous

Birth canal: Narrow, bone-walled passageway from the womb through the cervix, the vagina, and the vulva, through which the baby travels during birth

Bone mineral density (BMD) test: X-rays of the bones that detect osteoporosis

Breech birth: Birth in which the baby is born upside down with the feet first instead of the head

Cervical cancer: Cancer cells in the cervix

Cervical cap: Barrier method that blocks the sperm from entering the cervix

Cervical polyps: Growths on the lower part of the uterus

Cervical shield: Barrier method that blocks sperm from entering the cervix

Cervix: Ring of muscle at the end of the uterus that allows sperm to enter the uterus, and menstrual blood and babies to go through into the vagina

Cesarean delivery (or C-section): Surgery in which a fetus is delivered through the mother's abdomen and uterus

Chlamydia: Sexually transmitted infection caused by bacteria

Cilia: Hairs on the linings of some organs

Clitoris: Organ located just above the vagina

Conception: Moment when fertilization begins in the fallopian tubes

Contraceptive sponge: A disc that covers the cervix and blocks sperm

Cysts: Lumps filled with fluid

Diagnostic mammogram: X-ray exam of the breasts used to check for breast cancer when a lump has been found

Diaphragm: Barrier method that blocks the sperm from entering the cervix

Dilation and evacuation (D&E): Surgical abortion that uses suction to empty the uterus

Dysmenorrhea: Painful menstrual periods

Ectopic pregnancy: High-risk pregnancy in which the fetus grows outside the uterus, usually in the fallopian tubes

Embryo: The ball of cells formed by cell division following fertilization of an ovum

Emergency contraception pill: Medication that prevents pregnancy up to 5 days after unprotected sex

Endometrial cancer: Cancer of the endometrium, the innermost lining of the uterus

Endometriosis: Disease in which tissue from the uterus grows somewhere else—for example, in the ovaries

Endometrium: The innermost lining of the uterus

Epidural block: An injection in the spine during delivery

Estrogen: Hormone responsible for female sex characteristics

Expressing (of breast milk): Pumping out the milk from the breast

Fallopian tubes: Pair of tubes that connect each ovary to the uterus

Female condom: Thin sheath worn by a woman inside her vagina to keep sperm out

Female reproductive system: Body system that gives females the ability to make ova

Fertilization: The meeting in the fallopian tube of a sperm that has "swum" up from the vagina and an ovum

Fetus: An unborn baby, from the embryo stage (the end of the eighth week after conception) until its birth

Fibroadenoma: Lump in the breast that feels like a marble and moves around easily

First trimester: Week 1 to week 12 of pregnancy

Genital herpes: Sexually transmitted infection caused by a virus

Gestational diabetes: Diabetes in pregnant women, brought about by the hormone changes of pregnancy

Gonorrhea: Sexually transmitted infection caused by bacteria

Gynecological exam: Examination in which the health care provider palpates (feels) and checks the appearance of the breasts and the abdomen area

Gynecologic oncologists: Obstetrician-gynecologists with additional training in gynecologic cancer

Gynecologist: Physician with a specialty that focuses only on the reproductive care of women

Gynecology: Branch of medicine that deals with the functions and diseases specific to the female reproductive system

Hormone injection: Injection that causes changes in the cervix to keep sperm from joining with the ovum

Hormone replacement therapy (HRT): Treatment in which a woman takes hormones that help with menopause symptoms

Human papillomavirus (HPV): A virus that infects the genitals

Hysterectomy: Surgical removal of the uterus, and often the ovaries, cervix, and fallopian tubes

Implantable rod: Rod put in the arm of a female patient to prevent pregnancy

Implantation: The attaching of the fertilized ovum into the lining of the uterus

Induced labor: Labor stimulated by the use of medication

Infertility: The inability of a woman to get pregnant after at least 1 year of trying (or 6 months if a woman is 35 or older); also, repeated miscarriages

Intraductal papillomas: Wart-like growths near the nipple

Intrauterine device (IUD): A device that is inserted into the uterus to prevent pregnancy

Labia: Folds of external skin that surround the outside of the vagina

Laparotomy: Surgical removal of the ovaries, uterus, fallopian tubes, supporting ligaments, and possibly pelvic and lymph nodes

Lobules: Glandular tissues in each breast that hold clusters of milk-producing mammary glands

Lumpectomy: Surgical removal of cancerous tumors

Male condom: Thin sheath placed over an erect penis to keep sperm out of a woman's body

Mammary glands: Milk-producing glands in each breast

Mammogram: X-ray exam of the breasts to look for changes that are not normal

Manual vacuum aspiration: Surgical abortion that uses suction to empty the uterus

Mastectomy: Surgical removal of part or all of the breast

Medical abortion: Abortion caused by a chemical that blocks a hormone needed for pregnancy

Menarche: First menstruation

Menopause: The point when a woman has not had a period for 12 months in a row and is no longer producing female sex hormones

Menstruation: The process in which an unfertilized ovum passes out of the body along with blood and tissues from the uterus

Miscarriage, or spontaneous abortion: Unplanned loss of a pregnancy

Mutual monogamy: Having sex with one partner who has been tested for and is not infected and, this partner agreed to be sexually active only with you

Natural family planning/rhythm method: Not having sex, or using a barrier method

Nipple: Opening located near the tip of each breast

Obstetrician: Physician with a specialty that focuses on women during and shortly after pregnancy and that is also concerned with the health of the fetus

Obstetrics and gynecology (OB-GYN): Medical specialty in which gynecologists are also obstetricians

Oral contraceptive: Series of pills that cause changes in uterus and cervix to keep sperm from joining the ovum

Ova (singular ovum): Female eggs

Ovaries: Glands in the uterus that produced undeveloped female ova and female sex hormones

Pap test: Test done to find changes in the cells of the cervix

Patch: Skin patch that releases hormones that keep sperm from joining with the ovum

Pelvic exam: An examination in which the health care provider checks the size, mobility, shape, position, surface, texture, and tenderness of the uterus and ovaries

Perimenopause: The time before menopause

Placenta: A temporary sac-shaped organ in the uterus that holds and attaches the fetus to the uterus during pregnancy

Polycystic ovary syndrome (PCOS): Condition in which a woman's ovaries or adrenal glands make more male hormones than normal, causing ovarian cysts

Postmenopause: The period following menopause, which lasts the rest of a woman's life

Preconception care: Medical care for a woman before she considers becoming pregnant

Preeclampsia: High blood pressure and the buildup of protein in the urine of pregnant women

Premature ovarian failure: Condition in which the ovaries stop functioning before natural menopause

Premenstrual syndrome (PMS): Physical and emotional discomfort before menstrual periods

Prenatal care: Medical care during pregnancy

Preterm: Term for infants born before 37 weeks

Preterm labor: Labor that begins before 37 weeks

Progesterone: Hormone that helps with the development of the fetus

Puberty: The stage when ovaries start to make female sex hormones

Pubic lice: Parasitic insect that causes itching in the genital area

Reproduction: When ova become fertilized by sperm

Screening mammogram: X-ray exam of the breasts to detect breast cancer when the woman has no symptoms

Second trimester: Week 13 to week 28 of pregnancy

Sexually transmitted infection (STI): Infection passed from person to person through sexual contact

Spermicide: Chemical jelly, foam, cream, or suppository put into the vagina to kill sperm

Spinal block: An injection directly into the spinal fluid during delivery

Sterilization implant: Nonsurgical method of sterilizing women

Stillbirth: Loss of pregnancy after the 20th week

Surgical abortion: Abortion procedure in which the lining of the uterus is removed

Surgical sterilization: Surgery that closes the fallopian tubes by cutting, tying, or sealing them

Syphilis: Sexually transmitted infection caused by bacteria

Third trimester: Week 29 to week 40 of pregnancy

Trichomoniasis: Infection with trichomonas, a protozoan organism

Umbilical cord: Cord that runs from an opening in the fetus's stomach and connects to the placenta in the mother's uterus

Uterine fibroids: Tumors that grow within the wall of the uterus

Uterus, or womb: Organ where a fetus develops until its birth

Vagina: A muscular tube that connects the cervix to the outside of the woman's body

Vaginal candidiasis: Condition caused by too much of a fungus in the vagina

Vaginal ring: Flexible ring that releases hormones that keep sperm from joining with the ovum

Vaginitis: Inflammation of the vagina

Vulva: The area including both the labia and the clitoris

Weaning: Switching a baby's diet from breast milk or formula to other foods and fluids

Withdrawal: Removal of the penis from the vagina before ejaculation

CHAPTER ACTIVITIES

1. Work in pairs to list birth control methods. Once you have made your list, identify negatives and positives for each method. To continue this activity, you will role-play. One student is a health educator, and the other is a client deciding among birth control choices.

2. Form small groups to discussed the different ways a pregnancy can be terminated. Possible topics for discussion are: What are two opposing viewpoints on abortion? What states have the strongest abortion restrictions? Which have the fewest? Is the morning-after pill a form of abortion?

3. There are five main areas of information that people need to know to protect themselves from STIs. Create an informational sheet about one of the more common STIs and include these five areas:

    a. *Transmission.* How does the STI pass from one person to another?

    b. *Symptoms.* How does someone tell if he or she has the STI?

    c. *Treatment.* How is this STI treated? Is it curable? What happens if it goes untreated?

    d. *Prevention.* How can someone prevent getting the STI?

    e. *Responsibility.* What should people do if they find out they have this STI?

4. Draw a time line of the stages of your life. The purpose of the time line is to identify how your sexuality will change at specific ages, such as at 25, 40, 60, and 80.

5. You work as a community health educator at an urban health center. Your job responsibility is to conduct a breast cancer screening awareness campaign for diverse populations. Write a two-page paper on how you will develop and implement this campaign for a target audience, such as women who are African American, Native American, or Mexican American.

Bibliography and Works Cited

American Cancer Society. (2016). The American Cancer Society guidelines for the prevention and early detection of cervical cancer. Retrieved from http://www.cancer.org/cancer/cervicalcancer/moreinformation/cervicalcancerpreventionandearlydetection/cervical-cancer-prevention-and-early-detection-cervical-cancer-screening-guidelines

American Congress of Obstetricians and Gynecologists. (2015). Pelvic inflammatory disease (PID). Retrieved from http://www.acog.org/Patients/FAQs/Pelvic-Inflammatory-Disease-PID

American Congress of Obstetricians and Gynecologists. (2016). Pap smear (Pap test): Resource overview. Retrieved from http://www.acog.org/Womens-Health/Pap-Smear-Pap-Test

American Osteopathic Association. (2013). Visiting the gynecologist. Retrieved from http://www.osteopathic.org/osteopathic-health/about-your-health/health-conditions-library/womens-health/Pages/visiting-the-gynecologist.aspx

American Sexual Health Association. (2016). Menopause. Retrieved from http://www.ashasexualhealth.org/sexual-health/womens-health/menopause/

American Society for Reproductive Medicine. (2016). Sexually transmitted infections. *ReproductiveFacts.org.* Retrieved from http://www.reproductivefacts.org/topics/detail.aspx?id=1725

Centers for Disease Control and Prevention. (2014). Ovarian cancer. Retrieved from http://www.cdc.gov/cancer/ovarian/pdf/ovarian_facts.pdf

Centers for Disease Control and Prevention. (2015). Unintended pregnancy prevention. Retrieved from http://www.cdc.gov/reproductivehealth/unintendedpregnancy/index.htm

Centers for Disease Control and Prevention. (2016a). Bacterial vaginosis – CDC fact sheet. Retrieved from http://www.cdc.gov/std/bv/STDFact-Bacterial-Vaginosis.htm

Centers for Disease Control and Prevention. (2016b). Genital HPV infection – fact sheet. Retrieved from http://www.cdc.gov/std/hpv/stdfact-hpv.htm

Centers for Disease Control and Prevention. (2016c). Infertility FAQs. Retrieved from http://www.cdc.gov/reproductivehealth/infertility/index.htm

Centers for Disease Control and Prevention. (2016d). Pregnancy. Retrieved from http://www.cdc.gov/pregnancy/index.html

Centers for Disease Control and Prevention. (2016e). Sexually transmitted diseases (STDs). Retrieved from http://www.cdc.gov/std/

Endocrine Society. (2016). Polycystic ovary syndrome (PCOS). Retrieved from http://www.hormone.org/diseases-and-conditions/womens-health/polycystic-ovary-syndrome

Foundation for Women's Cancer. (2016). Uterine/endometrial cancer. Retrieved from http://www.foundationforwomenscancer.org/types-of-gynecologic-cancers/uterine/

National Breast Cancer Foundation. (2015). About breast cancer. Retrieved from http://www.nationalbreastcancer.org/about-breast-cancer/?gclid=CLiKlqGY38wCFUxZhgodj_gLig

National Cervical Cancer Coalition. (2016). Cervical cancer overview. http://www.nccc-online.org/hpvcervical-cancer/cervical-cancer-overview/

Office of Women's Health. (2014). Breastfeeding. Retrieved from http://www.womenshealth.gov/breastfeeding/index.html

Office of Women's Health. (2015a). Endometriosis. Retrieved from http://www.womenshealth.gov/publications/our-publications/fact-sheet/endometriosis.html

Office of Women's Health. (2015b). Uterine fibroids fact sheet. Retrieved from http://womenshealth.gov/publications/our-publications/fact-sheet/uterine-fibroids.html

Office of Women's Health. (2015c). Vaginal yeast infection. Retrieved from http://www.womenshealth.gov/publications/our-publications/fact-sheet/vaginal-yeast-infections.html

Ovarian Cancer National Alliance. (2016). About ovarian cancer. Retrieved from http://www.ovariancancer.org/about/

Planned Parenthood Federation of America Inc. (2016). Birth control. Retrieved from https://www.plannedparenthood.org/learn/birth-control/.

Society for Assisted Reproductive Technology. (2016). A patient's guide to assisted reproductive technology. Retrieved from http://www.sart.org/Patients_Guide/

Susan G. Komen for the Cure. (2013). Facts for life: Benign breast conditions. Retrieved from http://ww5.komen.org/uploadedfiles/Content_Binaries/806–377a.pdf

US National Library of Medicine. (2016a). Cervical polyps. *MedlinePlus.* Retrieved from https://www.nlm.nih.gov/medlineplus/ency/article/001494.htm

US National Library of Medicine. (2016b). Painful menstrual periods. *MedlinePlus.* Retrieved from https://www.nlm.nih.gov/medlineplus/ency/article/003150.htm

US National Library of Medicine. (2016c). Female reproductive system. *MedlinePlus.* Retrieved from https://medlineplus.gov/femalereproductivesystem.html#bp_91_a

US Preventive Services Task Force. (2012). Cervical cancer: Screening. Retrieved from https://www.uspreventiveservicestaskforce.org/Page/Document/UpdateSummaryFinal/cervical-cancer-screening

CHAPTER 19

MUSCULOSKELETAL SYSTEM AND RELATED DISEASES

CHAPTER OBJECTIVES

- Summarize the function and structure of the musculoskeletal system.

- Compare differences between the axial and appendicular skeletons.

- Describe three different types of muscles.

- Discuss five major symptoms of musculoskeletal diseases.

- Explain testing and diagnosis of musculoskeletal diseases.

- Explain muscle strain, tendonitis, and sprains.

- Describe causes of back pain.

The musculoskeletal system is a complex mesh of bones, muscles, and other connective tissues. The bones give support to our bodies and help form our shape. Although light, bones are strong enough to support our entire weight. Muscles help with movement as well as with body functions. They are found in most places in the body. As a connective tissue, muscles support as well as separate different types of tissues and body organs. They can even move substances throughout the body.

Function of the Musculoskeletal System

The musculoskeletal system has many functions, but its primary ones are to support the body, allow motion, and protect organs. Other functions include blood production and fat storage.

This system includes not only bones but also connective tissues. Connective tissues—muscles, tendons, and ligaments—bind tissues and organs together. Together, bones and connective tissues carry and hold the body. Without the musculoskeletal system, the body would have no form or structure. It gives the body height and mass, facial features, hand characteristics, and athletic ability.

Structure of the Musculoskeletal System

The *musculoskeletal system* includes muscles, cartilage, ligaments, and other connective tissues that connect the bones. *Bones* support the body's weight and work with muscles to maintain body posture and to create movements. Without bones to pull against, muscles could not make us sit, stand, walk, or run.

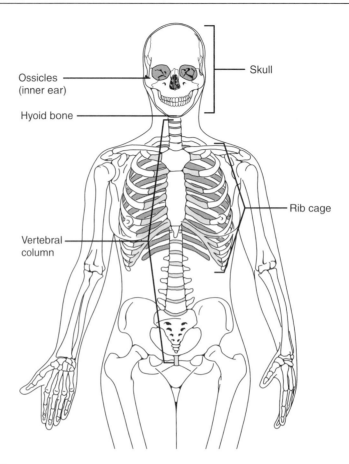

Ossicles
(inner ear)

Hyoid bone

Vertebral
column

Skull

Rib cage

Figure 19.1 Axial Skeleton
Note. Adapted from *Musculoskeletal System,* by R. Bear and D. Rintoul, 2014. Retrieved from the OpenStax-CNX website, http://cnx.org/content /m47521/1.3/

Skeleton

When the skeleton of a fetus first forms, it is made of *cartilage,* which is like a smooth covering that cushions and protects bones. Within a few weeks, ossification begins. *Ossification* is the process by which calcium, sodium, and other minerals, as well as a protein called collagen, replace the cartilage.

Humans are born with about 300 to 350 bones. Why no exact number? Although we have more bones when we are younger, many bones fuse together as we grow. As a result, an average adult skeleton has roughly 206 bones.

There are two distinct parts to the skeleton: the axial and the appendicular. The *axial skeleton* forms the body's central alignment and core (see Figure 19.1). The function of the axial skeleton is to support and protect the brain, spinal cord, and internal organs.

The axial skeleton provides a surface to which certain muscles attach. These muscles move the head, neck, and trunk, as well as perform respiratory movements. The axial skeleton has 80 bones, including the skull, the inner ear bones, the hyoid bone of the throat, the spinal column, and the rib cage. The rib cage comprises 12 pairs of ribs and the sternum.

The *appendicular skeleton* hangs from the axial skeleton and has 126 bones (see Figure 19.2). This skeleton comprises the bones of the upper limbs and lower limbs. The upper limbs are the arms, forearms, and hands, and their function is to grasp and move objects. The lower limbs—thighs, legs, feet—allow us to walk and run. The appendicular system also includes two bone girdles. One is the *pectoral or shoulder girdle* that attaches the upper limbs to the body. The other is the *pelvic girdle,* which attaches the lower limbs to the body. See Table 19.1 for a more detailed description of the axial and appendicular components.

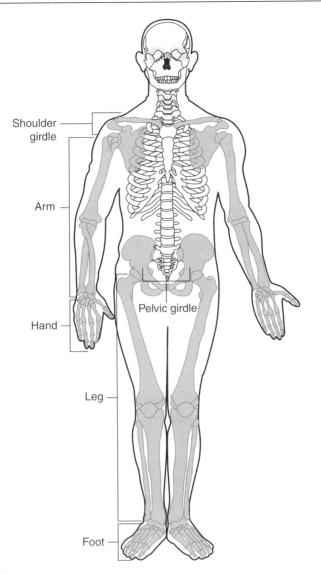

Shoulder
girdle

Arm

Hand

Pelvic girdle

Leg

Foot

Figure 19.2 Appendicular Skeleton
Note. Adapted from *Musculoskeletal System,* by R. Bear and D. Rintoul, 2014. Retrieved from the OpenStax-CNX website, http://cnx.org/content
/m47521/1.3/

There are differences between male and female skeletons. It is a myth that women have an extra pair of ribs, but they do tend to have slimmer bones, a narrower rib cage, a wider pelvic girdle, and a more rounded skull.

Bones

Bones have a wide range of tasks, including giving the body shape, protection, balance, and mobility. The average weight of a bone is less than an ounce, and each bone connects to at least one other. Bones are considered organs because they have blood, nerves, and bone tissue. Bone building occurs throughout a person's lifetime; the body constantly renews and reshapes the bones' living tissue.

There are different shapes to bones: long, short, flat, irregular, and sesamoid (see Figure 19.3). *Long bones,* found in the arms and legs, help skeletal muscles activate movement. These bones are longer than they are wide and have a shaft and two ends. They tend to be straight, giving them more strength than a curved bone. A honeycomb structure within these bones reduces their weight while increasing strength.

Long bones have yellow and red bone marrow. *Bone marrow* is an important part of blood production. Yellow marrow has fatty connective tissue and is in the marrow cavity. During times of

Table 19.1 Description of the Axial and Appendicular Skeletons

Axial Skeleton	Appendicular Skeleton
Skull—bones that support structures of the face and protect the brain. The skull has 22 bones, which are divided into two types: cranial bones and facial bones. Eight cranial bones form the cranial cavity. The cranial cavity houses the brain and is where muscles of the head and neck attach. Fourteen facial bones form the face, provide cavities for the sense organs, protect the entrances to the digestive and respiratory tracts, and serve as attachment points for facial muscles.	*Upper limbs*—30 bones in three regions: arm (shoulder to elbow), forearm, and wrist and hand.
Ossicles of the middle ear—six tiny bones transmit sounds from the air as vibrations. They are the smallest bones in the body.	*Lower limbs*—thigh bone, kneecap, and leg, ankle, and foot bones. These bones are thicker and stronger than those of the upper limbs because of the need to support the weight of the body and the forces from locomotion.
Hyoid bone of the throat—lies below the jawbone in the front of the neck. It acts as a movable base for the tongue.	*Pectoral* or *shoulder girdle*—bones that help attach the upper limbs to the axial skeleton. The shoulder girdle includes the collarbone and shoulder blades.
Spinal column—surrounds and protects the spinal cord, supports the head, and is an attachment point for the ribs and muscles of the back and neck. The adult vertebral column has 26 bones: 24 vertebrae and the sacrum and coccyx bones.	*Pelvic girdle*—attaches to the lower limbs of the axial skeleton. It is responsible for bearing the weight of the body and for locomotion.
Rib cage—ribs, sternum, vertebrae, and cartilage enclose and protect the organs of the thoracic cavity, including the heart and lungs. The rib cage also provides support for the shoulder girdles and upper limbs, and serves as the attachment point for the diaphragm, back muscles, chest, neck, and shoulders.	

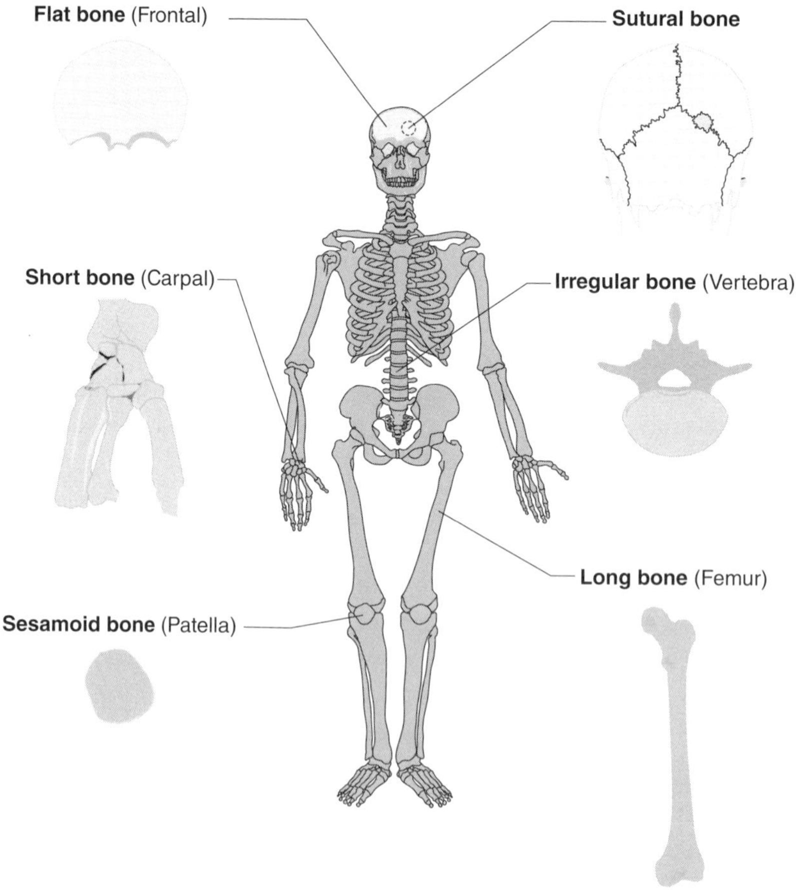

Figure 19.3 Shapes of Human Bones

Note. Adapted from Bruce Blaus (Own work) [CC BY 3.0 (http://creativecommons.org/licenses/by/3.0)], via Wikimedia Commons

starvation, the body uses the fat from yellow marrow for energy. Red marrow in some bones is a place for blood cell production—about 2.6 million red blood cells per second.

Short bones, such as those in the wrist and ankle, are the same width and length, giving them a cube-like shape. *Flat bones* (e.g., the shoulder blades) provide a place for the large skeletal muscles to anchor and activate movement. *Irregular bones,* because of their complex shapes, are not grouped with other bones. These bones may have short, flat, notched, or ridged surfaces (e.g., ribs and hipbones). *Sesamoid bones* are small, flat bones and look like sesame seeds. These bones arc inside tendons and near joints at the knees, hands, and feet.

Regardless of the shape, all bones have the same structure. This structure has two types of material—compact or spongy. *Compact bone* is the solid, hard, strong outside part of the bone; it looks like ivory. Holes and channels run through it, carrying blood vessels and nerves from the bone's outer membrane. *Spongy bone* looks like a sponge and is inside the compact bone. It is made up of tiny pieces of bone and is where red and white blood cells are produced.

Joints

A *joint* is the area where two or more bones are attached for the purpose of permitting body parts to move. Joints help the body move in different ways, and they are classified by their range of movement. For example, the joints of the skull are called *sutures*; they protect the brain. They have tissues that are fused together, allowing for no movement, and are called *immovable joints.*

Partially movable joints, such as those in the spine, move a little, and they are linked by cartilage. The bones of the spine, or *vertebrae,* have some movement. Each vertebra moves in relation to the one above and below it, and together these movements help the spine be flexible.

Synovial joints move in a variety of directions and are the main joints of the body. The hip, shoulders, and elbows are examples of synovial joints. They are filled with *synovial fluid,* which lubricates joints and helps them move. There are three kinds of synovial joints:

- *Hinge joints* allow movement in one direction (e.g., the knees)

- *Pivot joints* allow a twisting motion (e.g., the head moves from side to side)

- *Ball-and-socket joints* allow for the most movement, both rotation and in several directions (e.g., the hips and shoulders)

Most joints have ligaments and cartilage. *Ligaments* are long straps of muscle tissue that connect bones at a joint. Cartilage cushions and protects bones where they would otherwise rub directly onto each other. Cartilage is a smooth, flexible, rubbery substance that allows movement to occur with minimal friction. A thin coat covers the caps of the long bones, and thick pads cushion knees and other joints that perform major movements.

Teeth

Teeth are the hardest structures in the body. Made of calcium and other minerals, teeth also have a tough enamel coating. The upper and lower jaw bones anchor the teeth. We have two sets of teeth, *primary* and *permanent.* Primary teeth, or baby teeth, begin to grow through the gum line at about 4 months of age. They drop out and are replaced by the permanent teeth starting at about 6 years. The adult mouth has 32 permanent teeth that are in pairs on each side of the mouth.

Inside the tooth there is *pulp,* a living tissue that includes nerves and blood vessels, which nourish the tooth. Hollow *roots* grow deep into the jaw bones; their canals have nerves and blood vessels that supply the pulp.

Chips and cracks in the enamel occur through accidents and over time, causing damage. With damage, the enamel loses its ability to protect the tooth from bacteria. The bacteria destroy the tooth's cap and expose the pulp, causing one or more *cavities.*

Muscles

Bones do not work alone; they get help from muscles. There are more than 650 muscles in the body; they make up half of a person's body weight. *Muscles* pull on joints to create movement, and help give the body shape. Movement occurs when muscles shorten, pulling the bones with them. Muscles work in pairs; when one shortens, the corresponding muscle lengthens. Muscle fibers and special nerve cells are the cause of movement. Within each fiber, there are nerve cells that send impulses from the nervous system to the fibers, causing movement. Some fibers remain in partial contraction, providing muscle tone that supports posture. Other muscle fibers contract and relax, providing muscle strength. Muscles have other functions, such as helping the heart to beat, lungs to breathe, and blood to flow.

There are three kinds of muscle. *Skeletal muscles* attach to bone by tendons, mostly in the legs, arms, stomach, chest, neck, and face. These muscles are *striated* and have horizontal stripes. The functions of skeletal muscles are to provide movement, support, posture, and heat. They are also known as *voluntary muscles* because you can control their movement. For movement to happen, skeletal muscles pull against the bones they are attached. They can shorten quickly, but they tire easily and need rest.

Smooth muscle is also made of fibers, but looks smooth, not striated. We usually can't control our smooth muscles, so they are referred to as *involuntary*. They are controlled by the nervous system. Smooth muscles are inside the walls of internal organs; they help with nonstop movement of such organs as the esophagus, stomach, and bladder.

Smooth muscles are also found in the walls of blood vessels, where they squeeze blood flow through the vessels to help maintain blood pressure. Smooth muscles take longer to contract than skeletal muscles, but they can stay contracted for a long time because they don't tire easily.

Cardiac muscles are found only in the heart and are involuntary. The walls of the heart's chambers have these muscles to keep the heart pumping blood and to maintain blood circulation. Cardiac muscles work by shortening and relaxing nonstop to force blood out of the heart as it beats.

Connecting tissue, such as tendons, ligaments and fasciae, also join the bones and muscles. *Tendons* join muscle to bone. Ligaments connect bones to each other. Sheet-like *fasciae* cover the muscles and connect muscle to muscle. Fasciae also connect to skin and are a covering for groups of muscles, blood vessels, and nerves.

Common Diagnostic Tests and Procedures for Musculoskeletal Diseases

Diseases of the musculoskeletal system cause mostly movement problems. When movement problems become serious, then they are treated by specialists. *Orthopedics* is a surgical subspecialty that treats musculoskeletal problems. *Orthopedists, or orthopedic surgeons,* are physicians trained in orthopedics and may further specialize in sports medicine or rehabilitative medicine. Rheumatologists also treat musculoskeletal diseases, such as rheumatoid arthritis and osteoporosis.

Osteopaths, or osteopathic doctors (DOs) are physicians who study osteopathy. *Osteopathy* focuses on how the musculoskeletal system influences other body systems. An osteopathic physician uses musculoskeletal manipulation along with preventive care, medication, and surgery. They also use all the other medical treatments used by MDs and are licensed by all state medical boards in the same way as MDs.

Podiatrists are surgical subspecialists in foot diseases. They provide care for foot issues (e.g., calluses and ingrown toenails). Podiatrists also treat foot and ankle injuries as well as diseases, such as diabetes, that show signs and symptoms in the feet. They also prescribe special shoes and inserts to treat chronic foot pain. Podiatrists may further specialize in sports medicine, geriatrics, or diabetic foot care.

Physical therapists (PTs) are rehabilitation specialists who treat musculoskeletal issues, including recovery from joint surgery, limb amputation, and neuromuscular diseases. Along with treating patients, PTs teach them body strengthening exercises and injury prevention.

Signs and Symptoms

There are five major symptoms of musculoskeletal diseases: pain, swelling, redness, warmth, and stiffness. Pain is the major symptom—that is, aching or throbbing as opposed to sharp, which usually means nerve pain. Musculoskeletal pain is identified by five factors: location, relationship to organs, frequency (how often), duration (how long), and response to treatment.

Stiffness or moving with difficulty is a symptom unique to the musculoskeletal system. Information about the time of day that the stiffness affects the patient helps in making a diagnosis. The pattern of stiffness is also part of the diagnosis: Where is it? Does it go away? Does it get worse? Does it stay in one place, or does it move around?

Diagnostic Tests

There are diagnostic tests beyond blood tests and X-rays that identify and treat musculoskeletal problems:

- *Arthroscopy*—procedure that uses a scope used to see surfaces of bones at the joint, find tears, and determine causes of inflammation

- *Arthrography*—X-ray procedure in which an iodine solution is injected into the joint area and used to determine the cause of joint pain

- *Bone scan*—test in which a radioactive element is put into the patient's bloodstream; how and where the element builds up in the bone helps diagnose bone tumors and other diseases

- *Electromyography (EMG)*—test in which small, thin needles are put into muscles to make recordings of the electrical activity

- *CT scan*—scan that combines X-rays with computer technology and is used if there is a suspected tumor, fracture, or trauma

- *Flexibility tests*—tests that measure range of motion in a joint

- *Joint aspiration*—removal of joint fluid through a syringe, which reduces swelling and relieves pressure; is used as both diagnostic test and treatment

- *Palpation*—as part of the physical examination, touching and feeling joints to determine inflammation or identify growths

- *Muscle biopsy*—cutting out a muscle tissue sample for lab analysis

Joint Replacement Surgery

Joint replacement is one of the most frequently performed surgeries in the United States (American Academy of Orthopaedic Surgeons, 2016). *Joint replacement surgery* removes a damaged joint and puts in a new one. Knees and hips are the most commonly replaced; other joints replaced include shoulders, fingers, ankles, and elbows. Often surgeons do not remove the whole joint but instead replace only damaged parts.

The goal of joint replacement is to relieve pain caused by cartilage damage. The pain may be so severe that a person stops using the joint, which weakens the muscles that surround it. The weakened muscles cause even more movement difficulty. A physical examination, laboratory tests, and X-rays show the extent of damage to the joint. Total joint replacement may be necessary if other treatment options do not relieve the pain.

The new joint, or *prosthesis,* is made of plastic, metal, or both. It may be uncemented or cemented into place. An uncemented prosthesis is designed so that bones will grow into it. This type of prosthesis is for younger, more active people and those with good bone quality. The cemented prosthesis holds the new joint to the bone. This type of prosthesis is for older people with less mobility or with weak bones.

More than one million Americans have a knee or hip replaced each year (American Academy of Orthopaedic Surgeons, 2016). Total knee replacement is recommended when joint damage and pain do not improve with nonsurgical treatment. It is also recommended when lack of movement in the knee joint affects quality of life. Factors that increase risk of knee damage that requires knee replacement include being athletic before the age of 55, being obese, and having certain diseases (e.g., osteoarthritis) (American Academy of Orthopaedic Surgeons, 2016).

Hip replacement surgery removes the head of the thighbone or femur. The femur's ball-and-socket joint is replaced with artificial implants, a procedure that relieves pain and improves movement in the hip joint.

With joint replacement, about 90% of patients have rapid reduction in pain and enjoy improved movement (American Academy of Orthopaedic Surgeons, 2016). Although most joint replacement surgeries are successful, they can fail, requiring more surgery.

Joint replacement can give a patient years of pain-free living that would not have been possible otherwise. Younger joint replacement patients may need a second joint replacement surgery. Most older patients, however, can expect their total joint replacement to last a decade or more.

Diseases of the Musculoskeletal System

Many health problems can affect the musculoskeletal system, potentially causing severe pain, weakness, and even paralysis. Musculoskeletal diseases occur because of injury, overuse, infections, medications, genetics, and inflammation.

Muscle Strain, Tendonitis, and Sprains

A *strain* is the overstretching or tearing of a muscle or tendon. Muscle strains occur when a person twists or pulls muscles and tendons that haven't warmed up or that are engaging in a new activity. Strains can happen suddenly or develop over days or weeks. Back and hamstring muscle strains are the most common. Many people get strains playing sports or lifting heavy objects. Symptoms include pain, muscle spasms, swelling, and trouble moving. If a muscle or tendon is completely torn, it is often very painful and makes movement difficult.

Tendonitis is inflammation of a tendon, which occurs when there is repeated stress on the tendon. Tendonitis is a common sports injury and is painful. Because tendons have a poor blood supply and take time to heal—up to 6 weeks or more—the pain and movement difficulty can last for some time. Some common forms of tendonitis are named after the sports that increase their risk—for example, tennis elbow and swimmer's shoulder.

A *sprain* is the overstretching or tearing of a ligament and is caused by falling, twisting, or getting hit. There may be a pop or a tearing sound when the injury occurs. Ankle and wrist sprains are common; the symptoms include pain, inflammation, bruising, and lack of joint movement. A sprain can be mild, moderate, or severe.

Treatments are the same for strains and sprains. The first treatment goal is to reduce inflammation and pain by resting the injured area, icing it, wearing a bandage that compresses the area, and anti-inflammatory medication. Later treatment includes exercise and physical therapy that prevents stiffness and increases strength. Treatment for severe strains and sprains includes steroid injections and surgery.

To prevent strains and sprains, people should avoid exercising or playing sports when tired or in pain. They should also warm up before playing a sport, wear protective equipment when playing, and run on flat surfaces.

Bone Fracture

A *bone fracture*, or broken bone, may crack, snap, or shatter. The soft tissue surrounding the break may also be injured. Most bone fractures are injuries from falls, direct hits to the body, child abuse, or vehicle crashes. Diseases such as osteoporosis or bone tumors can also result in fractures.

There are different types of bone fractures. If the broken bone punctures the skin, then it is an *open or compound fracture.* Once the skin breaks, infection in both the wound and the bone can occur, causing serious health problems. Overuse that comes from long walks or running can cause small cracks in the bone known as *stress fractures.* Symptoms of a fracture are an out-of-place limb or joint, swelling, bruising, or bleeding. Other symptoms include intense pain, numbness, and inability to move a limb.

Most fractures need emergency medical care. Sometimes it is hard to tell the difference between a dislocated joint (a separation of two bones where they meet at a joint) and a fractured bone; however, both are medical emergencies, and the first aid steps are the same (US National Library of Medicine, 2015). Even when a broken bone is not a medical emergency, it still requires medical attention.

Treatment for bone fractures depend on the type of fracture and the specific bones involved and can include a cast, splint, or brace that keeps the bone from moving until it heals. If the fracture is complicated, then metal pins and plates will hold it in place while the bone heals. Pins are set into the bone through the skin above and below the fracture. These connect to a ring or a bar outside the skin that holds the pins in place. After the bones have healed, the pins are removed.

Fractured bones usually take at least 4 weeks to heal, although casts may come off earlier to prevent stiffness. The pain usually stops after a time, but the fracture might not heal enough to handle the stresses of normal activity. Even after the cast, splint, or brace is removed, the patient may need to limit movement until the bone heals. Physical therapy may be necessary after the bone has healed.

Proper diet and exercise can prevent some fractures. A diet rich in calcium and vitamin D along with weight-bearing exercises help keep bones strong.

Osteoporosis

Osteoporosis causes bones to become spongy and break. It also causes the spine to crumble and collapse. Patients with osteoporosis most often break bones in the hip, spine, and wrist. Osteoporosis is a "silent" disease because bone loss occurs without signs or symptoms. Unfortunately, a patient may not know that he or she has osteoporosis until a strain or fall causes a bone to break.

In the United States, more than 40 million people either have osteoporosis or are at high risk (NIH Osteoporosis and Related Bone Diseases–National Resource Center, 2016). Both men and women of any age can have osteoporosis, but it is most common in older women. This has to do with the fact that bone hardness and strength depend on calcium. Older women are especially vulnerable to osteoporosis because menopause causes a woman's ovaries to stop producing estrogen, a hormone that helps maintain proper calcium levels in bones. Insufficient calcium causes bone loss.

There are other risk factors for osteoporosis besides being an older woman. Some of these factors cannot be changed; others can. Risk factors that cannot be changed include body size (small, thin women are at greater risk) and ethnicity (particularly White and Asian women). Family health history is also a risk factor that cannot be changed: osteoporosis tends to run in families.

Risk factors that can be changed include sex hormone levels, eating disorders, calcium and vitamin D intake, certain medications, and regular exercise. Patients can also be at risk for osteoporosis if they use tobacco products and misuse alcohol.

A *bone mineral density test* is used to diagnose osteoporosis. This test checks both bone strength and whether current treatments are making bones stronger. Treatment for osteoporosis includes a diet rich in calcium and vitamin D, an exercise plan, and medications.

Scoliosis

Every person's spine curves a little. A certain amount of curve is necessary for people to move and to walk. However, up to 5 people out of 1,000 have *scoliosis,* which causes the spine to curve sideways (National Institute of Arthritis and Musculoskeletal and Skin Diseases Information Clearinghouse, 2014d). Curves are often S-shaped or C-shaped. Scoliosis usually starts when the spine is growing, in childhood or during adolescence, but people of all ages can develop it.

A birth defect, disease, or injury can cause scoliosis. It might also run in families. But in most people, there is no known cause. When the cause is unknown, the condition is referred to as *idiopathic scoliosis,* which is the most common type. It first appears in children ages 10 to 12 and in their early teens. Girls are more likely than boys to have idiopathic scoliosis.

Health care providers use the patient's health and family history, a physical examination, and other tests to diagnose scoliosis. An X-ray of the spine enables the health care provider to measure the curve and see its location, shape, and pattern.

Scoliosis does not usually cause symptoms, but there are readily noticed signs:

- Shoulder, shoulder blade, hip, or breast that is higher than the other

- Shoulder blade that sticks out farther than the other

- Skin fold on one side of the waist

When there are symptoms, they can involve back pain and heart problems. There can also be trouble breathing, particularly if the spinal curves do not allow the lungs enough room to work correctly.

Treatment is different for each person. Mild scoliosis does not need treatment—only observation, meaning that the health care provider checks the patient every few months to see if the curve is getting better or worse. Treatment for severe scoliosis depends on such factors as the patient's age, degree of the curve, and type of scoliosis. The treatment is usually a combination of bracing or surgery. Bracing means that the patient wears a brace to stop a curve from getting worse.

Surgery is used when the bracing is not enough. It corrects a curve or stops it from getting worse when the patient is still growing. Surgery involves fusing together bones in the spine or putting in a metal rod or other device. The metal rod or other device stays in the body and helps keep the spine straight after surgery.

Unfortunately, exercise programs do not keep scoliosis from getting worse. Chiropractic treatment, electrical stimulation, and nutritional supplements have not been shown to be effective treatments over time (National Institute of Arthritis and Musculoskeletal and Skin Diseases Information Clearinghouse, 2014d).

Paget's Disease

Paget's disease causes bones to grow too large and weaken, making them vulnerable to fractures. The disease can affect any bone in the body, but most patients have it in their spine, pelvis, skull, or leg bones. It does not spread to other bones, nor does it affect the entire skeleton. Paget's disease leads to other health issues, including arthritis, hearing loss, heart disease, and bone cancer.

About one million people in the United States have Paget's, making it the second most common bone disease (NIH Osteoporosis and Related Bone Diseases–National Resource Center, 2014). It occurs mainly in older people and those of Northern European descent. Men are more likely than women to have Paget's. It is not fully understood what causes this disease, but a viral infection and family history of this disease are risk factors.

Paget's disease does not affect everyone in the same way. The symptoms range from mild to severe. Most patients do not even know they have the disease because the symptoms are so mild. Paget's disease is often diagnosed when an X-ray is done for another reason. If Paget's disease is suspected, then it is diagnosed with X-rays, blood tests, and a bone scan. Early diagnosis and treatment prevent some symptoms from getting worse.

Some patients with this disease do have severe signs and symptoms that slowly develop. These include pain, enlarged bones, broken bones, and damaged cartilage. If Paget's disease is in the leg bones, then the patient may also have bowed legs. The spine may curve if the disease is in the bones of the spine.

Paget's disease is treated with medication and sometimes surgery for broken bones, malformed bones, or severe arthritis. A special diet rich in calcium and vitamin D and exercise can relieve symptoms.

Treatment reduces signs and symptoms, but is not a cure. The outlook for patients with Paget's disease is good if treatment is started early. If treatment is given before there are major changes in the affected bone, the outlook is even better.

Bone Tumor

A *bone tumor* is an abnormal growth within a bone. These tumors are either benign (noncancerous) or malignant (cancerous). Benign bone tumors are more common than malignant ones. Both benign and malignant tumors increase in size and destroy healthy bone tissue. However, unlike malignant tumors, benign tumors do not spread and are rarely life threatening. Some patients with benign bone tumors find that the tumors go away over time. In many cases, benign tumors just need observation. Other patients with these tumors need medication or surgery to remove the tumor.

The health care provider takes a health history and performs a physical examination to diagnose a bone tumor. Additional tests include blood tests, bone biopsy, bone scan, X-rays, and MRI.

The exact cause of bone tumors is unknown. Some possible causes include family history of cancer, genetic defects, radiation exposure, or an injury. In most cases, however, the cause is unknown.

Bone cancer is a malignant tumor that destroys bone tissue. Cancer that begins in bone is different from cancer that begins somewhere else in the body and spreads to bone. Cancers that start in the bones are called *primary bone tumors, or sarcomas,* and are rare. Primary bone cancers start in bone, muscle, blood vessels, fat tissues, and in some other tissues. They can develop anywhere in the body.

Multiple myeloma is the most common primary bone cancer. It is a malignant tumor in bone marrow, and any bone can have it; it tends to involve the entire skeleton. Multiple myeloma affects about 20,000 Americans each year. It is also responsible for the deaths of 10,000 Americans each year. Most cases involve patients between the ages of 50 and 70 years old, and it is more common in men than women (American Cancer Society, 2016).

Cancers that start in another part of the body and spread to the bone are *secondary bone tumors* and are more common (American Academy of Orthopaedic Surgeons, 2015a). The cancers that most often spread to the bone are cancers of the breast, kidney, lung, prostate, and thyroid. These forms of cancer usually affect older people.

The most common symptom of bone cancer is pain in the area of the tumor. Other symptoms depend on the location and size of the cancer. These symptoms include bone fractures from a small injury or a swelling at the tumor site.

Treatment for bone cancer depends on where the cancer started. Surgery is the main treatment for bone cancer, but other treatments include amputation, chemotherapy, and radiation therapy. Bone cancer can return after treatment, so regular follow-up visits by the patient are necessary.

The prognosis (outcome) depends on the type of bone tumor. The prognosis is good for people with benign bone tumors. However, some benign tumors can turn into cancer. Most patients with early stages of bone cancer can be cured, but it does depend on the type, location, and size of the cancer, and other factors.

Joint Pain

Joint pain affects one or more joints, and it can negatively impact a person's daily activities. Many types of injuries and diseases cause joint pain. In this chapter, the discussion of joint pain is limited to select common diseases.

Arthritis

Joint tissues begin to wear down and start to degenerate as we age. *Degeneration* is a weakening that causes swelling, pain, and loss of movement in the joints. If a patient feels pain and stiffness or has trouble moving around, he or she might have arthritis. *Arthritis* is one of the most common and disabling diseases of the musculoskeletal system. Although there are many different types of arthritis, the three most common are osteoarthritis, rheumatoid arthritis, and gout.

Osteoarthritis   Changes in both joint tissues and the opposing bones cause *osteoarthritis,* which is the most common type of arthritis (National Institute of Arthritis and Musculoskeletal and Skin Diseases Information Clearinghouse, 2014c). It is often related to aging, being overweight, or an injury. It can be present in any joint, but usually it affects the hands, knees, hips, or spine. Osteoarthritis breaks down cartilage. When you lose cartilage, then the bones rub together. Over time, this rubbing damages the joint.

No single test can diagnose osteoarthritis, so most health care providers use several methods, including health history, physical examination, X-rays, and lab tests. Treatment includes exercise, medications, and sometimes surgery.

Rheumatoid Arthritis   Osteoarthritis affects only joints and not internal organs. By contrast, *rheumatoid arthritis* affects other parts of the body besides joints. The second most common form of arthritis, rheumatoid arthritis is a more serious form of osteoarthritis (US National Library of Medicine, 2016a). It is an autoimmune disease that causes the body to make antibodies against joint tissues. These antibodies cause chronic inflammation. The result of this chronic inflammation is severe joint damage, pain, and loss of movement. See Chapter 11 for a detailed description of rheumatoid arthritis.

Gout   *Gout* is one of the most painful forms of arthritis. It occurs when too much *uric acid* builds up in the body, leading to deposits of uric acid crystals. These deposits, which look like lumps under the skin, are found in joints, often in the big toe. They also form in the kidney, as kidney stones.

For many people, the first attack of gout occurs in the big toe, causing it to be painful, red, stiff, and swollen. Gout can also affect ankles, knees, wrists, fingers, and elbows. Stressful events, alcohol or drugs, or another illness can trigger a gout attack. Early attacks usually get better within 3 to 10 days, even without treatment. The next attack may not occur for months or even years.

People are at risk for gout if they have a family history of the disease, are male, and are overweight. Exposure to lead, an organ transplant, use of certain medications, and alcohol misuse are also risk factors.

Health care providers ask the patient about symptoms, health history, and family history to diagnose gout. They may also draw a sample of fluid from an inflamed joint to look for the crystals associated with gout. Gout is usually treated with *nonsteroidal anti-inflammatory drugs (NSAIDs)* (e.g., aspirin). NSAIDS are medications that reduce pain, fever, and inflammation.

Some ways to prevent gout include having a healthy, balanced diet and drinking plenty of water. Exercising regularly and maintaining a healthy body weight can also prevent gout.

Temporomandibular Joint (TMJ) Dysfunction

The *temporomandibular joint (TMJ)* connects the jaw to the side of the head. When it works well, it lets a person talk, chew, and yawn. *TMJ dysfunction,* however, causes pain in the joint and muscles around and in the jaw. There also may be a change in how the upper and lower teeth fit together.

The pain from TMJ dysfunction is felt every time a person swallows, yawns, talks, or chews. The pain can be sharp or dull and constant. Pain in the chewing muscles or jaw joint is the common symptom, but pain can also radiate elsewhere, such as the side of the head, cheek, ear, and teeth. TMJ dysfunction can cause spasms in the muscles attached to the skull, face, and jaws. Other symptoms include jaw muscle stiffness, locking of the jaw, and painful clicking or popping in the jaw joint when opening or closing the mouth. Symptoms start without reason in most cases.

The exact cause of TMJ dysfunction is unknown, but there are risk factors associated with the condition, including trauma to the jaw, teeth grinding, gum chewing, stress, improper bite, and arthritis. It is estimated that TMJ dysfunction affects over 10 million Americans and appears to be more common in women than men (TMJ Association, 2015).

Diagnosis of TMJ dysfunction begins with a health history and physical examination, including an assessment of the patient's bite. An early diagnosis can respond to simple remedies, such as eating soft foods, not chewing gum, and avoiding clenching the jaw. In cases of joint injury, ice packs reduce swelling. Relaxation techniques, NSAIDs, and muscle relaxants can also offer relief. Aggressive treatments for more advanced cases are rare; these include wearing a mouth splint to prevent wear and tear on the joint, improving the alignment of the upper and lower teeth, or surgery.

Back Pain

Back pain ranges from a dull, constant ache to a sudden, sharp, and crippling *spasm,* or muscle contraction. The pain can happen fast like with lifting heavy objects. It can also happen over time and cause changes to the spine. Regardless of why back pain happens or how it feels, you know it when you have it. The chances are so high that if you don't have back pain now, you will someday. In any 3-month period, about 25% of US adults have at least 1 day of back pain (National Institute of Arthritis and Musculoskeletal and Skin Diseases Information Clearinghouse, 2014b). It is one of the most common health problems. Although anyone can have back pain, there are risk factors, including the following:

- *Age.* Back pain is more common with age.
- *Fitness level.* Back pain is more common among people with a low fitness level.
- *Diet.* An unhealthy diet combined with lack of exercise can lead to obesity, which puts stress on the back.
- *Work.* Jobs that demand heavy lifting or pulling can strain the back. Desk jobs can also cause back pain.
- *Cigarette smoking.* Although not a direct cause of *sciatica,* which is pain in the back area that radiates to the hip and down the leg due to pressure on the sciatic nerve, smoking can affect circulation, which in turn affects the health of the nerves.

Back pain can also be a symptom of a health problem, not just a diagnosis itself. The following are health problems associated with back pain:

- *Mechanical problems.* A mechanical problem occurs when the spine moves in certain ways. The most common mechanical problem is *degenerative disc disease* (DDD), or slipped disc. DDD occurs when discs between the spine's vertebrae break down with age.

- *Injuries.* Spine injuries (e.g., fractures) or severe injuries from accidents or falls cause either acute or chronic pain. Fractured vertebrae are often the result of osteoporosis.

- *Diseases.* Scoliosis, kidney stones, and arthritis are examples of diseases that cause back pain.

- *Infections and tumors.* Infections and tumors in the vertebrae can cause back pain.

- *Stress.* Emotional stress can make back muscles tense and cause pain.

Regular exercise is one of the best ways to prevent back pain, along with eating a healthy diet. A healthy diet helps maintain a healthy weight, which prevents stress and strain put on the back. Keeping good posture, supporting the back, and avoiding heavy lifting can also prevent back pain.

It is not necessary to see a health care provider for back pain in most cases. The pain usually goes away with or without treatment. It may, however, be necessary to see a health care provider if there is numbness or severe pain, or pain following an injury.

Diagnosing the cause of back pain requires a health history and a physical examination. The health care provider may also order medical tests, such as X-rays, MRI, CT scan, and blood tests.

Treatment for back pain depends on whether the pain is acute or chronic. Pain that comes on fast and leaves just as fast is acute pain. Acute pain is the most common type of back pain, and it does not last longer than 6 weeks. Chronic pain is much less common; it can come on fast or slow, but it stays for a long time. In general, chronic pain lasts longer than 3 months.

Acute back pain usually gets better without treatment. Over-the-counter pain medication can relieve symptoms. By contrast, treatment for chronic back pain falls into two types: one that needs surgery and one that does not. For most cases, back pain does not need surgery. For a small number of cases, surgery is necessary to ease the pain and prevent further problems. Examples of diagnoses that may entail surgery include:

- *Herniated or ruptured discs.* When the outer coating of the discs is damaged, the discs' liquid leaks, irritating nearby nerves. This causes nerve pain down the leg as well as muscle spasms.

- *Spinal stenosis.* Stenosis is a narrowing of the spinal canal through which the spinal cord and spinal nerves run. The narrowing puts pressure on the nerves and spinal cord. This pressure causes difficulty in walking, pain, numbness in the legs, and loss of bladder and bowel control.

- *Vertebral fractures.* Fractures caused by trauma to the vertebrae result in severe back and leg pain.

Shoulder Problems

The shoulder joint has bones that are held in place by muscles, tendons, and ligaments. Tendons hold the shoulder muscles to bones. They help the muscles move the shoulder. Ligaments hold the three shoulder bones to each other and make the shoulder joint stable. The breakdown of these soft tissues results in shoulder problems.

Using the shoulder too much causes soft tissue to break down faster as people get older. Doing manual labor or playing sports also causes shoulder problems. Shoulder problems occur in people of all ages, races, and ethnic backgrounds.

Pain can be felt in one small spot, in a large area, or down the arm. It can also be felt as it travels along the nerves to the shoulder. The most common shoulder problems are

- *Dislocation.* If the shoulder is twisted or pulled hard, the ball at the top of the bone in the upper arm pops out of its socket. To treat a dislocation, the ball of the upper arm is pushed back into the socket.

- *Separation.* This occurs when ligaments between the collarbone and shoulder blade are torn. The injury is often caused by a blow to the shoulder or by falling on an outstretched hand. Treatment for a *shoulder separation* includes a sling to keep the shoulder in place. Surgery is necessary if tears are severe.

- *Rotator cuff disease.* This is another term for tendonitis of the shoulder. *Bursitis* occurs when the *bursa*, a fluid-filled sac that protects the shoulder joint, becomes inflamed. (Various other joints in the body also have bursae.) Bursitis occurs with certain diseases or with certain sports or jobs. Tendonitis and bursitis can appear alone or at the same time. Treatment includes medications, ultrasound, injections, or surgery.

- *Rotator cuff tear.* Muscles around the shoulder joint rotate the shoulder. These muscles move the shoulders, upper arms, and hands. The tendons of these muscles also help strengthen the shoulder joint. A *rotator cuff tear* occurs when tendons tear and become inflamed from frequent use, an injury, or aging. Sports or jobs with repeated overhead motion also damage the rotator cuff. Some tears are not painful; others are very painful. Treatment depends on age, health, and the severity of the injury. It can include medication, injections, ultrasound, or surgery.

- *Frozen shoulder*—Movement of the shoulder is stopped. Causes of frozen shoulder can be lack of use, rheumatic diseases, or lack of fluid that helps the shoulder joint move. Treatment includes medications, injections, or surgery.

- *Fracture.* Fractures are often caused by a fall or a blow to the shoulder. Treatment includes having a health care provider put the bones into their original position, wearing a sling, medications, or surgery.

- *Arthritis.* Arthritis of the shoulder is one of two types: osteoarthritis or rheumatoid arthritis. Osteoarthritis of the shoulder is treated with NSAIDs. Patients with rheumatoid arthritis may need physical therapy, steroid medications, or surgery.

Health care providers diagnose shoulder problems by taking a health history, and doing a physical examination. Other tests include X-rays, ultrasound, and MRI. Treatment depends on the type of shoulder problem. Regardless of the problem, however, the first line of treatment is *RICE* (rest, ice, compression, and elevation):

- *Rest:* Don't use the shoulder for 48 hours

- *Ice:* Put an ice pack on the injured area

- *Compression:* Put even pressure, or *compression,* on the painful area to reduce swelling

- *Elevation:* Keep the injured area above the level of the heart

Knee Problems

The knee is a synovial hinge joint formed between three bones: the femur, tibia, and patella (kneecap). Knees provide support and flexibility, and allow the legs to bend and straighten. The flexibility that knees provide allows us to stand, walk, run, crouch, jump, and turn. When a knee problem affects daily activities such as walking, it can have a major impact on a person's life.

Knees are complex: bones, cartilage, muscles, ligaments, and tendons allow knees to move. Each part is at risk for disease and injury. If one part is injured, the knee hurts and can't move. Anyone at any age, including children, can have knee problems.

Knee problems usually occur because of injuries—for example, a direct blow or sudden movements that strain the knee. *Meniscal injuries* are often caused by sports. The meniscus, cartilage in the knee, is injured by rotating the knee while bearing weight. A partial or total tear occurs when a person quickly twists the upper leg while the foot stays still, as in turning to hit a baseball. If the tear is tiny, the meniscus stays connected to the front and back of the knee. If the tear is large, the meniscus hangs by a thread of cartilage.

When patients injure their meniscus, they feel pain when the knee is straight. If there is mild pain, patients can still move, but with severe pain, there is less movement. Swelling begins soon after the injury if there is blood vessel damage. After any injury, the knee may click, lock, or give way. Untreated meniscus injuries can sometimes be painful months or years later. Symptoms of a meniscal injury disappear on their own or can return and need treatment.

If the tear is minor and symptoms go away, then the health care provider may recommend a muscle-strengthening program. If the tear is major, then surgery may be needed, with recovery taking several weeks.

Injured ligaments can also cause knee problems. The two knee ligaments that are usually injured are the anterior and posterior cruciate ligaments (ACL and PCL, respectively). The ACL is stretched or torn by a sudden twisting motion; the PCL is usually injured by a direct impact. Treatment for knee ligament injuries includes RICE, strengthening exercises, or a brace. Surgery is the recommended treatment for severe injuries.

A common tendon injury is a *torn tendon*. Tendons tear when they are overused, as happens during some sports. The tendon stretches like a worn-out rubber band and becomes inflamed. Torn tendons can also occur when a person tries to break a fall. Treatment for tendon injuries includes RICE, NSAIDs, strengthening exercises, or surgery.

Joint-related diseases—osteoarthritis, rheumatoid arthritis, and gout—can result in knee problems. These diseases cause pain, swelling, and stiffness, with possible lasting knee damage.

Health care providers diagnose knee problems by taking a patient's health history and doing a physical examination. Diagnostic tests such as X-rays, bone scan, MRI, and biopsy are used to support a diagnosis.

Repetitive Stress Injuries (RSIs)

Repetitive stress injuries (RSIs) are a result of repeating the same movements that put stress on a particular part of the body. This stress causes inflammation, muscle strain, and tissue damage.

An example of an RSI is *carpal tunnel syndrome,* or pain of the wrist and hand. The carpal tunnel is a narrow tunnel formed by bones and other tissues in the wrist. This tunnel protects the nerve that moves the thumb and the first three fingers on each hand.

Doing the same hand movements repeatedly leads to carpal tunnel syndrome, which means that tissues in the carpal tunnel get inflamed and press against the nerve. That pressure makes the fingers, wrist, palm, and forearm painful or numb. Another symptom is trouble gripping objects.

Carpal tunnel syndrome is most common in those whose jobs require the wrists to be held bent, such as when working with computers. It can also be caused by an injury to the wrist or by a disease (e.g., rheumatoid arthritis). Women are more likely to develop carpal tunnel syndrome than men, and it can be hereditary.

Carpal tunnel syndrome is usually not serious. The pain goes away, and there is no lasting damage to the hand or wrist with treatment. Treatment includes resting the wrist or changing how patients use their hands. Patients may wear a splint on the wrist to keep the wrist from moving. Ice, massage, and stretching exercises help as well as NSAIDs. In more severe cases, surgery may be needed, or a health care provider can inject the wrists with steroids to reduce swelling and pain.

Fibromyalgia

Fibromyalgia is a complex chronic pain disorder that affects people physically, mentally, and socially. It causes muscle pain in the whole body. Patients with fibromyalgia have "tender points" at specific places on the neck, shoulders, back, hips, arms, and legs. These points hurt when touched.

The primary symptom of fibromyalgia is widespread body pain. Patients can have other symptoms, such as fatigue, sleep disorders, problems with thinking and memory, irritable bowel syndrome, migraines, anxiety, depression, and environmental sensitivities.

Fibromyalgia is often considered an arthritis-related disease, but it is not a true form of arthritis. It does not cause inflammation or damage to the joints, muscles, or other tissues the way arthritis does. However, fibromyalgia does cause significant pain and fatigue, and can interfere with a person's daily activities.

The cause, diagnosis, and treatment of fibromyalgia are not clear despite ongoing research. The cause is linked to a number of risks, such as genetics, stressful events, infection, other diseases, or physical trauma. There has also been increased attention to the role of the central nervous system and how it processes pain as an underlying cause of fibromyalgia.

It is estimated that five million or more Americans have fibromyalgia, and as many as 80–90% of them are women (National Fibromyalgia Association, 2015). It is the most common cause of generalized musculoskeletal pain in women; however, men and children also can be affected.

Those with fibromyalgia sometimes struggle for years before being correctly diagnosed. A reason for this delay is that pain and fatigue are also symptoms of other diseases, such as Lyme disease. Therefore, health care providers often rule out other possible causes of these symptoms before diagnosing fibromyalgia. In addition, there is no lab or imaging test used to diagnose the condition. A health care provider who understands the complexities of this disease can make a diagnosis based on two factors:

1. The patient has a history of widespread musculoskeletal pain.

2. The patient has tender points. The body has 18 places that are possible tender points. For a fibromyalgia diagnosis, a patient must have 11 or more tender points where she feels pain with touch.

Fibromyalgia is difficult to treat and a multidisciplinary health care team approach is often required. The team includes a physician, a physical therapist, and other providers for pain management. Treatment for fibromyalgia requires pain and sleep management as well as psychological support. Medications may help relieve some—but not all—symptoms. Other treatments that may help are complementary approaches, such as massage, meditation, yoga, and acupuncture.

Fibromyalgia is chronic and can last a lifetime, but it is not a progressive disease. It is never fatal, and it does not cause damage to the joints, muscles, or internal organs. Fibromyalgia does improve over time for some patients. Ways to manage symptoms are to get enough sleep and exercise and to try a complementary approach.

Chapter Summary

- The musculoskeletal system has many functions. Primary functions include supporting the body, allowing motion, and protecting organs. Other functions are blood production and fat storage.

- Bones work together with muscles to maintain body posture and to create movement. Without the skeleton to pull against, muscles could not make us sit, stand, walk, or run.

- Stiffness is a symptom unique to the musculoskeletal system. Health care providers need to know when, where, and how long the stiffness occurs in order to make a diagnosis.

- Joint replacement surgery is used for severe joint problems. This surgery removes a damaged joint and puts in a new synthetic one. Knees and hips are the most commonly replaced joints.

- In any given 3-month period, about 25% of US adults have at least 1 day of back pain, making it one of the most common health problems.

REVIEW QUESTIONS

1. What are the major differences between compact bone and spongy bone?

2. Identify the three kinds of muscles and explain the function of each.

3. What are similarities and differences among the three most common types of arthritis?

4. What is osteoporosis? Why does it develop? What are the symptoms and complications that can result from osteoporosis?

5. What are repetitive stress injuries (RSIs)? How does a person get carpal tunnel syndrome?

6. What are the differences among muscle strain, tendonitis, and sprains?

7. List and describe two diseases of the muscular system and list two ways people can keep their muscles healthy.

8. Explain the differences between primary and secondary bone tumors.

9. What is degenerative disc disease, and how is it treated?

10. Why is fibromyalgia difficult to diagnose?

KEY TERMS

Appendicular skeleton: The part of the skeleton that hangs from the axial skeleton and has upper and lower limbs

Arthritis: General term for disabling diseases of the musculoskeletal system

Arthrography: Diagnostic test used to determine the cause of unexplained joint pain

Arthroscopy: Procedure that uses a scope to see surfaces of bones at the joint, find tears, and determine causes of inflammation

Axial skeleton: The part of the skeleton that forms the body's central alignment and a longitudinal central axis

Ball-and-socket joint: Type of synovial joint that allows for the most movement, both rotation and in several directions

Bone cancer: Cancerous tumor that destroys bone tissue

Bone fracture: The cracking, snapping, or shattering of a bone

Bone marrow: Substance inside bone that helps in blood cell production

Bone mineral density test: Test used to diagnose osteoporosis

Bones: Organs that give the body shape, protection, balance, and mobility

Bone scan: Diagnostic test used to diagnose bone tumors and other bone problems

Bone tumor: Abnormal growth within a bone

Bursa: Fluid-filled sac that protects the shoulder joint and various other joints in the body

Bursitis: Inflammation of the bursa

Cardiac muscle: Type of muscle that is found only in the heart

Carpal tunnel syndrome: Type of repetitive stress injury with pain in the wrist and hand

Cartilage: Smooth covering over joints that supports bones and protects them where they would otherwise rub directly onto each other

Cavity: Tooth damage caused by bacteria

Compact bone: The hard outside part of the bone

CT scan: Diagnostic test that combines X-rays with computer technology

Degeneration: In the context of joint problems, weakening that causes swelling, pain, and loss of movement in the joints

Degenerative disc disease (DDD): Breakdown of the discs between the vertebrae, usually caused by age

Dislocation: In the context of shoulder problems, condition in which the ball at the top of the bone in the upper arm pops out of its socket

Electromyography (EMG): Diagnostic test used to identify muscular diseases

Fasciae: Fibers that cover muscles, connect muscle to muscle and then to skin as well as cover groups of muscles, blood vessels, and nerves

Fibromyalgia: Condition that causes muscle pain throughout the body and fatigue

Flat bones: Bones that provide a place for the large skeletal muscles to anchor and activate movement

Flexibility test: Diagnostic test used to measure the range of motion in a joint

Frozen shoulder: Shoulder that is unable to move

Gout: Type of arthritis in which there is too much uric acid buildup in the body

Herniated or ruptured disc: Disc of the spine whose outer coating is damaged

Hinge joint: Type of synovial joint that allows movement in one direction

Idiopathic scoliosis: Sideways curvature of the spine with an unknown cause

Immovable joint: Bone joint that allows no movement

Involuntary muscles: Muscles whose movement is controlled by the nervous system

Irregular bones: Bones—such as the vertebrae—that have complex shapes and are not grouped with other bones

Joint: The area where two or more bones are attached for the purpose of permitting body parts to move

Joint aspiration: Diagnostic test and treatment that removes joint fluid

Joint replacement surgery: Surgery in which a damaged joint is removed and replaced

Ligament: Muscle fiber that cushions and protect bones and that ties joints together

Long bones: Bones in the arms and legs that help skeletal muscles activate movement

Meniscal injury: Injury caused by rotating the knee while bearing weight

Multiple myeloma: Cancerous cells in the bone marrow

Muscle biopsy: Diagnostic test that cuts out a muscle tissue sample

Muscles: Tissue fibers that pull on the joints to activate movement

Musculoskeletal system: Mesh of bones, muscles, and other connective tissue that gives support and shape to the body and enables the body to move and perform tasks

NSAIDs: Nonsteroidal anti-inflammatory drugs

Open or compound fracture: Fracture in which the broken bone punctures the skin

Orthopedics: Surgical subspecialty that studies and treats musculoskeletal problems

Orthopedists, or orthopedic surgeon: Physician with a specialty in musculoskeletal problems

Ossification: Process in which cartilage is replaced by calcium, sodium, collagen, and other minerals

Osteoarthritis: Disease that causes disabling changes in joint tissues and opposing bones

Osteopath, or osteopathic doctor (DO): A physician who studies and is trained in osteopathy, using musculoskeletal manipulation along with medication and surgery

Osteopathy: Type of medical training that focuses on the influence that the musculoskeletal system has on other body systems

Osteoporosis: Bone disease that causes bones to break and become spongy

Paget's disease: Disease that causes bones to grow too large and to weaken

Palpation: Diagnostic test that uses touch and is done to identify the location of growths

Partially movable joint: Bone joint that moves a little

Pectoral or shoulder girdle: Group of bones that attaches the upper limbs to the body

Pelvic girdle: Group of bones that attaches the lower limbs to the body

Permanent teeth: Adult teeth

Physical therapist (PT): Rehabilitation specialist who treats musculoskeletal issues

Pivot joint: Type of synovial joint that allows a rotating motion

Podiatrist: Surgical subspecialist trained in foot care and diseases

Primary bone tumor, or sarcoma: Cancer that starts in the bones

Primary teeth: Baby teeth

Prosthesis: In the context of joint replacement surgery, a new joint that is made of plastic, metal, or both

Pulp: Living tissue inside a tooth

Repetitive stress injury (RSI): An injury that occurs when too much stress is repeatedly placed on a part of the body

Rheumatoid arthritis: Type of arthritis in which the body makes antibodies against joint tissues

RICE: Treatment for shoulder (and other musculoskeletal) problems: rest, ice, compression, and elevation.

Rotator cuff tear: Tearing and inflammation of the shoulder tendons caused by frequent use, an injury, or aging

Sciatica: Back pain that radiates to the hip and down the leg due to pressure on the sciatic nerve

Scoliosis: Sideways curvature of the spine

Secondary bone tumor: Cancer that starts in another part of the body and spreads to the bone

Sesamoid bones: Bones that are small and flat and look like a sesame seed

Short bones: Bones with the same width as length, giving them a cube-like shape

Shoulder separation: Condition in which the ligaments between the collarbone and the shoulder blade are torn

Skeletal muscle: Muscle that attaches to bone and provides movement, support, posture, and heat

Smooth muscle: Muscle fiber that looks smooth, not striated, and is slow to become tired

Spasm: Muscle contraction

Spinal stenosis: Narrowing of the spinal canal

Spongy bone: A part of the bone that looks like a sponge and is inside the compact bone

Sprain: The overstretching or tearing of a ligament

Strain: The overstretching or tearing of a muscle or tendon

Stress fracture: Small crack in a bone

Striated muscle: Muscles fiber that has horizontal stripes, tightens quickly, and tires easily

Sutures: Bone joints of the skull

Synovial fluid: Fluid in joints that lubricates them to move easily

Synovial joints: Bone joints that move in a variety of directions

Tendon: Cord-like tissue that allows muscles to pull on bones

Tendonitis: Inflammation of the tendon caused by repeated stress

Temporomandibular joint (TMJ) dysfunction: Pain in the joint and muscles around and in the jaw

Torn tendon: Tendon damaged by overuse

Vertebrae (singular vertebra): Bones of the spine

Vertebral fracture: Fracture caused by trauma to a vertebra

Voluntary muscle: Muscle whose movement can be controlled by the person

CHAPTER ACTIVITIES

1. Working in groups of four with enough butcher block paper or a large sheet of paper that is the length of an adult human body, draw the axial and appendicular human skeletons and identify major bones.

2. Conduct 10-minute interviews with two people who have fractured a bone (past or present). If possible, select interviewees who fractured their bone at different ages. For example, interview someone who fractured a bone in his or her 20s and then interview someone who had a fracture at an older age (e.g., in his or her 50s). Ask the interviewees to describe the type of fracture and the healing process. Did they wear a cast, use a wheelchair, or walk with crutches? How did they adapt to limited mobility while doing daily activities like washing, eating, and sleeping? What recommendations do the interviewees have for patients with a fractured bone? After you have conducted the two interviews, write a two- to three-page reflection paper on your impressions of what it requires to heal a bone fracture, in the context of the aging process; that is, how is it different to have a fracture when someone is younger versus when someone is older?

3. Take photographs or bring in pictures of artwork (painting or sculpture) that show muscles, and label the picture.

4. Pair up with another student and create a crossword puzzle with 30 terms from the Key Terms section. After you've completed your crossword, exchange it with another team in the class and solve the one you receive.

5. You have been hired as a health coach for fibromyalgia patients. Your task is to develop a 1-day workshop for 10 participants on complementary approaches to pain management. With a partner, develop a 7- to 10-slide PowerPoint presentation that describes complementary pain management techniques. At the end of the presentation, lead a class activity that demonstrates one of the pain management techniques described in your presentation.

6. You are hired by an urban senior center as a health educator. Your task is to present 1-hour workshops for 10 to 15 participants. The workshops highlight complementary approaches to back pain management. Select a complementary approach, such as yoga, meditation, or acupuncture, and develop an evidence-based workshop presentation.

Bibliography and Works Cited

10 facts about the skeleton: An overview of the skeletal system. (2016). *Visible Body/Learn Site.* Retrieved from http://learn.visiblebody.com/skeleton/overview-of-skeleton

American Academy of Orthopaedic Surgeons. (2012). Bone health basics. Retrieved from http://orthoinfo.aaos.org/topic.cfm?topic=A00578

American Academy of Orthopaedic Surgeons. (2015a). Bone tumor. Retrieved from http://orthoinfo.aaos.org/topic.cfm?topic=A00074

American Academy of Orthopaedic Surgeons. (2015b). Cervical radiculopathy (pinched nerve). Retrieved from http://orthoinfo.aaos.org/PDFs/A00332.pdf

American Academy of Orthopaedic Surgeons. (2016). Joint replacement. Retrieved from http://orthoinfo.aaos.org/menus/arthroplasty.cfm

American Cancer Society. (2016). What is bone cancer? Retrieved from http://www.cancer.org/cancer/bonecancer/detailedguide/bone-cancer-what-is-bone-cancer

Miller, S. B. (1990). An overview of the musculoskeletal system. In H. K. Walker, W. D. Hall, & J. W. Hurst (Eds.), *Clinical methods: The history, physical, and laboratory examinations* (3rd ed., Chapter 158). Boston, MA: Butterworth. Available from http://www.ncbi.nlm.nih.gov/books/NBK266/

National Fibromyalgia Association. (2015). About fibromyalgia. Retrieved from http://www.fmaware.org/about-fibromyalgia/

National Institute of Arthritis and Musculoskeletal and Skin Diseases Information Clearinghouse (2014a). Questions and answers about shoulder problems. Retrieved from http://www.niams.nih.gov/Health_Info/Shoulder_Problems/default.asp

National Institute of Arthritis and Musculoskeletal and Skin Diseases Information Clearinghouse. (2014b). What is back pain? Retrieved from http://www.niams.nih.gov/Health_Info/Back_Pain/back_pain_ff.asp

National Institute of Arthritis and Musculoskeletal and Skin Diseases Information Clearinghouse. (2014c). What is osteoarthritis? Retrieved from http://www.niams.nih.gov/Health_Info/Osteoarthritis/osteoarthritis_ff.asp

National Institute of Arthritis and Musculoskeletal and Skin Diseases Information Clearinghouse. (2014d). What is scoliosis? Retrieved from http://www.niams.nih.gov/Health_Info/Scoliosis/scoliosis_ff.asp

National Institute of Neurological Disorders and Stroke. (2012). Carpal tunnel syndrome fact sheet. Retrieved from https://www.ninds.nih.gov/Disorders/Patient-Caregiver-Education/Fact-Sheets/Carpal-Tunnel-Syndrome-Fact-Sheet#3049_2

NIH Osteoporosis and Related Bone Diseases–National Resource Center. (2014). What is Paget's disease of bone? Retrieved from http://www.niams.nih.gov/Health_Info/Bone/Pagets/pagets_disease_ff.asp

NIH Osteoporosis and Related Bone Diseases–National Resource Center. (2016). Osteoporosis and arthritis: Two common but different conditions. Retrieved from http://www.niams.nih.gov/Health_Info/Bone/Osteoporosis/Conditions_Behaviors/osteoporosis_arthritis.asp

TMJ Association. (2015). TMD basics: The basics of the jaw joint. Retrieved from http://www.tmj.org/Page/34/17

US National Library of Medicine. (2015). Broken bone. *MedlinePlus.* Retrieved from https://www.nlm.nih.gov/medlineplus/ency/article/000001.htm

US National Library of Medicine. (2016a). Arthritis. *MedlinePlus.* Retrieved from https://www.nlm.nih.gov/medlineplus/arthritis.html

US National Library of Medicine. (2016b). Fibromyalgia. *MedlinePlus.* Retrieved from https://medlineplus.gov/fibromyalgia.html

CHAPTER 20

INTEGUMENTARY SYSTEM AND RELATED DISEASES

CHAPTER OBJECTIVES

- Review the structure and function of the integumentary system.

- Give examples of how the integumentary system works with other body systems.

- Explain how aging affects the integumentary system.

- List and define terms used to describe basic skin lesions.

- Discuss common diseases of the skin, hair, nails, and oil glands.

- Describe differences among the four degrees of burns.

- List and describe three types of skin cancer and related prevention strategies.

Skin and its related organs—hair, nails, glands, and nerves—make up the *integumentary system* (IS). The main function of the skin is to protect against external factors, such as bacteria, chemicals, and temperature. Hair helps with heat and cooling and protects against ultraviolet (UV) rays. Nails protect the end of fingers and toes from injuries. Sweat glands regulate temperature and remove waste. Oil glands give moisture to the skin and hair. Nerves feel pain, sensation, pressure, and temperature.

Dermatology is the branch of medicine that studies the IS. A *dermatologist* is a physician who specializes in treating diseases and injuries of the IS. Some dermatologists have additional training in a specialty—for example, cosmetic surgery.

Function of the Integumentary System

The IS protects and regulates the body's internal activities. The skin's main function is to protect the body's tissues, bones, and organs from injury. It acts as a barrier to keep the body away from environmental risks like viruses, bacteria, and chemicals. Skin not only provides protection but also stores fat and water, removes waste, regulates body temperature, and produces vitamins and hormones. Without skin, we could not feel touch, pressure, pain, heat, and cold. To perform these functions, the IS works with other body systems (see Table 20.1).

The IS not only works with other body systems but also helps maintain *homeostasis*, or a stable equilibrium. An example of how the skin keeps homeostasis is that although you sweat, at the same time, it keeps body fluids from drying out. Skin

Table 20.1   Integumentary System's Relationship With Other Body Systems

System	How the Integumentary System (IS) Interacts
Urinary	IS helps rid water and waste. IS limits fluid loss through skin.
Musculoskeletal	IS synthesizes vitamin D.
Reproductive	IS covers external sexual organs and provides sexual sensations.
Respiratory	IS hairs guard the opening to the nasal cavity.
Cardiovascular	IS cells cause changes to blood flow.
Endocrine	IS synthesizes vitamin D, needed for hormones.
Lymphatic	IS provides physical barriers to stop germs from entering the body. IS helps trigger the immune response.
Immune	Immune cells live in the skin and help keep germs, chemicals, and other toxins away from internal organs.
Digestive	IS works with the digestive system by absorbing vitamin D. Digestive system also helps with healthy skin functioning.
Nervous	Skin helps with the sense of touch. The nervous system depends on skin's nerve cells to sense the outside world.
Circulatory	IS works with the circulatory system in the delivery of medication through *skin patches*. This type of medication delivery helps in treating chronic diseases.

acts as an early warning system if there is something wrong elsewhere in the body. The skin's texture, temperature, and color indicate health problems, such as infections.

Structure of the Integumentary System

The IS is the largest body system because skin is the largest organ. There are also special nerves that enable skin to be a sensory organ. Skin makes up to 15% of body weight, with a surface area of 22 square feet. Its color, thickness, and texture vary throughout the body. For example, skin on the face is different from skin on the feet.

There are two general types of skin. One type is thin and hairy, and is found on most parts of the body. The second type is thick and hairless, and is found only on the parts of the body that are used heavily: the palms of the hands and the soles of the feet.

The skin includes hair, nails, sweat glands, lymph, and fatty tissues (see Figure 20.1). Other parts of the skin and their function include the following:

*   *Blood vessels*—arteries and veins that carry nutrients and blood to skin cells and carry away waste products

*   *Hair shaft*—part of the hair that is above the skin

*   *Sensory nerves*—nerves that sense and send sensations to the nervous system

*   *Hair follicles*—tube-shaped covers that surround the part of the hair that is under the skin

*   *Oil glands*—small glands that release oil onto hair follicles

Skin has two layers that cover a third fatty layer (see Figure 20.1). These three layers differ in function, thickness, and strength. The *epidermis* is the top layer, the part that we can see; it protects the body. It gets oxygen and nutrients from the lower layers. The epidermis lacks blood vessels and can be either thick or thin, depending on the body part. As noted earlier, thick skin is only on the palms of the hands and soles of the feet. The rest of the body has thin skin, with the thinnest covering the eyelids.

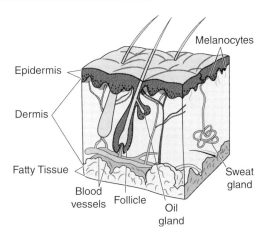

Figure 20.1 Skin

Note. Adapted from "Skin Anatomy," by Don Bliss, National Cancer Institute, Visuals Online, [Public domain]. Retrieved from https://visualsonline.cancer.gov/details.cfm?imageid=4604

The epidermis makes the pigment *melanin*, which gives skin its color and protects against the sun's ultraviolet rays. *Keratin* is a protein that is also made in the epidermis, and it protects against chemicals and infections.

The *dermis* is the middle and thickest layer; it makes up most of the skin. The main functions of the dermis are to regulate temperature and to supply the epidermis with blood. Other functions include removing waste, fighting infection, storing water, and supplying nutrients to the epidermis.

The dermis has hair follicles, nerve endings, blood vessels, lymph vessels, muscle cells, and oil and sweat glands. Strong fibers called *collagen* and *elastin* are in the dermis and give skin its strength and flexibility. The nerve endings in this layer are responsible for the sense of touch.

The *subcutaneous layer*, or hypodermis, is the skin's bottom layer. It is made up of fat and connective tissue that has nerves and blood vessels. The roots of oil and sweat glands as well as hair follicles are in this layer. The subcutaneous layer's main functions are to help the body stay warm and to protect inner organs from impact. A major part of this layer is *adipose tissue*, or fat tissue, that stores surplus energy. Blood vessels, lymph vessels, nerves, and hair follicles also go through the subcutaneous layer. This layer's thickness varies throughout the body and is different in each person.

Skin has tiny glands that secrete sweat and oil, which decrease acid on the skin's surface and kill germs. *Sebaceous glands*, or oil glands, lubricate hair and skin and stop bacterial growth. They secrete the oil *sebum*, which gives skin and hair moisture, protects them from friction, and acts as water-proofing. Oil glands are all over the body, but are mostly on the scalp, face, chest, and genitals.

Sweat glands open at the surface through *skin pores,* tiny holes in the skin. The body has about three million sweat glands, and they help the body cool off. Some types of sweat glands are part of the nervous system and are all over the body; other types are just in the armpits and groin. Sweat glands make sweat which is a solution for bacteria to break down and create "body odor". Sweat becomes smelly when bacteria break it down as food.

One of the major sources of body water loss is sweat. Sweat helps maintain homeostasis because it cools the skin surface and lowers body temperature. It also provides protection from environmental hazards by watering down harmful chemicals that touch the skin.

Hair is almost everywhere on the human body and has two distinct structures. The first is the *hair shaft,* which projects above the skin surface and is visible. The second is the *hair root,* which grows up from the base to the surface. Hair growth begins inside a tube called the *hair follicle* (see Figure 20.1). Hair follicles are small cavities in the epidermis and are lined with cells that make proteins that form hair. An oil gland, a capillary bed, a nerve ending, and a small muscle are all part of each hair follicle. One hair grows out of each follicle, and follicles are found throughout the body, except on the palms, soles, and lips. The only living part of hair is in the follicle. Genes control certain characteristics of hair, such as baldness, color, and texture.

The function of hair is to protect the scalp from UV light, cushion blows to the head, and insulate the skull. It also protects body openings, such as the nostrils, ears, and eyes, preventing entry of foreign objects. Hair can provide an early warning sign with goose bumps (raised hairs) that may help prevent injury.

A nail comes out of the nail bed. Nails are made of dead cells that contain the protein keratin. Cells in the nail bed link together and form the nails on fingers and toes. Nails protect exposed tips and limit injury.

Aging and the Integumentary System

With aging, skin begins to grow smaller and to function less effectively. The dermis and epidermis begin to thin, and the fat tissues of the subcutaneous layer can lose density. The skin loses its elasticity and becomes drier because of less active oil glands. Nerve endings become less sensitive. Sags and wrinkles are common, along with skin injuries and infections that heal more slowly and become more difficult to treat. Sweat glands and blood vessels become less active, too, reducing the skin's ability to respond to heat. All of these changes in structure put the skin at risk for damage. Skin repairs are slow, taking twice as long as those of a young adult.

Skin has less protection against UV rays with aging. Sensitivity to the sun increases. It is sun damage that is responsible for most of what happens to skin as we age, including wrinkles, irregular color, spots, and rough texture. Along with the skin and glands, hair also is affected by aging. It thins and loses melanin, which causes the hair to become gray or white. Hair follicles stop functioning altogether or only make finer hairs.

When the IS becomes less active due to aging, some people develop cosmetic concerns, resulting in billions of dollars spent on beauty products. However, aging and cosmetic concerns often foster beauty myths. Table 20.2 lists some examples of beauty myths.

Table 20.2 Beauty Myths

Drinking lots of water keeps skin looking young.	Water does help clean the kidneys and decrease appetite. But short of bloating and temporarily getting rid of some wrinkles, water doesn't do much for the skin's complexion.
Soap is bad for the skin.	Traditional true soap did contain a mix of animal fats and oils that caused drying. There are newer soaps to clean the skin in a milder way than true soap.
It's too late to start using sunscreen.	It is never too late to start protecting skin from the sun. The increasing effect of the sun is what's damaging, and you can stop some of its impact. There is clinical evidence that once you start protecting the skin, it can repair itself. This is a slow process, however, taking years to have significant results.
Scalp massage can reduce hair loss.	There is no scientific evidence that supports this claim. Supporters of massage claim that an increase in scalp circulation can help hair get nutrients needed for healthy hair growth. Yet the scalp already has a significant amount of blood flow.
You can shrink a pore.	The size of skin pores is determined by a person's genes. Once you reach puberty, the pores become their adult size. They can become overly large if clogged with bacteria. Antiaging creams (e.g., Retin-A brand) can break up the bacteria clogging the skin and return pores to their normal size.
Dry skin causes wrinkles.	The sun causes 80% of lines and wrinkles. The other 20% are caused by facial expressions, such as smiling. However, if someone is dehydrated, the skin does seem more wrinkled. Also, as one ages, the skin makes less oil.
Everyone needs a moisturizer.	Moisturizer is needed only if there is red, scaly, or itchy, dry skin.
A facelift can reverse the aging process.	A facelift does not reverse the aging process. It just gives the appearance of tighter skin.

Common Signs, Symptoms, and Diagnostic Tests for Integumentary Diseases

IS diseases can range from being mild enough to affect only how a person looks to being severe enough to interfere with daily activities, but the great majority are not life threatening. Even when the signs and symptoms are mild, however, these diseases cause stress due to changes in appearance or to constant itching and pain. Unlike diseases of other body systems, integumentary diseases are usually visible because they cause changes to the skin. Skin texture becomes dry or moist; there might be scabs or blisters; the skin may become red with bruises or *rashes*. These types of skin changes are known as *lesions*.

Visible changes to the IS can indicate the presence of a disease that involves one or more of the body's systems. Circulatory and respiratory diseases cause *cyanosis*, a bluish skin tone. Diseases involving the liver cause *jaundice*, a yellow skin tone. *Pallor*, a whiter, pale skin, may mean anemia. Swelling and redness of the skin may be an allergic response by the immune system.

Examination of lesions, along with a physical examination and a health history, helps a provider make a diagnosis. Lesions are identified based on their size, location on the body, shape, number, color, and texture. Table 20.3 describes types of skin lesions.

Table 20.3 Types of Skin Lesions or Skin Changes

Abrasion	Scrape or superficial wound
Abscess	Cavity filled with pus
Cellulite	Dimpled fat
Comedo	A blackhead or whitehead caused by buildup of oil
Crust or scab	Dried blood, pus, or fluids on the surface of the skin; a scab forms where the skin has been damaged
Cyst	Closed sac on the surface of the skin filled with fluid or solid material
Edema	Fluid buildup that causes swelling
Erythema	Redness
Fissure	Small, deep, linear crack or tear in the skin
Hive or wheal	Swelling in the skin that creates a soft, spongy area that appears suddenly and then disappears within 24 hours; hives are allergic reactions to drugs, insect bites, or some other irritant that touches the skin
Macule	Flat, discolored spot of any shape—for example, freckles, flat moles, and some rashes
Nodule	Solid and thick bump that is usually round
Papule	Solid small bump like a pimple without pus—for example, warts, insect bites, and some skin cancers
Pruritus	Itching
Pustule	Raised fluid-filled spot that has pus—for example, a whitehead
Rash	Temporary flair-up
Scales	Areas of dead cells that form a flaky, dry patch, as in psoriasis
Scar	Area where normal skin has been replaced by scar tissue
Ulcer or erosion	Eating away of tissue as with a bedsore
Vesicle; bulla	Small, fluid-filled sac—for example, a blister; a bulla is a larger vesicle

There are times when a physical examination and a health history are not enough to make a diagnosis. A final diagnosis does take time because many skin diseases look alike. It requires identifying possible causes and evaluating responses to treatment. If more information is required, then a *biopsy*, or small skin sample, is removed from a lesion for laboratory analysis. A biopsy enables the provider to determine whether it is a noncancerous or cancerous growth. In the case of skin cancer, a biopsy as part of the diagnosis can also serve as a treatment.

Skin Injuries, Bruises, and Burns

Injuries

A skin injury is damage or harm to the skin. Accidents, falls, hits, weapons, sharp objects, heat, and more cause skin injuries. In the United States, millions of people injure themselves every year. An injury can be unintentional or intentional. An *unintentional injury* occurs by accident—for example, falling off a ladder. An *intentional injury* occurs because a person wanted to inflict the injury as with a gunshot wound. Injuries range from minor to life threatening. They happen anywhere, any time, and to anyone.

Skin is the part of the body that is most exposed to the world, so it is especially at risk for an injury. *Wounds* are injuries that break the skin or other body tissues and include abrasions, incisions, lacerations, and punctures (see Table 20.4). They often occur because of an accident, but surgery can also be a cause. Minor wounds usually are not serious, but they need to be kept clean to avoid infection. If the wound is infected, if it is deep or does not heal, if bleeding does not stop, or if dirt is difficult to remove, then medical attention is needed.

It takes several steps for wounds to heal. First, a blood clot forms and stops the blood flow. After the blood clot forms, different types of cells help in the healing. Stem cells and immune cells prevent infection. For the first few days, a wound may be inflamed and painful.

As the body heals, a scab forms over the wound on the outside in order to protect the damaged skin underneath. New tissue forms under the scab: the skin makes collagen to reconnect broken tissue while the body repairs damaged blood vessels.

When the healing is complete, the scab dries up and falls off, leaving behind the repaired skin. There is often a scar that looks different from normal skin. Scars are caused by two proteins: elastin, which gives skin its flexibility, and collagen, which gives it strength. When the elastin and collagen bind together, they make a scar.

Table 20.4   Types of Wounds

Wound	Description
Abrasion	Made when the skin is rubbed or scraped off, as with rope burns. This kind of wound becomes infected easily because dirt and germs get caught in the tissues.
Incision or cut	Made by sharp objects like knives and razors. Incisions tend to bleed freely because the blood vessels are cut cleanly and without ragged edges. Of all types of wounds, cuts are the least likely to become infected, as the free flow of blood washes out the germs that cause infection.
Laceration	Caused by a tear, not a cut. Lacerations have ragged, irregular edges and torn tissues underneath. These wounds are made by blunt rather than sharp objects. Dirt, grease, or other materials are often ground into the tissue with these wounds, causing infection.
Puncture	Caused by objects that go deep into the tissues while leaving a small skin opening. Wounds made by nails, needles, wire, and bullets are usually punctures. Small puncture wounds do not bleed freely; larger ones can cause internal bleeding. The risk of infection is high with puncture wounds.

Bruises

When an injury crushes small blood vessels but does not break the skin. the vessels break open and leak blood under the skin. The mark on the skin caused by the blood trapped under the surface is a *bruise.* Bruises are often painful and swollen and can appear on skin, muscle, and bone.

It can take months for a bruise to fade, but most last about 2 weeks. They begin as a red color, then turn blue and yellow before returning to normal. To reduce bruising, a person can put ice on the injured area and raise it above the heart. A health care provider needs to be seen if the patient bruises for no reason or if the bruise looks infected.

Burns

A *burn* is skin damage caused by fire, radiation, electricity, chemicals, and other heat accidents. A burn caused by hot water or steam is called a *scald.*

In the United States, there are approximately 4,000 deaths a year from fire and burns. There are also 25,000 patients hospitalized in burn centers each year along with 600,000 burn injuries treated in emergency rooms.

Risk factors for burns include cooking with an open flame and wearing loose clothing while cooking. Smoking, alcohol use, poor electrical and chemical safety, and unsupervised children are also risk factors.

Burns cause death to skin cells. When skin cells die, there may be loss of fluid, causing dehydration. Renal (kidney) and circulatory failure may also occur, which can be fatal.

The severity of burns is measured by two factors: the amount of area damaged and the layers of skin affected (see Figure 20.2). *First-degree burns* (e.g., a mild sunburn) are superficial and affect only the

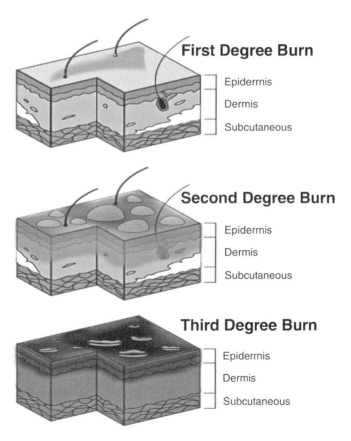

Figure 20.2 Types of Burns
Note. Adapted from K. Aainsqatsi (original uploader) at English Wikipedia (Original text: K. Aainsqatsi) [GFDL (http://www.gnu.org/copyleft/fdl.html) or CC-BY-SA-3.0 (http://creativecommons.org/licenses/by-sa/3.0/)], via Wikimedia Commons

epidermis. Although the skin may be painful and swollen, there are no blisters and no scarring. This type of burn heals within a week.

Second-degree burns go deeper and affect the epidermis and some of the dermis. These burns cause swelling, redness, and blistering. The amount of blistering depends on the depth of the burn. Blisters heal within 10 to 14 days if there are no problems, but deeper second-degree burns can take up to 3 months to heal. With this type of burn, scarring is common, and the burn site needs to be kept clean and sterile to prevent infection.

Third-degree burns are serious because they affect all three layers of the skin. These burns destroy the tissue, affect the nerve ending, and make the skin look white, red, or black. A third-degree burn can also destroy sweat and sebaceous glands, hair follicles, and blood vessels.

Fourth-degree burns are the worst type of burns. They affect muscle and cause bone damage. Oddly, third- and fourth-degree burns are usually not as painful as lesser burns because the nerve pain receptors are destroyed.

The swelling and blistering associated with burns cause loss of fluid from damaged blood vessels. In severe cases, such fluid loss causes shock. To prevent shock, burn patients receive intravenous (IV) fluids and nutrients to stop dehydration and allow the body to repair tissues and replace lost proteins. Burns also cause infection due to the damage they cause to the skin's barrier. To prevent infection, burn patients are given antibiotic skin creams.

The body cannot repair the skin following a third- or fourth-degree burn because tissues used for repair are damaged. These burns need IV fluids, pain management, and surgical removal of dead skin and tissue. In severe burn cases, amputation may be necessary.

Once skin is removed, then skin grafting may be part of treatment. *Skin grafting* is a procedure in which healthy skin from an unaffected part of the body is used to repair destroyed skin. *Autografting* is the use of the patient's own skin. *Heterografting* is required when the patient has suffered large areas of burn and has little healthy skin to graft. Skin for heterografting comes from the patient's own cells that are taken to a laboratory where they grow and form into skin tissue. Synthetic materials can also be made to look and act like skin. Skin can also be grafted from a donor, such as a family member or even from a dead body. Patients with skin grafts need intensive care before and after procedures. Skin grafting requires many surgeries because large areas of skin cannot be replaced all at once. Another problem is that grafts are often rejected by the burn victim's body.

Physical therapy and other treatments are used to aid burn recovery. Physical therapy helps prevent problems—for example, contracture. *Contracture* is a condition in which the skin and tissues are so burned that it is difficult and painful for the patient to move.

A few decades ago, burns covering half the body were often fatal. Today, many patients with burns covering 90% of their bodies can survive, although they may have permanent disabilities and scars (American College of Emergency Physicians, 2016).

Prevention strategies for burn injuries include not smoking. If a person does smoke, he or she should never smoke in bed and should avoid smoking while drinking alcohol. Other strategies include supervising children carefully, following electrical and chemical safety rules, and being careful around open flames.

Diseases of the Integumentary System

Some diseases of the integumentary system cause discomfort but are not life threatening; others can be deadly. Bacteria, viruses, fungi, or genetic factors cause many of these diseases. Such risk factors as direct contact with infected persons, hygiene, stress, and sun exposure influence their development.

Dermatitis

Dermatitis is a general term that describes inflammation of the skin. Although dermatitis has different causes and forms, it usually involves an itchy rash with swollen, red skin. Affected skin may blister, ooze, and develop a crust. The common forms of dermatitis are as follows:

- *Eczema*—usually starts in infancy. A rash that appears inside the elbows, behind the knees, and the front of the neck. When scratched, the rash leaks fluid and crusts over.

- *Contact dermatitis*—appears on different body areas. A body area gets a rash because it came into direct contact with something that either irritated the skin or caused an allergic reaction. This rash burns, stings, itches, and blisters.

- *Seborrheic dermatitis*—rash with yellowish scales that appears on the scalp or on the face. It causes dandruff and is seen in those with oily skin or hair. In infants, it is called *cradle cap*.

Dermatitis is usually not life threatening or contagious, but it is uncomfortable. Scratching the rash causes open sores that can become infected and spread to other parts of the body. The following are factors that increase risk for certain types of dermatitis:

- *Age.* Dermatitis occurs at any age, but eczema usually begins at infancy.

- *Allergies and asthma.* Those with a personal or family history of hay fever or asthma are more likely to have eczema.

- *Occupation.* Jobs that require handling certain metals or chemicals can cause contact dermatitis.

Medications help with dermatitis symptoms, but treatment does depend on the cause. Steroid creams, wet compresses, and avoiding skin irritants are the basis of most treatments. *Light therapy*, exposing skin to controlled amounts of light, also may help.

Psoriasis

Psoriasis, an autoimmune disease, causes raised, red, scaly skin patches on any part of the body, but mostly on elbows, knees, or scalp. The patches itch and sting. A provider can diagnose psoriasis by doing a physical examination and looking for scales with well-defined edges.

Psoriasis is like eczema, but there are differences. One difference is that psoriasis has well-defined edges, whereas the edges of eczema are less well defined. Psoriasis also looks thicker and more inflamed when compared to eczema. Another difference is that eczema appears on the body trunk, whereas psoriasis usually does not.

Psoriasis is caused by a combination of genes and exposure to triggers. Some of the triggers are stress, skin injuries, and infections. What triggers one patient's psoriasis may not trigger it for another patient.

Psoriasis can show on the eyelids, ears, mouth, hands, and feet. The skin at each of these sites is different and requires specific treatments. Psoriasis can be mild, moderate, or severe; most patients have the mild form. The severity of psoriasis is determined by signs and symptoms and by how much it affects a patient's quality of life. For example, psoriasis can have a serious impact on one's daily activities even if it is only in a small area. It can also be a sign of other diseases, such as diabetes, heart disease, and depression.

Treatment for mild psoriasis is over-the-counter or prescription creams and shampoos. Moderate to severe psoriasis needs not only creams and shampoos but also light therapy and systemic medications. *Systemic medications* are prescription drugs that work throughout the body.

Hives

Hives are raised skin blisters and lesions. Sometimes known as *welts*, hives can be of different shapes and sizes and look like tiny red or skin-colored spots or large interconnected bumps. They can be on any part of the body and often cause itching. Hives are not serious and go away within 24 hours for most patients (American Academy of Dermatology, 2016b). New hives may appear as old ones fade, so hives can last for a few days or longer. Hives that last less than 6 weeks are called acute hives. Allergic reactions, temperature extremes, illnesses, and stress can cause acute hives. Chronic hives last more than 6 weeks, and determining the cause can be difficult.

Symptoms of hives are an itch that can also sting. In some cases, hives cause swelling around the eyes, lips, hands, feet, or throat. In severe cases, the throat and airway can swell, making breathing or swallowing difficult, and emergency medical care is required.

Some patients always get hives in the same area on their body because they have a trigger. Examples of triggers are some medications, too much sunlight, certain foods, infections, insect bites, animals, and pollen.

A provider can make the diagnosis for hives just by looking at the skin, but finding the cause is difficult. To find the cause, a provider reviews the patient's health history, asks questions, and does a physical examination. Allergy tests, blood work, and a skin biopsy may also be necessary to complete the diagnosis.

The best remedy for hives is to avoid triggers. For mild or moderate hives, a treatment of over-the-counter antihistamines can relieve symptoms. Sometimes hives go away on their own, but in other cases, they can come and go for years.

Rosacea

Rosacea is a chronic skin inflammation causing red cheeks, nose, chin, or forehead. In some cases, rosacea can also be on the neck, chest, scalp, or ears. In many rosacea patients, the eyes can feel itchy and look bloodshot.

The redness becomes more intense over time and stays longer. Eventually, tiny blood vessels on the face become visible. If rosacea is untreated, bumps, patches and pimples develop, and in severe cases, the nose becomes swollen and bumpy from excess tissue. The signs and symptoms can be different from one person to the next, but rosacea usually goes away and then returns.

Rosacea is a common but poorly understood disorder of the facial skin that is estimated to affect well over 16 million Americans—and most of them don't know it. According to a National Rosacea Society survey (2016), 95% of rosacea patients had known little or nothing about its signs and symptoms prior to their diagnosis.

Although rosacea can affect anyone, those with fair skin are at greatest risk. The disease is more often diagnosed in women, but men tend to have the more severe symptoms. It usually begins between the ages of 30 and 60. It is not infectious, nor is it contagious.

Although there is no cure for rosacea and the cause is unknown, treatment can control signs and symptoms. Medications are given to treat bumps and pimples as well as reduce facial redness. When needed, *laser treatment,* which is intense pulsed light directed onto the skin, is given. Other procedures remove visible blood vessels and correct skin thickness on the nose.

A gentle skin-care routine can help control rosacea after treatment along with limiting exposure to triggers like sunlight, alcohol, spicy foods, and stress.

Acne

Acne is the medical term for pimples, and it affects the skin's oil glands. Inside the hair follicle, sebum, an oily and waxy substance, carries dead skin cells to the surface of the skin. A thin hair also grows through the follicle and out to the skin. Sometimes, the hair, sebum, and skin cells clump together into a plug. The bacteria in the plug cause swelling, and when the plug starts to break down, a pimple grows.

Pimples develop on the face, chest, and back, and there are different types. *Whiteheads* stay under the surface of the skin, *blackheads* stay on the skin's surface and look black, and *pustules* are red at the bottom and have pus on top.

Acne is the most common skin disease and affects about 40 million to 50 million Americans (National Institute of Arthritis and Musculoskeletal and Skin Diseases, 2014). People of all races and ages can get acne, but it happens mostly in teenagers and young adults. Nearly 85% of people have acne at some point in their lives, and it usually starts in puberty.

The cause is unknown, yet there are many myths about acne. Dirty skin, stress, chocolate, and greasy foods do not cause acne in most people. There are, however, risk factors that might cause acne:

- Hormone increase in teenage years
- Starting or stopping birth control pills
- Certain medications
- Hormone changes during pregnancy
- Family health history
- Greasy makeup

Acne treatment tries to heal pimples, stop new pimples from forming, and prevent scarring. Providers treat acne using different types of medications, including pills and creams. Isotretinoin is an oral medication that has been effective against severe acne. It can cause serious side effects and birth defects, however. Taking isotretinoin during pregnancy can cause miscarriage and life-threatening malformations in the baby. For these reasons, there are strict rules in the United States for providers, pharmacists, and patients regarding the prescription and use of isotretinoin. This medication was sold under the brand name Accutane, but that is no longer available in the United States.

Impetigo

Impetigo is a contagious skin infection. It starts when bacteria get into a lesion (e.g., a cut or scratch). Impetigo is more common in children than adults, and especially those ages 2 through 6. The cause is usually staph bacteria, but it also can be strep bacteria. The types of strep bacteria that cause impetigo are usually different from those that cause strep throat.

This bacterial skin infection spreads by direct contact with lesions or nasal discharge from an infected person. It usually takes 1 to 3 days from the time of infection until symptoms show. Symptoms start with red blisters surrounded by red skin. The blisters can be anywhere on the body, but mostly are on the face, arms, and legs. They fill with pus, then break open after a few days. Usually many blisters break open at the same time, then meet together, break open again, and form red patches with yellow scabs. The scabs are itchy, but scratching them only spreads the blisters. A provider looks for skin blisters to diagnose this infection. If the impetigo is from strep bacteria, then antibiotics are prescribed to be taken orally or applied to the infected area.

Impetigo blisters heal with little or no scarring if properly treated. Left untreated, impetigo might get better on its own, but there is a risk that it will continue to spread and scar.

Cellulitis

Normal skin has bacteria living on it, and when there is a break in the skin, the bacteria cause a skin infection. *Cellulitis* is a skin infection caused by staph and strep bacteria. It most often appears on the lower parts of the body, but any part of the body can become infected.

Risk factors for cellulitis include cracks in the skin between the toes, skin injuries, or wounds. Insect, animal, and human bites are also risk factors, as are skin ulcers.

Symptoms of cellulitis are fever, drowsiness, rash, and sweating. Skin in the infected area becomes red, hot, swollen, and painful. To diagnose cellulitis, the provider takes a health history and performs a physical examination to check the affected area. Diagnostic tests include blood tests and a fluid culture from the affected area.

Treatment for cellulitis is oral antibiotics, and the infected area must remain still and raised. If signs and symptoms are severe, then hospitalization may be necessary. Cellulitis usually goes away after taking antibiotics for 7 to 10 days, with longer treatment in more severe cases. If left untreated, cellulitis causes infections, inflammation of the heart, and shock.

People can prevent cellulitis by washing their hands frequently, cleaning small cuts, and keeping the skin moist to prevent cracking.

Methicillin-Resistant *Staphylococcus Aureus*

Some germs that live on the skin and in the nose are staph bacteria. Usually, staph bacteria do not cause problems, but sometimes they get inside the body through a skin lesion and cause an infection.

Staph infections are treated with antibiotics. However, when antibiotics do not kill the infection, it means that the bacteria are "resistant" to those antibiotics. That is, the antibiotics do not work against the infection. This type of resistant staph infection is *methicillin-resistant* Staphylococcus aureus *(MRSA)*.

MRSA was first identified in the 1960s and was found in hospitals and nursing homes. There are two main reasons why MRSA exists. First, antibiotics were given to patients when antibiotics were not needed. Second, patients were not taking antibiotics as directed. By the late 1990s, there was a new type of MRSA. This type, unlike the older type, is more common among children and adults who do not have medical problems.

There are different ways a person is infected with MRSA. One way is *healthcare-associated,* which means that the person got the infection in a health care setting (e.g., a hospital). Another way is *community-associated,* which means that the person got the infection in a community setting (e.g., a school). This infection spreads by skin-to-skin contact or by touching an object that has the bacteria on it. If one person in a family has MRSA, the rest of the family can get it.

MRSA causes infections in different parts of the body and can range from mild to severe to even life threatening. Most often, MRSA causes only a minor skin infection that has pimples and boils, but it can be life threatening if it reaches the bloodstream. Once MRSA enters the bloodstream, it can infect the bones, lungs, heart, and brain.

Anyone can get MRSA although it is more common in patients with a weak immune system and those in long-term health care settings. MRSA infections in these patients tend to be severe and in the bloodstream. Symptoms of severe MRSA infections are pneumonia and chest pain. MRSA can also infect healthy people, such as athletes, children in day care, prisoners, members of the military, and people with tattoos.

A MRSA infection is a red, swollen, and painful skin area with draining pus; it may look like a boil. These symptoms are more likely to occur if the skin has been cut or rubbed raw. Symptoms are also more likely in areas where there is more body hair.

The only way to tell the difference between MRSA and other staph infections is with lab tests. Lab tests can also help the provider decide which antibiotic should be used for treatment, if any.

Draining a skin infection and good skin care may be the only treatment needed for mild MRSA infection that has not spread. Severe MRSA infections, by contrast, are difficult to treat. The MRSA infections hardest to treat are those in the lungs or blood. MRSA infections are also difficult to treat in patients who already have a weakened immune system. MRSA-related pneumonia and blood infections are associated with high death rates.

The best way to prevent the spread of staph infection, including MRSA, is frequent hand washing. Other prevention steps are to keep cuts clean, cover cuts with a bandage until healed, and avoid sharing personal items. It is also important to contact a provider if a skin infection does not heal.

Tinea

Fungi can cause infection in humans. *Tinea,* or ringworm, are a group of fungi that cause skin, hair, and nail infections. As the fungus grows, it spreads out in a circle, leaving normal-looking skin in the middle. This makes it look like a ring, and at the edge of the ring, the skin is lifted and looks red and scaly. To some people, the infection looks as though a worm is under the skin, but a worm does not cause this infection.

Tinea infections spread by direct contact with an infected person or animal. Damp surfaces, doorknobs, clothing, bedding, and towels also spread the infection.

Symptoms usually appear between 4 and 14 days following exposure. Tinea can appear anywhere on the body, and these infections are named for the part of the body they infect:

- *Tinea corporis* (ringworm)—small, itchy red spots that grow into large rings almost anywhere on the arms, legs, or chest. Anyone who has skin contact with infected humans or domestic animals can get ringworm.

- *Tinea capitis* (scalp ringworm)—ringworm on the head. The hair is destroyed, leaving bald patches. It is contagious and often epidemic among school-age children.

- *Tinea cruris* (jock itch)—ringworm of the groin, skin folds, inner thighs, or buttocks. This rash is itchy and painful. It mostly occurs in men, especially if they wear athletic equipment.

- *Tinea pedis* (athlete's foot)—ringworm of the feet. It appears on the toes and the soles of the feet. The skin becomes itchy, red, blistered, and cracked. It can also spread to the hands and nails. Infected nails become discolored and thick, and crumble.

Sometimes people do not even know they have tinea and get better without any treatment; others have a serious infection that causes cellulitis. Other skin problems can look like tinea, but those need different treatments. To diagnose tinea, providers scrape a small amount of the irritated skin, hair, and nail onto a glass slide, then examine the slide under a microscope. A more precise test is to send a specimen of the patient's skin, hair, or nail to a lab to determine the type and cause of the tinea infection.

Treatment depends on the location of the tinea infection, but it usually involves antifungal medication. Tinea infections usually do not leave scars after the fungus is gone.

Tinea infections can affect anyone, but they occur more often among those with weakened immune systems. Ringworm is common in people who play sports and in those who have close contact with animals. Outbreaks of infections occur in schools, households, and institutional settings.

Good hygiene, such as keeping the skin clean and dry, is the best defense against tinea. People should avoid sharing personal items and check pets for signs of skin disease. Beauty salons and barbershops should disinfect instruments after each use. Making sure that shared exercise equipment (e.g., a treadmill) is clean before using is also important. Prevention steps are always necessary against tinea infection, and if people do not protect against tinea, they can get it again, even after treatment.

Fungal Nail Infection

Fungal nail infection occurs when a fungus grows in and around a fingernail or toenail. These infections occur mostly in adults, are more common in toenails than in fingernails, and often follow fungal infection of the feet.

People who frequent public swimming pools or gym shower rooms often have these infections, as do those who sweat a lot. Risk factors for fungal nail infection include having

- Manicures or pedicures with tools used on other people
- Moist skin for a long time
- Minor skin or nail injuries or a deformed nail
- Immune system problems

Symptoms are nail changes such as brittleness, change in nail shape, and thickness, as well as yellow streaks on the side of the nail. A provider can look at the nails to see if there is a fungal infection, and a diagnosis is confirmed by looking at nail scrapings under a microscope.

Fungal nail infections are hard to treat. Over-the-counter creams and ointments generally do not help, but laser treatments may work. Prescription antifungal medicines may also help, but only in about half the cases. In severe cases, the nail is removed. But even when treatment is effective, the fungus can return. The most promising way to get rid of fungal nail infections is with the growth of new, noninfected nails. Nails grow slowly, however, and it may take up to a year for a new nail to grow. Good hygiene—avoiding sharing manicure and pedicure tools, keeping skin clean and dry, and taking proper care of nails—helps prevent fungal infections.

Lice

Lice are wingless parasitic insects found on heads and bodies. They move by crawling; they cannot hop or fly. Lice spread mostly by close person-to-person contact. Dogs, cats, and other pets do not transmit human lice. There are three types of human lice, all of which live on human blood.

Head Lice

Head lice live close to the human scalp and are most common among children. Head lice are not dangerous and do not transmit disease, but they do spread easily. They can cause bacterial skin infections from too much scratching.

There are three stages in the life of head lice. *Nits,* or eggs, attach to the hair shaft and are yellow or white; they are often mistaken for dandruff, but cannot be brushed off. Baby lice are found on the scalp or in the hair. Adult lice are found behind the ears and near the neckline.

Transmission is through direct head-to-head contact with someone who already has head lice. Such contact occurs among children during school, at home, and on playgrounds. Sometimes lice are transmitted by contact with infested clothing, combs, brushes, or towels.

Anyone can get head lice, and it has nothing to do with cleanliness. There are an estimated 6 million to 12 million cases of head lice infestation each year in the United States among children 3 to 11 years of age (American Academy of Dermatology, 2016a). Some studies suggest that girls get head lice more often than boys. In the United States, head lice are much less common among African Americans than among persons of other races (American Academy of Dermatology, 2016a). The head lice found most often in the United States have claws that are better at grasping the shape and width of some types of hair than that of others.

The main sign and symptom of head lice is itchy sores on the scalp. In addition, sleep becomes difficult because lice are more active in the dark. People with head lice should see a provider as soon as possible. All household members and other close contacts also need to be checked. Treatment choices are over-the-counter and prescription medications, including shampoos. To stop the spread, family bedding, clothing, and towels need to be washed in hot water. Personal articles should be disinfected or thrown away.

Body Lice

Body lice are similar to head lice, but live and lay eggs on clothing. They move only to feed on the skin. Body lice spread by direct contact with a person who is infected with body lice. Body lice infestation can also spread by contact with articles—clothing, bedding, or towels—that have been in contact with an infected person. People of all races can become infected, but those who live in crowded places and lack access to good hygiene—for example, homeless people and survivors of natural disasters—are most susceptible. The lice spread fast and cause other diseases, such as bacterial infections.

Signs and symptoms are a rash and an itchy feeling. The itching leads to scratching, causing sores and bacterial skin infections. When someone has body lice for a long time, bitten areas of the skin can become thick and dark, especially in the midsection of the body.

A provider can diagnose body lice by finding eggs and crawling lice in the seams of clothing or feeding on the skin. Body lice are usually large enough to be seen with the naked eye.

Good hygiene and access to regular changes of clean clothes are the only treatment needed to get rid of body lice. Sometimes the infested person is also treated with medication that kills lice. If lice are on clothing, beds, or towels, these items need to be washed in hot water or destroyed.

Pubic Lice

Pubic lice, or crabs, live on the hair in the pubic area. They are also found on coarse hair elsewhere on the body—eyebrows, eyelashes, beard, or armpits. Crabs attach themselves to more than one hair and do not crawl as quickly as head and body lice.

Signs and symptoms of crabs include visible lice and itching in the genital area. A provider can diagnose crabs by finding one during a physical examination. Pubic lice are usually large enough to be seen with the naked eye. A patient who has crabs should be checked for other sexually transmitted infections.

Crabs spread through sexual contact, so all sex partners from within the previous month need to be informed of the risk for crabs and receive treatment. Patients should avoid sexual contact with their sex partners until they and their partners have been treated. Over-the-counter and prescription medications are available treatments.

Scabies

Scabies is a skin infestation with the human *mite.* The scabies mite has eight legs, is light brown in color, and is almost invisible to the naked eye. These mites dig into the skin, where they live and lay their eggs. A patient infected with scabies usually has at least 12 mites at any given time (American Academy of Dermatology, 2016d).

Scabies is passed from person to person through close skin-to-skin contact. Most adults who have scabies got it through sexual contact, but sometimes this infection can be passed on without sexual contact. What is interesting is that even though infected parents can pass scabies on to their child or vice versa because of close contact, it is unusual for schoolchildren to pass scabies to each other.

Scabies affects as many as 300 million people worldwide (American Academy of Dermatology, 2016d). People of all races and social classes can get scabies, but it spreads fast in crowded conditions (e.g., nursing homes and prisons). Child-care centers are also sites for scabies outbreaks.

Crusted scabies, or Norwegian scabies, is a severe form of scabies that infects people with a weak immune system, who are elderly, or who have a disability. Patients with crusted scabies have thick crusts of skin that contain large numbers of scabies mites. Crusted scabies is highly contagious and spreads fast through direct skin-to-skin contact as well as through contact with clothing, bedding, and furniture. Patients with crusted scabies may not show signs and symptoms of scabies but they need prompt medical attention to prevent future outbreaks.

The major sign and symptom of scabies are a rash and itching. The rash has tiny blisters and scales and can be difficult to see. The itching is worse at night, and scratching the rash causes infected skin sores. Much of the body or only certain parts (e.g., fingers, penis, waist, and buttocks) can be infected. Signs and symptoms can take as long as 3 to 4 weeks to appear, and an infected person can spread scabies during this time.

Diagnosis of scabies is based on the rash and itching and on the patient's health history. A provider confirms the diagnosis by scraping the top layers of skin and examining the sample under a microscope for mites. It is important to note that a patient can still have scabies even if mites are not found.

Prescription cream medications help get rid of scabies. Patients with crusted scabies need oral and cream prescription medications as part of their treatment. In some cases, family members and close contacts of a person with scabies need treatment to prevent future infections.

Bedsores

A *bedsore*, also called a pressure sore or pressure ulcer, is an area of the skin that breaks down. It breaks down because something keeps pressing against the skin and reduces blood flow. Bedsores are a deep-tissue injury, with red skin that gets worse over time. There can be blisters or open sores in the area; they eventually turn purple and can be painful and feel mushy. Bedsores often develop on the skin that covers bony areas, such as the hips, shoulders, and tailbone.

Patients are likely to get a bedsore if they are malnourished, use a wheelchair, or are bedridden. Those who cannot move parts of their body without help are also at risk for bedsores. Older adults are at most risk due to the aging process, which can cause limited mobility, urinary and bowel incontinence, and fragile skin. About three million people in the United States have bedsores.

A provider can see the size and depth of the bedsore by doing a physical examination. Bleeding or fluids in the sore indicate a severe infection, and the area around the sore can show spreading tissue damage or infection. The provider may also order blood tests to check for overall health and may take tissue cultures. Bedsores are categorized into stages, Stage 1 being the earliest stage and Stage 4 the worst.

Bedsores develop in a short time (2 to 6 hours) and are often difficult to treat (US National Library of Medicine, 2016b). The goals of treatment are cleansing, removing pressure from the affected area, and using special bandages. Sometimes surgery is necessary to close large sores.

Stage 1 and Stage 2 bedsores heal within several weeks to months if there is immediate and ongoing care of the wound. Stage 3 and Stage 4 bedsores are the most difficult to treat. The treatment goal for these bedsores is to reduce the pressure while the patient is bedridden, in a wheelchair, or unable to change body position. Pillows, foam cushions, and lotions can help reduce that pressure. If the patient is on bed rest or cannot move, a caregiver does a daily full-body examination of the patient and checks for blisters, sores, or craters.

If not treated, bedsores become a source of pain, disability, and infection. The following are some of the complications from bedsores:

- *Sepsis* can occur when bacteria enter the bloodstream via broken skin and spread throughout the body.

- Joint infections cause damage to cartilage and tissue.

- Cancer develops in chronic, nonhealing wounds.

Position changes of the body are key to preventing bedsores. These changes need to be made every 2 hours and need to avoid placing stress on the skin. Body positions in particular need to lessen pressure on vulnerable areas. Other steps include using pillows and foam that relieve pressure. Clean and dry skin, a healthy diet, no smoking, and daily exercise also prevent bedsores.

Skin Tumors

Skin tumors, or growths, are abnormal cells that grow together. People often think that a skin tumor means cancer, but most tumors are not cancerous. Tumors are usually classed as benign (non-cancerous) or malignant (cancerous). Benign growths, such as moles, are rarely a threat to life and do not invade surrounding tissues or spread to other parts of the body.

People can have many benign skin tumors. They are easily seen and are diagnosed by a physical examination and the patient's health history. To determine the type of tumor or if there is a possibility of skin cancer, then a skin biopsy becomes necessary. In a skin biopsy, all or part of the abnormal-looking growth is cut from the skin and viewed under a microscope by a pathologist to check for signs of cancer.

Benign tumors that show symptoms are usually managed with surgical removal. If the skin tumor is malignant, however, it can be *skin cancer* and may be life threatening. Skin cancer can be removed, but it sometimes grows back even larger than before. It also can invade nearby tissue and spread to other parts of the body.

To understand the common types of skin cancer, it helps to know about the different types of cells in the epidermis (see Figure 20.3). The epidermis is mostly made of *squamous cells.* Below these cells and deeper in the epidermis are *basal cells. Melanocytes* are cells scattered among the basal cells; they are the deepest in the epidermis. Melanocytes make the *pigment,* or color, found in skin. When skin is exposed to UV rays, melanocytes make more pigment and cause the skin to darken.

When skin cancer cells do spread, they break away from the original growth and enter blood or lymph vessels. Once in these vessels, the cancer cells can travel to other organs throughout the body. Skin cancers are named after the type of cells in the epidermis that become malignant. The following are three common types of skin cancer:

• *Melanoma* begins in melanocytes. Melanoma can develop on any skin surface and is more likely than other skin cancers to spread to different parts of the body. Melanoma is rare in people with dark skin.

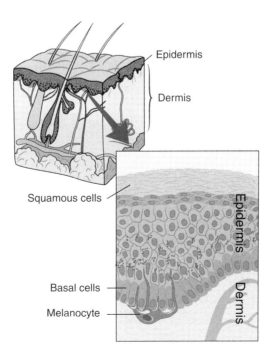

Figure 20.3 Epidermis Cells
Note. Adapted from the National Cancer Institute, Visuals Online. [Public domain]

- *Basal cell skin cancer* begins in basal cells. This cancer usually develops in places that have been in the sun, particularly for people with fair skin. It rarely spreads to other parts of the body.

- *Squamous cell skin cancer* begins in squamous cells. For those with dark skin, it is found in places that are not in the sun; for those with fair skin, it is found in places that have been in the sun. It sometimes spreads to other parts of the body.

One of every three cancers diagnosed in the United States will be skin cancer, for a total of more than 700,000 new cases per year. According to the National Cancer Institute (2016), melanoma alone causes one American to die almost every hour. The risk is greatest in the summer, because the sun's UV rays are the main cause of skin cancer. Fortunately, the most common types of skin cancer have a cure rate of more than 95% if they are detected and treated early. Even better, almost all skin cancers can be prevented simply by protecting the skin from UV rays.

Risk factors depend on the type of skin cancer; however, all of the skin cancers share some risk factors:

- Sunlight.

- Personal health history. Those who have had skin cancer in the past are at increased risk for other skin cancers.

- Skin that burns easily. Fair skin, blue or gray eyes, red or blond hair, or having many freckles increases the risk.

- Use of sunlamps and tanning booths.

- Family history of skin cancer.

- Certain diseases and medications. Diseases that cause the immune system to weaken and some medications make the skin more sensitive to sunlight.

The key symptom of skin cancers is a change on the skin. This change may be a new growth or a sore that does not heal. Cancer can also develop in an old growth.

Not all skin cancers share the same signs and symptoms. For example, the first sign of melanoma is a change in the shape, color, size, or feel of an existing mole. It can also appear as a new mole. Using the "ABCDE" of skin cancer helps identify signs and symptoms.

- *Asymmetry.* The shape of one half does not match that of the other half.

- *Border.* Edges are often jagged or uneven instead of smooth and even.

- *Color.* The mole is in mixed shades of tan, brown, or black instead of a single shade (often a single shade of brown).

- *Diameter.* There is an increase in size over time, and the mole usually becomes larger than the size of a pencil eraser.

- *Evolving.* When a mole starts to evolve or change in any way—in size, shape, color, elevation, or another trait—or any new symptom arises, such as bleeding, itching, or crusting, the patient needs medical attention.

Many melanomas show all of the ABCD signs; others show only one. With advanced melanoma, mole texture may change; that is, skin on the surface looks scraped and bleeds. It may also become hard, itchy, or painful.

To diagnose skin cancer, the provider takes a health history and conducts a physical examination. During the physical examination, the skin all over the body is checked for unusual growths. If the provider suspects that a skin spot is cancer, then the patient has a biopsy. If the biopsy shows skin cancer, the provider determines the stage of the disease by the size of the growth, how deep it has grown, and whether the cancer has spread. If the cancer has spread, blood tests and imaging tests are used in the diagnosis.

Treatment for skin cancer depends on the type, stage, size, and location of the tumor. It also depends on the general health and health history of the patient. In most cases, the goal of treatment is to remove the cancer completely. Sometimes all of the skin cancer can be removed in the early stage and then no more treatment is needed. Treatment for malignant melanoma is complicated, but surgery can be effective in the early stages. Sometimes, chemotherapy or radiation therapy may be a better treatment option.

The best way to prevent skin cancer is to protect against the sun by wearing sun-blocking clothing, sunglasses, and hats, and using sunscreen lotions with a sun protection factor (SPF) of at least 15. In addition, a person should regularly perform a full-body self-exam of the skin to check for any changes in moles and for sores that do not heal.

Chapter Summary

- The integumentary system has many functions, including protecting organs and tissues. It also helps excrete wastes and regulate temperature.

- Skin is a vital organ that covers the entire outside of the body, forming a protective barrier against germs and injuries from the environment.

- Aging affects the integumentary system's structure and function.

- Most diseases of the integumentary system are not life threatening. They can be mild and affect only how a person looks, or they may be severe enough to affect daily activities.

- In the United States, millions of people injure themselves every year. An injury is unintentional when it happens by accident; it can instead be intentional, when a person wanted to cause the injury.

- One of every three cancers diagnosed in the United States each year is skin cancer. The risk is greatest in the summer because UV rays from the sun are the main cause of skin cancer.

REVIEW QUESTIONS

1. What are the basic functions of the integumentary system?

2. What are the three layers of the skin?

3. How is skin color determined?

4. What is the difference between sebaceous glands and sweat glands?

5. A sunburn may cause redness, blisters, and pain. What degree of burn is it when there are blisters?

6. How does aging affect the integumentary system?

7. What are the ABCD warning signs of skin cancer?

8. What are the different types of tinea described in this chapter?

9. How are bedsores prevented?

10. What are the two main types of MRSA?

KEY TERMS

Acne: Disease of the skin's oil glands

Adipose tissue: Part of the subcutaneous layer that stores surplus energy as fat

Autografting: Use of the patient's own skin for a skin graft

Basal cells: Cells that lie below the squamous cells and are deeper in the epidermis

Basal cell skin cancer: Cancer that begins in the basal cell layer of the skin

Bedsore: Area of the skin that breaks down

Biopsy: Small piece of skin removed for examination under a microscope

Blackhead: Type of pimple that is on the skin's surface and looks black

Body lice: Type of lice that live and lay eggs on clothing, and move only to feed on the skin

Bruise: Mark on the skin caused by blood trapped under the surface

Burn: Injury that occurs when the skin is damaged by fire or other heat accidents

Cellulitis: Common skin infection caused by staph or strep bacteria

Collagen: Fibers found in the dermis that give skin its strength and flexibility

Contact dermatitis: Dermatitis caused by coming into direct contact with something that either irritates the skin or causes an allergic reaction

Contracture: Condition in which the skin and tissues are so burned that it is painful for the patient to move

Cradle cap: Seborrheic dermatitis in infants

Crusted scabies: Severe form of scabies

Cyanosis: Bluish skin tone

Dermatitis: General term that describes an inflammation of the skin

Dermatologist: Physician who specializes in treating the integumentary system

Dermatology: Branch of medicine that studies the integumentary system

Dermis: Middle layer of the skin

Eczema: Type of dermatitis with red, itchy rash

Elastin: Fibers found in the dermis that give skin its strength and flexibility

Epidermis: Top skin layer

First-degree burn: Superficial burn that affects only the epidermis

Fourth-degree burn: Burn that affects muscle and causes bone damage

Fungal nail infection: Infection that occurs when a fungus grows in and around a fingernail or toenail

Hair follicle: A tube-like structure where hair growth begins

Hair root: Part of the hair that grows up from the base to the surface of the skin

Hair shaft: Part of the hair that projects above the skin surface and is visible

Head lice: Type of lice that live close to the human scalp

Heterografting: Skin graft that uses skin formed from tissue grown from the patient's cells or from synthetic materials, or that uses skin from a donor

Hives: Raised red bumps on the skin that itch

Homeostasis: Stable equilibrium in the body

Impetigo: Common and contagious skin infection that starts when staph or strep bacteria get into a lesion

Integumentary system (IS): Body system made up of skin and its related organs—hair, nails, glands, and nerves

Intentional injury: Injury caused by a person who wanted to cause it

Jaundice: Yellow skin tone

Keratin: Protein made in the epidermis

Laser treatment: Procedure in which intense pulsed light is directed onto the skin

Lice: Parasitic insects that feed on human blood and are found on people's heads and bodies, including the pubic area

Light therapy: Exposing the skin to controlled amounts of artificial or natural light

Melanin: Skin pigment made in the epidermis

Melanocytes: Cells that are scattered among the basal cells and that are responsible for skin color

Melanoma: Cancer that begins in the melanocytes

Methicillin-resistant *Staphylococcus aureus* (MRSA): Antibiotics-resistant staph infection

Nits: Head lice eggs that attach to the hair shaft and are yellow or white

Pallor: Whiter, pale skin tone

Pigment: Color found in skin

Pimple: Lesion in which hair, sebum, and skin cells clump together into a plug, causing bacteria to swell the skin

Plaques: Raised red patches on the skin

Psoriasis: Autoimmune disease that causes raised, red, scaly patches on the skin

Pubic lice: Type of lice that live on the hair in the pubic area

Pustule: Type of pimple that is red at the bottom and has pus on top

Rashes: Temporary skin lesions that have many causes, including infections

Rosacea: Chronic inflammation of facial skin, causing red cheeks, nose, chin, or forehead

Scabies: Infestation of the skin by the human mite

Scabies mite: Small insect that digs into the skin, where it lives and lays its eggs

Scald: A burn caused by hot water or steam

Sebaceous glands: Skin glands that secrete oil to lubricate hair and skin and stop bacterial growth

Seborrheic dermatitis: Red rash with yellowish scales, usually on the scalp

Sebum: Oil secreted by the skin's sebaceous glands

Second-degree burn: Burn that affects the epidermis and some of the dermis

Sepsis: Serious infection that occurs when bacteria enter the bloodstream through broken skin and spread throughout the body

Skin cancer: Malignant skin tumor

Skin grafting: Procedure for repairing damage from severe burns, which involves taking healthy skin from another part of the body and replacing the burned skin

Skin lesions: Various types of changes to the skin, such scabs, blisters, bruises, and rashes

Skin patch: Medication patch placed on the skin

Skin pores: Tiny holes in the skin

Skin tumor: Group of abnormal cells that grow together

Squamous cells: Flat cells of the surface of the epidermis

Squamous cell skin cancer: Cancer that begins in the squamous cells

Subcutaneous layer: Bottom layer of the skin

Sweat glands: Glands in the skin that excrete sweat to help the body to cool off

Systemic medications: Prescription drugs that work throughout the body

Third-degree burn: Burn that affects all three layers of the skin

Tinea: Fungi that cause skin, hair, and nail infections

Tinea capitis: Type of tinea that causes itchy, red spots that are usually on the head

Tinea corporis: Type of tinea that causes small red spots that grow into rings almost anywhere on the arms, legs, or chest

Tinea cruris: Ringworm of the groin, skin folds, inner thighs, or buttocks

Tinea pedis: Ringworm of the feet, which appears on the toes and the soles of the feet

Unintentional injury: Injury that occurs by accident

Welts: Raised bumps on the skin

Whitehead: Type of pimple that stays under the surface of the skin

Wound: Injury that breaks the skin or other body tissues

CHAPTER ACTIVITIES

1. Find a partner to make a three-dimensional model of the skin. Use any materials you want, including paper, cloth, or plastic (creativity a plus). Once the model is completed correctly, research common myths related to maintaining healthy skin.

2. In small groups, discuss the pros and cons of getting a tattoo. Those who have had a tattoo might be willing to share their experiences with the rest of the class. As part of the discussion, identify tattoo safety precautions and talk about tattoo removal.

3. There is a head lice outbreak at the local elementary school. You're the school health educator and need to develop a head lice prevention campaign for students. What would be three or four prevention strategies for each of the target populations: students, teachers, administrators, and parents?

4. The US surgeon general has warned that tanning is a "major public health concern." Discuss the risks and benefits of tanning. How is indoor tanning that much more dangerous than natural light? Identify five ways to protect against UV rays.

5. Search the Web for images of a famous person who had cosmetic surgery (before and after) and then write a one- to two-page reflective paper on whether or not cosmetic surgery helped the famous person look younger, or just different. Be ready to debate the merits and consequences of cosmetic surgery.

Bibliography and Works Cited

American Academy of Dermatology. (2016a). Head lice: Overview. Retrieved from https://www.aad.org/public /diseases/contagious-skin-diseases/head-lice

American Academy of Dermatology. (2016b). Hives. Retrieved from https://www.aad.org/public/diseases/itchy -skin/hives

American Academy of Dermatology. (2016c). Impetigo. Retrieved from https://www.aad.org/public/diseases /contagious-skin-diseases/impetigo

American Academy of Dermatology. (2016d). Scabies. Retrieved from https://www.aad.org/public/diseases /contagious-skin-diseases/scabies

American College of Emergency Physicians. (2016). Emergencies A-Z: Burns. *EmergencyCareForYou.* Retrieved from http://www.emergencycareforyou.org/Emergency-101/Emergencies-A-Z/Burns/

Baddour, L. M. (2016). Patient education: Skin and soft tissue infection (cellulitis) (Beyond the basics). *UpToDate.* Retrieved from http://www.uptodate.com/contents/skin-and-soft-tissue-infection-cellulitis-beyond-the-basics ?view=print

Centers for Disease Control and Prevention. (2010). Scabies frequently asked questions (FAQs). Retrieved from http://www.cdc.gov/parasites/scabies/gen_info/faqs.html

Centers for Disease Control and Prevention. (2015). Ringworm. Retrieved from http://www.cdc.gov/fungal /diseases/ringworm/index.html

Centers for Disease Control and Prevention. (2016). Methicillin-resistant *Staphylococcus aureus* (MRSA). Retrieved from http://www.cdc.gov/mrsa/index.html

Mayo Clinic. (2016). Dermatitis. Retrieved from http://www.mayoclinic.org/diseases-conditions/dermatitis -eczema/basics/definition/con-20032183

National Cancer Institute. (2016). Skin cancer (including melanoma)—patient version. Retrieved from http:// www.cancer.gov/types/skin

National Institute of Arthritis and Musculoskeletal and Skin Diseases. (2014). What is acne? Retrieved from http://www.niams.nih.gov/Health_Info/Acne/acne_ff.asp

National Institute of General Medical Sciences. (2016). Burns fact sheet. Retrieved from https://www.nigms.nih .gov/Education/Pages/Factsheet_Burns.aspx

National Psoriasis Foundation. (2016). About psoriasis. Retrieved from https://www.psoriasis.org/about-psoriasis

National Rosacea Society. (2016). All about rosacea. Retrieved from http://www.rosacea.org/

Nemours Foundation. (2016). Skin, hair, and nails. *KidsHealth.* Retrieved from http://kidshealth.org/en/parents /skin-hair-nails.html

US National Library of Medicine. (2014). Fungal nail infection. *MedlinePlus.* Retrieved from https://www.nlm .nih.gov/medlineplus/ency/article/001330.htm

US National Library of Medicine. (2016a). Excema. *MedlinePlus.* Retrieved from https://medlineplus.gov /eczema.html

US National Library of Medicine. (2016b). Pressure sores: Also called: Bed sores, decubitus ulcers, pressure ulcers. *MedlinePlus.* Retrieved from https://medlineplus.gov/pressuresores.html

Wolters Kluwer. (2016). Patient education: Dermatitis (The basics). *UpToDate.* Retrieved from https://www. uptodate-com.ezproxy.springfield.edu/contents/dermatitis-the-basics

CHAPTER 21

THE BRAIN AND MENTAL HEALTH DISORDERS

CHAPTER OBJECTIVES

- Summarize differences between mental health and mental health disorders.
- Discuss three causes of mental health disorders.
- Give examples of mental health care providers.
- List and describe biological and mental health treatments.
- Explain signs and symptoms, etiology, and treatment of common mental health disorders.

The brain controls thoughts, memory, speech, and movement as well as regulates organ function. When the brain is healthy, it is capable of running complex body systems, but when it is unhealthy, mental health disorders can develop.

Most people don't realize how common mental health disorders are in the United States. They are so common that nearly all Americans at some time in their lives are affected by these disorders, whether in themselves, in a family member, or in a loved one.

Mental Health and Mental Health Disorders

Mental health and mental health disorders are different psychological states. *Mental health* includes emotional, psychological, and social well-being. It affects how we think, feel, and behave at every stage in our lives. It determines how we relate to others, make choices, and enjoy life.

A *mental health disorder* or mental illness refers to a brain disorder that alters a person's thinking, feelings, and behavior. With these disorders, there are changes in the brain's physiology and chemistry. There are different types of mental health disorders, and each changes a person in distinct ways.

People often are sad or angry during difficult times. A mental health disorder is different: such symptoms as sadness and anger are long lasting. In other words, a mental health disorder is characterized by ongoing and lasting signs and symptoms that affect a person's daily activities.

Differences between mental health and mental health disorder are not always clear. For example, if you are afraid of flying, does it mean you have a mental health disorder, or are you simply afraid? Part of the reason why making the distinction is difficult is that no one test shows that something is wrong. A mental health disorder diagnosis depends on specific signs and symptoms, and they need to involve three areas:

- *Thinking* that turns into *delusions,* or beliefs that do not change even when there is strong conflicting evidence
- *Feelings* of deep and ongoing sadness or anger
- *Behavior* that is out of the ordinary or not socially acceptable

Causes of Mental Health Disorders

What causes mental health disorders is not completely understood. There are disciplines that study brain biology and its relation to thoughts, feelings, and behaviors. These disciplines include psychiatry, psychology, and neuroscience. A multidisciplinary approach allows for a better understanding of the complex influences that biology and genetics, psychology, and the environment have on mental health disorders.

Some mental health disorders are partly due to chemistry issues that interfere with communication between the brain's nerve cells. Everything we do depends on the brain's nerve cells communicating with one another. When there is a communication gap between these nerve cells, then chemical changes occur in the brain that affect mental health.

Some mental disorders are caused by neurotransmitters in the brain. *Neurotransmitters* are chemicals that send messages between nerve cells. Mental health disorders occur when neurotransmitters and nerve cells are not working together, which means that messages can't reach the brain. The following are three main types of neurotransmitters:

- *Serotonin* controls such functions as mood, appetite, and sleep.
- *Dopamine* controls movement and helps the flow of information to the brain. It is linked to thoughts, emotions, and reward systems in the brain.
- *Glutamate* plays a role during early brain development and helps with learning and memory.

Other causes of mental health disorders go beyond just brain chemistry and can be genetic, biological, psychological, or environmental. These factors interact with each other and not only increase risk for developing a disorder but also can determine if it is mild or severe. Other factors include brain defects or a serious brain injury. A problem during early fetal brain development or at the time of birth can also cause certain disorders. Poor nutrition, exposure to toxins, or having a serious chronic disease like cancer can cause a disorder.

Common Signs and Symptoms of Mental Health Disorders

A diagnosis of a mental health disorder is based not just on signs and symptoms but also on how it affects daily activities. Most disorders rarely appear without warning, and it is often family, loved ones, or the person himself or herself who recognize that something is wrong. There are many signs and symptoms, and they vary depending on the disorder. The following are examples of signs and symptoms:

- Feeling sad or having suicidal thoughts
- Excessive fears, anger, or violence
- Low energy and problems sleeping
- *Hallucinations* (experiences of visual images, voices, or sounds that do not exist outside the mind)

- Inability to do daily activities

- Alcohol or drug abuse

- Strange behavior and beliefs

- Extreme mood swings

- Lack of personal hygiene

- Trouble relating to situations and to people

- Confused thoughts and speech

- Withdrawal from friends and activities

- Physical problems

- Increased sensitivity to sights, sounds, smells, or touch

- Extreme feelings of guilt

- Feeling isolated or alone

- Changes in eating habits

- Changes in sex drive

One or two symptoms does not predict a disorder. However, if a person has several together over time and they are causing major issues with daily activities, then a disorder may be developing. If this is the case, then the person should talk to a mental health care provider. If there are suicidal thoughts or attempts, or violent thoughts and behaviors, emergency medical care is needed. Untreated, signs and symptoms can progress to a psychotic episode. During a psychotic episode, the person appears to be out of touch with reality, develops delusions and hallucinations, and has confused thoughts and speech. A psychotic episode can start slowly, and, if left untreated, can last for extended periods of time.

Diagnosis and Treatment of Mental Health Disorders

A person must be evaluated by a mental health care provider to be diagnosed with a disorder (see Table 21.1). Family physicians, internists, and pediatricians are also qualified to diagnose common disorders, such as depression or anxiety disorders. In many cases, depending on the symptoms, a person may be referred to a psychiatrist. Psychiatrists are physicians with additional training in the field of mental health disorders. They evaluate patients' mental health along with their physical state, prescribe medications, and offer psychotherapy. In most states, only psychiatrists and other physicians can prescribe medications as treatment for mental health disorders.

Each mental health disorder has specific symptoms, and for a person to receive a diagnosis, a qualified mental health care provider must conduct a psychological evaluation. A *psychological evaluation* identifies several symptoms that the person shows; but, unfortunately, it does not lead to knowing the cause or the best treatment.

Mental health care providers gather information through an interview during which they ask the patient about symptoms, when they began, and how they affect daily activities. Often, providers will interview the patient's family members or loved ones to get more detailed information about symptoms.

The *Diagnostic and Statistical Manual of Mental Disorders (DSM)*, published by the American Psychiatric Association, also helps with the diagnosis. In the *DSM*, there is a general description and a list of symptoms of each disorder. Providers use the *DSM* to confirm that the patient's symptoms match those of a specific disorder.

Besides the psychological evaluation, a patient also has a physical examination and laboratory tests to determine if there is a health issue that is contributing to the symptoms.

Table 21.1   Examples of Mental Health Care Providers

Psychologist	These professionals specialize in psychology, a science that deals with the mind, mental processes, and behaviors. The term *psychologist* is used for those who have a doctoral degree, advanced training, and licensing and certification. Psychologists work in private practice, hospitals, and other health care settings. They cannot prescribe medications except in New Mexico and Louisiana.
Psychotherapist	*Psychotherapist* is a general term that can refer to psychologists, social workers, or others who provide psychotherapy. Some, however, have no formal training.
Social worker	Most social workers have a master's degree in social work (MSW). However, to provide mental health services, they must have advanced training and be licensed by their state. Licensed clinical social workers (LCSW) may provide psychotherapy in private practice, hospitals, and other health care settings.
Psychiatric nurse	These nurses are licensed registered nurse (RNs) with extra training in mental health. Under the supervision of physicians, they may offer mental health assessments and psychotherapy. Advanced practice registered nurses (APRNs) have at least a master's degree in mental health nursing. In general, they can diagnose and treat mental health disorders. In many states, they prescribe medications and can practice independently, without a physician's supervision.
Mental health counselor	Most mental health counselors have at least a master's degree, have several years of supervised work experience, and are licensed or certified. Licensure and certification require extra schooling, experience, and training. Counselors may work in private practice, hospitals, and other health care settings.
Marriage and family therapist	These therapists evaluate and treat disorders within the context of the family. They typically have a master's or doctoral degree. After additional experience under supervision, they take an exam to become licensed or certified.
Pastoral counselor	These are trained mental health care providers who also have religious training. They provide therapy in a spiritual context. Certification and licensing varies. They may work in pastoral counseling centers or other community settings.
Psychoanalyst	Psychoanalysis refers to specific treatment, developed by Sigmund Freud, that explores the unconscious. Anyone can be called a psychoanalyst, because it is not a legal term. However, many psychoanalysts have extensive training and are usually physicians, psychologists, or social workers.

After the patient's health is determined and the disorder diagnosed, the provider develops a treatment plan. Most disorders cannot be cured, and damage done may be permanent, but treatment can lessen symptoms.

Working together, patient and provider together decide on the best treatment options. Treatment options depend on symptoms, personal choices, medication side effects, and other factors. In some cases, a disorder can be so severe that a patient cannot make treatment decisions. If this is the case, the provider, family members, or loved ones may guide the treatment until the patient is able to make decisions.

Treatment options include either biological treatments (e.g., medication) or mental health treatment (e.g., psychotherapy). Biological and mental health treatments affect the disorder in different ways. For those with a more serious disorder, a combination of treatments is the most effective.

Medications for mental health disorders can be taken for a few days, a few years, or a lifetime, depending on the disorder. If a patient has been prescribed medications, the provider continually monitors the patient's health for side effects. If there are side effects, then the provider changes the dose or switches to a different medication. The best medications depend on patients' particular diagnosis, their situation, and how their body responds. Although medications do not cure a disorder, they can relieve symptoms and can also help make other treatments more effective.

One of the most widely used medications is *antidepressants.* Antidepressants are the third most frequently taken medication of any kind in the United States, and it is estimated that up to 10% of the population takes antidepressants to relieve symptoms (National Institute of Mental Health, 2016b). *Antianxiety medications* help reduce the symptoms of anxiety or panic attacks. They may also help reduce *insomnia,* or the inability to sleep. *Mood-stabilizing medications* treat and prevent the highs and lows of bipolar disorder. *Antipsychotic medications* treat psychotic disorders, such as schizophrenia. They can also treat clinical depression and the highs of bipolar disorder. Unfortunately, antipsychotics do not always make the symptoms go away completely, or forever. To stop symptoms from coming back, many patients need to take antipsychotic medication for the long term even if they feel better.

Patients with a disorder sometimes do not want to take their medications; among other reasons, they may not like the side effects, or they may be in denial about their illness. The failure of patients with severe disorders to take medications is a serious and common problem with psychiatric care. It often leads to relapse of symptoms, rehospitalizations, homelessness, incarceration, victimization, or episodes of violence.

Psychotherapy is often used along with medication. *Psychotherapy* is a general term used to describe treatment based on patients talking about their personal issues with a therapist. During psychotherapy, patients learn about their moods, feelings, thoughts, and behavior. With the knowledge gained, patients then learn coping skills to deal with their disorder. The aim of therapy is to understand and express feelings, help change negative attitudes and behavior, and promote healthy ways of coping. As mentioned earlier, for many disorders, medication (to relieve symptoms) and psychotherapy (to help patients cope) are used together.

There are different types of psychotherapy, including short term, long term, individual, and group. It can take place one-on-one, in a group, or with family members. Each type of psychotherapy has its own approach to improving mental health. It can often be successfully completed in a few months, but in some cases, long-term treatment is needed.

Brain stimulation therapies involve touching the brain directly with electricity, magnets, or implants to treat depression and other disorders. *Electroconvulsive therapy (ECT)* has the longest history of use as brain stimulation therapy. ECT, or shock therapy, is generally used for situations in which medications and psychotherapy haven't worked. The patient is given an electric charge that is applied to the brain, causing a small seizure. In its early days, ECT was painful and resulted in short- and long-term memory loss. Today, ECT is much less painful and has been effective in treating clinical depression and bipolar disorder.

Self-help groups are run by patients of the mental health care system or their families. These groups offer the chance to meet informally with other people who understand the same issues and challenges of dealing with a specific disorder. Self-help groups reduce a sense of isolation and provide opportunities to learn from others' experiences.

Sometimes a disorder is so severe that a patient needs care in a psychiatric hospital or a residential treatment program. These health care settings are recommended when patients cannot care for themselves or when they are in immediate danger of harming themselves or others. Options include 24-hour inpatient care or residential treatment. These settings offer a temporary supportive place to live. There are intensive outpatient treatment programs that offer ongoing mental health supervision, but the patient lives elsewhere.

Most Americans with a disorder who receive treatment do recover and lead productive lives. It is unfortunate, however, that up to half of all people with disorders, and 90% of those who have a substance use disorder, do not get the treatment they need. Most disorders do not improve on their own; in fact, if left untreated, they may get worse over time and cause long-lasting problems. Shame, fear, denial, and lack of services often prevent people from seeking help. But early treatment does make a difference and can lessen symptoms.

Common Mental Health Disorders

Having a mental health disorder at some time in your life is not that unusual. It is a myth that disorders are things that happen only to people whose lives are very different from yours (see Figure 21.1). In fact, disorders are common in the United States: about one in four people develops a disorder during his or

Myth	Mental health disorders are rare and only affect certain types of people.

- **Fact:** Mental disorders are common:

  One in 10 young people experienced a period of clinical depression

  One in 20 Americans lived with a serious disorder, such as schizophrenia or major depression

Myth	People with mental health disorders are violent.

- **Fact:** The majority of people with mental health disorders are no more likely to be violent than anyone else. Most people with mental disorders are not violent. In fact, people with severe disorders are over 10 times more likely to be victims of violent crime than the general population.

Myth	People with mental health disorders cannot handle the stress of having a job.

- **Fact:** People with mental health disorders are just as productive as other employees. Employers who hire people with disorders report good attendance as well as motivation, good work, and job tenure the same as or greater than other employees.

Myth	Character weakness causes mental health disorders and people can snap out of it if they try hard enough.

- **Fact:** Mental health disorders have nothing to do with being weak and most people need help to get better. Many factors contribute to mental health disorders, including biological, psychological, and environmental.

Myth	Therapy is a waste of time. Why bother when you can just take a pill?

- **Fact:** Treatment for mental health disorders depends on the individual and can include medication, therapy, or both.

Myth	I can't do anything for a person with a mental disorder.

- **Fact:** Family and loved ones can make a difference. Only 38% of adults with a mental health disorder and less than 20% of children and adolescents receive needed treatment. Family and loved ones can be important influences to help someone get the treatment and services they need.

Figure 21.1 Myths and Facts About Mental Health Disorders

Note. Adapted from "Dispelling Myths on Mental Illness," by the National Alliance on Mental Illness, 2015. Retrieved from http://www.nami.org/Blogs/NAMI-Blog/July-2015/Dispelling-Myths-on-Mental-Illness

her lifetime. And one in four families has at least one member who is currently suffering from a disorder (National Alliance on Mental Illness, 2016c). National data show that disorders are so common that even if you have not had a disorder, you probably know someone with one and do not even realize it. This is because many people with a disorder are active and productive members of our communities.

US statistics on mental health disorders show how widespread this health problem is (see Figure 21.2). According to the Substance Abuse and Mental Health Services Administration (SAMHSA, 2015), these disorders are the leading cause of disability among people ages 15 to 44. And about 26% of adult Americans have a mental health disorder in any given year. Even more alarming, half of all people who have a disorder probably suffer from another one at the same time.

The onset of disorders is almost entirely before the age of 25, with about 12 million children under the age of 18 having disorders in the United States. Half of all disorders show first signs before a person turns 14 years old. The National Alliance of Mental Illness (2016c) states that one in five young people

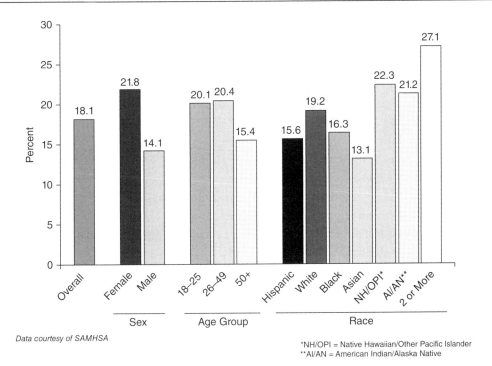

Figure 21.2 Prevalence of Any Mental Illness Among US Adults (2014)

Note. From Substance Abuse and Mental Health Services Administration, 2015

has a mental disorder at any given time, but less than 20% of these young people get the treatment they need.

There are seven general areas of mental health disorders discussed in this chapter:

1. *Neurodevelopmental disorders* occur because of a problem with the growth and development of the brain or central nervous system.

2. *Anxiety disorders* cause stress, but a person can still think rationally and function socially.

3. *Mood disorders* are characterized by emotional states that are outside the bounds of normal ups and downs of happiness and sadness.

4. *Substance use disorder* occurs when a person needs alcohol or other drugs to function normally. Stopping the substance use causes withdrawal symptoms.

5. *Psychotic disorders* are characterized by a loss of contact with reality; patients experience delusions, paranoia, or hallucinations.

6. *Personality disorders* cause emotional instability and unhealthy behavior.

7. *Eating disorders* are characterized by behaviors that involve an obsession with food, weight, and appearance.

These seven areas of mental disorders have one thing in common: they lead to harmful behaviors that are seen to be unusual and disturbing.

Neurodevelopmental Disorders

Neurodevelopmental disorders start in childhood and are most likely due to abnormal brain and nervous system development. The abnormal development causes problems with cognition, learning, communication, and behavior. There are many different types of neurodevelopmental disorders. This chapter's discussion is limited to attention deficit hyperactivity disorder and autism spectrum disorder.

Attention deficit hyperactivity disorder (ADHD) is one of the most common mental health disorders of childhood. According to the American Psychiatric Association (2015a), 10% of US children ages 5–17 years were diagnosed with ADHD or ADD. (Both terms refer to the same disorder.) The disorder is usually first diagnosed in childhood and often lasts into adulthood. In recent years, there has been popular concern and debate in regard to the increasing number of children being diagnosed with ADHD. Although the number of children diagnosed with ADHD is increasing, it remains unclear as to why.

Children, teens, and adults of all backgrounds can have ADHD. Boys are four times more at risk than girls. It is unclear what causes ADHD, although genes may play a role. Like many other disorders, ADHD may be a result of a combination of factors in addition to genetics, such as low birth weight, brain injuries, exposure to toxins, and childhood trauma.

Symptoms of ADHD can appear in some children as early as 2 or 3 years of age. These symptoms include difficulty paying attention and controlling behavior, and being overactive, or hyperactive. It is normal for all children to have these behaviors sometimes. But for children with ADHD, the behaviors are more severe and occur often.

To receive a diagnosis of ADHD, a child must have symptoms for 6 months or longer and to a degree that is greater than other children of the same age. These children struggle with paying attention and focusing on one thing; they forget things and switch from one activity to another. They seem not to listen when spoken to and find it difficult to follow instructions. Those with difficulty controlling behavior act or speak without regard for consequences. They can talk nonstop and are always in motion. Those with ADHD also struggle with low self-esteem, troubled relationships, and poor performance in school. Symptoms sometimes lessen with age. However, some people never completely outgrow their ADHD symptoms.

Many other disorders (e.g., anxiety and depression) have symptoms similar to those of ADHD. To complicate matters further, there is no single test to diagnose ADHD; several steps are required. One step is a physical examination, including hearing and vision tests. The examination rules out other health problems. Another step is for parents, teachers, and others who know the child to fill out a checklist for rating ADHD symptoms. The final step is to take a health history of the child from parents, teachers, and sometimes the child. Adults with ADHD are evaluated by a licensed mental health care provider. Part of this evaluation includes having the patient take an adult ADHD test. For a diagnosis, an adult must have ADHD symptoms that began in childhood and continued throughout adulthood.

Although treatment does not cure ADHD, it does reduce symptoms and improves functioning. Treatment includes medication, therapy, or a combination of both. An often used medication for treating ADHD is a stimulant. Although it may seem strange to treat ADHD with a stimulant, it does have a calming effect on those with ADHD and improves the ability to focus, work, and learn. Medication also improves physical coordination. As for psychotherapy, *behavioral therapy* is most often used. This therapy helps patients control their behavior. Treatment plans include close monitoring, follow-ups, and any needed adjustments, but no single treatment is the answer for every patient. The good news is that with treatment, most ADHD patients can lead productive lives.

Autism spectrum disorder (ASD) begins early in life and affects the structure and function of the brain and nervous system, causing behaviors that often result in social, behavior, and communication problems. Autism is referred to as a "spectrum" disorder because people with ASD experience a range of symptoms with differing degrees of severity. ASD affects how a person acts and interacts, how he communicates, and how he learns. For example, people with ASD have problems talking to others and avoid eye contact; they may repeat behaviors, or they may say the same sentence again and again. Some ASD patients are mildly impaired by their symptoms; others have a severe disability and need help with daily activities.

Symptoms of ASD begin as early as age 2 and usually last throughout a lifetime. ASD is present in all ethnic, race, and socioeconomic groups. The Eunice Kennedy Shriver National Institute of Child

Health and Development (2016) estimates that 1 out of 68 children in the United States has been identified as having ASD, with males 4.5 times more likely to have ASD than females. The causes are not known, but both genetics and environment probably play a role. Some people have expressed concern that ASD might be linked to the vaccines children receive, but studies have shown that there is no link between receiving vaccines and developing ASD.

ASD is an umbrella term for several disorders, the two most common being autistic disorder and Asperger syndrome. *Autistic disorder, or autism*, is the most severe form of ASD, the key symptom being impaired social interaction. In infancy, a baby with autism can be unresponsive to people or focus only on one thing for long periods of time. Children with autism may fail to respond to their names and often avoid eye contact. They have difficulty understanding what others are thinking or feeling. Autistic children do not understand social cues, such as tone of voice, eye contact, and facial expressions.

Some autistic children engage in repeated movements such as rocking and twirling. They may do self-abusive behaviors, such as biting or head-banging. These children also tend to start speaking later than other children and may refer to themselves by their name instead of "I" or "me." They often do not know how to play with other children. For many children, symptoms of autism do improve with treatment and with age.

Adolescents with autism may become depressed or experience behavior problems. Their treatment may need changes as they age, and they usually need services into adulthood. However, many are able to work and live independently within a supportive environment.

Asperger syndrome (AS) is a high-functioning form of autism. Those with AS have difficulty establishing and maintaining social relationships. They are likely to engage in repetitive actions and have limited interests and activities. The main difference between autism and AS is that children with AS do not have speech or cognitive delays. Other differences are that children with AS:

* Acquire language at a normal or even faster than normal rate in infancy and childhood
* Are rigid in their thinking
* May do well at visual tasks like drawing but have difficulty with written work
* Are often clumsy

There are two steps to an ASD diagnosis. The first step is a developmental screening with a provider who conducts a physical examination and testing. Children who show some developmental problems need a follow-up evaluation. The second step is an evaluation by a team of mental health care providers including child psychologists.

There is growing concern about labeling a young child with ASD. However, the sooner intervention begins, the better the outcome. Early intervention such as educational and behavioral services do prevent more severe disabilities associated with ASD and can improve the child's IQ, language, and everyday skills. There is no cure for ASD, and it can last a lifetime. However, treating it early, using school-based programs, and getting proper health care can increase the child's ability to improve and learn new skills.

Anxiety Disorders

Everybody knows what it is like to feel anxious. Fear and anxiety are a normal response to stress, and they can be helpful in some situations because they motivate a person to act and solve problems. However, people who feel too much anxiety, or feel it too often, experience an opposite effect: Their lives are restricted, and they are unable to solve problems. People with an *anxiety disorder* have fears that are not based on fact and that make them feel anxious most of the time without any reason, or their anxiety stops them from doing daily activities and gets worse over time. Sometimes the anxiety arises only once in a while, but is so intense that it can't be controlled.

Anxiety disorders are the most common mental health disorders and affect more than one in five American adults each year (Anxiety and Depression Association of America, (2014). More women than men have anxiety disorders, and they can affect children and teens with symptoms starting around age 6 (National Institute of Mental Health, 2016d). Anxiety disorders cannot be prevented, but they are treatable; unfortunately, two thirds of patients with this disorder never receive treatment (National Institute of Mental Health, 2016d).

Anxiety disorders last for at least 6 months and get worse if not treated. The cause is not known, but there are risk factors including genetics, brain chemistry, personality, and life events. Anxiety disorders often coexist with other disorders. Sometimes these other disorders, such as depression, often need treatment first before a person is treated for anxiety.

There are different types of anxiety disorders, and each has specific symptoms, but they all share excessive, irrational fear. The following anxiety disorders are discussed in this chapter:

- Generalized anxiety disorder
- Obsessive-compulsive disorder
- Panic disorder and phobias
- Posttraumatic stress disorder

Generalized Anxiety Disorder

We all worry about things like health or personal problems, but those with *generalized anxiety disorder (GAD)* have excessive and unrealistic worry. For example, a person with GAD thinks things will always go wrong. At times, this anxiety is so intense that it keeps people from engaging in daily activities. GAD starts slowly and can begin at any age, though the risk is highest between childhood and middle age. It affects 3% of the US population, and women are twice as likely to have GAD as men (Office of Women's Health, 2015).

It is diagnosed when a person worries excessively about a variety of everyday problems for at least 6 months. Symptoms may get better or worse at different times, and often are worse during times of stress. A person with GAD has trouble relaxing and sleeping, and is irritable. GAD can cause headaches, pain, and twitching. When the anxiety level is mild, those with GAD can function socially and can work; but when it is more severe, many have difficulty carrying out the simplest tasks. Other disorders (e.g., depression) are often diagnosed along with GAD.

GAD sometimes runs in families, but it is uncertain why some people have it while others do not. Stress and environmental factors may also cause GAD. This disorder is usually treated with psychotherapy or with antianxiety medications and antidepressants. *Cognitive behavioral therapy (CBT)*, a type of psychotherapy, is helpful in treating GAD because it teaches people different ways of thinking, behaving, and reacting to situations and helps them feel less anxious.

Obsessive-Compulsive Disorder

Obsessive-compulsive disorder (OCD) causes a person to have repeated, unwanted thoughts or behaviors that seem impossible to control. OCD causes anxiety and gets in the way of doing daily activities. The frequent, repeated unwanted thoughts become *obsessions*. To try to control obsessions, people with OCD repeat certain behaviors; these repeated behaviors are called *compulsions*.

OCD starts during childhood or adolescence for many patients, with most being diagnosed by about age 19. It sometimes runs in families, but it is unknown why some people have it while others don't. About two million people, or 2% of the US population, has OCD; 50% of these cases are severe (National Institute of Mental Health, 2016d). OCD patients often have other mental disorders, such as depression.

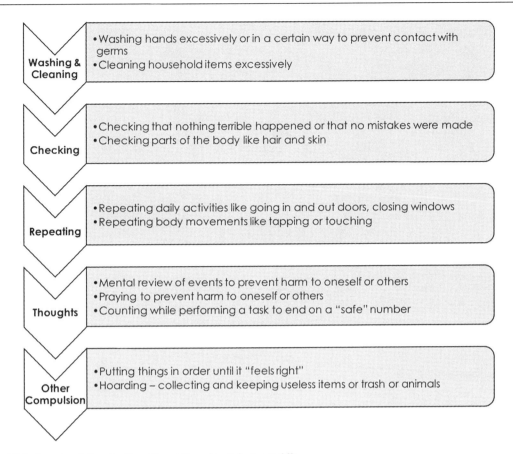

Figure 21.3 Examples of Obsessive Thoughts and Compulsive Behaviors in OCD

Signs and symptoms can come and go and be better or worse at different times. (See Figure 21.3 for examples of obsessive thoughts and compulsions.) Patients with OCD:

- Have repeated thoughts about different things, such as fear of germs. They can be obsessed with certain behaviors, such as violence or sexual acts.

- Repeat the same behaviors over and over, such as counting objects and checking locks. They often keep useless items, which is known as *hoarding*.

A patient needs to spend at least 1 hour a day on obsessive thoughts and compulsive behaviors to receive a diagnosis of OCD. The thoughts and behaviors cause anxiety and get in the way of daily activities. Patient with OCD do not get pleasure from the obsessions and compulsions, but they do get some relief from the related anxiety. This disorder then creates a cycle of obsessions and compulsions based on relieving anxiety (see Figure 21.4).

Several parts of the brain are involved in OCD, so it is treated with more than one approach, including psychotherapy, medication, or both. Cognitive behavioral therapy (CBT) is useful for treating OCD because it helps OCD patients manage obsessive thoughts and compulsive behaviors to feel less anxious. Some patients with OCD do better with CBT; others do better with antidepressants or a combination of both. OCD is treatable, but it often coexists with depression and other anxiety disorders, which can complicate treatment. Most patients who seek treatment do experience improvement. Unfortunately, if not treated properly, OCD can be disabling.

Panic Disorder and Phobias

A *panic disorder* causes *anxiety attacks,* which are sudden and repeated attacks of fear that last for several minutes or longer. The person experiences a fear of disaster or of losing control even when

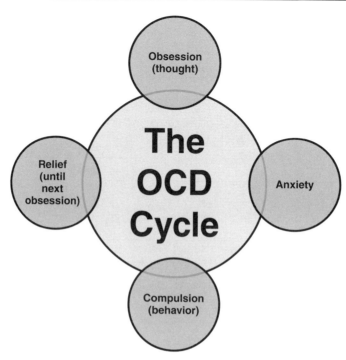

Figure 21.4 The OCD Cycle

there is no real danger, and may have a strong physical reaction during these attacks. The attacks happen anytime and anywhere and can be so intense that many people have anxiety over future attacks.

Anxiety attacks create feelings of intense fear that reach a peak within minutes. An attack can cause chest pain, sweating, shaking, shortness of breath, or even fear of death. People can think that they are having a heart attack or stroke, losing their mind, losing control, or dying. Although most attacks average a couple of minutes, they sometimes last as long as 10 minutes.

About six million American adults have panic disorder in a given year (National Institute of Mental Health, 2016d). Usually developing around age 24, panic disorder is twice as likely to affect women as men. The disorder often coexists with other mental and physical disorders, including depression and asthma.

New places, crowds of people, or flying may make us a bit anxious or even frightened. We might try to avoid these situations, but most of us can control our everyday anxiety. Those with *specific phobias*, however, feel that they must avoid certain situations or objects even though they know there is no danger. Having phobias disrupts daily routines, limits work, and strains relationships. Their onset is usually sudden, and they may occur in situations that did not cause any phobia in the past. The following list contrasts examples of everyday anxiety with those of specific phobias:

Everyday Anxiety	Specific Phobia
Feeling dizzy when climbing a tall ladder	Refusing to go to your best friend's wedding because the reception is being held on the 13th floor of a hotel
Worrying about taking off in an airplane during a snowstorm	Avoiding a family vacation because it requires air travel
Feeling nervous around your neighbor's pit bull	Avoiding leaving your house for fear of seeing a dog

Specific phobias focus on animals, insects, germs, heights, public places, and flying, to name a few. The most common phobia is fear of animals and reptiles (e.g., snakes). Other phobias are *claustrophobia* (fear of closed spaces) and *acrophobia* (fear of heights).

Some people stop going to places where they had a panic attack, in fear of it happening again. These people have *agoraphobia* and avoid public places where they feel that they can't escape when they suffer severe panic. About one in three people with panic disorder has agoraphobia (Anxiety and Depression Association of America, 2016). These people's world becomes smaller and smaller as they try to prevent the next panic attack. Agoraphobia can make it so that some people cannot leave their home or go places.

Some people have *social phobia*, in that they fear and avoid interpersonal interactions. A person with social phobia fears being watched or humiliated while doing a daily activity in front of others. This makes it difficult for them to go to work or to socialize. The most common social phobia is the fear of speaking in public. Social phobias usually develop after puberty and can be lifelong if left untreated.

Those suffering from panic attacks or specific phobias often don't know they have a treatable disorder. Although treatment is different for each person, several approaches have proved effective for most patients, including psychotherapy, medication, or a combination of both. Treatment can take a few months or more depending on the person and the phobia, and can be more complicated if the person suffers from other disorders, such as clinical depression.

Posttraumatic Stress Disorder

When someone experiences a traumatic event, a healthy response is an intense emotional reaction. Those with *posttraumatic stress disorder (PTSD)*, however, have an intense emotional reaction long after a traumatic event. A *traumatic event* is a terrifying and life-threatening experience. These events include combat, violence, or a car crash where there was a possibility of serious bodily harm. Car crashes are the leading cause of PTSD (Wolters Kluwer, 2016c). Although PTSD is often linked to veterans, it can affect anyone who has experienced a traumatic event, including children. It is not known why certain events cause PTSD in some people but not in others. Genes, emotions, family setting, and past emotional trauma may all influence a PTSD response.

The body has a normal physical response to a traumatic event in that it releases stress hormones and chemicals. After a traumatic event, the body stops the physical response, and stress hormones and chemicals return to normal levels. For those with PTSD, however, the body keeps releasing stress hormones and chemicals long after the traumatic event.

PTSD symptoms start soon after the traumatic event or not appear until months or years later. Symptoms also can come and go over many years. If the symptoms last longer than a month and interfere with daily activities, then it could be PTSD. Whether or not someone gets PTSD depends on many things, such as how bad the traumatic event was, whether there was an injury, or whether there was a death of a family member.

About 5.2 million adults in the United States are diagnosed with PTSD in a given year, but less than 50% receive treatment (Wolters Kluwer, 2016c). About 10% of women develop PTSD in their lives, compared to 5% of men. The signs and symptoms of PTSD differ from person to person, but there are four general types of symptoms:

1. *Reexperiencing*—having thoughts, dreams, and feelings as though the event is happening again

2. *Avoidance*—avoiding places, people, or activities that are reminders of the event

3. *Negative thoughts and feelings*—experiencing, for example, anger outbursts that are often unpredictable and irrational

4. *Hyperarousal*—being startled easily and on the lookout for danger

As mentioned earlier, a diagnosis can be made if symptoms of PTSD last for more than a month. The provider may also do a mental health exam, a physical examination, and blood tests to look for other health problems, such as depression, that may influence PTSD signs and symptoms. In many cases, treatments for PTSD lessen other health problems because they are often related.

The two main types of PTSD treatment are psychotherapy and medication, and they may be combined. Antidepressant medications are generally used to help control anger and sadness. How long PTSD lasts depends on patients' ability to follow their treatment plan and overcome their experience. Treatment can last for 6 to 12 weeks and sometimes longer.

Mood Disorders

Mood disorders are characterized by constant and extreme changes in emotions caused by biochemical imbalances in the brain. Mood disorders affect about 7% or 19.3 million US adults and rank among the top 10 causes of disability (Depression and Bipolar Support Alliance, 2016a). Children and adolescents can also have mood disorders. The two mood disorders discussed in this chapter are clinical or major depression and bipolar disorder.

Clinical Depression

A person has *clinical depression* when he or she has depressed moods for no obvious reason and, in severe cases, has suicidal thoughts.

Although it is normal for people to feel sad sometimes during their lives, those with clinical depression have specific symptoms daily for 2 weeks or more. Clinical depression is marked by long-lasting changes in mood, thought, and behavior. These symptoms make it difficult to perform daily activities, cause the loss of pleasure, complicate other health problems, and can lead to suicide. The following list contrasts sadness and clinical depression:

Sadness	Clinical Depression
Normal reaction to life events	Illness
Affects only mood	Affects mood, thoughts, and bodily functions
Temporary signs and symptoms	Persistent signs and symptoms
Usually no suicidal thoughts	Can result in suicide
Requires a good listener or psychotherapy and time to heal or grieve	Requires medical treatment and psychotherapy

Clinical depression is not a sign of weakness but rather an imbalance in brain chemicals. The following are signs and symptoms of clinical depression:

- Long periods of sadness with aches and pains
- Alcohol or other drug abuse
- Inability to concentrate
- Feelings of guilt or hopelessness
- Changes in appetite and sleep patterns
- Irritability, anger, or anxiety
- Lack of energy and interest
- Suicidal thoughts

There is no single cause for clinical depression, but genetics, environment, diseases, brain chemistry, and trauma can play a role. Patients of all ages, races, ethnic groups, and social classes have clinical depression. Although it can occur at any age, clinical depression usually develops between the ages of 25 and 44 and more often in women than in men (Depression and Bipolar Support Alliance, 2016b).

For some patients, clinical depression is intense and occurs in episodes that last for weeks at a time. For others, it takes the form of *dysthymia*, a form of clinical depression that is less severe but lasts at low levels for years.

There is no cure for clinical depression, but of all the mental health disorders, it is one of the most treatable. With proper treatment, about 80% of patients have significant improvement. Treatment for clinical depression can include medication, psychotherapy, or a combination of both. Unfortunately, though treatment is usually successful, less than half of those with this disorder get the services they need (Depression and Bipolar Support Alliance, 2016b).

Antidepressant medications are prescribed for clinical depression, but trying several types may be necessary to see improvement and avoid side effects. For mild to moderate clinical depression, psychotherapy can sometimes be effective without medication. Psychotherapy alone, however, may not benefit those who are severely depressed. A provider may recommend hospitalization for severe clinical depression if side effects from medication leave a patient unable to do daily activities. In addition, if the patient is violent to self or to others or has attempted suicide, then treatment requires a safe environment.

Bipolar Disorder

The symptoms of bipolar disorder are different from the normal ups and downs that everyone goes through. *Bipolar disorder*, or manic depression, is characterized by a cycle of depression (low) followed by a normal mood and then mania (highs). The symptoms are extreme changes in mood, thought, energy, and behavior. The changes in mood, or mood swings, can last hours, days, weeks, or even months. Every experience of a mood swing is called an *episode*. For example, the overexcited state is a *manic episode*, when a person is hyperactive and in a happy state. Manic individuals feel important and have increased energy. These episodes also cause nonstop talking and an increase in risky behaviors.

There are different types of bipolar disorder, and each is identified by the degree of depression or mania. Most patients with bipolar disorder experience moods with "high" and "low" swings. The swings can be severe, ranging from extreme energy to despair. The severity of the mood swings and the way they affect daily activities distinguish bipolar mood episodes from clinical depression. The following list describes the symptoms of bipolar disorder:

Highs of Bipolar Disorder	Lows of Bipolar Disorder
Overly happy and self-confident	Long periods of sadness
Anger and aggressive behavior	Changes in appetite and sleep patterns
Decreased need for sleep	Anger, worry, anxiety
Grandiose thoughts, inflated sense of self-importance	Negative attitude and social withdrawal
Fast-paced speech and racing thoughts	Loss of energy, health problems
Impulsive behavior, poor judgment, easily distracted	Feelings of guilt and worthlessness
Reckless behavior	Inability to make decisions
Delusions and hallucinations	Thoughts of suicide

Mixed mania is characterized by both a manic and a depressive episode at the same time. Those who have had mixed mania often describe it as the worst part of bipolar disorder.

Nearly six million adult Americans have bipolar disorder, and most cases are severe (Mental Health America, 2016a). It usually begins in early adulthood, but often first appears as depression. It can, however, start in early childhood or later in life. An equal number of men and women develop this disorder, but men tend to begin with a manic episode, whereas women have a depressive episode. Bipolar disorder is found among all ages, races, ethnic groups, and social classes. It tends to run in families and may have a genetic link. Abnormal brain structure and function may also cause it. It is the sixth leading cause of disability in the world (Mental Health America, 2016a). Like clinical depression, bipolar disorder needs to be managed. There is no cure, and it lasts a lifetime. Those who have bipolar disorder can suffer for years before it is diagnosed and treated, and only a little over half of patients with this disorder receive treatment. Treatment includes psychotherapy and mood stabilizing medications.

Mood Disorders and Suicide

Some patients with mood disorders get so sad that they think about suicide. Suicide or self-inflicted injury is the most dreaded complication of mood disorders. Up to 15% of patients who are hospitalized with mood disorders commit suicide. Suicide is the 10th leading cause of death among Americans (Centers for Disease Control and Prevention [CDC], Division of Violence Prevention, 2016). According to the CDC's National Center for Health Statistics (NCHS, 2016), suicide causes the death of more than 41,000 Americans each year, more than double the number of deaths caused by homicide. It is the second leading cause of death among 15- to 34-year olds (NCHS, 2016).

Suicide deaths, however, are only part of the problem. More people survive suicide attempts than die, with an estimated 12 attempted suicides for every 1 suicide death (Suicide Prevention Resource Center, 2016). There are more than 376,000 people who harm themselves every year and are treated in emergency rooms (NCHS, 2016). Many have serious self-inflicted injuries, including brain damage or organ failure.

Suicide affects everyone, but some groups are at higher risk than others. Men are four times more likely than women to die from suicide. However, three times more women than men report attempting suicide. In addition, suicide rates are highest among middle-aged and older adults.

Suicide is a complex behavior that has no single cause, but there are risk factors that put a person at risk: mood disorders, access to lethal weapons, previous suicide attempt(s), substance abuse, and family history of suicide or violence. With proper treatment, most patients who have attempted suicide do feel better and recover.

There are behaviors that may indicate that a person is at immediate suicide risk. The following three symptoms taken together are warnings for prompt medical attention:

• Talking about wanting to die or to kill oneself

• Looking for a way to kill oneself, such as buying a gun

• Talking about feeling hopeless or having no reason to live

Substance Use Disorder

A *substance use disorder* is characterized by the need for alcohol or other drugs to function normally. Abruptly stopping the drugs leads to withdrawal symptoms. There are close to 21 million adults in the United States who are diagnosed with substance use disorder (SAMHSA, 2015). Substance use disorder is related to mood disorders because a person's mood, thoughts, and behavior changes in dramatic ways.

This disorder causes noticeable changes to the brain and the body as well as to what a person thinks and does. The changes lead to *addiction*, which means that the body becomes physically and psychologically dependent on drugs. Because drugs become necessary to function on a daily basis, people with this disorder develop obsessive-compulsive thoughts that weaken their ability to control behaviors despite the consequences.

Sometimes, a person can have a diagnosis of both a mental health disorder and substance use disorder; this is referred to as a *dual diagnosis*. For example, close to 30% of people with substance use disorder also have clinical depression (SAMHSA, 2015). Almost nine million people in the United States have a co-occurring disorder, but, unfortunately, only about 7% receive treatment for both disorders (US National Library of Medicine, 2016).

Sometimes the mental health disorder develops first and causes people to abuse drugs to feel better, or sometimes the substance use disorder begins first. Whatever happened first, a downward spiral starts in which the patient uses drugs to relieve symptoms. Although substance use disorder can co-occur with other disorders, this does not mean that one caused the other. In fact, knowing which came first or why is difficult because:

- A substance use disorder can cause symptoms similar to those of another disorder
- Some genetic factors put a person at risk for both substance use and other disorders
- Stress and trauma can lead to both substance use and other disorders

Dual diagnosis requires an intervention that identifies and treats both disorders, but it can be difficult to treat due to complex influences. Both mental health disorders and substance use disorders are influenced by biological, psychological, and social factors. Other reasons for the difficulty may be inadequate provider training and overlap of symptoms. In any case, the consequences of untreated dual diagnosis include higher risks for homelessness, incarceration, diseases, suicide, or early death.

Several types of psychotherapies show promise for treating dual diagnosis. The psychotherapies are tailored to each patient based on age, the drug abused, and other factors. Some psychotherapies are more effective for adolescents; others are better for adults. Some are for families, for groups, or for individuals.

Patients with dual diagnosis often receive a combination of psychotherapy and medication for treatment. The patient must stop using all alcohol or other drugs before treatment can start. Stopping the use causes *withdrawal,* which is the body's response to not having the drug; this is a medical emergency that requires detoxification. *Detoxification* is the withdrawal of the drug abruptly from the body in a place where there is medical support. It can be done on an inpatient or outpatient basis.

There are several treatment choices for those who are trying to avoid *relapse,* or the return to using again. These choices include supportive housing that offers services to those in recovery. Examples of supportive housing include residential treatment facilities, sober houses, or group homes. Other patients may choose to return home to their family or loved ones who can offer support during recovery. Continued support is important because most patients with substance use disorder do relapse into addiction at some point in their lives. Some patients find support in self-help groups such as Alcoholics Anonymous, which can be essential to their recovery.

Psychotic Disorders

Psychotic disorders cause abnormal thinking and perceptions. They are different from an anxiety disorder because the person loses contact with reality. *Psychosis*, the major symptom of this disorder, causes a person to have hallucinations or delusions. Genes, environmental factors, and certain diseases (e.g., brain cancer) cause a psychotic disorder. People with bipolar or substance use disorder may not have a dual diagnosis of psychotic disorder, but they can have psychotic episodes.

Schizophrenia is a serious psychotic disorder that affects the way a person thinks, acts, and sees the world. This disorder affects a person's brain structure, making it difficult to function normally, show emotions, and develop relationships. Hallucinations, delusions, and speech and movement problems are all symptoms of schizophrenia. "Voices" are the most common type of hallucination for a schizophrenic. Other symptoms can be lack of pleasure in life, antisocial behavior, depression, paranoia, speaking in strange ways, and loss of memory.

Many schizophrenics are unaware that their symptoms are warning signs of something wrong. Their lives may be unraveling, yet they believe that they are fine. They can feel that they're blessed with special powers that others can't understand. In the extreme, schizophrenia can cause someone to withdraw into *catatonic* behavior and not move or respond to others.

Schizophrenia affects about 1 in 100 people in the United States; more than two million people currently suffer from this disorder (National Institute of Mental Health, 2016c). Most schizophrenics develop symptoms between the ages of 16 and 30. It affects men and women equally regardless of ethnic or racial group; however, it tends to be more severe in men than in women (National Institute of Mental Health, 2016c).

Causes of schizophrenia are not fully known, but it may be a result of the interaction between genes and the environment. Genes can put a person at risk and then environmental factors trigger the disorder. For example, the greatest risk is to both have a first-degree relative (e.g., a parent) with the disorder and undergo an environmental stress like physical abuse during childhood.

Schizophrenia is only influenced by genes, not determined by it. Although it runs in families, about 60% of schizophrenics have no family members with the disorder (National Institute of Mental Health, 2016c). In addition, those who have the genes associated with schizophrenia don't always develop the disease.

Diagnosis of schizophrenia includes a physical examination, laboratory tests, and psychological evaluation. Although it is chronic and there is no cure, patients with schizophrenia can live independent lives with psychotherapy, life skills support, and antipsychotic medications.

A common problem is that schizophrenic patients often stop taking their medications because of issues with judgment or dislike of the medications' side effects. However, when patients with schizophrenia stop taking their medication, there are long-term effects:

Damage to relationships. Relationships suffer because patients often isolate themselves and are suspicious of others.

Interference with daily activities. Eating, bathing, and other daily activities become difficult, if not impossible because of delusions and hallucinations.

Substance abuse. Patients often abuse alcohol or other drugs in an effort to self-medicate. They may also be heavy smokers; smoking can interfere with the effectiveness of prescribed medications.

Suicide risk. Patients with schizophrenia are at high risk for suicide attempts. They are especially likely to attempt suicide during psychotic episodes, during periods of depression, and in the first 6 months after the start of treatment.

Personality Disorders

Personality is a set of specific traits, behavior, and patterns that make up a person's character. How we look at the world, our thoughts, emotions, and behaviors, are all part of our personality. A person with a healthy personality copes with normal stress and has little or no trouble forming relationships. A person is said to have a *personality disorder* when he or she has a long-term pattern of thoughts, emotions, and behaviors that are different from those considered normal in his or her culture. This pattern leads to difficulty with relationships and an inability to cope with normal stress. About 9% of the adult population in the United States has a personality disorder (American Psychiatric Association, 2016). There are no differences in gender, culture, or race associated with personality disorders.

Patients with a personality disorder have trouble with other people. They tend to be rigid and do not respond to the changes and demands of life. These patients feel that their behavior is normal, but they have a narrow view of the world and find it difficult to be social. Personality disorders usually begin in adolescence or early adulthood and can continue throughout adulthood; however, they become less obvious by middle age.

The cause of personality disorders is not fully understood. Some research suggests that what happens in childhood strongly influences the development of these disorders. Other research suggests that genes are the cause. For some patients, the cause is a combination of genetics and the environment.

There are different types of personality disorders, each with its own set of behaviors. Personality disorders are usually categorized into three clusters in terms of their associated behaviors:

- *Cluster A:* odd or weird thinking and behavior

  Example: *Paranoid personality disorder* causes a person to see the behavior of others as threatening. Patients with this disorder are untrusting and unforgiving, and have angry outbursts. They may also be jealous and secretive, and can be emotionally cold or withdrawn. Those with this disorder see others as unfaithful or as liars.

- *Cluster B*: dramatic, emotional, or strange behavior

  Example: *Antisocial personality disorder* causes a person to act out and ignore normal rules of social behavior. These individuals are impulsive, irresponsible, and mean-spirited. They feel no remorse about the effects of their behavior on others. The antisocial personality has a history of legal problems, aggressive behavior, and violent relationships. Those with this disorder are at high risk for substance use disorder because it helps them relieve tension and boredom.

- *Cluster C:* anxious, fearful behavior

  Example: People are given a diagnosis of *dependent personality disorder* when they have a history of dependent behavior, relying on others to make decisions for them. Because they feel so helpless, these individuals constantly need support and advice when making even small decisions. These patients are easily hurt by others' words and behaviors. Because they lack self-confidence, people with dependent personality disorder rarely do things by themselves. This disorder usually begins in early adulthood and occurs more often in women than in men.

When personality disorder symptoms become extreme, persist over time, and interfere with daily activities, then diagnosis and treatment are necessary. The diagnostic process includes a physical examination, lab tests, and a psychological evaluation. If left untreated, personality disorder symptoms eventually get worse.

There are different treatment options available for these disorders. Treatment may include psychotherapy or medication. Some psychotherapies focus on specific behaviors associated with personality disorders, such as the inability to form or maintain relationships. Medications can relieve some of the symptoms, including anxiety.

Eating Disorders

Eating disorders are a group of disorders characterized by disturbed or abnormal thoughts and behaviors related to one's body, foods, and eating habits. These thoughts and behaviors lead to physical, psychological, and social problems. If left untreated, eating disorders cause severe medical and behavior problems, including death. In any given year, more than five million Americans have an eating disorder (National Eating Disorders Association, 2016). These disorders usually start in adolescence and tend to affect mostly females. They can be chronic and often difficult to treat. In addition, eating disorders can often coexist with other anxiety or personality disorders, which makes treatment that much more challenging.

Eating disorders are marked by extremes. A person changes his or her eating habits, severely reducing food intake or overeating. Although changes in eating habits may at first be minor, at some point, the urge to eat less or more spirals out of control.

There are three types of eating disorders. *Anorexia nervosa* is self-starvation. *Bulimia nervosa* is binge eating followed by *purging* (vomiting), fasting, or excessive exercise. *Binge eating* is uncontrolled overeating and does not include purging to prevent weight gain, unlike bulimia.

Anorexia nervosa symptoms include extreme thinness and denial of being thin. A person with this disorder has a distorted body image, fear of weight gain, and food obsessions. If female, her menstrual cycle may stop due to extreme weight loss. Anorexic patients often have thinning bones, brittle hair and nails, and irregular heart rate. They can also have anemia, muscle weakness, constipation, dehydration, and hair loss. To prevent weight gain, an anorexic eats only tiny meals or abuses laxatives. In severe cases, some symptoms of anorexia can become life threatening without treatment. Anorexic patients, for example, are 18 times more likely to die early compared to people of similar age in the general population (National Eating Disorders Association, 2016). One in ten cases leads to death from starvation, other medical problems, or suicide (Wolters Kluwer, 2016a).

A person with bulimia is of normal weight, but has a distorted body image. These individuals have an intense fear of weight gain and will binge-eat. Binge-eating means eating large amounts of food fast or eating large amounts of food when not hungry. This symptom is coupled with behaviors that prevent weight gain, including self-induced purging, using laxatives, fasting, or excessive exercise. Other symptoms are decaying teeth, chronic sore throat, and kidney and stomach problems.

Binge eating disorder is characterized by repeated episodes of binge-eating for at least 2 days a week for 6 months. Unlike other eating disorders, binge eating disorder does not include purging, excessive exercise, or fasting. People with this disorder are overweight and have anxiety over their shape and size. Other symptoms include feelings of guilt and shame about eating. These symptoms lead to more binge eating, anxiety, and clinical depression, as well as health problems.

Eating disorders are caused by a complex interaction of genetic, biological, behavioral, psychological, and social factors. Although females are much more at risk for eating disorders, males can also be affected. Men and boys account for up to 15% of patients with anorexia or bulimia and 35% of those with binge eating disorder (National Eating Disorder Association, 2016). Males with eating disorders can have *muscle dysmorphia,* which is an extreme concern with being more muscular.

Eating disorders are treatable. Treatment is most successful when the eating disorder is diagnosed early and tailored to individual needs. Adequate nutrition, reducing excessive exercise, and stopping purging are part of most treatment plans. Specific forms of psychotherapy and medication are effective for milder forms of eating disorders. However, for the more severe cases, specific treatments have not yet been found.

Chapter Summary

- Mental health disorders can develop when the brain is not functioning correctly. At some time in their lives, nearly all Americans are affected by a mental health disorder, either in themselves, in a family member, or in a loved one.

- Mental health disorders change a person's thinking, feelings, and behavior. These changes affect the person's ability to cope with everyday activities.

- Mental health disorders rarely appear without warning. Many times, it is family, loved ones, or the patients themselves who recognize that something is wrong.

- The causes of mental health disorders are not fully understood. There are disciplines—psychiatry, psychology, and neuroscience—that study brain biology and its relationship to thoughts, feelings, and behaviors.

- Treatment depends on the type of mental health disorder. The most common forms of treatment are medication, psychotherapy, or a combination of both.

REVIEW QUESTIONS

1. What are the differences between mental health and mental health disorders?

2. What are the four long-term effects when a schizophrenic stops taking her or his medications?

3. List and explain four types of mental health providers identified in this chapter.

4. Describe the different symptoms associated with sadness versus clinical depression.

5. Summarize differences among the three eating disorders discussed in this chapter.

6. How is bipolar disorder different from clinical depression?

7. What are three clusters of personality disorder?

8. List myths related to mental health disorders. Explain why they are myths.

9. What are warning signs that a person has suicidal thoughts?

10. Describe the differences between hallucinations and delusions.

KEY TERMS

Acrophobia: Specific phobia of heights

Agoraphobia: Specific phobia of public places

Addiction: Physical and psychological dependence on alcohol or another substance

Anorexia nervosa: Self-starvation

Antianxiety medication: Medication used to treat anxiety disorders and insomnia

Antidepressants: Medications prescribed for clinical depression

Antipsychotic medication: Medication used to treat psychotic and bipolar disorders as well as depression

Antisocial personality disorder: Disorder that causes a person to act out his or her conflicts and ignore normal rules of social behavior

Anxiety attack: Sudden attack of fear that lasts for several minutes or longer

Anxiety disorder: Disorder characterized by fears that are not based on fact and that interfere with daily activities

Asperger syndrome (AS): High-functioning form of autism

Attention deficit hyperactivity disorder (ADHD): Neurodevelopmental disorder whose symptoms include difficulty in paying attention, controlling behavior, and being overactive (hyperactive)

Autism spectrum disorder (ASD): Neurodevelopmental disorder that changes the structure and function of the brain and nervous system and causes social, communication, and behavior problems

Autistic disorder, or autism: Most severe form of autism spectrum disorder

Behavioral therapy: Therapy with an emphasis on teaching children to control their behaviors

Binge eating: Eating large amounts of food when not hungry

Bipolar disorder: Disorder in which a person has a cycle of depression, normal mood, and then mania

Bulimia nervosa: Binge-eating followed by purging, fasting, or excessive exercise

Catatonic: State in which a person with schizophrenia does not move or does not respond to others

Claustrophobia: Specific phobia of closed spaces

Clinical depression: Condition in which a person has depressed moods for no obvious reason, and may even have thoughts of suicide

Cognitive behavioral therapy (CBT): Type of psychotherapy that teaches people different ways of thinking, behaving, and reacting to situations and helps them feel less anxious

Compulsions: Efforts to control obsessions, which take the form of repeated behaviors

Delusions: Beliefs that do not change even when there is strong conflicting evidence or facts

Dependent personality disorder: Disorder that causes a person to have a pattern of dependent behavior, relying on others to make decisions for him or her

Detoxification: Withdrawal of alcohol or another substance abruptly from the body in a place where there is support

Diagnostic and Statistical Manual of Mental Disorders (DSM): Book published by the American Psychiatric Association that helps in the diagnosis of a mental disorder

Dopamine: Neurotransmitter that controls movement and is linked to the brain's reward systems

Dual diagnosis: Diagnosis of a mental health disorder and substance use disorder

Dysthymia: Type of clinical depression that is less severe but can last at low levels for years

Eating disorders: Group of disorders characterized by disturbed or abnormal thoughts and behaviors related to one's body, foods, and eating habits

Electroconvulsive therapy (ECT): Treatment procedure in which the patient is given an electric charge to the brain

Episode: Mood swing

Generalized anxiety disorder (GAD): Disorder characterized by excessive and unrealistic worry

Glutamate: Neurotransmitter that plays a role during early brain development

Hallucination: An experience of visual images, voices, or sounds that do not exist outside the mind

Hoarding: Keeping useless items

Hyperarousal: Feeling of being on edge, startling easily, and being on the lookout for danger, common after a traumatic event

Insomnia: Inability to sleep

Manic episode: Episode during which a person with bipolar disorder is hyperactive and in a happy state

Mental health: Emotional, psychological, and social well-being

Mental health disorders, or mental illness: Wide range of mental health problems that cause ongoing changes in a person's thinking, feelings, and behavior

Mood disorders: Group of disorders characterized by extreme emotions that are outside the normal range

Mood-stabilizing medication: Medication used to treat bipolar disorder

Muscle dysmorphia: Extreme concern with becoming more muscular

Neurodevelopmental disorder: Disorder that cause problems with cognition, learning, communication, and behavior

Neurotransmitter: Brain chemical that helps brain nerve cells communicate with each other

Obsessions: Frequent and repeated unwanted thoughts

Obsessive-compulsive disorder (OCD): Anxiety disorder in which a person has repeated unwanted thoughts or behaviors

Panic disorder: Disorder characterized by sudden and repeated anxiety attacks that last for several minutes or longer

Paranoid personality disorder: Disorder that causes a person to see the behavior of others as threatening

Personality: Set of specific traits, behavior, and patterns that make up a person's character

Personality disorder: Group of disorders that cause a person to have a long-term pattern of thoughts, emotions, and behaviors that are different from those considered normal in his or her culture

Posttraumatic stress disorder (PTSD): Disorder that causes a person to have an intense emotional reaction long after a traumatic event

Psychological evaluation: Evaluation conducted by a qualified provider to identify mental health disorder symptoms

Psychosis: Major symptom of a psychotic disorder in which a person has hallucinations or delusions

Psychotherapy: General term used to describe a form of mental health treatment based on a patient talking about his or her issues with a therapist

Psychotic disorders: Groups of severe mental disorders that cause abnormal thinking and perceptions, which leads to a person's losing contact with reality

Psychotic episode: Event during which the patient experiences delusions and hallucinations, with confused thoughts and speech

Purging: Vomiting

Relapse: The return to using alcohol or another substance after detoxification

Schizophrenia: Psychotic disorder that affects the way a person acts, thinks, and sees the world

Self-help groups: Groups run by patients of the mental health care system or their families. and their families who meet informally to discuss issues and challenges of dealing with a specific disorder

Serotonin: Neurotransmitter that helps control many brain functions

Social phobia: Specific phobia of interpersonal interactions

Specific phobias: Fears and avoidance of certain situations or objects even when there is no danger

Substance use disorder: Disorder in which a person needs alcohol or another substance to function normally

Traumatic event: A terrifying and life-threatening experience

Withdrawal: Body's response to not having alcohol or other substance(s) to which it is addicted

CHAPTER ACTIVITIES

1. Form groups of three or four. Each of you writes down three symptoms of a mental health disorder. Then discuss and compare your selected mental health disorder and related symptoms with the rest of your group. The group members then select a mental health disorder that can be viewed differently depending on the culture. For example, how are substance use disorders viewed in the United States, as opposed to China? As a follow-up, you can discuss examples of ways that mental health disorders are stigmatized in the United States. What are ways to raise awareness about and remove stigma associated with mental health disorders?

2. Mental health disorders are diagnosed based on how they affect daily activities. In small groups, brainstorm what daily activities are affected by these disorders.

3. In an independent project, explore and write a report about a career that specializes in mental health. As part of the assignment, conduct at least one interview with a mental health care provider.

4. In teams of two, brainstorm both appropriate and inappropriate ways of talking about, and behaving toward, people with mental health disorders.

5. In pairs, create a PowerPoint that answers the following questions: How are mental health disorders similar to other diseases? How are they different? What are examples of complementary or alternative treatments for mental health disorders? Present and discuss your PowerPoint in class.

Bibliography and Works Cited

American Psychiatric Association. (2015a). Help with ADHD. Retrieved from https://www.psychiatry.org/patients-families/adhd

American Psychiatric Association. (2015b). Warning signs of mental illness. Retrieved from https://www.psychiatry.org/patients-families/warning-signs-of-mental-illness

American Psychiatric Association. (2016). Get help with personality disorders. Retrieved from https://www.psychiatry.org/patients-families/personality-disorders

American Psychological Association. (2016). Understanding psychotherapy and how it works. Retrieved from http://www.apa.org/helpcenter/understanding-psychotherapy.aspx

Anxiety and Depression Association of America. (2014). Understanding the facts of anxiety disorder and depression is the first step. Retrieved from http://adaa.org/understanding-anxiety

Anxiety and Depression Association of America. (2016). Understanding the facts: Specific phobias. Retrieved from http://www.adaa.org/understanding-anxiety/specific-phobias

Attention Deficit Disorder Association. (2016). Adult ADHD test. Retrieved from https://add.org/adhd-test/

Centers for Disease Control and Prevention. (2013). Mental health basics. Retrieved from http://www.cdc.gov/mentalhealth/basics.htm

Centers for Disease Control and Prevention, Division of Violence Prevention. (2016). Suicide prevention. Retrieved from http://www.cdc.gov/violenceprevention/suicide

Depression and Bipolar Support Alliance. (2016a). About mood disorders. Retrieved from http://www.dbsalliance.org/site/PageServer?pagename=education_mood_disorders

Depression and Bipolar Support Alliance. (2016b). Depression. Retrieved from http://www.dbsalliance.org/site/PageServer?pagename=education_depression

Eunice Kennedy Shriver National Institute of Child Health and Development. (2016). Autism spectrum disorder (ASD): Condition information. Retrieved from http://www.nichd.nih.gov/health/topics/autism/conditioninfo/Pages/default.aspx

Mental Health America. (2016a). Bipolar disorder. Retrieved from http://www.mentalhealthamerica.net/conditions/bipolar-disorder

Mental Health America. (2016b). Personality disorder. Retrieved from http://www.mentalhealthamerica.net /conditions/personality-disorder

National Alliance on Mental Illness. (2015). Dispelling myths on mental illness. Retrieved from http://www.nami .org/Blogs/NAMI-Blog/July-2015/Dispelling-Myths-on-Mental-Illness

National Alliance on Mental Illness. (2016a). Know the warning signs. Retrieved from http://www.nami.org /Learn-More/Know-the-Warning-Signs

National Alliance on Mental Illness. (2016b). Types of mental health professionals. Retrieved from http://www .nami.org/Learn-More/Treatment/Types-of-Mental-Health-Professionals

National Alliance on Mental Illness. (2016c). Mental health by the numbers. Retrieved from http://www.nami .org/Learn-More/Mental-Health-By-the-Numbers

National Center for Health Statistics. (2016). Suicide and self-inflicted injury. Retrieved from http://www.cdc .gov/nchs/fastats/suicide.htm

National Eating Disorders Association. (2016). Types & symptoms of eating disorders. Retrieved from http:// www.nationaleatingdisorders.org/types-symptoms-eating-disorders

National Institute of Diabetes and Digestive and Kidney Diseases. (2016). Binge eating disorder. Retrieved from https://www.niddk.nih.gov/health-information/health-topics/weight-control/binge-eating-disorder/Pages /overview.aspx

National Institute of Mental Health. (2016a). Brain stimulation therapies. Retrieved from http://www.nimh.nih .gov/health/topics/brain-stimulation-therapies/brain-stimulation-therapies.shtml

National Institute of Mental Health. (2016b). Mental health medications. Retrieved from http://www.nimh.nih .gov/health/topics/mental-health-medications/mental-health-medications.shtml

National Institute of Mental Health. (2016c). Schizophrenia (Easy-to-read). Retrieved from http://www.nimh .nih.gov/health/publications/schizophrenia-easy-to-read-12-2015/index.shtml

National Institute of Mental Health. (2016d). Understanding anxiety disorders: When panic, fear and worries overwhelm.`NIH News for Health. Retrieved from https://newsinhealth.nih.gov/issue/Mar2016/Feature1

Office of Women's Health. (2015). Anxiety disorders. Retrieved from http://www.womenshealth.gov/publications /our-publications/fact-sheet/anxiety-disorders.html

Substance Abuse and Mental Health Services Administration. (2015). Mental and substance use disorders. Retrieved from http://www.samhsa.gov/disorders/

Suicide Prevention Resource Center. (2016). About suicide. Retrieved from http://www.sprc.org/basics

US Department of Health and Human Services. (2016). What is mental health? MentalHealth.gov. Retrieved from https://www.mentalhealth.gov/basics/what-is-mental-health/index.html

US National Library of Medicine. (2016). Substance use disorder. *MedlinePlus*. Retrieved from http://www.nichd .nih.gov/health/topics/autism/conditioninfo/Pages/default.aspx

Wolters Kluwer. (2016a). Patient education: Anorexia nervosa (The basics). *UpToDate*. Retrieved from https:// www.uptodate-com.ezproxy.springfield.edu/contents/anorexia-nervosa-the-basics?source=see_link

Wolters Kluwer. (2016b). Patient education: Bulimia nervosa (The basics). *UpToDate*. Retrieved from https:// www.uptodate-com.ezproxy.springfield.edu/contents/bulimia-nervosa-the-basics

Wolters Kluwer. (2016c). Patient education: Post-traumatic stress disorder (The basics). *UpToDate*. Retrieved from https://www.uptodate-com.ezproxy.springfield.edu/contents/post-traumatic-stress-disorder-the-basics? source=see_link